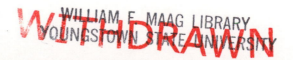

# BIOLOGICAL ANTHROPOLOGY AND AGING

# BIOLOGICAL ANTHROPOLOGY AND AGING

*Perspectives on Human Variation over the Life Span*

Edited by

DOUGLAS E. CREWS
*The Ohio State University, Columbus, Ohio*

RALPH M. GARRUTO
*National Institutes of Health, Bethesda, Maryland*

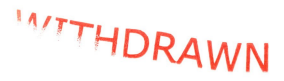

New York   Oxford
OXFORD UNIVERSITY PRESS
1994

Oxford University Press

Oxford   New York   Toronto
Delhi   Bombay   Calcutta   Madras   Karachi
Kuala Lumpur   Singapore   Hong Kong   Tokyo
Nairobi   Dar es Salaam   Cape Town
Melbourne   Auckland   Madrid

and associated companies in
Berlin   Ibadan

Library of Congress Cataloging-in-Publication Data
Biological anthropology and aging : perspectives on human variation
over the life span / Douglas E. Crews and Ralph M. Garruto, editors.
p.   cm.   Includes bibliographical references and index.
ISBN 0-19-506829-7
1. Aging.   2. Physical anthropology.   I. Crews, Douglas E.
II. Garruto, Ralph M.
QP86.B516   1994
612.6′7—dc20                                   93-11232

9 8 7 6 5 4 3 2 1

Printed in the United States of America
on acid-free paper

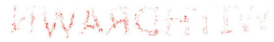

# Foreword

PAUL T. BAKER

Studies of aging and the aged have increased dramatically during the past decade. While progress in describing the process of aging has partially motivated this interest, the major stimulus has been the rapidly rising percentage of people of over 60 years of age in the populations of the world. While total life expectancy is rising in almost all countries, only the developed countries are showing a significant increase in life expectancy for individuals over 60. Even so it is the increase in life expectancy in this group that has caused national economic planners to be concerned and inspired the general public with hope for a longer and healthier "old age".

A severely reductionist approach to the study of human biological problems as exemplified by those applied in the past to the study of infectious disease has contributed in a major fashion to the increased life expectancies of most populations. Today the rapid discoveries associated with biochemical and molecular genetics and gene mapping are yielding exciting prospects for understanding our biology and some of our health problems. However, strictly reductionist approaches to the study of general life processes such as growth and aging must, for a full understanding of the process, be balanced by more integrative strategies common to such disciplines as epidemiology, human population genetics, social sciences, and biological anthropology. This volume, written primarily by researchers with a background in biological anthropology, provides a view of aging which differs significantly from previous publications.

Biological anthropologists and other specialists included under the broad title of human population biologists have in recent decades been the major contributors to the development of human physical growth norms. This group has also provided much of the standardized norms for gross physical characteristics such as height, weight, and fatness in adult populations throughout the world. These norms include the limited data we have about the morphological changes which occur in old age. Indeed one of the earliest studies of morphological change in old age was a 1941 study of the older male population of Ireland by anthropologists E. A. Hooton and C. W. Dupertuis.

During the past three decades the focus of biological anthropology has expanded from a descriptive science to one emphasizing process and causality. The unified theory of evolution forms the theoretical basis of the discipline

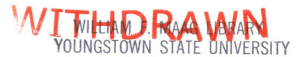

while individual practitioners have specialized in diverse aspects of the human biological sciences including genetics, primatology, nutrition, physiology, immunology, and neurology. As a consequence of these subdisciplinary specializations, this book provides a unique perspective on the human aging process.

Of particular import are the insights gained by the focus on population and individual variability. For example, from an evolutionary and genetic perspective it appears that as a species we probably do not have any specific genes that limit our life span. However, both as populations and individuals we do have genes and gene combinations which contribute to early death and aging disabilities. Of course phenotypic manifestations are always the product of a lifelong interaction between the genetic information and the environmental context. Thus, varying either the environment or the genes will modify the phenotype.

This basic axiom of genetics suggests that it is not an easy task to create either the genes or the environment that will improve longevity and health in older individuals. In spite of the difficulties, the life expectancies of the old have been increased, and the quality of life and functional capabilities have been improved. Much of this progress has been achieved by traditional approaches which treat the disorders as they appear. However, as developed in this book, a more integrated approach dependent upon assessing the genetic structure of both populations and individuals along with a continuous study of and intervention in lifetime environments will be necessary if the aging populations of the world are to become more productive and reasonably healthy.

# Prologue: Human Aging—A Paradigm of Transdisciplinary Research

## DOUGLAS E. CREWS AND RALPH M. GARRUTO

This volume represents an attempt by a small group of biological anthropologists, human population biologists, and gerontologists to summarize and evaluate critical information and theoretical perspectives on human biological aging, longevity, and senescence. It is intended to acquaint scholars, students, and practitioners in both anthropology and gerontology with the usefulness of evolutionary, adaptive, and ecological perspectives for understanding both individual and population variation in patterns of aging, while detailing how traditional anthropological research designs (comparative, cross-cultural, longitudinal, and holistic) are a logical necessity for studying the great diversity in human biological aging. Although much of the potential usefulness of biological anthropology/human population biology to gerontology remains unrealized, the contributors to this volume articulate numerous research strategies for study of problems in aging using traditional and emerging anthropological methods.

One reason that the value of biological anthropology and human population biology to biological gerontology has not been more fully realized may be that clinicians and biomedical researchers still perceive biological anthropologists as primarily anatomists and fossil hunters rather than as the evolutionary biologists, geneticists, ethnogerontologists, human ecologists, and epidemiologists that modern biological anthropologists have become. As interdisciplinary and transdisciplinary features of biological anthropology and human population biology have come to dominate anthropological research on modern human variation during recent decades (Baker, 1982; Baker and Garruto, 1992) and as the great diversity and variation in aging among human populations, in naturalistic and experimental animal models, and in prokaryotic organisms has become well-documented (Arking, 1991; Gavrilov and Gavrilova, 1991; Rose, 1991), synthesis between these two research areas has become inevitable. The major focus of this new synthesis is human variation over the life span. The extent to which biological anthropologists and human population biologists have been successful in exploiting this niche for scientific inquiry along with future applications of their methods to biological gerontology are the subject of the contributions to this volume.

Biological anthropologists and human population biologists have long been interested in adaptive systems, social, cultural, ecological, genetic, and life-history parameters that produce human biological variation and allow humans to maintain homeostasis and to grow, develop, and reproduce in the wide variety of environmental, sociocultural, and ecological settings in which they find themselves. Today their quest increasingly includes examinations of the consequences of adaptation and evolutionary inertia on human physiological variation in the later years. The concept of heterogeneity in older persons is a centerpiece of anthropological inquiry into the aging processes. In contrast to previous emphases on patterns of human growth and development, this new focus is on life span, individual patterns of change with age, and the causes and consequences of age-related disease.

This volume is divided into several sections reflecting current themes in biological aging research. This prologue serves to introduce the area of biological anthropology and aging, while the first substantive chapter serves to describe aging in a worldwide context. These are followed by a section on Evolutionary Biology of Aging and Senescence. In the third section, Populations. Environment and Morbidity issues are examined. The last section examines Methods for Aging Research and Ongoing Programs available to fund aging research. Lastly, the epilogue briefly reviews the thematic issues raised by the contributors to this volume as they seek to merge biological anthropology and biological gerontology in the study of human biological variation in later life.

This prologue reacquaints readers, particularly non-biological anthropologists, with the general concepts, methods, and research perspectives used in biological anthropology and human population biology and summarizes highlights of later chapters. The Prologue is followed by Miles and Brody's introductory overview documenting worldwide trends in lifespan, survivorship, patterns of disability, and morbidity and mortality. Miles and Brody also briefly examine cross-cultural variation observed in demographic, health, and clinical characteristics of the elderly. They succinctly review data showing recent increases in the absolute and relative number of elderly worldwide, trends and shifts in a number of age-related diseases—heart disease, stroke, cancer, osteoporosis—gains in life span, delays in mortality among persons aged 65 and older, and declining health status of the oldest old that presents as frequent comorbidity from several chronic degenerative diseases, thus setting the stage for the remaining sections and contributions to this volume.

The second theme addresses the Evolutionary Biology of Aging and Senescence. Wood, Weeks, Bentley, and Weiss review the theoretical population biology of aging to identify the most plausible evolutionary models and to present their implications for two views of life span—as a programmed maximum (gerontological model) and as an artifact of competition among causes of death in a particular environment and genotype (epidemiological model). Focusing on the fact that with any degree of organismal complexity senescence is an inherent property, Wood *et al.* review available data on the evolution of aging. They review two basic evolutionary mechanisms through which senescence will likely evolve: age-specific gene action and antagonistic pleiotropy, as recently reviewed by Rose (1991). Wood and colleagues review empirical evidence in support of an evolutionary model of aging and explore the implications and applicability of this model for understanding human aging. An important component of their contribution is the inclusion of a thorough examination of the life history of reproduction and fecundity, and of the associations of these processes with longevity and aging. Their examination and explication of an evolutionary, physiological, and simple model for human female menopause is particularly enlightening. Wood and colleagues conclude that we age and die because the benefits of maintaining a complex organism are offset by the costs of curtailing reproduction to provide for that maintenance.

The next chapter by Turner and Weiss presents a review of genetic theories of aging, anthropological genetics and aging, and an examination of genetic epidemiology and biomarkers of longevity in humans. Among the important points made by the authors are that, based upon the massive amount of data collected on aging organisms, most genetic theories of aging receive both support and criticism. In their view, aging is related to complex gene–environment interactions at the cellular and molecular level. Turner and Weiss support the notion that both invertebrate and vertebrate models can provide meaningful insights into human aging. They conclude that if longevity has a heritable component, it is very small, and that long life most likely depends on not having genes that lead to an early death. In the end, Turner and Weiss call for more use of anthropological perspectives to examine intra- and interpopulation human variability in terms of allozymes, histocompatibility loci, oncogenes, and susceptibility genes for chronic disease. They concur with the general hypothesis that as the force of natural selection fades with increasing age it is inevitable that functional performance of adults should also deteriorate. In Chapter 4, Katz and Armstrong explore several factors of perennial interest to biological anthropologists and human population biologists—evolution, language, the X-chromosome, and marriage systems—and explore their associations with longevity. After reviewing recent research developments, they show that in certain systems of cousin marriage, grandmothers have an enhanced probability of making social investments in their grandchildren who are most likely to share their X-chromosomes. This may help to explain the cultural evolution of mating systems and in part the evolution of X-linked loci that have specific influences on longevity—such as the X-linked steroid sulfatase locus.

The next major theme, Populations, Environment and Morbidity, begins with a review of primate gerontology and its relationship to human aging. DeRousseau concentrates on the importance of "adaptability" defined as "the interaction between genes and environment," for models of both aging and evolution. She suggests that the environment may be just as influential on an adult's range of variability and aging as are its genes, a theme echoed by several authors in this volume. DeRousseau finds one inescapable conclusion: based on contrasts of data from captive and natural populations, environment has a major impact on the primate life cycle. DeRousseau documents the adaptability of non-human primate life stages and overall life histories, and then, based on her review of data, contends that age-related disorders in non-human primates are strongly influenced by "life style." She concludes that ongoing research is paving the way for comparative studies of adaptability and examination of the significance of life-cycle adjustments in response to environmental pressures and constraints among primates, including humans.

The later chapters in this section deal with aging and age-related chronic diseases in human populations. Crews and Gerber invoke the concepts of antagonistic pleiotropy and thrifty genotypes to explore associations between chronic degenerative diseases, aging, and longevity. They propose that multiple "thrifty genotypes" with "antagonistic pleiotropy," i.e., early-acting benefits and late-acting problems, may have been incorporated into the hominid gene pool over evolutionary time and examine possible mechanisms that may be associated with selected diseases. The authors propose that changing sociocultural environments and ecological settings have revealed detrimental late-acting effects of genes with antagonistic pleiotropy in recent generations as an epidemic of chronic degenerative diseases and present several hypotheses for future testing of these theoretical concepts.

In the next chapter, Mayer weaves numerous conceptual threads from the foregoing chapters that have relevance to an understanding of aging and the human immune system into a tapestry of immune system aging. He divides his approach across four conceptual areas: human biological diversity, biocultural perspectives, ontogeny and gerontology, and evolutionary models of human immunosenescence. Mayer is particularly careful to make clear distinctions between immune system aging, which is universal, progressive, cumulative, and irreversible, and immunosenescence, which includes processes that are pathogenic, dysfunctional, and detrimental. He concludes that, although decreases in immune function occur with age, these changes are not readily explained by a single common mechanism or event. He further notes that equally diverse immunological phenomena increase or show no change with increasing age.

Strong and Garruto continue the theme of Populations, Environment, and Morbidity by examining neuronal aging and age-related disorders of the human nervous system. Like many contributors to this volume, they also examine age changes from a life span perspective by discussing neuronal proliferation and regression during development as well as during senescence. Their major contention is that the human nervous system is a dynamic structure capable of considerable plasticity throughout the human life span and that the process of neuronal degeneration has a long temporal sequence, one that begins early in life, whether initiated *in utero*, during infancy, childhood, adolescence or even later, but long before the onset of clinical disease. Strong and Garruto also suggest that concomitant with neuronal aging, late onset neurological disorders with long latency and slow progression may represent disease syndromes rather than single disease entities, and put forth their concept of a neurodegenerative disease continuum. Finally, they discuss several examples of age-related neurodegenerative diseases in traditional non-Western populations that provide common links between anthropology, gerontology, and neurology.

The next four contributions in this section examine nutrition and aging and changes in bone, fat, lipid, and blood pressure over the adult years. Stini provides a detailed review of intraindividual variations in diet and nutritional requirements across the life span. He suggests that failure to accommodate changing nutritional requirements during the aging process can contribute to early senescence, morbidity, and mortality. Stini finds that older individuals are highly idiosyncratic and express a great degree of individuality in what they eat. Such dietary idiosyncracy is related to a multiplicity of factors including physiological changes that reduce taste sensitivity, mechanical loss of teeth, changes in nutritional intake due to socioeconomic, behavioral and biological factors, difficulties in digestion, and alterations in stomach and intestinal microflora. Stini's contribution is followed by that of Plato, Fox, and Tobin, who continue the theme by describing skeletal aging. Skeletal changes during human growth and development represent a traditional area of inquiry for biological anthropologists, but in more recent years post-maturity bone changes have been studied cross-culturally and longitudinally. Plato, Fox, and Tobin explicitly use a human life span perspective to view skeletal aging as a process of slow nonuniform change through time that ultimately leads to decreasing levels of adaptability and performance. Conversely, skeletal growth and development may be viewed as processes that are relatively fast, beneficial to the individual, and that lead to improved performance. Plato and colleagues also discuss bone loss (and its measurement) leading to clinical signs of osteoporosis and related pathologies, as well as cross-cultural variability in skeletal aging by race, nationality, and sex. Last, they discuss the influence of reproductive characteristics (estrogen levels, menopause) on bone mass and fracture rates. This is particularly interesting and relevant in light of the possible evolutionary biology of bone mineralization and loss discussed by Crews and Gerber.

Garn's review of changing patterns of weight, fat, fat placement, lipids, and blood pressure over the adult life span continues the theme of Populations Environment, and Morbidity. Garn reviews reports of great variability in these aspects of body morphology and physiological variation cross-culturally and with age, sex, socioeconomic status, and educational level. Garn argues that adult increases in fatness are secondary to a positive energy balance in an ecological setting of diminished voluntary physical activity and decreased basal energy production that remain uncompensated for by alterations in food intake. After considering the extent of variation in weight, fat, lipids, and fat changes over the later years of life, Garn examines possible genetic contributions to this variation and finds grandparent–grandchild correlations for fatness close to genetic expectancy (unlike correlations of life span). His chapter is followed by that of James and Pecker who examine age changes in blood pressure, a variable that is very difficult to measure accurately and is of questionable relevance cross-sectionally. They view blood pressure regulation as a complex, dynamic system with multiple interacting fail-safe mechanisms that produce a dynamic physiological variable we call blood pressure. They view the key to understanding age-related change in blood pressure as a problem of how well regulatory mechanisms compensate for one another. In an ideal system the net effect of such compensation throughout most of adult life is no change in blood pressure, because homeostatic mechanisms act to maintain the vascular system. Using this model, increased blood pressure occurs only when compensatory functions have been lost or altered. James and Pecker do not consider the weight of evidence as supporting the conclusion that blood pressure increases with normal aging. Rather, they believe that increases in blood pressure occur only when some aspect of regulation is lost and homeostatic compensation does not occur. Finally, they warn against studies that use cross-sectional rather than longitudinal measurements. Because these studies often use a single measurement of such a highly variable trait, they do not allow for differential adaptation and development cross-culturally. Furthermore, these studies fail to control for attrition due to morbidity and mortality across the life span.

Among the long-term interests of biological anthropologists and human population biologists are studies of human plasticity, adaptability, and the maintenance of homeostasis. Beall presents a thorough review of human adaptation in older age groups to three major environmental stressors—heat, cold, and hypoxia. Using a conceptual model of adaptation to environmental stress, Beall examines whether the homeostatic state differs at different stages in the life cycle or whether adaptive systems change in their temporal course or degree of response over the human life cycle. She finds strong evidence for adult age changes and age differences in physiological responses to these major stressors. In general, such responses are less efficient, show a larger range of variation, and include increasing numbers of individuals whose adaptive responses are poor or have failed with increased age. These findings support the hypothesis of relaxed natural selection at older ages. Beall stresses the need for more study of the oldest old, more documentation of age-related changes in traditional anthropological populations residing under conditions of extreme stress and in acculturating groups undergoing modernization. She calls for developing research designs to separate effects of social factors, disease, and dysfunctional biological changes from age processes in the adaptation of older individuals to their environment.

The final theme discusses Methods for Aging Research and Ongoing Programs. The contribution by Brant and Pearson from the Gerontology Research Center of the National Institute on Aging uses innovative mathematical modeling to examine individual variability in longitudinal patterns of change. They use individual differences in patterns of aging as individual-level natural experiments and illustrate their model using original longitudinal data on changes in hearing thresholds. Their chapter concludes with a "mixed effects model" that allows an integrated estimate of the average longitudinal patterns of aging in the population as well as of individual variation from the average. Mixed effects modeling will allow researchers to move away from oversimplified views of "normal aging" to estimates and descriptions of cross-sectional, longitudinal, and individual patterns of aging, thereby better describing the overwhelming diversity of the aging processes. The second chapter on this theme addresses issues of reconstructing aging and longevity from fossil and skeletal materials, a process that provides the basic data for examining evolutionary as well as recent trends in life span, longevity, and mortality. Loth and İşcan review morphological indicators of age in skeletal remains and address issues relating age estimates to paleodemography and paleogerontology. They present both old and new skeletal aging techniques and then discuss one of the most recent and, in their view, most accurate methods of assessing age using the sternal extremity of the rib. The authors then proceed to examine Neanderthal remains using the rib phase technique. To Loth and İşcan, interpretation of age is a matter that can be tested and refuted; however, implications for paleodemography and paleogerontology drawn from these age estimates is quite another matter and subject to problems of temporal, racial, and geographic variation, as well as overall representivity, because of the general lack of skeletal materials relative to the total number of individuals who have ever lived. In addition, they compare results obtained using the rib phase technique on an archaeological sample to those obtained using modern forensic remains.

In the last chapter to this volume, Eveleth provides an uncommon view of the role of the National Institute on Aging in funding anthropological studies of aging. From her unique perspective it is obvious that research areas of interest to our discipline are scattered throughout the Institute's current initiatives without a specific "anthropology" focus. It is this lack of an anthropological focus that has probably had a major affect on the low level of funding for bioanthropological studies from the Institute, although with their new initiative on cross-cultural aging and slow recognition of the relevance and importance of biological anthropology to aging, this funding pattern may change. Finally, the overall importance of her chapter is that it provides biomedical anthropologists (and gerontologists) with a concise, up-to-date review of the National Institute on Aging funding priorities as well as an examination of some of the major goals of the National Institute on Aging. In the Epilogue, the scientific relevance of transdisciplinary approaches to aging research is discussed, including the common challenges facing both biological anthropology and biological gerontology.

Based on the materials presented by the contributors to this volume, it is clear that they view biological anthropology as a major force in unraveling the complexity of biological aging. Although covering a diverse range of subject matter, the authors consistently demonstrate how traditional theories and tools of anthropology—evolutionary biology, adaptation and natural selection, human variation, plasticity, life-span perspectives, and holistic and comparative cross-cultural research—are necessary tools for gerontology and aging research. Furthermore, the contributors to this volume provide ample illustrations of the value of anthropological perspectives and reveal numerous areas where future research could benefit from this perspective. It is left to the reader to determine how well these directions are articulated, to interpret for themselves the usefulness of biological anthropology in the study of human aging, and to conclude whether or not biological anthropology and aging represent a paradigm of transdisciplinary research.

## REFERENCES

Arking, R. (1991) *Biology of Aging: Observations and Principles*. Englewood Cliffs, NJ: Prentice Hall.
Baker, P. T. (1982) Human population biology: a viable transdisciplinary science. *Human Biology* **54**, 203–220.
Baker, P. T. and Garruto, R. M. (1992) Health transitions: examples from the western Pacific. *Human Biology* **64**, 785–789.
Gavrilov, L. A. and Gavrilova, N. S. (1991) *The Biology of Life Span: A Quantitative Approach*. New York: Harwood Academic Publishers (Revised and updated English edition, edited by V. P. Skulachev, translated by John and Linda Payne).
Rose, M. R. (1991) *Evolutionary Biology of Aging*. New York: Oxford University Press.

# Acknowledgments

We would like to express our appreciation to the anonymous reviewers who devoted their time and efforts to comment usefully on the individual chapters included in this volume. In addition, we are thankful to Ms Lori Fitton for her help in preparing the final submission.

# Contents

14. Modeling the Variability in Longitudinal Patterns of Aging          373
    *L. J. Brant and J. D. Pearson*
15. Morphological Indicators of Skeletal Aging: Implications for
    Paleodemography and Paleogerontology                               394
    *S. R. Loth and M. Y. İşcan*
16. Role of the National Institute on Aging                            426
    *P. B. Eveleth*

    Epilogue: Human Aging—The Scientific Relevance of
    Transdisciplinary Approaches                                       434
    *R. M. Garruto and D. E. Crews*

    Index                                                              437

# Contributors

DAVID F. ARMSTRONG
Gallaudet University
800 Florida Avenue NE
Washington DC 20002

PAUL T. BAKER
Evan Pugh Professor Emeritus
Department of Anthropology
The Pennsylvania State University
409 Carpenter Building
University Park PA 16802

CYNTHIA M. BEALL
Department of Anthropology
Case Western Reserve University
433 Yost Building
Cleveland OH 44106

GILLIAN R. BENTLEY
Department of Anthropology
Northwestern University
Evanston IL 60208

LARRY J. BRANT
Gerontology Research Center
National Institute of Aging
4940 Eastern Ave
Baltimore MD 21224

JACOB A. BRODY
School of Public Health
University of Illinois at Chicago
2121 W Taylor St.
Chicago IL 60612-7260

DOUGLAS E. CREWS
Department of Anthropology and
    Department of Preventive Medicine
The Ohio State University
124 W 17th Ave
Columbus OH 43210

C. JEAN DEROUSSEAU
Department of Anthropology
University of Miami
Box 248106
Coral Gables FL 33124

PHYLLIS B. EVELETH
Office of Extramural Affairs
National Institute on Aging, NIH
Gateway Building, Suite 2C218
Bethesda MD 20892

KATHLEEN M. FOX
Department of Epidemiology and
    Preventive Medicine
University of Maryland at Baltimore
School of Medicine
660 W Redwood St
Baltimore MD 21201-1596

STANLEY M. GARN
Center for Human Growth &
    Development
University of Michigan
300 N Ingalls
Ann Arbor MI 48109-0406

RALPH M. GARRUTO
Laboratory of Central Nervous
    System Studies
National Institutes of Health
Building 36, Room 5B-21
9000 Rockville Pike
Bethesda MD 20892

LINDA M. GERBER
Cardiovascular Center
Cornell Medical Center
520 East 70th St—Starr 4
New York NY 10021

MEHMET YAŞAR İŞCAN
Department of Anthropology
Florida Atlantic University
PO Box 3091
Boca Raton FL 333431-0991

GARY D. JAMES
Department of Medicine
The New York Hospital
Cornell Medical Center
525 E 68th St
New York NY 10021

SOLOMON H. KATZ
University of Pennsylvania
3700 Spruce St
Philadelphia PA 19104

SUSAN R. LOTH
Department of Anthropology
Florida Atlantic University
PO Box 3091
Boca Raton FL 33431-0991

PETER J. MAYER
Department of Radiation Oncology
S.U.N.Y. Health Science Center at
   Brooklyn
450 Clarkson Ave
Box 1212
Brooklyn NY 11203

TONI P. MILES
Biobehavioral Health Program
Director, Center for Special
   Populations and Health
The Pennsylvania State University
210 E. Henderson Bldg.
University Park PA 16802

JAY D. PEARSON
Gerontology Research Center
National Institute on Aging
4940 Eastern Ave
Baltimore MD 21224

MARK S. PECKER
Department of Medicine
The New York Hospital
Cornell Medical Center
525 E 68th St
New York NY 10021

CHRIS C. PLATO
Gerontology Research Center
National Institute on Aging
National Institute of Health
4940 Eastern Ave
Baltimore MD 21224

WILLIAM A. STINI
Department of Anthropology
University of Arizona
Tucson AZ 85721

MICHAEL J. STRONG
Department of Clinical Neurological
   Sciences
University Hospital
University of Western Ontario
London Ontario N6A 5A5

JORDAN D. TOBIN
Gerontology Research Center
National Institute on Aging
National Institute of Health
4940 Eastern Ave
Baltimore MD 21224

TRUDY R. TURNER
Department of Anthropology
University of Wisconsin—Milwaukee
Milwaukee WI 53201

STEPHEN C. WEEKS
Savannah River Ecological
   Laboratory
University of Georgia
Athens, GA 29802

KENNETH M. WEISS
Department of Anthropology
The Pennsylvania State University
409 Carpenter Building
University Park PA 16802

MARK L. WEISS
Department of Anthropology
Wayne State University
Detroit MI 48202

JAMES W. WOOD
Department of Anthropology
The Pennsylvania State University
409 Carpenter Building
University Park PA 16802

# I

# INTRODUCTION AND BACKGROUND

# Aging as a Worldwide Phenomenon

## TONI P. MILES AND JACOB A. BRODY

### INTRODUCTION

For the first time in the history of humanity, large numbers of persons are surviving to older and older ages. This dramatic shift in the age structure of human populations is a process which is now occurring almost universally in countries across the globe. The process of population aging is best studied using mortality and survival statistics. Each country has similarities and differences in these statistics, which make it possible for us to measure rates of population aging. For students of biological anthropology and human population biology, it is the variation in the details of these events that is of particular interest. The goal of this chapter is to illustrate the occurrence of aging worldwide and to familiarize the reader with associated trends in causes of death and health status.

For purposes of discussion in this chapter, a population refers to a group of persons functioning as a unit. Anthropological studies of free-living animal behavior generally define interbreeding social groups as the unit of analysis. In human population aging, countries are the functional unit. Fertility and mortality statistics are the biological parameters used to describe unit function and are generally available through data-gathering organizations such as the United Nations (1955, 1988, 1991) or the World Health Organization. In the United States, population-level data are also available for individual racial and ethnic groups through the National Center for Health Statistics (NCHS) (1991). Trends in human population aging are studied by scientists called demographers. Demography is a science whose basic objectives are the analysis of variation and change in survival, migration and related factors affecting the size and age structure of human populations.

This chapter will concentrate on demographic factors leading to the currently observed increase in both absolute and relative numbers of older persons worldwide. During this century, owing to increased birth rates, demographers have documented an almost exponential increase in the overall size of the human population (United Nations, 1988). There has also been an increase in numbers of both middle-aged (45–64 years) and older (65 years and over) persons during the same period. This increase in the number of older

persons was not evenly distributed because each country has experienced
population aging at different rates (Torrey *et al.*, 1987; Kinsella, 1988). In the
following discussion, time-trend statistics demonstrating the relative or prop-
ortionate age distribution in several countries are presented to illustrate the
variability in rates of population aging. The increased survival by middle-aged
and older persons is primarily due to a lessening of the "forces of mortality" at
younger ages and a shift in the specific diseases which cause death (Omran,
1971; Olshansky and Ault, 1986). Statistics highlighting these mortality trends
are also presented. Finally, as a prelude to further discussions on evolutionary
aspects of population aging, data illustrating the population burden of chronic
disease and disability will be presented (see also Crews and Gerber, this
volume).

## WORLDWIDE GROWTH OF THE AGED POPULATION

An increase in the absolute number of persons aged 65 years and over is a
phenomenon that is occurring in both industrialized and nonindustrialized
nations (Torrey *et al.*, 1987; Kinsella, 1988; Miles and Brody, 1993). Since the
early part of this century, there has been a steady increase worldwide in the
numbers of persons aged 45–64 years as well as those 65 years and over. There
were 290 million persons aged 65 years and over worldwide in 1985 (United
Nations, 1988). By the year 2005, this number will increase to an estimated 410
million persons (Torrey *et al.*, 1987).

During the second half of the 20th century, population aging—an increase
in the proportion of the population aged 65 years and over—was also occurring
in most countries. Figure 1-1 shows historical and projected trends in

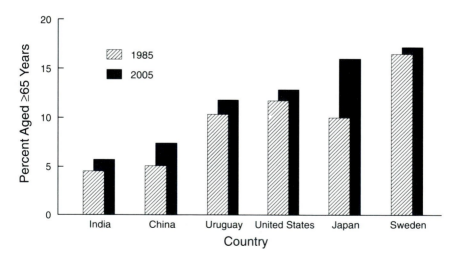

**Figure 1-1**   Global aging: percentage of persons aged 65 years and over in selected
countries, 1985 and 2005. Source: *Torrey et al.* (1987).

population aging for both industrialized (Sweden, United States, and Japan) and nonindustrialized (India, China, and Uruguay) countries. This shift in age structure for each country has been achieved at varying speed by low birth rates coupled with the lowest mortality rates in human history. In many cases (Japan is the most notable example) there has been a low birth rate coupled with a rapid decline in premature mortality (death before age 65 years). Speed of population aging can be expressed in the amount of time each country will take to double the size of its current population over the age of 65 years. Japan will take only 26 years to double its proportion of elderly from 7% to 14% (1970–1996), while that same process will take 115 years in France, and 66 years in the United States (Torrey et al., 1987). The continued growth of this population segment creates its own set of imperatives which are felt by each country to varying degrees now and in the years to come. Countries such as Japan, India, and China will experience the greatest growth in the proportion of the population aged 65 years and over (Figure 1-1).

## DEMOGRAPHIC FACTORS OF GROWTH

Wherever the phenomenon of population aging has occurred, shifts in the diseases which cause the most deaths are also observed (Omran, 1971; Olshansky and Ault, 1986). Over time there is usually a decline in the number of deaths from diseases with a rapid onset such as infections and accidents, accompanied by an increase in deaths from diseases with a longer clinical course such as cancer, heart disease and stroke (see also Crews and Gerber, this volume). Figure 1-2a and 1-2b illustrate this trend for the period 1900 through 1988 in the United States. In the US, deaths due to infectious diseases (tuberculosis, influenza, pneumonia) have declined dramatically since 1900 (Figure 1-2a). Diarrhea mortality has also declined and the greatest impact of this decline was on infants under age 1 year. For example, tuberculosis mortality rates have fallen from 194 per 100,000 in 1900 to 0.7 per 100,000 in 1986 (data not shown; NCHS, 1991). During the same period mortality due to chronic diseases such as cancer increased (Figure 1-2b) from 64 per 100,000 in 1900 to 194.7 per 100,000 in 1986 (NCHS, 1991). Mortality rates due to suicide remained constant throughout the period. Shifting mortality and population aging can also be stated this way: in 1900, 4.1% of the US population were aged 65 years or older and the life expectancy of a child born that year was 47.3 years (Siegel and Davidson, 1984). At that time infectious diseases such as tuberculosis, pneumonia, and diarrhea were major causes of death (NCHS, 1953). By 1980, 11.3% of the population was over age 65 years, the life expectancy at birth had increased to 73.7 years, and the leading causes of death had shifted to heart disease and cancer (NCHS, 1991).

In all human populations the first year of life is a period of high mortality risk. The increase in numbers of older persons worldwide can be partially attributed to improved survival among infants during the first year of life. Figure 1-3a shows the time trends in infant mortality rates for two countries and two racial groups in the US. Despite different rates of population aging, all

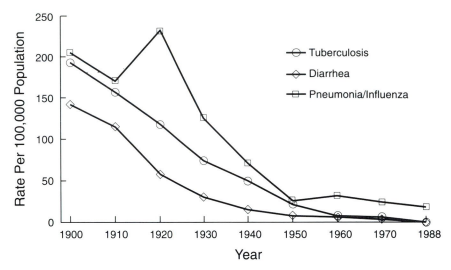

**Figure 1-2a** Time trends in US causes of death, 1900–1988: declining trends in tuberculosis, influenza/pneumonia and diarrhea mortality. Sources: Vital and Health Statistics (NCHS), 1953; Health United States, 1990.

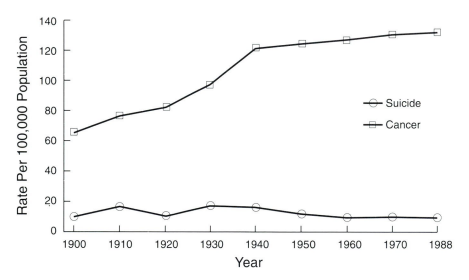

**Figure 1-2b** Time trends in US causes of death, 1900–1988: emerging trends in cancer and suicide mortality. Sources: Vital and Health Statistics (NCHS), 1953; Health United States, 1990.

four groups show the trend of decreasing infant mortality rates over time characteristic of an aging population. Sweden is a highly industrialized country and has been experiencing population aging since the 1800s while in India, population aging is limited to the later half of the 20th century (Kinsella, 1988). In the next century, India will have the largest number of persons over the age of 65 of all countries—an estimated 49 million persons aged 65 years and over by the year 2005 (Kinsella, 1988). Between 1900 and 1940, US children under age 1 experienced a 66% decline in death rates (Bogue, 1985). Despite the well-documented differences between US Blacks and Whites in measures of economic and health-care status, declines in infant mortality during the 1900s occurred for both groups—leading to growth in the numbers of Black and White older adults in the US (McKenney, 1979; Siegel and Davidson, 1984).

Another demographic trend contributing to population aging is increased survival among females. In all countries where population aging is occurring, females of all ages are experiencing marked declines in mortality rates (Omran, 1971; Fingerhut, 1982). Maternal mortality in the post-partum period has traditionally been a major contributor to low female life expectancy (Omran, 1971). Figure 1-3b shows the time trends in maternal mortality rates for US Blacks and Whites, and in Sweden. Although the rates vary across the groups, all show marked declines in maternal mortality over time which is also characteristic of an aging population.

A third demographic factor leading to the growth of the older population is delayed mortality among persons aged 65 years and over (Fingerhut, 1982; Olshansky and Ault, 1986). In 1985 for the most developed countries, the percentage of deaths occurring among persons under age 65 ranged from 20–30% of the year's total (Brody and Miles, 1990). If present trends continue, by the year 2020 all countries in the developed world will have less than 20% of deaths occurring prior to age 65 years. The increased survival of the current cohorts of older persons can be attributed to improved nutrition, better sanitation practices, and improved health care. Figure 1-4 shows the average remaining years of life in selected countries of females at three ages—65, 75, and 85 years. Average remaining years is a measure which describes both individual and group aspects of survival. For the individual, it can be interpreted as the average number of additional years a person that exact age can be expected to survive. For a group of individuals of the same age, it can be interpreted as an estimate of the number of years half the members of that group will survive. For example, in 1950, a person aged 65 years in Japan was expected to survive an average of 4.9 additional years. By 1985 in Japan, a person planning the health-care resource needs for the 13 million persons aged 65 years could expect that half this number, some 7.5 million persons, would survive to age 82 years (NCHS, 1987; United Nations, 1988; Feeney, 1990). It is worth noting that in the groups shown in Figure 1-4, females currently aged 85 years in 1985 have between 5.3 (Japan) and 7.3 (US Blacks) average remaining years.

## INCREASED MORBIDITY WITH ADVANCED AGE

In the period preceding death, declining health status and increasing numbers of co-morbid chronic diseases and conditions is the predominant pattern of morbidity in most industrialized nations among older persons (Brody and Miles, 1990; Olshansky et al., 1991). Whether or not this pattern represents

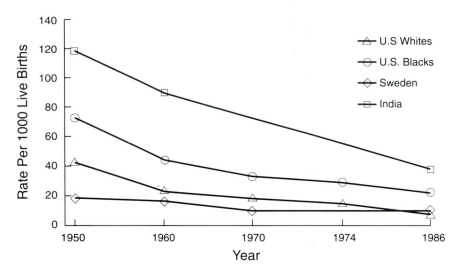

**Figure 1-3a** Time trends in infant mortality, 1950–1986: US Blacks, US Whites, Sweden, and India. Markers indicate time points for which data are available. Sources: NCHS (1991), UN Demographic Yearbook (1955–1991).

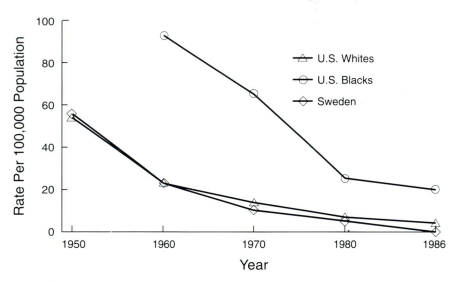

**Figure 1-3b** Time trends in maternal mortality: 1950–1986, US Blacks, US Whites, and Sweden. Markers indicate time points for which data are available. Sources: NCHS (1991), UN Demographic Yearbook (1955–1991).

normal aging and can be expected to continue in future populations of aged persons is the subject of controversy among researchers (Fries, 1980; Katz *et al.*, 1983; Schneider and Brody, 1983; Brody and Schneider, 1986; Olshansky *et al.*, 1990, 1991). The population burden of late-life morbidity can be envisioned in two ways. One way focuses on issues relevant to the specific

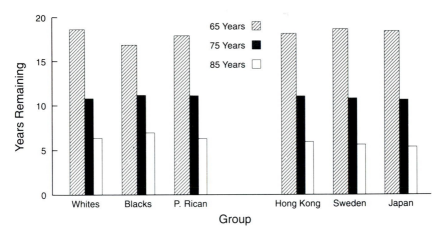

**Figure 1-4**  Average remaining years, females at age 65, 75, and 85 in 1985: US groups—Whites, Blacks, Puerto Ricans; Hong Kong, Sweden, and Japan. Source: NCHS (1987).

organ system involved and associated sequela of disease. When morbidity is viewed this way, similarities in disability emerge among persons affected by diseases which have very different biological mechanisms. A second way of understanding the burden of morbidity can be obtained from examining the experience of persons aged 85 years and over—the oldest old (see Suzman and Riley (1985) for an in-depth discussion of this segment of the population). By taking this perspective on morbidity, factors which may be universal to human aging across populations begin to emerge.

To illustrate the notion that homogeneous patterns of disability can be observed among older persons with diseases that have biologically heterogeneous mechanisms, consider the morbidity associated with skeletal aging—most notably osteoarthritis and osteoporosis (see Plato *et al.* (this volume) for an in-depth discussion of skeletal aging). Damage to muscles, bones, and joints is the final common pathway leading to pain, limited mobility, and loss of independence in both disorders (Mauer, 1979; White *et al.*, 1986; Lawrence *et al.*, 1990). In the US, arthritis is the most prevalent of chronic diseases among persons 45–64 years as well as among those 65 years and over, and most commonly involves the back, knees, and hips (Cunningham and Kelsey, 1984; Miles *et al.*, 1993). Osteoporotic vertebral and hip fractures are responsible for a significant proportion of the morbidity and mortality experienced by persons aged 65 years and older (Cummings *et al.*, 1985). Risk factors for the development of either osteoarthritis or osteoporosis have been linked to biological characteristics such as bone density (Dalen and Lamke, 1975; Bloom and Pogrund, 1982, Dequeker *et al.*, 1982, 1983; Mazess, 1982), body weight (Wootton *et al.*, 1982; Davis *et al.*, 1988, 1990), and other genetic factors (Smith *et al.*, 1973, Sowers *et al.*, 1986) as well as environmental exposures (Miles and Furner, 1991) which vary tremendously across human populations.

The reciprocal nature of biological risk factors for developing either osteoarthritis or osteoporosis makes the study of morbidity associated with skeletal aging across human populations a complex undertaking. Clinical studies indicate that these two diseases rarely occur in the same individual (Dequeker et al., 1982). Dequeker and colleagues (1983) describe this dichotomy in the following comparison of patients with the two disorders: osteoarthritic patients generally had a greater body weight, skeletal size, and grip strength than patients with osteoporosis of similar age, sex, height, and racial group. Bone density is also being studied as a contributor to these differences in body habitus. Low bone density is a well-recognized risk factor for osteoporotic hip fracture. Several investigators have proposed that high bone density may increase an individual's risk of knee osteoarthritis (Felson, 1988). In all populations studied, common biological determinants of bone density include sex, age, family genetics, early childhood nutrition (Miles and Furner, 1991), current physical activity (Dalen and Olsson, 1974; Smith et al., 1984), and current diet (Anderson and Tylavsky, 1984). Skeletal pathology of the lower back, hips, and knees—whether it is due to osteoporotic fractures or osteoarthritic erosion of joints—leads to chronic pain, impaired mobility, and loss of independent function. Research identifying the degrees to which individual factors contribute to the diseases of skeletal aging—osteoarthritis as well as osteoporosis will be an area of fruitful inquiry in the future (see also Plato et al., this volume).

The circumstances of persons aged 85 years and over can be used to illustrate universal features of morbidity and its impact on late life. Members of this group commonly experience a triad consisting of co-morbid medical conditions, poor physical function, and declining health prior to death (Olshansky et al., 1991). An examination of the cross-national variation in this pattern among 85 year olds, imposed by disease and disability, is not currently possible because comparable data do not exist. We can, however, examine morbidity and disability data available from four geographically distinct communities of older adults in the US (see Cornoni-Huntley et al., 1986, 1990) for a complete description of the communities). The Established Populations for Epidemiologic Studies of the Elderly (EPESE), initiated by the National Institute on Aging in 1984, were designed to provide information on the health and well-being of a sample of non-institutionalized, community-based older adults (see Eveleth, this volume) for a further discussion of National Institute of Aging research initiatives).

The burden of chronic conditions among the oldest-old is an issue of public health concern. Many of the diseases and conditions listed in Table 1-1 do not cause death but can impose serious limitations in functioning. For both the individual and society, the problems created by having one or more chronic diseases are related to the amount of time a person *lives* with those diseases. The restrictions in physiology associated with diseases deplete reserves and can ultimately cause an individual to lose independence in late life (Guralnik et al., 1989a, 1989b). Consider as an example, disorders referable to the cardiovascular system such as hypertension, heart attack, and stroke which are highly

**Table 1-1**  Prevalence rates for selected chronic conditions among females aged 85 years and over, by site, EPESE populations, 1984.[a]

|  | Sites | | | | |
|---|---|---|---|---|---|
| Conditions | East Boston | New Haven | Iowa | North Carolina (Blacks) | North Carolina (Whites) |
| Hypertension | 41.3 | 35.7 | 49.5 | 59.1 | 50.7 |
| Stroke | 10.3 | 6.2 | 8.7 | 9.0 | 16.9 |
| Angina | 1.4 | 3.4 | 3.6 | 10.1 | 7.2 |
| Heart attack | 12.5 | 9.3 | 12.8 | 19.8 | 14.4 |
| Diabetes | 13.6 | 8.3 | 8.7 | 13.7 | 14.3 |
| Cancer | 7.6 | 15.1 | 17.4 | 8.2 | 16.1 |
| Hip fracture | 9.8 | 14.4 | 11.8 | 4.0 | 17.1 |
| Hearing[b] impairment | 22.8 | 29.4 | 23.8 | 36.3 | 30.3 |
| Visual[c] impairment | 84.8 | 95.7 | 98.3 | 89.9 | 92.6 |
| Urinary[d] incontinence | 41.3 | 30.0 | 40.5 | 51.6 | 48.1 |

[a]Source: Cornoni-Huntley (1986, 1990).

[b]Percentage reporting difficulty. Question: "(With/without) a hearing aid, can you usually hear and understand what a person says without seeing his face if that person talks in a normal voice to you in a quiet room?"

[c]Percentage reported wearing eyeglasses/contact lenses or both. Question: "Do you wear eyeglasses/contact lenses or both?"

[d]Percentage reporting "some, most, or all" of the time. Question: "How often do you have difficulty holding your urine until you get to a toilet?"

prevalent in each of the EPESE communities among the oldest old. Persons with cardiovascular disease—particularly hypertension—now live longer due in part to improved medical care. During the past 40 years, hypertension-induced stroke mortality in the adult US population has declined dramatically while in the same period hypertension prevalence rates have increased (Osfeld, 1980). This may account for the high prevalence of hypertension in the EPESE communities, which ranges from 35.7% (New Haven) to 59.1% (North Carolina, Blacks).

Disability due to either impaired sensory perception or difficulty with activities of daily living (or some combination of both) appear to be a nearly universal feature of life for persons aged 85 years and over. Impairment in hearing and vision are non-fatal chronic conditions which place a considerable burden on persons aged 85 years and over (Table 1-2). Between 30 and 51.6% of persons in these communities report that they have difficulty holding urine "some, most, or all" of the time. Difficulty with stooping, moving objects large or small, or walking a half mile can make it impossible for a person to live independently. In the EPESE communities, between 58.9% (Iowa) and 70.7% (East Boston) reported being unable to walk a half mile without help. The focus of currently ongoing research is the identification of risk factors for the development of impairments and disability. By preventing or delaying the onset of these disabilities, the quality of life can be improved for older persons and their families.

**Table 1-2** Prevalence rates for disability in selected activities of daily living among females aged 85 years and over, by site, EPESE populations, 1984.[a]

| Activity | Sites | | | | |
|---|---|---|---|---|---|
| | East Boston | New Haven | Iowa | North Carolina (Blacks) | North Carolina (Whites) |
| Bathing[b] | 43.5 | 30.9 | 14.1 | 18.0 | 23.0 |
| Dressing[b] | 22.8 | 16.4 | 9.1 | 12.9 | 17.3 |
| Room walking[b] | 39.1 | 32.4 | 24.1 | 26.4 | 31.1 |
| Grooming[b] | 21.2 | 11.0 | 8.3 | 10.2 | 11.4 |
| Transferring[b] | 22.8 | 15.0 | 10.3 | 11.0 | 15.6 |
| Using toilet[b] | 18.5 | 9.7 | 10.3 | 11.7 | 15.2 |
| Eating[b] | 12.5 | 4.8 | 4.1 | 3.3 | 1.8 |
| Stairs[c] | 50.0 | 29.6 | 25.7 | 48.0 | 52.7 |
| Half mile walk[c] | 70.7 | 61.2 | 58.9 | 66.1 | 66.3 |
| Shoulder extension[d] | 44.4 | 25.9 | 34.9 | 44.4 | 33.8 |
| Small objects[d] | 43.1 | 20.2 | 36.9 | 54.7 | 40.2 |
| Large objects[d] | 77.8 | 48.1 | 69.2 | 82.9 | 72.3 |
| Sleeping[d] | 79.2 | 58.0 | 75.4 | 78.5 | 78.2 |

[a]Source: Cornoni-Huntley (1986, 1990).

[b]Question: "Other than when you might have been in the hospital, was there any time in the past 12 months in which you needed help from some person or from some equipment or device to do the activity." Percentage reporting *assistance needed/unable to do.*

[c]Question: "Are you *able* to walk stairs/walk half mile *without* help?" Percentage reporting *unable.*

[d]Question: "How much difficulty, if any, do you have (with activity)"? Percentage reporting *any* difficulty.

## SUMMARY

An increase in the absolute number of persons aged 65 years and over is a phenomenon that is occurring in both industrialized and nonindustrialized nations. The continued growth of this population segment creates its own set of imperatives which are felt by each country to varying degrees now and will continue to be felt in the years to come. The phenomenon of aging in most human populations is associated with several trends, such as a shift to heart disease, stroke, and cancer as the major causes of mortality, improved survival among infants, improved survival among females, and delayed mortality among persons aged 65 years and over. Declining health status and increasing numbers of co-morbid chronic diseases and conditions prior to death is the predominant pattern of morbidity in most industrialized nations among older persons. The problem created by having one or more chronic diseases is related to the amount of time a person lives with the diseases. Skeletal aging—most notably osteoarthritis and osteoporosis—are major causes of morbidity in late life. Cross-population studies of biological risk factors for these diseases will significantly enhance our understanding of the aging process.

## REFERENCES

Anderson, J. J. B. and Tylavsky, F. A. (1984) Diet and osteopenia in elderly caucasian women. In: *Osteoporosis: Proceedings of the Copenhagen Symposium on Osteoporosis June 3–8, 1984* (eds Christiansen, C., Arnaud, C. D., Nordin, B. E. C. *et al.*). Denmark: Department of Clinical Chemistry, Glostrup Hospital, pp. 299–304.

Bloom, R. A. and Pogrund, H. (1982) Humeral cortical thickness in female Bantu: its relationship to the incidence of femoral neck fracture. *Skeletal Radiology* **8**, 56–62.

Bogue, D. J. (1985) *The Population of the United States: Historical Trends and Future Projections*. New York: Macmillan, Inc.

Brody, J. A. and Miles, T. P. (1990) Mortality postponed and the unmasking of age-dependent non-fatal conditions. *Aging* **2**, 283–289.

Brody, J. A. and Schneider, E. L. (1986) Diseases and disorders of aging: an hypothesis. *Journal of Chronic Diseases* **39**, 871–876.

Cornoni-Huntley, J. C., Brock, D. B., Ostfeld, A. M., Taylor, J. O. and Wallace, R. B. (1986) *Established Populations for Epidemiologic Studies of the Elderly*. Bethesda, MD. NIH publication no. 86-2443.

Cornoni-Huntley, J. C., Blazer, D. G., Lafferty, M. E., Everett, D. F., Brock, D. B. and Farmer, M. E. (1990) *Established Populations for Epidemiologic Studies of the Elderly*. Bethesda, MD. NIH publication no. 90-495.

Cunningham, L. S. and Kelsey, J. L. (1984) Epidemiology of musculoskeletal impairments and associated disability. *American Journal of Public Health* **74**, 574–579.

Cummings, S. R., Kelsey, J. L., Nevitt, M. C. and O'Dowd, K. (1985) Epidemiology of osteoporosis and osteoporotic fractures. *Epidemiologic Reviews* **7**, 178–208.

Dalen, N. and Lamke, B. (1975) Bone mass in obese subjects. *Acta Medica Scandinavica* **197**, 353–355.

Dalen, N. and Olsson, K. E. (1974) Bone mineral content and physical activity. *Acta Orthopedica Scandinavica* **45**, 170–174.

Davis, M. A., Ettinger, W. H., Neuhaus, J. M. and Hauck, W. W. (1988) Sex differences in osteoarthritis of the knee: the role of obesity. *American Journal of Epidemiology* **127**, 1019–1030.

Davis, M. A., Neuhaus, J. M., Ettinger, W. H. and Mueller, W. H. (1990) Body fat distribution and osteoarthritis. *American Journal of Epidemiology* **132**, 701–707.

Dequeker, J., Goris, P. and Uytterhoeven, R. (1983) Osteoporosis and osteoarthritis (osteoarthrosis): anthropometric distinctions. *Journal of the American Medical Association* **249**, 1448–1451.

Dequeker, J., Burssens, A. and Bouillon, R. (1982) Dynamics of growth hormone secretion in patients with osteoporosis and in patients with osteoarthrosis. *Hormone Research* **16**, 353–356.

Feeney, G. (1990). *The Demography of Aging in Japan: 1950–2025*. Series no. 55, NUPRI research paper. Tokyo: Nihon University Population Research Institute.

Felson, D. T. (1988) Epidemiology of hip and knee osteoarthritis. *Epidemiologic Reviews* **10**, 1–28.

Fingerhut, L. (1982) *Changes in Mortality Among the Elderly, U.S., 1940–1978*. Vital Health Statistics series 3 no. 22. Hyattsville, MD: National Center for Health Statistics.

Fries, J. F. (1980) Aging, natural death and the compression of morbidity. *New England Journal of Medicine* **303**, 130–135.

Guralnik, J. M., LaCroix, A. Z. and Everett, D. F. (1989a) Comorbidity of chronic conditions and disability among older persons—United States. 1984. *Morbidity and Mortality Weekly Report* **38**, 1788–1891.

Guralnik, J. M., LaCroix, A. Z., Everett, D. F. and Kovar, M. G. (1989b) Aging in the eighties: the prevalence of comorbidity and its association with disability. *Advance Data from Vital and Health Statistics*, no. 170. Hyattsville, Maryland: National Center for Health Statistics.

Katz, S., Branch, L. G., Branson, M. H., Papsidero, J. A., Beck, J. C. and Greer, D. S. (1983) Active life expectancy. *New England Journal of Medicine* **309**, 1818–1224.

Kinsella, K. (1988) Aging in the third world. International Population Reports; series P-25, no. 79. Washington: US Bureau of the Census.

Lawrence, R. C., Everett, D. S. and Hochberg, M. C. (1990). Arthritis. In: *Health Status and Well Being of the Elderly* (eds Cornoni-Huntley, J.C., Huntley, R. R. and Feldman, J. J.). National Health and Nutrition Examination I Epidemiologic Followup Survey. New York: Oxford University Press, pp. 136–154.

Mauer, K. (1979) *Basic Data on Arthritis Knee, Hip, and Sacroiliac Joints in Adults 25–74 Years, United States, 1971–1975*. Vital Health Statistics series 11 no. 213. Hyatsville, MD: National Center for Health Statistics.

Mazess, R. B. (1982) On aging bone loss. *Clinics in Orthopedics* **165**, 239–252.

McKenney, N. D. R. (1979) *The Social and Economic Status of the Black Population in the United States*: An Historical View, 1790–1978. Series P-23, no. 80. Washington: US Bureau of the Census.

Miles, T. P. and Brody, J. A. (1993) International aging. In: *Health Statistics on Older Persons*. Hyatsville, MD: National Center for Health Statistics, Chapter 11, Series 3, no. 27, pp. 289–295.

Miles, T. P., Flegal, K and Harris, T. (1993) Musculoskeletal disorders—time trends, co-morbid conditions, self assessed health status and associated activity limitations. In: *Health Statistics on Older Persons*. Hyatsville, MD: National Center for Health Statistics, Chapter 10, Series 3, no. 27, pp. 275–288.

Miles, T. P. and Furner, S. E. (1991) Early life malnutrition and risk of hip fracture: identifying populations at risk. *Age & Nutrition* **2**, 137–140.

National Center for Health Statistics (1953) *Vital Statistics of the United States: Mortality, 1950*. Washington: US Government Printing Office.

National Center for Health Statistics (1987) *Health Statistics on Older Persons, US 1986* (eds Havlik, R. J., Liu, M., Kovar, M. G. *et al.*). Vital and Health Statistics, series 3, no. 25, DHHS publication no. (PHS) 87-1409. Washington: US Government Printing Office.

National Center for Health Statistics (1991) *Health United States, 1990*. Hyattsville, Maryland: Public Health Services.

Olshansky, S. J. and Ault, A. B. (1986) The fourth stage of the epidemiologic transition: the age of delayed degenerative diseases. *The Milbank Quarterly* **64**, 355–391.

Olshansky, S. J., Carnes, B. A. and Cassel, C. (1990) In search of methuselah: estimating the upper limits of human longevity. *Science* **250**, 634–640.

Olshansky, S. J., Rudberg, M. A., Carnes, B. A., Cassel, C. K. and Brody, J. A. (1991) Trading off longer life for worsening health. *Journal of Aging and Health* **3**, 194–216.

Omran, A. R. (1971) The epidemiologic transition: a theory of the epidemiology of population change. *The Milbank Memorial Fund Quarterly* **49**, 509–538.

Osfeld, A. M. (1980) A review of stroke epidemiology. *Epidemiologic Reviews* **2**, 136–152.

Schneider, E. L. and Brody, J. A. (1983) Aging, natural death and the compression of morbidity: Another view. *New England Journal of Medicine* **309**, 854–856.

Siegel, J. S. and Davidson, M. (1984) *Demographic and Socioeconomic Aspects of Aging in the United States*. Series P-23, no. 138. Washington: US Bureau of the Census.

Smith, D. M., Nance, W. E., Ke, W. K., Christian, J. C. and Johnston, C. C. (1973) Genetic factors in determining bone mass. *Journal of Clinical Investigation* **52**, 2800–2808.

Smith, E. L., Smith, P. E., Ensign, C. J. and Shea, M. M. (1984) Bone involution decrease in exercising middle-aged women. *Calcified Tissue International* **36**, 129–138.

Sowers, M. F., Burns, T. L. and Wallace, R. B. (1986) Familial resemblance of bone mass in adult women. *Genetic Epidemiology* **3**, 85–93.

Suzman, R., and Riley, M. W. (eds) (1985) The oldest old. *Milbank Memorial Fund Quarterly* **63**, 177–205.

Torrey, B. B., Kinsella, K. and Taeuber, C. M. (1987) *An Aging World*. International Population Reports, series P-25, no. 78. Washington: US Bureau of the Census.

United Nations (1955) *United Nations Demographic Yearbook 1954*, 6th issue, pp. 588–597.

United Nations (1988) *United Nations Demographic Yearbook 1986*, 35th issue, ST/ESA/STAT/SER ST/ESA/STAT/SER.R/16.

United Nations (1991) *United Nations Demographic Yearbook 1989*, ST/ESA/STAT/SER.R/19.

White, L. R., Cartwright, W. S., Cornoni-Huntley, J. and Brock, D. B. (1986) Geriatric epidemiology. *Annual Review of Gerontology and Geriatrics* **6**, 215–311.

Wootton, R., Bryson, E., Elsasser, U., Freeman, H., Green, J. R., Hesp, R., Hudson, E. A., Klenerman, L., Smith, T. and Zanelli, J. (1982) Risk factors for fractured neck of femur in the elderly. *Age and Ageing* **11**, 160–168.

# II
# EVOLUTIONARY BIOLOGY OF AGING AND SENESCENCE

# 2

# Human Population Biology and the Evolution of Aging

JAMES W. WOOD, STEPHEN C. WEEKS, GILLIAN R. BENTLEY
AND KENNETH M. WEISS

## INTRODUCTION

With some oversimplification, most current ideas about the mechanisms of
human aging can be dichotomized into two contrasting positions, which we will
call the *gerontological* (GR) and the *epidemiological* (EP) points of view.[1] In
the extreme GR view, the various aspects of aging reflect a single unitary
process that is programmed in a central way. We call this position "gerontological" because it has been a dominant paradigm within the field of
gerontology, at least until very recently (Finch, 1990). According to that
paradigm, it is meaningful to think of the life span as a single measurable
phenotype and to treat age patterns of fertility and mortality during the later
segments of life as controlled by one underlying mechanism that has evolved
and can be compared across species. Researchers who adopt this view spend
much of their time searching for common biological factors that may explain
several aspects of aging at once. From this perspective, linkages among
life-span events and processes (e.g., similar accelerations in risk with age
among different senescent diseases, or parallel declines in fertility and survival
with age) are a foregone conclusion.

The EP view, in contrast, holds that fertility and mortality are each
determined by several distinct, independent (or quasi-independent) physiological processes. We call this position "epidemiological" because of
epidemiologists' longstanding interest in independent competing causes of
death. In the EP view, life span is virtually an artifact: it is the outcome of
whatever collection of competing causes of morbidity and mortality happens to
be operating in a particular environmental setting, as well as of the ways in
which the risks of experiencing those various causes accelerate with age.
According to this view, natural selection does not act upon a unitary phenotype
such as life span or total reproductive output, but rather acts upon the separate

[1]We are grateful to James Vaupel for suggesting these terms.

underlying physiological processes involved in birth and death. From the EP perspective, the apparent coordination of fertility and mortality is not a foregone conclusion and requires special explanation. This is not to say that such coordination is inconsistent with the EP view, but only that it does not follow as a necessary corollary of that view. In a sense, life-course coordination is a more interesting phenomenon for those who adhere to the EP position than for die-hard supporters of the GR view.

One way to contrast these two views is to reduce them to their extreme predictions. In the EP view, if the environmental risk factors associated with all existing causes of death were eliminated, life expectancy could increase with little or no theoretical limit. In the GR view, complete elimination of the current causes of death would not extend life beyond its programmed maximum, usually assumed to be about 95–105 years for humans, but would merely allow a larger fraction of individuals to attain that maximum. In this latter view, causes of death that are now of great importance, such as cancer or cardiovascular disease, are not fundamentally related to the determination of the maximal life span.

In research on human aging, it has proven difficult to devise critical tests of the GR and EP views based solely upon empirical evidence. We suggest that an alternative way to evaluate the two views is to gauge how consistent they are with established theoretical models for the evolution of aging. In this paper, we review the theoretical population biology of aging with two basic aims in mind: (1) to identify the most plausible evolutionary models; and (2) to explore the implications of those models for the GR and EP views. In general, we argue that the EP view is more consistent with evolutionary theory than the GR view, a conclusion that has important implications for our understanding of human aging.

Unlike many treatments of aging in the biomedical literature, we define aging in terms of *fitness components* and therefore include senescent changes affecting not only mortality, but fertility as well. We believe that a complete theoretical treatment of human aging must include reproduction as well as morbidity and mortality. In keeping with established usage, the terms *fecundity* and *viability* will be used to refer to the biological capacity for reproducing and staying alive, respectively.

## MODELS FOR THE EVOLUTION OF AGING

### Does Senescence Require an Evolutionary Model?

The starting point for all evolutionary thinking about senescence is the intuition that senescence *per se* poses a special problem for natural selection. Since senescence can be defined as increasingly negative changes to fitness components with increasing age (Rose, 1991), how can such declining age-specific fitness be reconciled with evolution by natural selection? This question was first posed by Haldane (1941) and Medawar (1952) and has been taken up subsequently by most evolutionary biologists who have written on the

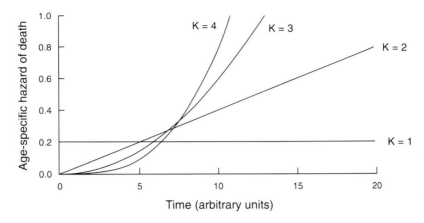

**Figure 2-1** A simple multi-hit model. Hits are assumed to occur with constant hazard λ, and a total of K hits results in death. Age-specific hazards of death are plotted for various values of K. Note that "senescence" (a hazard of death that increases with age) is an inherent feature of the model whenever K>1.

subject. All have built upon Medawar's original suggestion (embodied in his famous analogy of breaking test tubes) that the "natural" starting point for the evolution of senescence is a complete absence of senescence.

We suggest that the absence of senescence may be an inappropriate evolutionary "null" model, at least for metazoans. To take Medawar's analogy, a test tube has a constant hazard of mortality because it has a single component, the glass tube itself, and when that component breaks the entire "organism" may be regarded as dead; if the hazard of breakage is constant, then the hazard of death is also constant and no senescent increase in mortality occurs. In contrast, complex organisms are made up of multiple components with a high degree of redundancy and "parallel processing." Death in such an organism may not occur until several or all components in a given physiological system fail. Even if the hazard of failure *per component* is constant, the risk of death increases monotonically with age as long as more than one component must fail for death to occur.

This logic has been parameterized in the so-called *multi-hit* or *multi-stage model* of death (Elandt-Johnson and Johnson, 1980). In the simplest version of this model, first investigated by Nordling (1953), component failures ("hits") occur among $N$ components at risk of failure with a constant hazard λ, and $K$ hits result in death. The hazard function, $h(t)$, for death at age $t$ under this model is a simple Weibull function:

$$h(t) = K\omega t^{K-1}, \quad \omega > 0, K \geqslant 1 \tag{2-1}$$

where $\omega = N\lambda^K$. This function is plotted for various values of $K$ in Figure 2-1. As can be seen, the only case in which no senescent increase in mortality occurs is the one-component case $(K = 1)$, which corresponds to Medawar's test tube analogy. With any degree of organismal complexity $(K \geqslant 2)$, senescence is an inherent property of the system. While many, more complex multi-stage/multi-hit models have been proposed over the years (e.g., Whittemore and Keller, 1978; Weiss and Chakraborty, 1984, 1988; Moolgavkar, 1993), they all retain this same property; mortality rates increase monotonically with age whenever more than one hit must occur before death ensues.

Natural selection thus appears to be unnecessary to explain the *origin* of senescence, except indirectly by explaining the evolution of organismal complexity. What this idea leaves unexplained, however, is the tremendoous *differential delay* of senescence observed in different species: some species live a few days, others a hundred years. This differential is what we are really trying to explain with our evolutionary models, not the mere fact of senescence itself.

## The Basic Evolutionary Model

All successful models of aging begin with a single insight: in an age-structured population, phenotypic traits that are expressed late in life have a smaller impact on fitness (positive or negative) than those expressed early in life, simply because fewer individuals survive to display such traits. As a consequence, reductions in fertility and mortality, the two major components of fitness, are more nearly *selectively neutral* if they occur at late ages than if they occur at early ones. This insight was first discussed by Haldane (1941), Medawar (1952), and Williams (1957), and later formalized by Hamilton (1966), Charlesworth (1980), and others (Abugov, 1986; Abrams, 1991).

To understand the various formalizations, we first need to agree on a measure of fitness. Fisher (1930) originally equated fitness with the *Malthusian parameter* (*r*), the intrinsic rate of increase of a group of individuals sharing the same genotype. From stable population theory, *r* is found by solving the *Lotka–Euler renewal equation*,

$$\int_0^\infty \exp(-rt)S(t)f(t)\mathrm{d}t = 1 \qquad (2\text{-}2)$$

where $S(t)$ is the age-specific survival function (i.e., the probability of surviving from birth to age $t$) characteristic of the genotype, and $f(t)$ is the age-specific hazard of a live birth at age $t$ to individuals sharing the genotype. The survival function $S(t)$ is the outcome of all the preceding age-specific risks of death: if $q(t)$ is the probability of dying at age $t$ and $p(t) = 1 - q(t)$, then $S(t) = p(0)p(1)p(2) \ldots p(t-1)$. (The probability of death at age $t$ is related to the *hazard* of death as $q(t) = 1 - e^{-h(t)}$.) The Malthusian parameter, $r$, is calculated by incorporating known values of $S(t)$ and $f(t)$ into Equation 2-2 and solving for the dominant root. In this model, then, fitness is a function of age-specific survival and fertility, which seems intuitively correct.

Assuming for the moment that $r$ is an appropriate measure of fitness, one way to gauge the evolutionary impact of senescence is to perform a *sensitivity analysis* of Equation 2-2. In such an analysis, small changes or "perturbations" in either fertility or mortality are introduced at a particular age while all other components of the model are held constant, and the resulting change in fitness is computed. Hamilton (1966) performed such an analysis using a discrete-time form of Equation 2-2 and taking partial derivatives of $r$ with respect to $f(t)$ and $\ln p(t)$, yielding[2]

$$\partial r/\partial f(t) = \exp(-rt)S(t)/\sum_{a=1}^{\infty} a\exp(-ra)S(a)f(a) \qquad (2\text{-}3)$$

$$\partial r/\partial \ln p(t) = \left[ \sum_{a=t+1}^{\infty} \exp(-ra)S(a)f(a) \right] \bigg/ \left[ \sum_{a=1}^{\infty} a\exp(-ra)S(a)f(a) \right]$$
$$(2\text{-}4)$$

These equations are plotted using human data in Figure 2-2, showing that changes in survival and reproduction have a monotonically decreasing effect on fitness with increasing age. The fitness effects of changes in fertility begin to decline immediately after birth, while those of changes in survival begin to decline only after the age at first reproduction (approximately 19 years in the population illustrated in Figure 2-2). In other words, factors that reduce fertility or increase mortality will have a decreasing effect on overall fitness with increasing age. Since natural selection "recognizes" only those factors that affect fitness, selection intensity thus declines with age, as first suggested by Haldane (1941) and Medawar (1952). Note, however, that the partial derivatives in Figure 2-2 never become negative, although they can take on values negligibly different from zero. This fact indicates that there is never positive selection for senescence *per se*, but only that senescence is likely to be selectively neutral or nearly neutral if it occurs late enough.

Although Hamilton's analysis is widely regarded as providing the standard model for the evolution of senescence, there are several reasons to believe that $r$ may not always be a good measure of fitness. For example, Charlesworth (1974, 1976) has shown for both single and two-locus systems, that the Malthusian parameter approximates fitness only when: (1) selection is weak; (2) the population is near the selective equilibrium gene frequency; and (3) the population has attained its stable age distribution (i.e., the equilibrium age distribution associated with a constant set of age-specific fertility and mortality rates). In addition, non-random mating, density dependence, differences in selection coefficients between the sexes, and multiple loci can all cause the Malthusian parameter to depart markedly from the "true" value of fitness.

How, then, are the conclusions drawn from Hamilton's sensitivity analysis altered if alternative measures of fitness are used? An important recent analysis by Abugov (1986) has shown, first, that Hamilton's results always emerge as special cases of a more general treatment and, second, that the more general model produces large departures from Hamilton's results only in extreme circumstances (e.g., very intense selection or initial gene frequencies that are very far from equilibrium). In general, it appears that the primary *qualitative*

---

[2]Hamilton worked with $\ln p(t)$ rather than $p(t)$ or $S(t)$ purely for mathematical convenience.

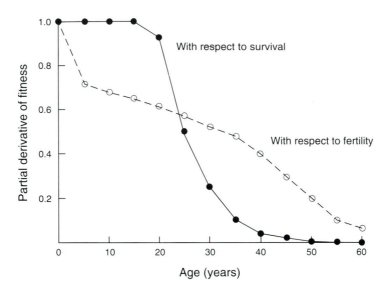

**Figure 2-2**   Results of Hamilton's (1966) sensitivity analysis of the Lotka–Euler renewal equation (Equations 2-3 and 2-4) plotted using data on males in the Gainj, a tribal population of highland Papua New Guinea. Data from Wood (1987).

conclusion drawn from Hamilton's work applies to a very close approximation regardless of the fitness measure used, namely, selection intensity declines monotonically with time since birth (for fertility) or time since the onset of reproduction (for mortality).

Hamilton's analysis provides the basic reason senescence *can* evolve, but does not specify the precise evolutionary mechanisms through which it *will* evolve. Two such mechanisms are now widely recognized (Rose, 1991): *age-specific gene action* (ASGA) and *antagonistic pleiotropy* (AP). In the ASGA model, which is the simpler of the two, senescence merely reflects the random accumulation of deleterious alleles that depress viability or fecundity but that are not expressed phenotypically until late in life (Edney and Gill, 1968). The AP model involves alleles with pleiotropic effects that differ in different segments of the life course, showing beneficial effects early in life but deleterious effects at later ages (Williams, 1957); because of the decline in selection intensity with age, small but early beneficial effects can more than offset large (even fatal) but late negative effects. One important difference between the AP and ASGA models is that selection will actively favor senescence (or rather permit it as a byproduct of favorable selection on a correlated character) only in the AP model; the ASGA model is essentially one of random genetic drift. It is important to stress, however, that the two models are in no way mutually exclusive. Either or both could be operating in any given instance (Service *et al.*, 1988). Moreover, population genetics models show that both mechanisms are plausible and consistent with genic selection (Charlesworth, 1980; Rose, 1984).

It is important to emphasize that these mechanisms are also consistent with multi-stage/multi-hit models of senescence. If, for example, the onset of reproduction were delayed, natural selection would favor delayed senescence associated, perhaps, with a higher value of $K$ in Equation 2-1 (i.e., greater system-component redundancy) or a lower value of $\lambda$ (a lower system-component failure rate). One can imagine, for some physiological systems, that $\lambda$ is a reflection of DNA repair mechanisms. Delayed senescence could be achieved by fine tuning such mechanisms so that the accumulation of age-specific deleterious mutations is effectively postponed until advanced ages.

## EMPIRICAL EVIDENCE FOR THE EVOLUTIONARY MODEL

### Fissile Versus Ovigerous Reproduction

One virtue of the evolutionary model is that it makes several testable predictions (for a detailed review, see Rose, 1991). The first involves a comparison of organisms that reproduce through fission (e.g., protozoa, some annelid worms, and cnidarians) with those that reproduce through ovigerous mechanisms (most higher plants and animals). In an organism with a clearly defined soma and germ line, senescence is expected to evolve because of reduced selection on fertility and survival at later stages in the organism's life history (Medawar, 1952; Williams, 1957; Edney and Gill, 1968; Rose, 1991). Fissile organisms do not have distinguishable somatic and germ cells and thus cannot be separated into distinguishable adults and offspring. Such organisms reset the developmental clock each time they split into equal-sized individuals and therefore do not have age classes or distinct parents and offspring. Thus, fissile organisms should not senesce. This prediction has recently been called "one of the strongest theoretical predictions in all of evolutionary biology" (Rose, 1991).

Although this prediction was clearly stated by Williams in 1957, there have been few studies designed specifically to test it (Rose, 1991). Bell (1984c) compared two fissile oligochaete worms to four ovigerous animals (two rotiers and two crustaceans) and found that all four of the ovigerous animals showed mortality rates that increased with age, whereas the two fissile animals showed no such increase in mortality. These results clearly support the evolutionary model of senescence. Comparative studies generally confirm the expected lack of senescence in fissile organisms. For example, Rose (1991) has brought together comparative data from vertebrates, invertebrates, protozoa, and plants, showing that organisms with a well-defined soma (e.g., vertebrates and arthropods) have mortality rates that increase with age. In contrast, organisms that reproduce through fission (e.g., many cnidarians, annelids, platyhelminths, and protozoa) or vegetatively (many plants) commonly have "endogenously unlimited life spans" (Rose, 1991). The only fissile organisms that do not show the expected lack of senescence are the ciliates (Bell, 1988). Accumulations of deleterious mutations in mitotically dividing cells have been postulated as an explanation for the loss of viability with time in ciliates (Bell, 1988). The differentiation of macro- and micronuclei in ciliates has also been proposed as an analog of the soma/germ line distinction in larger organisms (Rose, 1991). Neither of these explanations is entirely satisfactory and further work on senescence in ciliates seems in order.

### Correlations in Exogenous Mortality and the Rate of Senescence

One apparent prediction of the evolutionary model, first noted by Williams (1957), is that species of populations with high levels of "exogenous" mortality should be characterized by rapid senescence. (Here "exogenous" means extrinsic to the physiological state of the organism and thus independent of age.) The reason is that species with relatively high exogenous mortality are less likely to live to advanced ages, even in the absence of senescence. For example, in Figure 2-3 (top panel), species 1 experiences a level of exogenous mortality that is twice as high as that of species 2. As a consequence, the

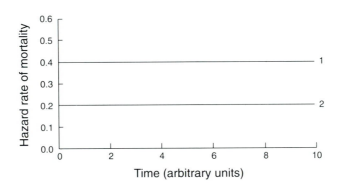

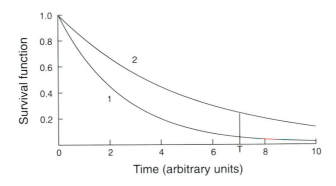

**Figure 2-3** Differing levels of exogenous mortality and their associated survival curves. Species 1 has a level of age-independent mortality that is twice as high as that of species 2 (top). As a result, far fewer members of species 1 survive to age $T$ (bottom). (If $\lambda_i$, the mortality hazard rate in species $i$, is constant and independent of age, then the corresponding probability of surviving to age $T$ is $S(T) = \exp(-\lambda_i T)$.) Over time, species 1 is expected to evolve a higher rate of senescence than species 2.

probability that an individual of species 1 survives to age $T$, say, is necessarily lower than the corresponding probability for a representative of species 2 (Figure 2-3, bottom panel). According to the evolutionary model, alleles with deleterious effects at age $T$ are more likely to evolve in species 1 than in species 2. Therefore, species 1 is expected to develop an earlier and more rapid onset of senescence than species 2.

Empirical tests of this prediction have yielded mixed results. As a general rule, life span is shorter in small animals than in large ones (Charlesworth, 1980; Peters, 1983; Calder, 1984; Reiss, 1989). If large animals have comparatively low exogenous mortality—if, for example, they are better able to thermoregulate or less prone to predation—this empirical generalization would support Williams' prediction. In a more specific test, Austad (1993) has found delayed senescence in a population of opossums living on a predator-free island. However, a recent reanalysis of 56 mammalian life tables (Promislow, 1992) has found no correlation between the observed senescence rate (defined as the slope of the regression of the log of age-specific mortality on age) and early adult mortality (a possible measure of exogenous mortality), and Finch (1990) has reviewed more general comparative evidence showing lack of such a correlation.

It could be argued that early adult mortality may be a poor measure of exogenous mortality since some senescent causes of death are already operating at those ages, albeit at very low levels. Gage and his colleagues (Gage and Dyke, 1986; Gage, 1989, 1990, 1991) have explored an alternative method for estimating exogenous mortality based on the so-called Siler competing hazards model:

$$h(t) = \alpha_1 \exp(-\beta_1 t) + \alpha_2 + \alpha_3 \exp(\beta_3 t) \tag{2-5}$$

This model specifies three components of $h(t)$, the hazard of death at age $t$. The first component represents "immature" mortality, modeled as an exponentially declining hazard with parameters $\alpha_1$ and $\beta_1$. The second is an age-independent component of mortality, equal to $\alpha_2$. Finally, senescent mortality is treated as an exponentially increasing hazard with parameters $\alpha_3$ and $\beta_3$. In this model, exogenous mortality is given by the value of $\alpha_2$, while the rate of senescence is equal to $\beta_3$. Recently, Gage fitted this model to 602 national-level human life tables by non-linear least squares; contrary to expectation, the correlation between the estimated values of $\alpha_2$ and $\beta_3$ for those populations was significantly *negative* ($r = -0.145$, $P < 0.01$).[3]

For two reasons, it is unclear if these results falsify the evolutionary model. First, differences among human populations are likely to represent purely environmental differentials rather than evolved characteristics. Such differences may, therefore, be uninformative about the evolutionary model. In addition, recent theoretical work suggests that the positive relationship between exogenous mortality and the rate of senescence postulated by

---

[3]We are grateful to Tim Gage for sharing these unpublished results with us.

Williams may not, in fact, be a necessary corollary of the evolutionary model, especially if fertility or mortality is independent of density (Abrams, 1991). Moreover, if fertility and mortality are *not* density independent, as is likely to be true of many human societies, then the expected relationship between exogenous mortality and senescence depends critically upon the age-structure of the density dependence (Abrams, 1991). Apparently, this is one area in which an uncritical use of the Malthusian parameter as a measure of fitness may be misleading.

On balance, then, neither theory nor empirical evidence on the correlation between exogenous mortality and aging has provided unequivocal support for (or refutation of) the evolutionary model. We suggest that both new models and new empirical methods will be necessary to clarify this particular issue.

## Age-specific Gene Action

A basic element of the evolutionary model is that natural selection is comparatively insensitive to deleterious traits that are expressed late in life (Medawar, 1952; Edney and Gill, 1968). Based on this idea, Rose (1991: 73) has suggested that "the additive genetic variance of age-specific life-history characters should increase with age." In general, traits that are correlated with fitness tend to have little if any additive genetic variance at genetic equilibrium (Mousseau and Roff, 1987; Falconer, 1989). By their nature, fertility and mortality are highly correlated with fitness—they *constitute* fitness—but the correlation is higher at early ages than at late ages. Therefore, the additive genetic variance (and therefore the strict-sense heritability) of senescent changes affecting fertility and mortality may often be higher than that of traits expressed early in life.[4]

Studies of *Drosophila* designed to test this prediction have proven ambiguous. One direct test of the prediction found no increase in additive genetic variance for daily fertility with increasing age in *D. melanogaster* (Rose and Charlesworth, 1980, 1981a, 1981b). However, a second experiment, again using *D. melanogaster*, showed a probable accumulation of genetic variation for male fertility with increasing age (Kosuda, 1985). In a long-term selection experiment, later fertility was shown to decrease after more than 100 generations of selection for early reproduction in *D. melanogaster* (Mueller, 1987; Bierbaum *et al.*, 1989), results that can be explained by the accumulation of age-specific alleles that affect later fecundity (Rose, 1991). In sum, though the data are scanty and all studies to date have been done on a single species,

---

[4]There are important exceptions to this generalization. In particular, traits whose fitness effects involve phenotypic trade-offs with other fitness components can retain substantial additive genetic variance at equilibrium (Bulmer, 1980; Falconer, 1989). In humans, it is not yet established that such trade-offs are involved in traits affecting mortality (see the paper by Crews and Gerber, this volume), but they may be quite common for traits affecting fertility (see, for example, Mauskopf and Wallace, 1984; Palloni and Tienda, 1986). In general, therefore, the heritability of such traits as age at menarche that affect early reproduction might be expected to be higher than that of traits like bone cancer or leukemia that affect early mortality. In a very general way, the empirical evidence appears to be consistent with this expectation (Treloar and Martin, 1990; Meyer *et al.*, 1991).

the results suggest a likely role for the accumulation of age-specific deleterious alleles in the evolution of senescence.

In humans, family studies suggest that the heritability of longevity *per se* may be low, contrary to expectation (Abbot *et al.*, 1978; Murphy, 1978; but see Sørensen *et al.*, 1988). However, Vaupel (1988) has shown mathematically that, even if children are perfectly correlated with their parents in "frailty" (i.e., the individual-level contribution to the age-specific hazard of death), the correlation in their ages at death will be small. This lack of a strong correlation reflects the fact that the variance in life span among people with different frailties is only slightly greater than that among people at the same level of frailty. Thus, total life span is unlikely to be an informative phenotype in family studies. Unfortunately frailty itself is unobservable, and it is at present unclear how to circumvent this problem (for an extended discussion, see Wood *et al.*, 1992a).

## Antagonistic Pleiotropy

A fourth testable prediction of the evolutionary theory of senescence concerns the selective trade-off between early and later portions of an organism's life history implied by the antagonistic pleiotropy model. Such a trade-off can be accomplished either by selection for genes with direct senescent effects or by selection for genes that exert indirect effects. Genes that cause direct effects would be those associated with a particular phenotype that is beneficial early but detrimental later in life. For example, a gene that promotes efficient uptake of cholesterol might be beneficial for early reproduction, since cholesterol is the precursor for steroid hormones, but the same gene might cause cardiovascular disease later in life. Such direct effects have received little attention in empirical research.

Genes causing an indirect effect on senescence would be those that redirect resources away from somatic maintenance and toward reproduction; such effects are implicit in the concept of the "cost of reproduction" (Williams, 1966; Bell, 1984a, 1984b; Reznick, 1985). Most empirical studies of the cost of reproduction can be divided into four classes (Reznick, 1985): phenotypic correlations, correlated responses to experimental manipulations, genetic correlations, and correlated responses to artificial selection.

Numerous studies have attempted to measure the cost of reproduction using phenotypic correlations (Reznick, 1985; Rose, 1991). These studies have produced mixed results. Some show a negative correlation between early reproduction and subsequent survival (Gowen and Johnson, 1946; Maynard Smith, 1958; Tinkle and Hadley, 1975; Clutton-Brock *et al.*, 1982; Hiraizumi, 1985), while others show no association or even a positive correlation between these two fitness components (van Dijk, 1979; Bell, 1984a, 1984b). This method of measuring the cost of reproduction has been criticized on the grounds that phenotypic correlations confound genetic and environmental sources of covariation when in fact only the former are relevant to the problem (Rose and Charlesworth, 1981a, 1981b; Reznick, 1985; Reznick *et al.*, 1986; Rose, 1991). Thus, the lack of consistent findings of a cost of reproduction in studies employing phenotypic correlations may not be damaging to the antagonistic pleiotropy model.

Attempts to measure the cost of reproduction through experimental manipulations have often yielded significant trade-offs between early reproduction and later survival (Reznick, 1985). These experiments are usually designed to measure phenotypic plasticity in life-history allocation patterns.[5] For example, some aspect of the experimental organism's life history (e.g., onset of reproduction) or some aspect of its environment (e.g., food availability) is artificially altered, and the correlation between reproduction and survival is estimated across treatment groups. Such studies have produced far more instances of negative correlation than either positive or no correlation (Reznick, 1985). While this method has also been criticized because it does not directly measure genetic correlations (Reznick, 1985; Rose, 1991), it may still be informative to study phenotypic plasticity in resource allocation and its effects on senescence.

Genetic correlations between traits are determined using quantitative genetic designs that measure the resemblances among relatives in breeding experiments (Falconer, 1989). Such designs are preferable to those estimating phenotypic correlations because they measure the "raw material" of evolutionary change, namely additive genetic variation (Rose and Charlesworth, 1981a, 1981b; Reznick, 1985; Reznick et al., 1986; Rose, 1991). Unfortunately, few experiments have directly measured the genetic correlation of early and late fitness characters, and of those that have, the results are equivocal. Some studies report no or even positive genetic correlations between age-specific fitness components (Giesel, 1979; Giesel and Zettler, 1980; Giesel et al., 1982; Bell, 1984a, 1984b; Lynch, 1984). Others have detected the expected negative correlations (Gowen and Johnson, 1946; Law, 1979; Rose and Charlesworth, 1981a; Hiraizumi, 1985; Friedman and Johnson, 1988; Hughes and Clark, 1988; Scheiner et al., 1989). Of the studies showing a positive genetic correlation, some have been criticized on the basis of experimental design (Rose and Charlesworth, 1981a, 1981b; Rose, 1984; Reznick, 1985; Rose and Service, 1985; Reznick et al., 1986; Clark, 1987). The main criticism is that estimation of genetic correlations from organisms in novel environments or using inbred lines tends to bias the results in the direction of positive values (Rose, 1984; Service and Rose, 1985). If the studies subject to this criticism are excluded, the case for antagonistic pleiotropy becomes much stronger. Nevertheless, empirical support is still weak in this area, and many more breeding experiments should be undertaken using a variety of organisms.

A fourth approach to estimating the cost of reproduction involves measuring correlated responses of fitness components to artificial selection. In this approach, laboratory strains are selected for either increased early fecundity or increased longevity, and simultaneous changes in life-history parameters not directly subject to selection are measured. This approach, like the previous

---

[5]*Phenotypic plasticity* refers to the range of phenotypes exhibited by a single genotype in a variety of environments. Such plasticity may allow organisms to respond immediately to different environmental conditions within a single individual's lifetime without requiring genetic change.

one, directly measures the underlying additive genetic variation affecting early and late fitness components (Falconer, 1989); it is arguably the best method for measuring reproductive costs (Rose, 1991), although it is not without short-comings (Reznick, 1985). Most of the studies that have adopted this approach have observed reduced early fertility and increased later mortality as responses to selection for increased longevity and for early onset of reproduction, respectively (Wattiaux, 1968; Sokal, 1970; Mertz, 1975; Law et al., 1977; Wallinga and Bakkar, 1978; Rose and Charlesworth, 1980, 1981b; Doyle and Hunte, 1981; Hutchinson and Rose, 1990). These experiments cover a wide range of organisms and thus provide strong support for the antagonistic pleiotropy hypothesis.

People, of course, cannot be subjected to these sorts of experimental manipulations. Consequently there is little evidence for antagonistic pleiotropy in humans. Recently, it has been suggested that women who are heterozygous for the allele for Huntington's chorea, a fatal neurological disease with late age of onset, experience enhanced fertility early in life (Albin, 1988). The empirical support for this idea is weak and, even if it were stronger, it would still amount to a phenotypic correlation rather than a genetic one. There have been a few studies of the cost of reproduction in specific human groups where aspects of the life history have been culturally or medically controlled to the extent that they are at least somewhat comparable to experiments. For example, predictions about the cost of reproduction are supported by data on eunuchs, showing that human castrates enjoy longer life spans and greater resistance to morbidity than intact human males (Hamilton, 1948; Hamilton and Mestler, 1969). Male eunuchs and intact males in Hamilton and Mestler's unique study (1969) showed significant differences in survival rates beginning at age 25; the estimated median age at death was 55.7 years for intact males and 69.3 years for eunuchs ($P < 0.01$). In addition, age at castration was important in predicting the age at death, with those males orchiectomized at 8–14 having a median life span of 76.3 years compared to a median life span of 68.9 years for men orchiectomized at 30–39 ($P < 0.003$). A small sample of oophorecto-mized women also showed significantly higher age at death than intact women ($P < 0.001$). Trade-offs between reproduction and longevity may also be studied in noncastrated but celibate human groups. Madigan's (1957) study of records for 9,813 men and 32,041 women in Catholic religious orders demonstrated that longevity was increased in both sexes within these nullipar-ous groups. Life expectancy at age 15 for celibate males was 54 years compared to 51.8 for non-celibate US males during the same period; life expectancy at 15 for celibate females was 56.6 compared to 55.1 for non-celibate US females.

While these studies of humans superficially appear to support the antagonis-tic pleiotropy model, they all suffer from two shortcomings, both reflecting the fact that true experimental control is impossible with humans. First, many of the groups studied (monks, nuns, and castrated individuals who are institu-tionalized for various mental impairments) are likely to be selective for a wide variety of traits and therefore differ from the general population not solely by their reproductive patterns. Consequently, it is unclear that their longer life spans are purely a result of celibacy. Second, all these comparisons represent phenotypic correlations, which, as we have seen, are a poor reflection of the underlying genetic correlations. In their contribution to the present volume, Crews and Gerber discuss whether negative pleiotropy is likely to be operating for many of the chronic degenerative diseases that currently dominate human patterns of senescent mortality; later in this paper, we will suggest one reproductive characteristic of humans for which a plausible case for antagonistic pleiotropy can be made.

Summarizing all these empirical studies, the evidence is generally favorable for the evolutionary model of senescence. There is strong support for the claim that organisms lacking a definable soma should not experience senescence, and there is also some evidence for an accumulation of late-acting deleterious mutations. Similarly, well-designed tests of antagonistic pleiotropy have generally confirmed the expected negative correlations between early and late fitness components. Taken together, these studies allow provisional acceptance of the idea that senescence is attributable to an accumulation of genes with deleterious age-specific effects, as well as genes exhibiting antagonistic pleiotropy, both reflecting a decline in selection intensity with increasing age.

## IMPLICATIONS OF THE EVOLUTIONARY MODEL FOR UNDERSTANDING THE MECHANISMS OF HUMAN AGING

Regardless of whether it incorporates age-specific gene expression, antagonistic pleiotropy, or multi-stage/multi-hit processes, the basic evolutionary model of aging has several important implications for our understanding of the mechanisms of human aging, implications to which most gerontologists have paid little attention. While the remainder of this paper is, in effect, an exploration of these implications, it will be useful to list them here first.

*Aging is not adaptive.* Although an outcome of natural selection, aging *per se* is not adaptive. It is, in effect, a failure of adaptation, but one that occurs so late in life that it has negligible effects on fitness—or else is associated with earlier increases in fitness that are sufficient to offset the failure of adaptation. One important implication of this view is that theories proposing an adaptive function for senescence—e.g., kin selection theories suggesting that the function of senescent mortality is to make resources available for offspring or that the function of the menopause is to give women an opportunity to take care of their grandchildren—are unnecessary.

*Phenotypes expressed late in life are selectively neutral or nearly neutral.* Perhaps the single most important implication of this conclusion is that apparent differences in maximal life span across species are unlikely to be of selective importance. Similarly, it is unlikely that the maximal life span is determined by an underlying developmental switch mechanism—as suggested by Dawkins' (1976) "killer gene" hypothesis—since such an elaborate mechanism could not have been assembled by natural selection.

*Aging is not a unitary process but a "mosaic" one.* The fact that several independent mechanisms (age-specific gene expression, antagonistic pleiotropy, multi-stage processes) are consistent with the basic evolutionary model of

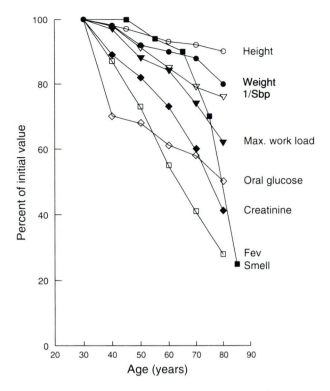

**Figure 2-4** Age-dependent changes in selected physiological and antomical systems in humans, showing the mosaic nature of human senescence. The value at each age is expressed as a percentage of the value at 30 years, taken to represent the optimal response. Sbp = systolic blood pressure; Fev = forced expiratory volume. Redrawn from Arking (1991), based on data from Shock (1972), Tobin (1981), Doty *et al.* (1984), and Rodenheffer *et al.* (1984).

aging strongly suggests that senescence is unlikely to be a unitary process. There is no reason that all these mechanisms cannot be operating simultaneously on different aspects of the phenotype. As a result, aging is likely to be "mosaic" in nature, involving any number of distinct physiological changes responding to different forms of selection. As shown in Figure 2-4, the physiological evidence on humans appears to be consistent with this viewpoint.

*Different aspects of aging should be only weakly coordinated in rate.* If attributable to genes with delayed expression rather than to antagonistic pleiotropy, the various senescent processes affecting different tissues and organ systems should display only weak coordination in their timing and rates across the life span. There will, however, be some degree of temporal coordination simply because all these senescent changes are expected to be delayed until after a common minimal age, and beyond that age they will tend to accelerate as age increases. However, there need not be any close correspondence in the rate of acceleration displayed by different senescent processes. Again, the changes summarized in Figure 2-4 appear to be consistent with this expectation.

*The only senescent changes expected to show a marked deviation from the weak coordination discussed above are those associated with antagonistic pleiotropy.* In particular, it is possible for such changes to occur substantially earlier than other forms of aging, because the fitness cost of an earlier age of onset is paid for by advantageous pleiotropic effects. This idea may provide a basis for identifying possible cases of antagonistic pleiotropy (see below).

*At least under some genetic models, phenotypic traits expressed late in life are expected to display greater additive genetic variance than those expressed early in life.* While there are some exceptions to this expectation, e.g., situations far from genetic equilibrium and traits subject to fitness trade-offs or frequency-dependent selection, in general we would expect senescent traits to have higher strict-sense heritabilities than similar traits with early phenotypic expression. Degenerative disease and menopause, for example, may have higher strict-sense heritabilities than childhood illnesses and menarche.

Taking these implications together, it seems clear that the epidemiological view of aging—that aging involves a multitude of different, poorly coordinated senescent processes—is far more consistent with evolutionary theory than the gerontological view that aging is regulated by a single underlying process. Paradoxically, though researchers supporting the GR view have generally been more inclined to discuss evolution explicitly, it appears that the EP view makes more evolutionary sense.

We turn now to a more detailed discussion of senescent changes in humans affecting, first, morbidity and mortality and, second, reproduction.

## MORBIDITY AND MORTALITY

In the extreme GR view, a single process underlies and controls the acceleration of mortality with age. If this process could be shielded from environmental perturbations, it would give rise to a rectangular survival function; that is, virtually all individuals would survive long enough to die at or near the species-specific maximum life-span potential (MLP). In this view, evolution of mortality patterns involves direct genic selection for the MLP *per se*, although within species the age pattern of mortality can be modified by accelerating or decelerating the rate at which vital processes move individuals toward the MLP. The EP view, in contrast, holds that rectangularization of the survival function is an illusory goal and that the MLP has little meaning as a phenotypic trait.

We suggest that the GR model of age-related mortality is oversimplified and that the EP model is likely to be more realistic. In view of their very different etiologies, it is unlikely that all causes of death accelerate with age at the same rate. Even if they did, natural selection would be unable to preserve the rate of acceleration very precisely because the acceleration occurs at precisely those segments of the life span to which natural selection is relatively insensitive. Mortality is better viewed as the outcome of whatever particular

**Table 2-1**   Mortality characteristics of selected mammalian species.[a]

| Taxon | Common name | IMR/year | MRDT (years) | MLP (years) |
|---|---|---|---|---|
| Artiodactyla | | | | |
|   *Hippopotamus amphibius* | Hippopotamus | 0.01 | 7 | >45 |
|   *Ovis dalli* | Dall mountain sheep | 0.05 | 1.5 | 15–20 |
| Chiroptera | | | | |
|   *Pipistrellus pipistrellus* | Pipestrelle bat | 0.36 | 3–8 | ≥11 |
|   *Myotis lucifugis* | Little brown bat | | | >32 |
| Carnivora | | | | |
|   *Canis familiaris* | Domestic dog | 0.02 | 3 | 20 |
| Perissodactyla | | | | |
|   *Equus caballus* | Horse | 0.0002 | 4 | >45 |
|   *Rhinosceros unicornis* | Indian rhinoceros | | | >50 |
| Proboscidea | | | | |
|   *Loxodonta africana* | African elephant | 0.002 | 8 | >70 |
| Rodentia | | | | |
|   *Mus musculus* | Mouse (female) | 0.01 | 0.3 | 4–5 |
|   *Rattus norvegicus* | Norway rat (male) | 0.002 | 0.3 | 5–6 |
|   *Peromyscus leucopus* | White-footed mouse | 0.001 | 0.5 | 7–8 |
| Primates | | | | |
|   *Macaca mulatta* | Rhesus monkey | 0.02 | 8 | >35 |
|   *Homo sapiens* | Human (female) | 0.0002 | 8 | >110 |

[a]IMR, initial mortality rate; MRDT, mortality rate doubling time; MLP, maximum life-span potential. All estimates must be regarded as crude approximations.
Source: Finch (1991).

collection of tissue- or organ-specific competing causes of death happens to be operating in a given population. This view has important implications for our ability to modify the MLP; indeed, in the EP view there is no MLP to modify.

Despite our skepticism about the GR view, there are several strands of evidence that have been offered as support for a unitary cause of aging. One of the most compelling is the simple observation that different species have different life-span characteristics (Table 2-1). These differences must have some kind of genetic basis and seem in some way to be coordinated; that is, the absolute age at which many senescent diseases strike is scaled approximately to the maximal observed life span of the species. Most cancers, for example, arise in humans at much later ages than they do in mice. Is this because evolution has involved recalibration of some underlying housekeeping genes affecting all causes of death simultaneously, or because selection has favored certain life-history characteristics so that genes leading to early death, from whatever cause, are simply eliminated?

## Consistent Phylogenetic Patterns

There is abundant evidence for consistent relationships between the average values of various morphological and physiological traits for different species and their average adult body size (Peters, 1983; Calder, 1984; Reiss, 1989).

These relationships are usually expressed as *allometric functions*, in which the regression of the trait on $M$ (adult body mass in kg) takes the form

$$\text{Trait} = aM^k \tag{2-6}$$

The power $k$ is often estimated to be about ¼. Such allometric relationships have been shown to fit aging and longevity quite well (see Finch, 1990, for an encyclopedic review). The apparent consistency of these relationships across taxa has suggested to many investigators that the life span has evolved in a coherent way, often assumed to imply the existence of a simple underlying mechanism for aging in basic mammalian physiology.

In addition to allometric relationships, many authors have noted that age patterns of mortality in a wide variety of species can be fit reasonably well at adult ages by a two-parameter Gompertz function:

$$h(t) = (\text{IMR})\exp[(\ln 2/\text{MRDT})t] \tag{2-7}$$

where IMR is the "initial mortality rate" (the rate characteristic of the age at which senescence begins, usually taken to be sexual maturity or, in humans, 15 years of age), and MRDT is the "mortality rate doubling time" (the time it takes senescent mortality to attain twice the IMR). Finch and his colleagues (Finch, 1990; Finch *et al.*, 1990) have argued that, while the IMR may primarily reflect environmental conditions, the MRDT is a genetically and evolutionarily meaningful parameter for comparing senescent pattern across higher vertebrate species.[6] Calder (1984) found that, across vertebrate species, the parameters of the Gompertz mortality function fit the same kind of allometric relationship to body mass as other phenotypic traits:

$$\text{IMR} = 0.0124M^{-0.56} \tag{2-8}$$

$$\text{MRDT} = 0.709M^{-0.27} \tag{2-9}$$

Both these regressions are significant in Calder's analysis. Note that a power of approximately ¼ relates $M$ to the MRDT, and the power 0.56 for IMR is perhaps not very different statistically from ¼.

It is unclear what to make of such regularities. Despite its wide use, the Gompertz function is not based on biological first principles; thus, its parameters may have little if any relationship to the actual biological processes related to aging. In addition, the function is often fitted to data that are of dubious reliability and based on small samples, especially those from non-human species. Although the Gompertz may often look superficially as if it fits the data well, many other survival models with monotonically increasing hazard rate functions (e.g., the Weibull, gamma, or linear-exponential) often fit the data more or less equally well (Figure 2-5). Such alternative models are, however, rarely tested against the Gompertz in comparative studies. Thus, the

---

[6]While Finch (1990) does not argue for a unitary cause of all senescence, he clearly believes that the MRDT is a phenotype subject to natural selection. It is less clear that he would make the same claim for the IMR.

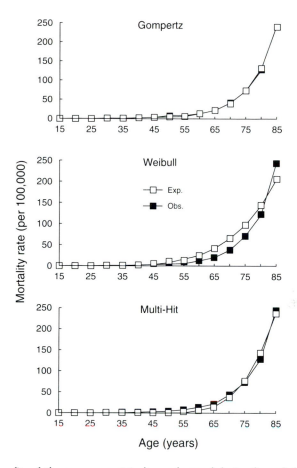

**Figure 2-5** The fit of three parametric hazards models to the adult mortality rates of women from Bulgaria (1987). Top panel shows the fit of a Gompertz function, $h(t) = a\exp(bt)$; middle panel shows a Weibull function, $h(t) = abt^{b-1}$; bottom panel shows the more elaborate multi-stage model of Weiss and Chakraborty (1984), $h(t) = ab\exp(-at)[1 - \exp(-at)]^{b-1}/\{1 - [1 - \exp(-at)]^b\}$. In each case, $t$ is age in years, and $a$ and $b$ are the fitted parameters. Despite the fact that the specifications differ markedly across models, all three models have two parameters and fit the data almost equally well. Data from United Nations (1991).

IMR and MRDT are summary measures derived from the untested fit of an atheoretical model to imperfect data, and may only approximately capture the age pattern of mortality for any particular species. In this light, it is unclear what would constitute a meaningful difference in the estimated allometric relationships.

## Characterizing a Species by its Maximum Life-span Potential

There is little doubt that there are characteristic limits to the life spans of different species. Mice do not live as long as most humans, and humans do not live as long as most bristlecomb pines. A common, superficially meaningful way to express these differences is in terms of the maximum life-span potential (Table 2-1). From a statistical point of view, however, the actual meaning of the MLP is quite obscure. In reality, the individuals making up a species die at different ages and from different causes. The MLP of the species is typically *estimated* as the maximum of the observed ages at death. What, then, was the life span "potential" of individuals who died at younger ages? Since this potential is unobservable as a general phenotypic trait, it must be estimated from a single data point: the age at death of whichever individual dies last. However, estimation of the MLP as the extreme value of a mortality sample makes the estimate dependent upon sample size: the larger the sample, the more likely we are to observe rare cases of very long-term survival (Weiss, 1989a). It is strange to characterize a distribution either by its extreme value (or any other single observation) or by a statistic that is intrinsically dependent upon sample size. In most standard statistical theory, it is the sampling variance of the estimate, not the estimate itself, that is sample-size-dependent.[7]

In addition to these statistical problems, the MLP confuses two distinct aspects of survival: (1) the maximum age at death among individuals subject to the *same* hazard function; and (2) the maximum among individuals subject to *differing* hazards. Among genetically identical imbred animals, the MLP may provide an estimate (albeit a poor one) of the former parameter, but in a natural population the oldest surviving member may be one with a rare genotype associated with unusually high viability, not at all representative of the other members of the species. Why should an individual with the rarest, most "resistant" multiple-locus genotype be chosen to represent the survival characteristics of an entire species? Doing so makes no more sense than using a person with cystic fibrosis who dies at age 20 to typify human mortality.

Comparisons across species can be made slightly more meaningful when some parametric survival function can be assumed, in which case the MLP can be defined as the age beyond which the predicted probability of survival is smaller than some arbitrarily chosen value, $p$. It follows from this definition that $t_{MLP} = S^{-1}(p)$, where $S^{-1}$ is the inverse survival function (Weiss, 1989a). For example, we might choose $p = 10^{-6}$ and thus define the MLP as the age beyond which the probability of survival is less than one in a million. Unfortunately, a $p$ value that is small enough to represent our intuitive notion of a MLP may often require projection of the assumed parametric survival function well beyond the data from which it is estimated. Thus, it is difficult to make a strong case for this definition of the MLP.

---

[7]The sample-size-dependence of the MLP may explain a common finding in the comparative study of life span, namely, that humans consistently fall above the allometric regression line relating MLP to body size (Finch, 1990). There has been considerable speculation among anthropologists about why this "special" longevity evolved in humans; for example, explanations have been offered invoking culture, language, or the advantage of having elderly "living libraries" who can help their younger kin in times of environmental stress. But the apparent excess longevity of humans is likely to be a statistical artifact. Human mortality statistics are based upon millions of observations, in contrast to most species for which dozens or hundreds of observations may be available. Our MLP is thus higher than expected at least in part because the sample size for humans is so enormous.

Authors who believe in the MLP differ on whether it is about 85 years in humans, the boundary towards which our survival curve has been moving during the past century (Manton and Stallard, 1984), or lies somewhere beyond age 85 (for discussions of this issue, see Weiss, 1989a, 1989b; Finch, 1990; Olshanky *et al.*, 1990). Regardless of the MLP chosen, the very idea of a MLP requires that its advocates identify the underlying mechanism determining the MLP. The history of gerontology is littered with discarded hypotheses about global mechanisms of aging, including somatic mutations, free radical damage, hormonal cascades, collagen cross-linkage, and the Hayflick limit on cell division cycles (Finch, 1990; Arking, 1991). While the supporters of such hypotheses have not yet completely given up, the data do not provide strong support for the claim that any of the mechanisms postulated to date is *the* cause of aging (Rose, 1991; Turner and Weiss, this volume). If a unitary cause of aging actually exists, our utter inability to identify the mechanism through which it works is very strange indeed.

According to some authors who believe in the reality of the MLP, our survival curve could be rectangularized if only we could eliminate all current causes of death through medical intervention and public health measures (Fries, 1980, 1987; for a critique, see Manton and Tolley, 1991). If this were to happen, an age to which *almost no one* has lived from the dawn of hominid evolution until now would become the age to which *almost everyone* lives. One implication of such a view is that the current survival pattern is largely an artifact of unrelated causes of "premature" deaths; that is, the known causes of death and processes of senescent decline are themselves unrelated to the underlying process that sets the MLP. This view is alarming because we know nothing whatsoever about what determines the MLP; thus, if the GR view is correct, none of our current biomedical knowledge has any bearing on the evolution of the human life span. If the EP view is correct, however, this problem evaporates, along with the very idea of a species-specific MLP.

## Characterizing a Species by its IMR and MRDT

An implication of the claim that a species can be characterized by a single set of IMR and MRDT values, is that there must be some sense in which the individual members of the species share the mortality characteristics summarized by those values, although this sense has rarely been made clear by gerontologists. The species-specific IMR and MRDT are summary measures based upon the overall mortality experience of a species. We would argue that such an aggregate approach may be misleading, precisely because the overall hazard is a composite of may separate hazards of death associated with different biological causes. What can we learn from the age patterns of *specific* causes of death?

The age-specific hazard functions for many causes of senescent death, especially chronic diseases of late onset, have similar shapes. In particular, although the *absolute* risks may vary among such causes by several orders of magnitude, the hazard rates for most adult ages can often be fit by a Gompertz function (note, however, that there are numerous exceptions and often the fit of the Gompertz is far from perfect; see Weiss, 1990). Thus, in humans at least, there appear to be regularities in age patterns across individual causes of death similar to those across species for total, all-cause mortality. Do these regularities support the hypothesis of a single, unitary cause of human aging?

Unfortunately, the IMRs for most causes of death in humans are so small (in the range 0–0.02) that meaningful comparisons are difficult, even with enormous samples. As can be seen from Tables 2-2–2-4, the standard deviation of IMRs across causes is often as great as or greater than the estimated mean IMR itself. The MRDTs, in contrast, are less variable and thus easier to compare. MRDT estimates from various causes of adult death in the general United States population (ages 15–84) are presented in Table 2-2. The estimated MRDTs for 26 causes vary from about 3.0 (atherosclerosis) to 33.1 (chronic liver disease and cirrhosis), a range that spans seven of the 11 mean MRDTs given for different mammalian species in Table 2-1. In other words, different causes of death appear to exhibit widely divergent doubling times within a single population. Consequently, characterization of a population (and, even more so, a species) by a composite mortality statistic like the all-cause MRDT is likely to misrepresent the true variation in cause-specific mortality.

Table 2-3 shows MRDTs for four cancers in various human populations representing the worldwide diversity of cancer risks. Presumably the differences in these values are attributable primarily to differential exposure to environmental risk factors, although genetic differences may also play a part. As before, the estimates of IMR prove to be unstable, especially in the case of prostate cancer for which the standard deviation substantially exceeds the mean value. The estimates of MRDT are somewhat more stable than those of IMR, although the variance in the former is still substantial. The range of estimates of MRDT for lymphatic leukemia across the nine populations (2.0–36.4) actually exceeds the range of the 26 separate causes of death in the United States. Thus, MRDTs within a cause but across populations can differ as much as MRDTs within a population but across causes. In light of this variation, how can the global MRDT for the human species as a whole possibly have any real biological meaning?

The estimated values of IMR and MRDT for all-cause mortality in 27 human populations are shown in Table 2-4. Once again, the variability of IMR values is too great to assign a meaningful single estimate. The average MRDT is $8.5 \pm 7.6$ (mean $\pm$ 2s.d.) for females (with a range of 4.8–19.8) and $9.8 \pm 9.0$ for males (range = 6.1–26.4). Thus, even when we ignore the within-population variation in MRDT associated with distinct causes (Tables 2-2 and 2-3), there remains considerable heterogeneity in the overall MRDT across populations. Since the data summarized in these tables are all from large samples (whole nations), sampling variation is unlikely to be an important reason for the apparent heterogeneity, and insofar as the heterogeneity is real, there is no single "species-specific" IMR or MRDT for humans.

The IMR and MRDT are rather abstract concepts. We can gain a more intuitive sense of their implications for the human life span by using them to

**Table 2-2**  Initial mortality rate (IMR) and mortality rate doubling time (MRDT) for a variety of causes in humans (United States, 1987).[a]

| Cause | IMR | MRDT |
|---|---|---|
| Major cardiovascular disease | 0.00 | 5.5 |
| Acute myocardial infarction | 4.05 | 8.3 |
| Diseases of the heart | 1.08 | 5.7 |
| Hypertensive heart disease | 0.09 | 6.8 |
| Atherosclerosis | 0.00 | 3.0 |
| Anemia | 0.00 | 4.3 |
| Diabetes mellitus | 1.01 | 9.4 |
| Asthma | 0.32 | 13.2 |
| Bronchitis, chronic and unspecified | 0.03 | 7.3 |
| Emphysema | 1.30 | 12.8 |
| Tuberculosis | 0.08 | 11.2 |
| Appendicitis | 0.00 | 7.1 |
| Ulcer of the stomach and duodenum | 0.01 | 5.8 |
| Malignant neoplasms, including neoplasms of lymphatic and hematopoietic tissues | 43.90 | 13.5 |
| Malignant neoplasm of the breast | 4.49 | 15.0 |
| Malignant neoplasm of digestive organs and peritoneum | 6.36 | 11.2 |
| Malignant neoplasm of the genital organs | 0.67 | 8.6 |
| Malignant neoplasms of lip, oral cavity, and pharynx | 1.25 | 17.5 |
| Malignant neoplasms of respiratory and intrathoracic organs | 26.88 | 19.7 |
| Malignant neoplasms of urinary organs | 0.86 | 10.6 |
| Leukemia | 0.63 | 10.4 |
| Cerebral thrombosis and unspecified occlusion of cerebral arteries | 0.00 | 4.5 |
| Intracerebral and other intracranial hemorrhage | 0.51 | 9.3 |
| Chronic liver disease and cirrhosis | 8.18 | 33.1 |
| Renal failure, disorders resulting from impaired renal function, and small kidney of unknown cause | 0.02 | 5.4 |
| Meningitis | 0.03 | 11.2 |
| Mean | 3.91 | 10.4 |
| Standard deviation | 9.80 | 6.2 |

[a]IMRs are given $\times 10^{-5}$.
Data Source: Public Health Service (1991).

predict the value of the MLP. Using the criterion $S(t_{MLP}) \leqslant 10^{-6}$, then if the Gompertz model is correct

$$t_{MLP} = \ln[1.0 + \alpha\ln(10^6)/IMR]/\alpha \qquad (2\text{-}10)$$

where $\alpha = (\ln 2)/MRDT$. As shown in Table 2-5, the range of inter-cause and inter-population variation in IMR and MRDT values summarized in Tables 2-2–2-4 implies MLP values that vary from less than 10 years to more than 150 years, far too inconsistent to provide convincing support for a unitary force underlying all of human senescence. Indeed, plotting the individual cause-specific survival functions based on their respective hazard functions shows clearly that *no* individual cause of death would by itself eliminate a cohort of

**Table 2-3**  Initial mortality rate (IMR) and mortality rate doubling time (MRDT) for a variety of cancers in nine countries (1974–1977).[a]

| Cancer | Country | IMR | MRDT |
|---|---|---|---|
| Colon cancer | Brazil | 338.17 | 12.8 |
| | Hungary | 390.28 | 21.2 |
| | Italy | 763.48 | 13.8 |
| | Japan | 335.22 | 15.0 |
| | Romania | 290.62 | 16.9 |
| | Spain | 284.15 | 11.7 |
| | Switzerland | 392.09 | 10.5 |
| | United Kingdom | 586.86 | 13.1 |
| | United States | 1036.86 | 14.4 |
| Mean | | 490.86 | 14.4 |
| Standard deviation | | 257.85 | 3.2 |
| Lymphatic leukemia | Brazil | 42.59 | 16.9 |
| | Hungary | 95.07 | 36.4 |
| | Italy | 127.02 | 13.6 |
| | Japan | 0.00 | 2.0 |
| | Romania | 124.38 | 28.5 |
| | Spain | 22.34 | 10.8 |
| | Switzerland | 1.31 | 6.1 |
| | United Kingdom | 19.11 | 9.3 |
| | United States | 89.12 | 12.3 |
| Mean | | 57.88 | 15.1 |
| Standard deviation | | 51.37 | 10.9 |
| Pancreatic cancer | Brazil | 315.03 | 17.5 |
| | Hungary | 392.35 | 32.1 |
| | Italy | 270.37 | 14.5 |
| | Japan | 266.84 | 15.8 |
| | Romania | 338.25 | 17.3 |
| | Spain | 218.91 | 18.2 |
| | Switzerland | 174.53 | 11.1 |
| | United Kingdom | 227.52 | 12.2 |
| | United States | 88.45 | 8.3 |
| Mean | | 254.69 | 16.3 |
| Standard deviation | | 90.86 | 6.8 |
| Prostate cancer | Brazil | 687.31 | 12.2 |
| | Hungary | 462.14 | 13.2 |
| | Italy | 491.81 | 10.3 |
| | Japan | 9.88 | 7.0 |
| | Romania | 500.23 | 13.3 |
| | Spain | 184.96 | 8.7 |
| | Switzerland | 427.88 | 9.1 |
| | United Kingdom | 388.45 | 10.1 |
| | United States | 2325.02 | 11.6 |
| Mean | | 608.63 | 10.6 |
| Standard deviation | | 672.51 | 2.1 |

[a]IMRs are given $\times 10^{-5}$.
Data Source: Waterhouse *et al.* (1982).

**Table 2-4** Initial mortality rate (IMR) and mortality rate doubling time (MRDT) for selected countries (1987).[a]

| Country | Females | | Males | |
|---|---|---|---|---|
| | IMR | MRDT | IMR | MRDT |
| Algeria | 90.37 | 10.4 | 200.32 | 12.8 |
| Argentina | 18.12 | 7.4 | 71.90 | 9.1 |
| Bulgaria | 3.59 | 5.7 | 20.15 | 7.0 |
| Brazil | 27.70 | 8.0 | 80.55 | 9.5 |
| Canada | 0.81 | 5.1 | 11.37 | 6.8 |
| Ecuador | 12.23 | 6.9 | 25.59 | 7.6 |
| Egypt | 145.95 | 9.6 | 294.40 | 12.0 |
| El Salvador | 11.47 | 6.6 | 13.37 | 6.3 |
| Fiji | 203.87 | 12.6 | 294.62 | 12.6 |
| Guatemala | 52.22 | 8.6 | 93.52 | 9.5 |
| Iceland | 0.47 | 4.8 | 8.04 | 6.5 |
| Iran | 163.45 | 16.9 | 441.84 | 19.5 |
| Italy | 0.67 | 5.0 | 9.73 | 6.5 |
| Japan | 0.39 | 4.8 | 5.05 | 6.1 |
| Malaysia | 49.25 | 8.8 | 84.14 | 9.3 |
| Mali | 170.59 | 13.7 | 208.85 | 13.6 |
| Mexico | 19.83 | 7.4 | 46.29 | 8.4 |
| Pakistan | 91.67 | 10.4 | 86.94 | 10.4 |
| Peru | 6.44 | 6.2 | 12.00 | 6.7 |
| Romania | 1.63 | 5.1 | 14.31 | 6.6 |
| Switzerland | 0.66 | 5.1 | 13.78 | 7.1 |
| Thailand | 97.89 | 10.8 | 163.65 | 11.4 |
| Tunisia | 71.66 | 9.9 | 89.51 | 10.1 |
| United Kingdom | 2.60 | 5.8 | 31.01 | 7.8 |
| United States | 7.40 | 7.4 | 23.85 | 7.6 |
| USSR | 7.16 | 6.4 | 64.13 | 8.7 |
| Zimbabwe | 103.12 | 19.8 | 318.60 | 26.4 |
| Mean | 50.42 | 8.5 | 101.06 | 9.8 |
| Standard deviation | 61.73 | 3.8 | 117.34 | 4.5 |

[a]IMRs are given $\times 10^{-5}$.
Data Source: United Nations (1991).


**Table 2-5** Sensitivity analysis of the Gompertz hazards model: values for MLP such that $S(t_{MLP}) \leq 10^{-6}$.

| MRDT (years) | IMR | | | |
|---|---|---|---|---|
| | 0.0001 | 0.001 | 0.01 | 0.1 |
| 1 | 17 | 13 | 10 | 7 |
| 4 | 58 | 45 | 32 | 19 |
| 8 | 100 | 82 | 55 | 30 |
| 12 | 155 | 116 | 76 | 38 |

individuals by an MLP of 85 or even 100 years; for most causes, an individual would have to be centuries old before his or her probability of survival were reduced to $10^{-6}$ (Weiss, 1981, 1985, 1989a; Olshansky *et al.*, 1990).

## The Common Shape Characteristics of Hazards from Diverse Senescent Causes

Despite the shortcomings of the GR view, the EP view in itself does not explain the common shape characteristics of different chronic diseases. Why does a model like the Gompertz fit such a wide variety of specific causes of death? Are different cells, tissues, and organs constructed so as to wear out in some similar way? It would scarcely appear so. Cancer is caused by somatic mutations accumulating in individual cells during life, and its onset is timed by the risks of mutation associated with mitosis and exposure to exogenous and endogenous mutagens. Heart disease is caused by the accumulation of fatty deposits on the interior walls of the coronary arteries. Renal failure is caused by the gradual accumulation of lesions in the glomeruli induced by elevated blood pressure or, in the case of diabetes, by the toxic byproducts of systemically impaired glucose metabolism. And yet, despite these profound differences in the underlying physiological mechanisms, the mortality hazards associated with these diverse diseases are all fitted reasonably well by the Gompertz model. If the EP view of aging is correct, this apparent commonality across causes requires explanation.

One possible explanation is that all these pathological processes are, in some sense, multi-stage or multi-hit processes. As noted above, the accumulation of damage in a complex system is likely to generate hazards of system failure that increase more or less exponentially with time, even if the failure rates of the system's individual components do not increase with time. Any mortality model with a hazard function that increases monotonically with age, including the Gompertz, should fit such a situation tolerably well.

Another explanation would rest on an increasing diversity of susceptibility levels with age among members of a cohort, reflecting their differing genotypes and experiences of exposure to environmental risk factors, or simply reflecting chance variation. Consider, for example, a cohort of individuals who are identical in their mortality risks at birth. As the cohort ages, different exposures will induce differences in susceptibility, and an increasing fraction of the cohort will enter the high-risk portion of the susceptibility distribution. The hazard of death at age $t$ will largely reflect the fraction of the cohort in that high-risk segment, and as the cohort ages this fraction will increase, causing a corresponding increase in the hazard. For example, differing exposures to environmental pollution, radon gas, and cigarette smoke among members of a cohort will produce an increasingly divergent distribution of cumulative lung damage and liability to develop emphysema, chronic obstructive pulmonary disease, lung cancer, and perhaps even pneumonia. Assuming that the distribution of damage at any age is approximately Gaussian and that the size of the tail of the distribution is related to risk, it can be shown that an approximately Gompertz hazard of death will be produced (Weiss, 1993).

Thus, to the extent that similar age-related increases occur in the liability distributions characteristic of different tissues, the mortality functions associated with those tissues can all exhibit Gompertz-like behavior without having any specific etiologic mechanisms in common.

While these models do not *prove* that the exponentially accelerating hazards associated with diverse diseases have independent causes, they do suggest that the observed patterns are consistent with such independence. Therefore, the common shape of those patterns does not necessarily imply a common underlying mechanism.

Just as completely unrelated causes of death may all exhibit Gompertz-like age patterns, an aggregate of different, but approximately Gompertz hazards will itself be approximately Gompertz. Elsewhere (Wood *et al.*, 1992b) we have shown that any number of independent, competing causes of death, each with its own Gompertz hazard, will produce an overall, all-cause Gompertz hazard function if the individual cause-specific hazards are small (as seems to be the case for most causes, at least in humans). Thus, a sum of approximately Gompertz, but individually small, hazards yields an approximately Gompertz aggregate mortality curve. Putting all these results together, the fact that the cause-specific mortality curves for many causes of death appear to share a common Gompertz form, and that total mortality from all causes shares the same functional form, appears to be completely uninformative about any possible unitary control of senescence.

## How, Then, Does Life Span Evolve?

If we adopt the EP view and abandon the search for a unitary cause of aging, it would appear that our current longevity characteristics have evolved through selection on genes affecting individual causes of death rather than the all-cause MRDT or MLP. This view of selection is consistent with our current understanding of genetic epidemiology, since the disease-related genetic variants thus far identified in humans do not appear to recalibrate global senescence, but rather affect quite specific traits—for example, members of a particular family may be at elevated risk for some specific disease such as breast cancer, heart disease, or diabetes.[8] In the absence of medical intervention, genes predisposing to an elevated risk of death from some specific cause may arise by mutation but will be removed selectively from the population unless they occur at a sufficiently late age to have a negligible impact on fitness.

Genetic studies of chronic disease risk factors, such as cholesterol levels or blood pressure, have found only a few genes that by themselves seriously affect the risk of death (Weiss, 1993). Once the effects of these major genes are

---

[8]One apparent exception is familial progeroid disease, including Hutchinson–Gilford syndrome and Werner's syndrome. These syndromes have traditionally been described as dramatic accelerations in overall aging. Recent research, however, indicates that the specific pathologies associated with progeroid disease, which are mainly restricted to connective tissue, have little if anything to do with most manifestations of normal aging (Brown, 1987; Arking, 1991: 226–227).

removed, there is usually some residual variation in risk attributable to a large number of "polygenes," each with small effect. For example, the polygenic component appears to explain about 25% of the observed variation in serum cholesterol levels (Sing and Boerwinkle, 1987). Such unidentified polygenes could, in principle, affect many different traits simultaneously and thus affect global aging; however, on an individual basis these genes should be nearly invisible to natural selection and are therefore unlikely to be involved in the evolution of a tightly controlled MLP.

While there are many unanswered questions about the evolution of the life span, certain key facts now seem well established. First, age-related changes in specific physiological traits affecting mortality vary greatly in absolute magnitude, both within and across human populations. Although some general shape characteristics are shared by many traits, these similarities in age pattern may be coincidental rather than a reflection of common causal factors. Looking at the individual traits, we can sometimes identify biological processes that explain much of the observed age pattern; those processes, however, are quite diverse, ranging from the detrimental effects of somatic mutations and cellular damage, to chemical degradation, to purely mechanical damage. No single etiologic model can account for all these changes except, perhaps, for the very general notion that the effects of deterioration accumulate more or less gradually and continuously over time. In general, senescent changes affecting mortality do not appear to involve the sudden switching on or off of genetically controlled enzymes, hormones, or repair mechanisms; moreover, evolutionary theory suggests that such elaborate physiological switches are very unlikely to evolve by natural selection. In view of what we know about the widely differing *proximate* causes of failure and degeneration, any underlying unitary control, if it exists, must involve a physiological mechanism that can coordinate all these distinct processes at once. Such a mechanism has never been identified.

## REPRODUCTION

From the present perspective, fecundity is fundamentally different from viability in that there are no competing causes of birth. However, while the modeling details will look quite different than in the case of mortality, fecundity can also be decomposed into several underlying physiological components (Wood, 1989). When such modeling is done, age patterns of fecundity appear to be dominated by a small number of more or less independent senescent changes, with little coordination in the rate of those changes. Thus, it is possible to view fertility from a perspective that is parallel to and consistent with the EP view of mortality.

Since the specific processes involved in reproductive senescence are quite distinct in males and females, it is necessary to review them separately for the two sexes.

## Male Reproductive Senescence

Until recently, efforts to portray human male reproductive senescence as a process independent of other pathogeric and eugeric changes remained ambiguous. Contradictory data emerged from studies of testosterone secretion, Leydig cell maintenance, hypothalamic–pituitary function, spermatogenesis, and sperm motility. What these ambiguities reveal is a high degree of heterogeneity among men in the processes of reproductive senescence (Sniffen, 1950; Neaves *et al.*, 1984). In particular, individual levels of general health as well as socioeconomic correlates can have significant confounding effects on the aging process (Harman and Tsitouras, 1980; Harman *et al.*, 1982; Tsitouras *et al.*, 1982).

Some studies of serum testosterone levels have reported no age-related decline (Harman and Tsitouras, 1980; Sparrow *et al.*, 1980; Nieschlag *et al.*, 1982; Neaves *et al.*, 1984). The weight of the evidence, however, now consistently points to lower secretion of testosterone in elderly men (Vermeulen *et al.*, 1972, 1989; Pirke and Doerr, 1973; Harman, 1978; Purifoy *et al.*, 1981; Zumoff *et al.*, 1982; Takahashi *et al.*, 1983; Deslypere and Vermeulen, 1984; Royer *et al.*, 1984; Bremner *et al.*, 1986; Montanini *et al.*, 1988; Tenover *et al.*, 1988), a decline in amplitude of the circadian rhythm in testosterone secretion (Marrama *et al.*, 1982; Deslypere and Vermeulen, 1984; Bremner *et al.*, 1986; Tenover *et al.*, 1988), and a gradual diminution of the circadian rhythm itself (Zumoff *et al.*, 1982; Bremner *et al.*, 1983; Deslypere and Vermeulen, 1984; Montanini *et al.*, 1988; Tenover *et al.*, 1988).[9] Based upon studies of elderly men with prostate cancer, Takahashi *et al.* (1983) suggest that declining testosterone levels are attributable to decreased production in the testicular mitochondria of its precursor, pregnenolone, leading to a reduction in steroidogenesis. Pirke *et al.* (1980) have also found a decline in pregnenolone in the testes of aging men.

---

[9]Conflicting results concerning whether testosterone declines or remains stable during senescence are probably attributable to several factors, including biases in subject selection since the health of older subjects may be of critical importance (Harman and Tsitouras, 1980; Sparrow *et al.*, 1980; Tsitouras *et al.*, 1982; Nieschlag and Michel, 1986). There may also have been insufficient attention to the circadian rhythm in testosterone release (Harman and Tsitouras, 1980; Winters and Troen, 1982; Bremner *et al.*, 1983, 1986). Other complications may reflect the effect of sexual activity in raising testosterone levels (Fox *et al.*, 1972; Kraemer *et al.*, 1976), as well as what appears to be a high degree of interindividual heterogeneity in testicular function with age (Sniffen, 1950; vom Saal and Finch, 1988). Recently, Nahoul and Roger (1990) have suggested that contradictory results are related to whether researchers measure total testosterone (protein-bound and free) or just free testosterone. Studies of total testosterone levels in elderly men probably reflect the confounding effect of a reduction in metabolic clearance that may obscure any real decline in plasma testosterone levels (Vermeulen *et al.*, 1972; Baker *et al.*, 1976). Studies evaluating levels of free testosterone are more consistent in showing declines with age (e.g., Harman and Tsitouras, 1980; Nieschlag *et al.*, 1982; Davidson *et al.*, 1983; Vermeulen *et al.*, 1989). An increase in testosterone-binding globulin in older men (Harman and Tsitouras, 1980; Sparrow *et al.*, 1980; Winters and Troen, 1982; Davidson *et al.*, 1983) could also explain the more consistent results in free as opposed to total testosterone. Given these discrepancies, however, Nahoul and Roger (1990) have suggested that measurement of bioavailable testosterone (free plus albumin-bound testosterone) is the most appropriate index of androgen activity.

Although declining testosterone production among elderly men implies reduced Leydig cell function, studies comparing Leydig cell numbers in younger and older men have yielded conflicting results. While some researchers have found a reduction in Leydig cell numbers (Kaler and Neaves, 1978; Neaves *et al.*, 1984; Nieschlag and Michel, 1986: 67), others have not (Sniffen, 1950; Sokal, 1964; Kothari and Gupta, 1974). In fact, Kothari and Gupta (1974) found evidence for Leydig-cell hyperplasia in the elderly subjects in their study. The finding that pathogeric changes can have significant effects on Leydig cells (Harbitz, 1973) has complicated resolution of this issue. There is also evidence for testicular atrophy and degeneration of the seminiferous tubules with aging (Harman *et al.*, 1982). Kothari and Gupta (1974) noted an age-related thickening of the tunica propria of the seminiferous tubules, which may be related to a decline in spermatogenesis.

In males, testosterone exerts a negative feedback on the release of luteinizing-hormone (LH) releasing hormone (LHRH) by the hypothalamus (Kaufman *et al.*, 1990), analogous to the negative feedback mechanism in the hypothalamic–pituitary–ovarian axis in women (see below). And men exhibit a rise in follicle-stimulating hormone (FSH) and LH levels with age similar to the menopausal pattern of gonadotropin secretion in women (Vermeulen *et al.*, 1972; Baker *et al.*, 1976; Harman, 1978; Sparrow *et al.*, 1980; Harman *et al.*, 1982; Nieschlag *et al.*, 1982; Davidson *et al.*, 1983; Takahashi *et al.*, 1983; Neaves *et al.*, 1984; Montanini *et al.*, 1988; Nahoul and Roger, 1990). There is thus a negative relationship between gonadotropin function and steroid function during senescence in both sexes. However, no study has yet been able to detect any alteration in LH pulse frequency or amplitude that might explain the higher LH levels observed in aging men (Rubens *et al.*, 1974; Snyder *et al.*, 1975; Winters and Troen, 1982). It therefore remains unclear what mechanism is responsible for the increase in gonadotropins or even whether the hypothalamic–pituitary axis is involved. Recently, Kaufman *et al.* (1990) have developed a mathematical model suggesting that the plasma half-life of immunoreactive LH is prolonged in older men, which could account for their higher plasma LH levels.

Declining androgen levels, increasing gonadotropins, and the apparently normal pulsatile production of LH would appear to indicate primary degeneration of testicular function with reproductive senescence. But other data point to an independent age-related reduction in hypothalamic-pituitary function (Vermeulen *et al.*, 1989). Various studies have found evidence of impaired hypothalamic LHRH signaling and a decrease in hypothalamic–pituitary sensitivity to feedback (Tenover *et al.*, 1988; Urban *et al.*, 1988; Kaufman *et al.*, 1990). For example, administration of exogenous LHRH to aging men results in delayed gonadotropin secretion (Harman *et al.*, 1982; Winters and Troen, 1982). Similarly, reaction to bioassay of the opioid antagonist naltrexone in elderly monks leads to decreased LH response in comparison with younger monks (Vermeulen *et al.*, 1989; Kaufman *et al.*, 1990).

An increased sensitivity of the hypothalamic–pituitary axis to the negative feedback control of androgens at later ages has been detected in bioassays.

Exogenously administered dihydrotestosterone has a significantly greater effect in lowering gonadotropin levels (both LH and FSH) in elderly men than in younger men (Winters *et al.*, 1984; Vermeulen *et al.*, 1989). In comparison, exogenous testosterone has a greater effect on LH but not FSH. The increased senescent response to androgens is thought to be mediated at the hypothalamic level by modified LHRH secretion.

There is a clear reduction in male libido and potency with age, with obvious implications for fertility (Verwoerdt *et al.*, 1969; Martin, 1977; Comfort, 1980; Davidson *et al.*, 1983). Tsitouras *et al.* (1982) noted a positive relationship between testosterone levels and the degree of sexual activity in 183 men ages 60–79 years. Using autopsy material, Neaves *et al.* (1984) found that spermatogenic function was also reduced in older men, with a significant negative correlation between FSH levels and sperm production. Spermatogenesis is therefore linked to the change in gonadotropin levels with age. However, Nieschlag *et al.* (1982; Nieschlag and Michel, 1986) found that spermatogenesis remained similar between younger and older men in their study, while sperm motility and seminal fructose was significantly lower in older subjects. These latter differences may be explained by decreasing sexual activity with age and a longer latency period rather than as a physiological symptom of senescence. Thus, the age-related decline in male fertility may reflect lower coital frequency rather than reduced sperm viability. Certainly, there exist cases of successful male reproduction at extremely advanced ages (Seymour *et al.*, 1935), reinforcing the notion of a high degree of individual variability among males.

There is some evidence suggesting that the paternal contribution to birth defects and fetal deaths increases with age, similar to the maternal pattern (Selvin and Garfinkel, 1976; Hook, 1986), although it has recently been shown that the genetic origin of trisomy 21 offspring is predominantly maternal (Antonarakis *et al.*, 1991). While it is possible that this reflects a higher incidence of fetal loss in cases of paternally derived trisomies (Antonarakis *et al.*, 1991), at present there is no direct evidence to support this possibility.

In sum, the emerging picture suggests that declining testosterone levels are one central feature of male reproductive senescence, and perhaps the only consistent feature. Superficially, this might appear to indicate a unitary cause for at least this one major form of aging. However, the studies reviewed above indicate that even this "central feature" may arise from a remarkable mutliplicity of etiologic processes.


## Female Reproductive Senescence

Reproductive aging in women appears to be dominated by three fairly well-characterized processes: (1) an increasing cumulative incidence of chromosomal aberrations and germinal mutations resulting in an elevated risk of fetal loss (Kline and Stein, 1987); (2) progressive depletion of primordial follicles in the ovary, resulting in less effective estradiol feedback control of the hypothalamic–pituitary–ovarian axis and ultimately in menopause (Richardson *et al.*, 1987); and, to a lesser extent, (3) reduced responsiveness of the pituitary and hypothalamus to feedback by ovarian steroids (Metcalf *et al.*, 1982).[10] In theory, these various age-related physiological changes should be manifested demographically as a decline in fecundability (the monthly probability of conception), an increase in the risk of fetal loss, and a final cessation of reproduction at the menopause. The available demographic and epidemiological evidence suggests that these changes occur at markedly different rates, consistent with the EP view of aging.

Despite statistical difficulties in estimating fecundability (Wood, 1989), most studies indicate a continuous decline with the female partner's age after about age 25 or 30 years (Bendel and Hua, 1978; Wood and Weinstein, 1988; Wood *et al.*, 1992b).[11] This demographic evidence is consistent with what is known about several age-related changes in female reproductive physiology. For example, ovarian function undergoes various alterations during later reproductive life, including changes in the length of the ovarian cycle, the likelihood of anovulatory cycles, and the prevalence of luteal insufficiency (Treloar *et al.*, 1967; Lenton *et al.*, 1984a, 1984b; Lipson and Ellison, 1992). In addition, since estimates of fecundability are based on *diagnosed* pregnancies, and some degree of subclinical fetal loss may occur prior to diagnosis (Wilcox *et al.*, 1988), changing levels of early fetal loss may also be implicated.

Despite the likely contribution of all these physiological factors, James (1979) has argued that the decline in fecundability at higher ages is caused primarily by declines in coital frequency reflecting increases in either age or marital duration. At least two recent analyses seem to contradict this claim (Schwartz and Mayaux, 1982; van Noord-Zaadstra *et al.*, 1991). In a study coordinated by the Fédération Française des Centres d'Etude et de Conservation des Oeufs et du Sperme, Schwartz and Mayaux (1982) analyzed the cumulative pregnancy rates of 2,193 French women who underwent artificial insemination with donor sperm. The husbands of these women all appeared to be completely sterile due to azoospermia, but there were no apparent

---

[10]Until recently, it was thought that a deteriorating uterine environment also plays a major role in female reproductive senescence; for example, it was hypothesized that sclerotic changes in the uterine blood supply, loss of cell elasticity, and increasing amounts of collagen in the endometrium and myometrium contributed to failure of implantation and increasing risks of spontaneous abortion with age (Woessner, 1963; Naeye, 1983; Gosden, 1985; Gostwamy *et al.*, 1988). While lower levels of estrogen and progesterone in postmenopausal woman are certainly responsible for adverse endometrial changes, it is unlikely that the uterus plays a primary role in the loss of female reproductive function. A recent study of women age 40–44 suffering from premature ovarian failure demonstrated the viability of the older uterus in maintaining pregnancy throughout gestation following initial artificial stimulation of the endometrium and transplantation of embryos from young oocyte donors (Sauer *et al.*, 1990). Similarly, Navot *et al.* (1991) have applied the techniques of donor–oocyte treatment to infertile but cycling women age 40+ whose previous attempts at *in vitro* fertilization with self-oocytes failed; women in this study achieved a 56% pregnancy rate using donated oocytes from younger women, compared to only 3.3% with their own oocytes.

[11]It is by no means clear that this is strictly an effect of the female's age since most studies do not control for any possible effect of the male partner's age. (In most human populations, the two are highly correlated.) This reflects a widespread tendency to treat fecundability as a characteristic of the female rather than the couple.

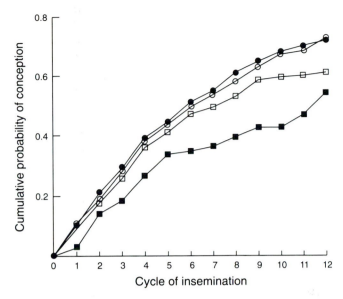

**Figure 2-6**   Cumulative pregnancy rates following artificial insemination with donor sperm in four age-groups of French women: ≤25 years (●), 26–30 years (○), 31–35 years (□), and ≥36 years (■). The heterogeneity chi-square for all four curves is highly significant ($P<0.01$). Controlled comparisons show that ages ≤25 and 26–30 do not differ significantly from each other, but both ages differ from the two older groups ($P<0.05$ in comparison with ages 31–35, $P<0.001$ in comparison with ages 36+). Redrawn from Schwartz and Mayaux (1982).

reproductive impairments in the women themselves. The attraction of this study in relation to James' hypothesis is that coital frequency was essentially invariant with age; in all the cycles analyzed, the women were inseminated at least once during the periovulatory segment of the cycle. Nonetheless, there remained significant differences in cumulative pregnancy rates when the data were classified by woman's age (Figure 2-6). In particular, the cumulative rates were consistently lower in women age 31 to 35 than in women age 30 or less, and sharply lower in women over 35. Since there was no attempt to match older women with older sperm donors, these differences are presumably attributable to age-related differences in the reproductive physiology of the women and not the men involved. A more recent study of 1,637 women undergoing artificial insemination with donor sperm in the Netherlands has produced almost identical results (van Noord-Zaadstra *et al.*, 1991). These two studies are of great importance in establishing that fecundability does indeed decline as a result of age-related changes in female reproductive physiology (see also Edwards *et al.*, 1984; Virro and Shewchuk, 1984; Romeu *et al.*, 1987).

Many studies suggest that the risk of fetal loss increases in women after age 25 or 30 (e.g., Wilcox and Gladen, 1982; Kline and Stein, 1987; Casterline, 1989; Santow and Bracher, 1989). For example, Selvin and Garfinkel (1976)

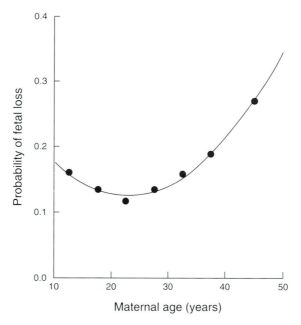

**Figure 2-7**   Age pattern of fetal loss in women from several populations in which induced abortion is not a competing risk. Circles represent pooled data from nine populations, each adjusted to yield an overall loss rate across all ages of 150 per 1,000 conceptions. Solid curve is a quadratic equation fitted to the pooled data by ordinary least squares ($r^2 = 0.998$). Redrawn from Wood and Weinstein (1988), based on data from Yerushalmy *et al.* (1956), Stevenson *et al.* (1958), Warburton and Fraser (1964), Potter *et al.* (1965), Shapiro *et al.* (1970), Naylor (1974), Resseguie (1974), and Leridon (1976).

performed a multivariate logistic regression analysis of over 1.5 million pregnancies registered in New York State between 1959 and 1967. After controlling for paternal age and gravidity, they found a highly significant effect of maternal age on the risk of fetal loss ($P < 0.001$). (Together, the three predictor variables explained approximately 41% of the variation in these data.) Further, maternal age was a more important predictor of fetal loss than paternal age in this study, although the regression coefficients for the two were surprisingly similar.[12]

Figure 2-7 summarizes data from nine studies of the risk of fetal loss by maternal age conducted in a variety of locales from North America, Europe, Asia, and the Caribbean. These studies were selected for two reasons: they included reasonably large samples of pregnancies, and they were conducted at periods and/or in locations that minimized contamination of the results by induced abortion, which is a competing risk for pregnancy termination. Despite

---

[12]Gravidity (pregnancy order) had an effect that was also similar in magnitude to those of maternal and paternal age. This apparent effect of gravidity probably reflects heterogeneity in risk among women, since two women of the same age may differ in gravidity precisely because one of them has experienced more losses.

variation among these studies in the overall level of fetal loss, all indicated a marked rise in the risk of loss after maternal age 30. Adjusting the results so that each study has the same overall risk of loss (arbitrarily set at 150 per 1,000 pregnancies) and pooling results across studies, we obtain the relationship shown in Figure 2-7. Interestingly, an analysis of data from a large prospective study (1,507 fetal deaths during the first 28 weeks of pregnancy in more than 3.25 million woman-days of observation) shows essentially the same relationship (Harlap *et al.*, 1980).

It has recently been suggested that the apparent elevation in the risk of fetal loss at later maternal ages is at least partly an artifact of heterogeneity in risk among women, combined with selective reproduction associated with fertility control (Wilcox and Gladen, 1982; Gladen, 1986; Santow and Bracher, 1989). In populations where most couples successfully use birth control, women who are still reproducing at, say, age 40 are likely to be a highly select subsample of all women; in particular, they may disproportionately represent those women who have not yet achieved their desired family size because of prior pregnancy loss. Thus, the apparent increase in the risk of fetal loss with maternal age may partly reflect two facts: (1) that the risk varies among women, and (2) that high-risk women are more likely to attempt to reproduce at later ages. If correct, this "heterogeneity/selectivity" hypothesis would require us to modify conventional views of an age-related increase in the risk of fetal loss.

Few studies have attempted to test the heterogeneity/selectivity hypothesis. In one study of 2,547 Australian women in which appropriate statistical controls for the number of previous losses were implemented, the rise in risk of loss with maternal age was much less marked than in other studies and did not begin until age 35 or 40 (Santow and Bracher, 1989). An alternative approach to the problem is to study fetal loss in a population without widespread birth control, where selectivity would not be expected to occur. Only one study to date, involving 7,363 pregnancies reported by Old Order Amish women from Illinois, Iowa, Missouri, and Wisconsin (Resseguie, 1974), has provided a sample large enough for statistical analysis. The results of this study are shown in Figure 2-8, along with those from a study of the general United States population in which case ascertainment was similar to the Amish study. In addition to lower rates of loss at all ages among Amish women (an interesting finding in its own right), the age curve of fetal loss appears to be much flatter in the Amish, suggesting little or no elevation in risk prior to about age 40, and only a small elevation after that age. A tentative conclusion would be that some, but not all, of the apparent increase in fetal loss at later maternal ages is artifactual.

The most obvious age-related decline in female reproductive capacity occurs at menopause, the final cessation of ovarian cycles. Prior to menopause, regular cycles are maintained by a complex regulatory system linking the hypothalamus, anterior pituitary gland, and ovaries (Wood, 1994). During the follicular (preovulatory) phase of the cycle, this regulatory system involves gradually increasing secretion of estrogen by the growing ovarian follicles. These follicles are stimulated by FSH secreted by the pituitary in response to hypothalamic gonadotropin-releasing hormone (GnRH). The process of fol-

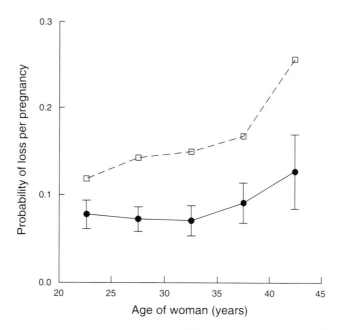

**Figure 2-8**  Age patterns of fetal loss. Solid line: probability of fetal loss per pregnancy (±95% confidence limit) by maternal age, estimated from 7,363 pregnancies reported by Old Order Amish women from Illinois, Iowa, Missouri, and Wisconsin. Broken line: age-specific probabilities of fetal loss estimated from 33,254 pregnancies among non-Amish US women at approximately the same period and ascertained through methods similar to those used in the Amish study. Data from Naylor (1974) and Resseguie (1974).

licular recruitment and the gradual dominance of an antral follicle are still not completely understood, but adequate estrogen secretion by the cohort of developing follicles (most of which will undergo atresia) is necessary to maintain this cyclic process. Following ovulation, the remnant granulosa cells from the ruptured follicle in the ovary transform themselves into the corpus luteum, which secretes progesterone during the luteal (postovulatory) phase of the cycle in preparation for potential implantation and gestation of a fertilized ovum. Given this sequence of events, luteal function and the secretion of progesterone depend upon follicular development itself, especially the adequacy of estrogen secretion during the follicular phase.

Central to this system is the so-called GnRH pulse generator, located in the hypothalamus. This neural plexus controls pulsatile secretion of the pituitary gonadotropins, LH and FSH, which in turn act upon the ovary to initiate follicular development and induce ovulation. Although the GnRH pulse generator has its own endogenous rhythm, its baseline, frequency, and amplitude can all be modified by changes in the plasma concentration of ovarian steroids—estrogen during the follicular phase and progesterone during the luteal phase. Crucial to maintaining regular cycles is the negative feedback of estradiol on the pulse generator during the early stages of the follicular

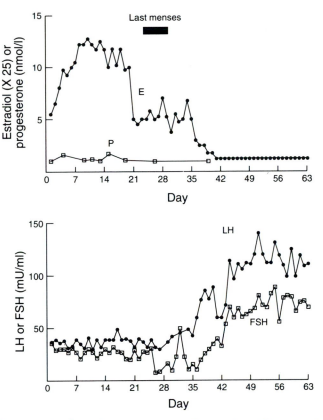

**Figure 2-9** Changes in the plasma concentrations of ovarian steroids (top) and pituitary gonadotropins (bottom) during the menopausal transition in a woman age 48 years. E = estradiol-17β (concentration multiplied by 25); P = progesterone; LH = luteinizing hormone; FSH = follicle-stimulating hormone. Note that the fall in estradiol induces the last menses and is followed by a marked rise in LH and FSH. Redrawn from van Look *et al.* (1977).

phase, followed by an abrupt change to positive feedback just before the mid-cycle surge in LH and FSH that triggers ovulation.

The salient feature of menopause is loss of estrogen feedback control of the GnRH pulse generator. The distinctive hormonal profile associated with this process is shown in Figure 2-9. The woman in this example experienced her last menses at age 48; it is clear from her negligible plasma progesterone levels that the cycle preceding her final menses was anovulatory. Following the last menses is a period of one or two weeks during which some estrogen is present, presumably reflecting one last round of partial follicular development. After this period, the levels of both estrogen and progesterone (if they are present at all) are well below the assay system's limits of detection, and they will remain that low for the rest of the woman's life. Coinciding with the decline in ovarian steroids is a marked elevation in LH and FSH, indicating that the hypothalamic–pituitary axis has been relieved of negative feedback by estrogen. From this point on, at least until very late in her life, this woman's gonadotropin levels will be high and quite variable, and she will experience ephemeral spikes of LH and FSH, apparently coinciding with the "hot flashes" of menopause (Tataryn et al., 1979; Meldrum et al., 1980). The combination of no detectable ovarian steroids and high gonadotropins is the unmistakable endocrine signature of menopause.

What accounts for the loss of estrogen regulation? The answer, baldly stated, is that the ovary runs out of eggs. More precisely, the remaining pool of viable primordial follices (i.e., those not yet lost to atresia or ovulation) apparently becomes too small to produce the amount of estrogen necessary to support further follicular development and feedback control of gonadotropin secretion (Baird, 1991; Jaffe, 1991). In contrast to males, the number of gametes produced by females is fixed during embryogenesis: the maximum number of oocytes, about seven million on average, is observed in the female zygote during the fifth month of gestation (Block, 1953; Baker, 1963). In addition, females experience an ongoing process of follicular loss, mostly through atresia. This process of follicular depletion also begins in utero and ends at menopause. At birth, the female fetus is endowed with approximately one million follicles, of which only 3–400,000 remain at puberty, and fewer than 0.01% are subsequently ovulated (Block, 1952, 1953; Baker, 1963).

A critical feature, therefore, of reproductive senescence in women is the decline in the pool of ovarian follicles with time. This results in diminishing levels of both estrogen and progesterone with successive cycles, and a corresponding elevation in gonadotropins (Sherman and Korenman, 1976; Sherman et al., 1976). The gross anatomy of the aging ovary reflects this process, with a gradual decrease in ovarian size as the follicular pool shrinks, and the growth of surface scars from the corpora albicans following each menstruation (Nicosia, 1986, 1987). The postmenopausal ovary weighs approximately two-thirds as much as the mature ovary.

The idea that follicular depletion is the primary mechanism driving menopause has been around for several decades, but it was long rejected because of autopsy estimates of the number of primordial follicles present in the ovaries of women at various ages (Figure 2-10). Based on a linear regression fit to the logarithm of these estimates (straight line in Figure 2-10, right panel), it appears that something like 5,000 viable follicles are still present at about age 50, too many, it would seem, to support the hypothesis that menopause is caused by follicular depletion. It appears, however, that the relationship between the log of the number of remaining follicles and age may not be linear, and indeed a quadratic regression fits the data better (curved line in Figure 2-10, right panel). According to this curve, far fewer than 1,000 primordial follicles, and perhaps as few as 100–200 or less, are still present at menopause. It should be noted, however, that the apparent curvilinearity in these data is largely attributable to the two lowest data points. Before age 40 the relationship with age does in fact appear to be log-linear, implying a constant rate of follicular loss; there may, however, be some acceleration in loss after age 40.

Until recently, autopsies have provided the only evidence for follicular

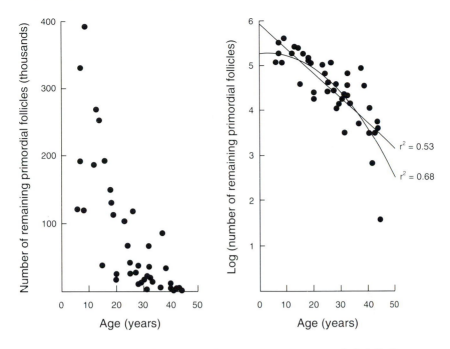

**Figure 2-10** Age-related changes in the number of primordial follicles per ovary based on cross-sectional autopsy data: linear plot (left panel) and semi-log plot (right panel). One ovary was selected at random from each subject. A quadratic regression (curved line) fits the semi-log data significantly better than a linear regression (straight line), suggesting near-depletion of follicles by the time of menopause. Data from Block (1952).

depletion in humans. The special nature of autopsy samples makes selectivity bias a concern, since women who undergo autopsy may not be representative of living women. Usually, moreover, nothing is known about the cycling status of autopsied women prior to their deaths, i.e., which ones were menopausal and which still cycling; consequently, the relationship between follicular depletion and cycling status remained obscure.

Recent evidence provides more direct support for the follicle depletion hypothesis. In a study of 17 women of known cycling status who underwent elective hysterectomy and oophorectomy at ages 45–55, Richardson *et al.* (1987) observed follicle reserves that differed significantly by cycling status ($P < 0.001$), ranging from 1,000 to 2,500 in cycling women, to a few hundred in perimenopausal women, to zero or one in postmenopausal women. There is some confounding by age in this study since regularly cycling women were slightly younger on average than perimenopausal women, who were in turn slightly younger than postmenopausal women. However, an analysis of covariance designed to adjust for these age differences still indicates a strong relationship between cycling status and the number of remaining follicles (Table 2-6).

**Table 2-6**  Analysis of covariance of the effects of cycling status (whether a woman is cycling normally, experiencing the irregular menses of the perimenopausal transition, or postmenopausal) and age on the number of remaining primary follicles in one ovary.[a]

| Source | Sum of squares | d.f. | Mean square | $F$ | $P$ |
|---|---|---|---|---|---|
| Cycling status | 5,608,198.06 | 2 | 2,804,099.03 | 9.628 | 0.003 |
| Age | 216,989.29 | 1 | 216,989.29 | 0.745 | 0.404 |
| Error | 3,785,996.39 | 13 | 291,230.49 | | |
| $R^2 = 0.64$ | | | | | |

[a]The sample consists of 17 women ages 45–55 undergoing elective hysterectomy and oophorectomy. Cycling status was determined by a menstrual history confirmed by plasma hormone levels. Women were classified as postmenopausal if they had experienced at least 1 year since the last menses. One ovary chosen at random from each woman was serially sectioned for determination of follicle number. In the analysis, cycling status is treated as a class variable, while age is treated as the continuous covariate.

Data source: Richardson et al. (1987).

These data, coming as they do from oophorectomies, may still be unrepresentative of normal women. However, the oophorectomies were elective, and none of the subjects had any prior condition with a known relationship to follicle number or follicular loss. In addition, Richardson et al. (1987) summarize evidence indicating that ovaries obtained through autopsy and oophorectomy yield similar estimates of the number of remaining follicles at each age. Each of these two sources of data may be biased, but they are very unlikely to be biased in the same way.

This study provides the clearest evidence to date of a causal relationship between follicular depletion and onset of menopause. In addition, when the results of this study are combined with the earlier autopsy data, they provide powerful evidence that the rate of follicular depletion is indeed accelerated after age 40, so that essentially no follicles are left at menopause (Figure 2-11). Menopause is thus the endpoint of a continuous process begun before birth, whereby an initial reserve of some seven million primordial follicles (and the oocytes they contain) is gradually diminished, principally through atresia. Entry into the menopausal transition is apparently not caused by the absolute exhaustion of this reserve; rather, the remaining pool of follices appears to fall below some threshold number necessary to sustain efficient estrogen regulation of gonadotropin secretion. Acceleration of follicular loss during perimenopausal life may well correspond to the crossing of that threshold. Not surprisingly, either the threshold or the estrogen produced by the remaining pool of follicles near the threshold appears to be subject to considerable stochastic variation. As a result, women's cycles tend to become extremely variable in length just before menopause (Treloar et al., 1967; Chiazze et al., 1968; Döring, 1969; Metcalf et al., 1982).

These biological considerations suggest a simple model for the etiology of menopause (Figure 2-12, upper left panel). Follicles are lost, primarily through atresia, at a more or less constant rate per follicle throughout prereproductive life and most of reproductive life. Eventually the number of remaining follicles

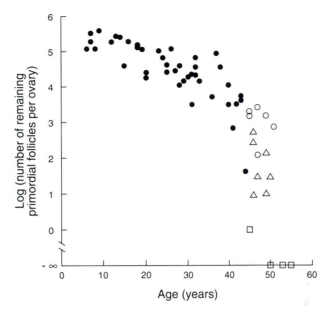

**Figure 2-11** A comparison of the relationship between age and primordial follicle number per ovary in Block's (1952) autopsy study of 43 girls and women ages 6–44 years (closed circles), with that in the Richardson *et al.* (1987) study of oophorectomy data from 17 women ages 45–55 years (open symbols: O, women who were experiencing regular menses; △ perimenopausal women; □, postmenopausal women). Since only one ovary was examined in the study of Richardson *et al.*, a single ovary was selected at random from each subject in Block's study. Insofar as these two data sets are comparable, follicular depletion appears to accelerate during the years preceding menopause.

crosses a threshold (broken line in Figure 2-12), below which the basal level of circulating estradiol is too low to maintain regular cycles. Once this threshold has been passed, cycles become extremely irregular and the rate of follicular loss increases until menopause (complete follicular depletion) occurs. Under this simple model, there are likely to be only three important sources of heterogeneity among women (Figure 2-12, upper right and bottom panels): differences in the size of the initial pool of follicles, differences in the rate of follicular loss, and differences in the level of the threshold. All three sources of heterogeneity are biologically plausible, and at least the first two are known to be important in determining differences among inbred strains of laboratory mice (Faddy *et al.*, 1983).

In sum, menopause is not a discrete trait that is simply "switched on" at some particular age, but rather the outcome of a continuous underlying process that unfolds over several decades of life. To miss this essential point is to make much the same mistake as treating life span itself as a unitary phenotypic trait related to a simple developmental switch. And in general, while there has been a tendency to emphasize the apparently sudden cessation in reproductive function at menopause, reproductive senescence in females is in fact a gradual

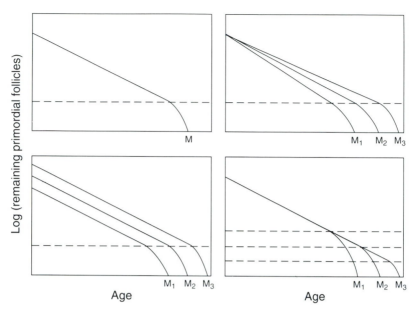

**Figure 2-12** A graphical model of menopause, emphasizing the fact that menopause is the final, discrete outcome of a continuous, decades-long process of follicular depletion (upper left panel). It is assumed that follicular loss occurs at a constant rate per follicle until a threshold is reached (broken line). Below that threshold, the remaining pool of follicles secretes too little estrogen early in the follicular phase to maintain regular cycles. Accelerated follicular depletion is hypothesized to result from the loss of efficient estrogen feedback on the hypothalamus and anterior pituitary gland. Menopause (M) occurs when the pool of remaining follicles is more or less completely exhausted. Under this model, variation among women in the age of menopause can result from heterogeneity in the rate of follicular loss (upper right panel), heterogeneity in the initial number of follicles (lower left panel), or heterogeneity in the level of the regulatory threshold (lower right panel). If acceleration in follicular depletion occurs during perimenopausal life, additional variation could result from heterogeneity in the rate of acceleration. From Wood (1994).

process. This is indicated by studies of the pattern of luteal progesterone release with increasing age in normal healthy women; after a period of peak luteal function at about ages 20–35 years, there is a slow but steady decline in luteal progesterone output until the menopause (Lipson and Ellison, 1992).

Demographic evidence mirrors these physiological processes. In many natural fertility populations, birth intervals tend to grow longer with maternal age after about age 30–35 (Wood, 1990). In addition, the mean age of women at their last birth in such populations (excluding women who die before age 50) is remarkably constant across populations at around age 40, with menopause occurring on average approximately 8–10 years later (Bongaarts and Potter, 1983; Wood, 1994). While partly attributable to lactational infecundability following the last birth, the approximate ten-year period of infertility preceding

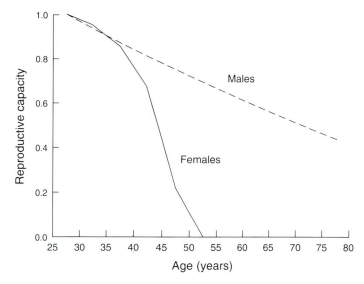

**Figure 2-13**  Reproductive senescence in human males and females, relative to ages 25–29 years. Reproductive capacity in males is taken as proportional to circulating testosterone concentration. (Data on salivary testosterone levels for 107 healthy US men ages 25–79 were kindly provided by Benjamin Campbell; line shown in figure is a quadratic regression fit to those data, standardized to equal one at age 27.5.) Female reproductive capacity is proportional to the value of fecundability expected if coital frequency were held constant while the physiological determinants of fecundability were allowed to vary by the female partner's age. The model from which expected fecundability was derived is described in Wood and Weinstein (1988); the predicted values are from Wood (1989).

menopause may be linked to the acceleration in follicular depletion and the associated decline in hypothalamic–pituitary–ovarian function that appears to occur during the final decade of female reproductive life.

## The Contrast in Male and Female Reproductive Senescence

One of the most striking features of human aging is the dramatic difference in the pace of reproductive senescence between males and females (Figure 2-13). Reproductive function in healthy women reaches its peak between ages 25 and 35, and remains fairly constant during this decade. Decline in oocyte quality and hormone production is evident from approximately 35 onwards, with a marked threshold at age 40. The mean age at menopause, with the total cessation of reproductive function, occurs on average at age 50 in Western women, but fecundability for the ten years preceding this event is very low. In contrast, reproductive senescence in men is a continuous process until death. In healthy men, senescent changes in reproductive function appear to have a negligible impact on potency and fertility, even at quite advanced ages. In addition, reproductive senescence in males, but not in females, occurs at a rate that is broadly similar to other senescent changes affecting the risk of death (compare Figures 2-4 and 2-13). Female reproductive senescence thus appears markedly accelerated relative to other forms of senescence.

The key feature explaining these differences lies in the differential process of gametogenesis and the ultimate depletion of primary follicles and oocytes in women. Because of follicular depletion, reproductive function ceases in women decades earlier than in men—indeed, at no age do men show a comparable total loss of reproductive capacity. Several authors have suggested that this "premature" loss of fecundity in women poses a particular problem for the evolutionary theory of aging, and have formulated special models to reconcile theory and observation. For example, it has been suggested that women are programmed to cease childbearing early so that they have time to rear their last child to maturity or even to help take care of their grandchildren (Hill and Hurtado, 1991). We suggest that such special pleading is unnecessary.

As detailed above, menopause is merely the endpoint of a decades-long process of follicular depletion. In addition, the mechanism that drives follicular depletion—namely, selection of follicles for partial development followed by atresia—plays an essential role in the neuroendocrine system that maintains regular ovarian cycles and results in the release of a single egg at mid-cycle (Baird, 1987). It is almost certain, therefore, that the rate of follicular depletion at early reproductive ages is under tight selective control since changes in that rate may disrupt normal ovarian function and ovulation. Moreover, this rate of depletion is maintained throughout reproductive life, except perhaps for the last few years before menopause when depletion appears to accelerate. In light of these considerations, we suggest that menopause is an incidental byproduct of selection for regular ovarian function and ovulation at earlier reproductive ages. If this suggestion is correct, the reduction in fitness at later, postmenopausal ages is presumably more than offset by the gain in fitness at earlier ages. In other words, we suggest that menopause is likely to have evolved through antagonistic pleiotropy.[13]

Despite the obvious difference between the sexes in the pace of gametogenesis, there remain important similarities between men and women in the processes of reproductive senescence. Both sexes exhibit an age-related decline in steroid production that is linked to degeneration of gonadal function, and both show a corresponding increase in gonadotropin levels. There are also intriguing data to suggest an independent alteration with aging in the hypothalamic–pituitary–gonadal axis, which some have suggested amounts to a "resetting" of the hypothalamic pulse generator (Tenover et al., 1988; Vermeulen et al., 1989; Kaufman et al., 1990). Finally, if the selectivity/ heterogeneity hypothesis proves to be correct, the acceleration in the risk of fetal loss with age in the two sexes would be extremely similar. In view of these similarities we suggest that, if only the effects of follicular depletion in females could be removed, reproductive function would decline with age at roughly similar rates in males and females. We also admit that this suggestion is likely to be untestable.

---

[13]Ellison (1992) has independently arrived at a similar hypothesis.

## MORTALITY AND FERTILITY VIEWED JOINTLY

The view of mortality and fertility outlined in the previous sections makes it possible to examine causal associations between the two. The progressive loss of reproductive capacity at later adult ages coincides with an accelerating increase in the risk of death. There are at least two possible explanations for this relationship: (1) all forms of aging reflect a single underlying clock (the GR view); and (2) a finite number of parallel senescent changes (germinal and somatic mutations, loss of receptors, sclerotic degeneration, etc.) occur at the cellular level in tissues affecting fecundity and in tissues affecting risks of morbidity and mortality, but no single aging process captures all these changes simultaneously (the EP view).

Based on current evidence, the second of these explanations appears more likely. As detailed above, reproductive senescence can be attributed to a fairly small number of independent processes, involving such things as declining steroidogenesis, an increasing cumulative incidence of genetic damage affecting the risk of fetal loss, sclerotic changes in the uterine blood supply and increasing amounts of collagen in the lining of the uterus, progressive depletion of ovarian follicles, and reduced responsiveness of the pituitary and hypothalamus to gonadal steroids. The point we wish to stress here is that many of these processes are exactly analogous to senescent changes occurring in other tissues that affect the risk of morbidity, loss of functionality, and mortality. For example, chromosomal rearrangements and somatic mutations, which are of central importance in the etiology of cancers, are similar in nature to changes occurring in germ cell lines and predisposing to fetal loss. Similarly, sclerotic changes affect all vascularized tissues and are important in the etiology of coronary heart disease and stroke. Depletion of ovarian follicles has its analogs in the aging of the brain and eye, since in all these cases certain cells (primordial oocytes, neurons, retinoblasts) cease proliferating early in development and then undergo continuous attrition through cell death.[14] And loss of hypothalamic–pituitary responsiveness to steroids involves changes, such as loss of receptors on the target cell surface, that also occur in chronic endocrine diseases such as certain forms of adult-onset non-insulin-dependent diabetes.

In sum, the fundamental mechanisms of reproductive aging are similar at the cell and tissue level to other aging processes occurring simultaneously in other tissues and reflected in increasing risks of disease, disability, and death. Thus, while there appears to be no single unitary aging process, there may be a delimitable number of independent processes, at least some of which may simultaneously affect both fecundity and viability. This hypothesis helps make sense of the recent finding that early menopause may be associated with shortened subsequent life span (Snowdon *et al.*, 1989). It would also allow for some degree of coordination in senescent processes while still being consistent with the EP view of aging. Indeed, we suggest that the EP view may allow a

---

[14]One possible difference here is that the rate of atresia is likely to be programmed, whereas the loss of other kinds of cells is probably stochastic.

more precise specification of the linkages between reproductive aging and the determinants of life span, and thus point to other ways in which the linkages can be estimated from empirical data. We further suggest that those linkages deserve to be a major focus of future research.

## Overview

As should now be clear, the EP and GR models imply very different views about the senescent phenotypes exposed to natural selection. Since the GR model assumes a single, unitary aging process, all phenotypic expressions of aging must be selected simultaneously. Under the EP model, in contrast, different manifestations of aging can, at least potentially, be decoupled to a large extent. We suggest, therefore, that the pattern of temporal coordination among different aspects of the aging process may provide the basis for distinguishing and testing these two very different views of aging. We also suggest that the studies reviewed in this paper are fairly consistent in showing that such coordination is loose and that at least some aspects of aging differ markedly in their timing from others. These findings are consistent with the EP model and inconsistent with the GR model. On this basis, the EP view appears to be more realistic.

This conclusion is comforting because it means that we actually know a great deal about the processes that determine the human life span. One of the more curious elements of the GR view is the idea that the maximal life span is set by a special developmental switch mechanism and, consequently, that known causes of morbidity and mortality induce "premature" death having nothing to do with the MLP. If such a switch exists, we know nothing whatsoever about it and therefore know nothing about the ultimate determinant of the life span. If there is no switch, we actually know quite a lot about aging.

Established evolutionary theory also supports the EP view—so much so, in fact, that the EP view could with equal appropriateness be called the EV ("evolutionary") view. Natural selection is not expected to favor tight coordination of senescent processes, nor is it expected to act on maximal life span as a unitary phenotype. Indeed, according to the standard evolutionary model, senescence occurs precisely because natural selection is blind (or at least near-sighted) to phenotypes expressed at later ages. From this perspective, maximal life span is very unlikely to be determined by a genetic switch mechanism since such a switch could by its nature have little if any fitness advantage. We age and die because the fitness benefits of maintaining a complex body against myriad insults diminish with age and finally approach zero. The intuitive view of aging—that "things fall apart"—is the correct one.

## ACKNOWLEDGMENTS

We thank Benjamin Campbell and Timothy Gage for sharing unpublished data with us. We also thank Steven Austad, Douglas Crews, Henry Harpending,

Darryl Holman, James Vaupel, Maxine Weinstein, and two anonymous reviewers for comments and suggestions. Partial support for this research was provided by NIA Training Grant 5 T32-AG00208-02 and by the Population Research Institute, Pennsylvania State University, which has core support from the NICHD (Grant 1-HD28263-01).

## REFERENCES

Abbot, M. H., Abbey, H., Bolling, D. R. and Murphy, E. A. (1978) The familial component in longevity: a study of offspring of nonagenarians: intrafamilial studies. *American Journal of Medical Genetics* **2**, 105–120.

Abrams, P. A. (1991) *Does Increased Mortality Favor the Evolution of More Rapid Senescence?* Research Report 91-05-4. Center for Population Analysis and Policy, Humphrey Institute, University of Minnesota, Minneapolis.

Abugov, R. (1986) Genetics of Darwinian fitness. III. A generalized approach to age structured selection and life history. *Journal of Theoretical Biology* **122**, 311–323.

Albin, R. L. (1988) The pleiotropic gene theory of senescence: supportive evidence from human genetic disease. *Ethologyl and Sociobiology* **9**, 371–382.

Antonarakis, S. E. and the Down Syndrome Collaborative Group (1991) Parental origin of the extra chromosome in trisomy 21 as indicated by analysis of DNA polymorphisms. *New England Journal of Medicine* **324**, 872–876.

Arking, R. (1991) *Biology of Aging: Observations and Principles*. Englewood Cliffs, NJ: Prentice Hall.

Austad, S. (1993) Retarded senescence in an insular population of Virginia opossums (*Didelphis virginiana*). *Journal of Zoology* **229**, 695–708.

Baird, D. T. (1987) A model for follicular selection and ovulation: lessons from superovulation. *Journal of Steroid Biochemistry* **27**, 15–23.

Baird, D. T. (1991) The ovarian cycle. In *Ovarian Endocrinology* (ed. Hillier, S. G.). Oxford: Blackwell Scientific, pp. 1–24.

Baker, H. W. G., Burger, H. G., De Kretser, D. M., Hudson, B., O'Conner, S., Wang, C., Mirovics, A., Court, J., Dunlop, M. and Rennie, G. C. (1976) Changes in the pituitary–testicular system with age. *Clinical Endocrinology* **5**, 349–372.

Baker, T. G. (1963) A quantitative and cytological study of germ cells in human ovaries. *Proceedings of the Royal Society of London*, Series B. **158**, 417–433.

Bell, G. (1984a) Evolutionary and nonevolutionary theories of senescence. *American Naturalist* **124**, 600–603.

Bell, G. (1984b) Measuring the cost of reproduction. I. The correlation structure of the life table of plankton rotifer. *Evolution* **38**, 300–313.

Bell, G. (1984c) Measuring the cost of reproduction. II. The correlation structure of the life tables of five freshwater invertebrates. *Evolution* **38**, 314–326.

Bell, G. (1988) *Sex and Death in Protozoa: The History of an Obsession*. Cambridge: Cambridge University Press.

Bendel, J. and Hua, C. (1978) An estimate of the natural fecundity ratio curve. *Social Biology* **25**, 210–227.

Bierbaum, T. J., Mueller, L. D. and Ayala, F. J. (1989) Density-dependent selection of life-history traits in *Drosophila melanogaster*. *Evolution* **43**, 382–392.

Block, E. (1952) Quantitative morphological investigations of the follicular system in women: variations at different ages. *Acta Anatomica 1* **4**, 108–123.

Block, E. (1953) A quantitative morphological investigation of the follicular system in newborn infants. *Acta Anatomica* **17**, 201–206.

Bongaarts, J. and Potter, R. G. (1983) *Fertility, Biology, and Behavior: An Analysis of the Proximate Determinants.* New York: Academic Press.

Bremner, W. J., Vitiello, M. and Prinz, P. N. (1983) The loss of circadian rhythmicity in blood testosterone with aging in normal men. *Journal of Clinical Endocrinology and Metabolism* **56**, 1278–1281.

Bremner, W. J., Matsumoto, A. M., Steiner, R. A., Clifton, D. K. and Dorsa, D. M. (1986) Neuroendocrine correlates of aging in the male. In: *Aging, Reproduction, and the Climacteric* (eds Mastroianni, L. and Paulsen, C. A.). New York: Plenum Press, pp. 47–57.

Brown, W. T. (1987) Genetics of human aging. *Reviews of Biological Research in Aging* **3**, 77–91.

Bulmer, M. G. (1980) *The Mathematical Theory of Quantitative Genetics.* Oxford: Clarendon Press.

Calder, W. A. (1984) *Size, Function, and Life History.* Cambridge, MA: Harvard University Press.

Casterline, J. B. (1989) Maternal age, gravidity, and pregnancy spacing effects on spontaneous fetal mortality. *Social Biology* **36**, 186–212.

Charlesworth, B. (1974) Selection in populations with overlapping generations. VI. Rates of change of gene frequency and population growth rate. *Theoreticall Population Biology* **6**, 108–133.

Charlesworth, B. (1976) Natural selection in age-structured populations. In: *Lectures on Mathematics in the Life Sciences* (ed. Levin, S. A.). Providence, RI: American Mathematical Society, pp. 69–87.

Charlesworth, B. (1980) *Evolution in Age-Structure Populations.* Cambridge: Cambridge University Press.

Chiazze, L., Brayer, F. T., Macisco, J. J., Parker, M. P. and Duffy, B. J. (1968) The length and variability of the human menstrual cycle. *Journal of the American Medical Association* **203**, 377–380.

Clark, A. G. (1987) Senescence and the genetic-correlation hang-up. *American Naturalist* **129**, 932–940.

Clutton-Brock, T. H., Guinness, E. F. and Albon, S. D. (1982) *Red Deer: Behavior and Ecology of Two Sexes.* Chicago: University of Chicago Press.

Comfort, A. (1980) Sexuality in later life. In: *Handbook of Mental Health and Aging* (eds Birren, J. E. and Sloane, R. B.). Englewood Cliffs, NJ: Prentice Hall, pp. 885–892.

Davidson, J. M., Chen, J. J., Crapo, L., Gray, G. D., Greenleaf, W. J. and Catania, J. A. (1983) Hormonal changes and sexual function in aging men. *Journal of Clinical Endocrinology and Metabolism* **57**, 71–77.

Dawkins, R. (1976) *The Selfish Gene.* New York: Oxford University Press.

Deslypere, J. P. and Vermeulen, A. (1984) Leydig cell function in normal men: effect of age, life-style, residence, diet and activity. *Journal of Clinical Endocrinology and Metabolism* **59**, 955–962.

Döring, G. K. (1969) The incidence of anovular cycles in women. *Journal of Reproduction and Fertility* (Suppl) **6**, 77–81.

Doty, R. L., Shaman, P., Applebaum, S. C., Gierson, R., Sikosorski, L. and Rosenberg, L. (1984) Smell identification: changes with age. *Science* **226**, 1441–1443.

Doyle, R. W. and Hunte, W. (1981) Demography of an estuarine amphipod (*Gammarus lawrencianus*) experimentally selected for high "*r*": A model of the genetic effects of environmental change. *Canadian Journal of Fish and Aquatic Science* **38**, 1120–1127.

Edney, E. B. and Gill, R. W. (1968) Evolution of senescence and specific longevity. *Nature* **220**, 281–282.

Edwards, R. G., Fishel, S. B., Cohen, J., Fehilly, C. B., Purdy, J. M., Slater, J. M., Steptoe, P. C. and Webster, J. M. (1984) Factors influencing the success of in vitro fertilization for alleviating human infertility. *Journal of In Vitro Fertilization Embryo Transfer* **1**, 3.

Elandt-Johnson, R. C. and Johnson, N. L. (1980) *Survival Models and Data Analysis*. New York: Wiley.

Ellison, P. T. (1992) *The Ecology of the Ovary*. Cambridge, MA: Harvard University Press.

Faddy, M. J., Gosdon, R. G. and Edwards, R. G. (1983) Ovarian follicle dynamics in mice: a comparative study of three inbred strains and an $F_1$ hybrid. *Journal of Endocrinology* **96**, 23–33.

Falconer, D. S. (1989) *Introduction to Quantitative Genetics*, 3rd edn. London: Longman.

Finch, C. E. (1990) *Longevity, Senescence, and the Genome*. Chicago: University of Chicago Press.

Finch, C. E., Pike, M. C. and Witten, M. (1990) Slow mortality rate accelerations during aging in some animals approximate that of humans. *Science* **249**, 902–905.

Fisher, R. A. (1930) *The Genetical Theory of Natural Selection*. Oxford: Clarendon Press.

Fox, C. A., Ismail, A. A. A., Love, D. N., Krikham, K. E. and Loraine, J. A. (1972) Studies on the relationship between plasma testosterone levels and human sexual activity. *Journal of Endocrinology* **52**, 51–58.

Friedman, D. B. and Johnson, T. E. (1988) A mutation in the age-1 gene in *Caenorhabditis elegans* lengthens life and reduces hermaphrodite fertility. *Genetics* **118**, 75–86.

Fries, J. F. (1980) Aging, natural death, and the compression of morbidity. *New England Journal of Medicine* **303**, 130–135.

Fries, J. F. (1987) Reduction of the national morbidity. *Gerontology Perspectives* **1**, 54–64.

Gage, T. B. (1989) Bio-mathematical approaches to the study of human variation in mortality. *Yearbook of Physical Anthropology* **32**, 185–214.

Gage, T. B. (1990) Variation and classification of human age patterns of mortality: analysis using competing hazards models. *Human Biology* **62**, 589–617.

Gage, T. B. (1991) Causes of death and the components of mortality: testing the biological interpretations of a competing hazards model. *American Journal of Human Biology* **3**, 289–300.

Gage, T. B. and Dyke, B. (1986) Parameterizing abridged mortality tables: the Siler three-component hazard model. *Human Biology* **58**, 275–291.

Giesel, J. T. (1979) Genetic co-variation of survivorship and other fitness indices in *Drosophila melanogaster*. *Experimental Gerontology* **14**, 323–328.

Giesel, J. T. and Zettler, E. E. (1980) Genetic correlations of life historical parameters and certain fitness indices in *Drosophila melanogaster*. $r_m$, $r$, diet breadth. *Oecologia* **47**, 299–302.

Giesel, J. T., Murphy, P. A. and Manlove, M. N. (1982) The influence of temperature on genetic interrelationships of life history traits in a population of *Drosophila melanogaster*: what tangled data sets we weave. *American Naturalist* **119**, 464–479.

Gladen, B. C. (1986) On the role of "habitual aborters" in the analysis of spontaneous abortion. *Statistics in Medicine* 5, 557–564.

Gosden, R. G. (1985) Maternal age: a major factor affecting the prospecting and outcome of pregnancy. *Annals of the New York Academy of Sciences* 442, 45–57.

Gostwamy, R. K., Williams, G. and Steptoe, P. C. (1988) Decreased uterine perfusion: a cause of infertility. *Human Reproduction* 3, 955–959.

Gowen, J. W. and Johnson, L. E. (1946) On the mechanism of heterosis. I. Metabolic capacity of different races of *Drosophila melanogaster* for egg production. *American Naturalist* 80, 149–179.

Haldane, J. B. S. (1941) *New Paths in Genetics*. London: Allen and Unwin.

Hamilton, J. B. (1948) The role of testicular secretions as indicated by the effects of castration in man and by studies of pathological conditions and the short lifespan associated with maleness. *Recent Progress in Hormone Research* 3, 257–322.

Hamilton, J. B. and Mestler, G. E. (1969) Mortality and survival: comparison of eunuchs with intact men and women in mentally retarded populations. *Journal of Gerontology* 24, 395–411.

Hamilton, W. D. (1966) The moulding of senescence by natural selection. *Journal of Theoretical Biology* 12, 12–45.

Harbitz, T. B. (1973) Morphometric studies of the Leydig cells in elderly men with special reference to the histology of the prostate. *Acta Pathologica Microbiologica Scandinavica* 81A, 301–313.

Harlap, S., Shiono, P. H. and Ramcharan, S. (1980) A life table of spontaneous abortions and the effects of age, parity, and other variables. In *Human Embryonic and Fetal Death* (eds Porter, I. H. and Hook, E. B.). New York: Academic Press, pp. 145–158.

Harman, S. M. (1978) Clinical aspects of aging in the male reproductive system. In: *The Aging Reproductive System* (ed. Schneider, E. L.). New York: Raven Press, pp. 29–58.

Harman, S. M. and Tsitouras, P. D. (1980) Reproductive hormones in aging men. I. Measurement of sex steroids, basal luteinizing hormone and Leydig cell response to human chorionic gonadotropin. *Journal of Clinical Endocrinology and Metabolism* 51, 35–40.

Harman, S. M., Tsitouras, P. D., Costa, P. T. and Blackman, M. R. (1982) Reproductive hormones in aging men. II. Basal pituitary gonadotropins and gonadotropin responses to luteinizing hormone-releasing hormone. *Journal of Clinical Endocrinology and Metabolism* 54, 547–551.

Hill, K. and Hurtado, M. (1991) The evolution of premature reproductive senescence and menopause in human females: an evaluation of the "grandmother hypothesis". *Human Nature* 2, 313–350.

Hiraizumi, Y. (1985) Genetics of factors affecting the life history of *Drosophila melanogaster*. I. Female productivity. *Genetics* 110, 453–464.

Hook, E. B. (1986) Paternal age and effects on chromosomal and specific locus mutations and on other genetic outcomes in offspring. In: *Aging, Reproduction, and the Climacteric* (eds Mastroianni, L. and Paulsen, C. A.). New York: Plenum Press, pp. 117–145.

Hughes, D. M. and Clark, A. G. (1988) Analysis of the genetic structure of life history of *Drosophila melanogaster* using recombinant extracted lines. *Evolution* 42, 1309–1320.

Hutchinson, E. W. and Rose, M. R. (1990) Quantitative genetic analysis of postponed aging in *Drosophila melanogaster*. In: *Genetic Effects on Aging II* (ed. Harrison, D. E.). Caldwell, MA: Telford Press, pp. 66–87.

Jaffe, R. B. (1991) The menopause and perimenopausal period. In: *Reproductive Endocrinology: Physiology, Pathophysiology and Clinical Management* (eds Yen, S. S. C. and Jaffe, R. B.). Philadelphia: Saunders, pp. 389–408.

James, W. H. (1979) The causes of the decline in fecundability with age. *Social Biology* **26**, 330–334.

Kaler, L. W. and Neaves, W. B. (1978) Attrition of the human Leydig cell population with advancing age. *Anatomical Record* **192**, 513–518.

Kaufman, J. M., Deslypere, J. P., Giri, M. and Vermeulen, A. (1990) Neuroendocrine regulation of pulsatile luteinizing hormone secretion in elderly men. *Journal of Steroid Biochemistry and Molecular Biology* **37**, 421–430.

Kline, J. and Stein, Z. (1987) Epidemiology of chromosomal anomalies in spontaneous abortion: prevalence, manifestation and determinants. In: *Spontaneous and Recurrent Abortion* (eds Bennett, M. J. and Edmonds, D. K. Oxford). Blackwell Scientific, pp. 29–50.

Kosuda, K. (1985) The aging effect on male and female Fischer 344 rats. *Mechanisms Ageing and Development* **48**, 191–198.

Kothari, K. L. and Gupta, A. S. (1974) Effect of ageing on the volume, structure and total Leydig cell content of the human testis. *International Journal of Fertility* **19**, 140–146.

Kraemer, H. C., Becker, H. B., Brode, H. K. H., Doering, C. H., Moos, R. H. and Hamburg, D. A. (1976) Orgasmic frequency and testosterone levels in normal human males. *Archives of Sexual Behaviour* **5**, 125–132.

Law, R. (1979) The cost of reproduction in annual meadow grass. *American Naturalist* **113**, 3–16.

Law, R., Bradshaw, A. D. and Putwain, P. D. (1977) Life-history variation in *Poa annua*. *Evolution* **31**, 233–246.

Lenton, E. A., Landgren, B.-M. and Sexton, L. (1984a) Normal variation in the length of the luteal phase of the menstrual cycle: identification of the short luteal phase. *British Journal of Obstetrics and Gynaecology* **91**, 685–689.

Lenton, E. A., Landgren, B.-M., Sexton, L. and Harper, R. (1984b) Normal variation in the length of the follicular phase of the menstrual cycle: effect of chronological age. *British Journal of Obstetrics and Gynaecology* **91**, 681–684.

Leridon, H. (1976) Facts and artifacts in the study of intrauterine mortality: a reconsideration from pregnancy histories. *Population Studies* **30**, 319–335.

Lipson, S. F. and Ellison, P. T. (1992) Normative study of age variation in salivary progesterone profiles. *Journal of Biosocial Sciences* **24**, 233–244.

Lynch, M. (1984) The limits of life history evolution in *Daphnia*. *Evolution* **38**, 465–482.

Madigan, F. C. (1957) Are sex mortality differentials biologically caused? *Milbank Memorial Fund Quarterly* **35**, 202–223.

Manton, K. C. and Stallard, E. (1984) *Recent Trends in Mortality Analysis*. Orlando, FL: Academic Press.

Manton, K. C. and Tolley, H. D. (1991) Rectangularization of the survival curve: implications of an ill-posed question. *Journal of Aging and Health* **3**, 172–193.

Marrama, P., Carani, C., Baraghini, G. F., Volpe, A., Zini, D., Celani, M. F. and Montanini, V. (1982) Circadian rhythm of testosterone and prolactin in the aging man. *Maturitas* **4**, 131–138.

Martin, C. E. (1977) Sexual activity in the aging male. In: *Handbook of Sexology* (eds Money, J. and Musaph, H.). Amsterdam: ASP Biomedical Press, pp. 813–824.

Mauskopf, J. and Wallace, T. D. (1984) Fertility and replacement: some alternative stochastic models and results for Brazil. *Demography* **21**, 519–536.

Maynard Smith, J. (1958) The effects of temperature and of egg-laying on the longevity of *Drosophila subobscura*. *Journal of Experimental Biology* **35**, 832–842.

Medawar, P. B. (1952) *An Unsolved Problem of Biology*. London: H. K. Lewis.

Meldrum, D. R., Tataryn, I. V., Frumar, A. M., Erlik, Y., Lu, K. H. and Judd, H. L. (1980) Gonadotropins, estrogens and adrenal steroids during the menopausal hot flush. *Journal of Clinical Endocrinology and Metabolism* **50**, 685–689.

Mertz, D. B. (1975) Senescent decline in flour beetle strains selected for early adult fitness. *Physiological Zoology* **48**, 1–23.

Metcalf, M. G., Donald, R. A. and Livesey, J. H. (1982) Pituitary–ovarian function before, during and after the menopausal transition: a longitudinal study. *Clinical Endocrinology* **17**, 489–494.

Meyer, J. M., Eaves, L. J., Heath, A. C. and Martin, N. G. (1991) Estimating genetic influences on the age-at-menarche: a survival analysis approach. *American Journal of Medical Genetics* **39**, 148–154.

Montanini, V., Simoni, M., Chiossi, G., Baraghini, G. F., Velardo, A., Baraldi, E. and Marrama, P. (1988) Age-related changes in plasma dehydroepiandrosterone sulphate, cortisol, testosterone and free testosterone circadian rhythms in adult men. *Hormone Research* **29**, 1–6.

Moolgavkar, S. H. (1993) Stochastic models of carcinogenesis. In: *Handbook of Statistics*, Vol. 8 (eds Rao, C. R. and Chakraborty, R.). New York: Elsevier/ North-Holland (in press).

Mousseau, T. A. and Roff, D. A. (1987) Natural selection and the heritability of fitness components. *Heredity* **59**, 181–197.

Mueller, L. D. (1987) Evolution of accelerated senescence in laboratory populations of *Drosophila*. *Proceedings of the National Academy of Sciences, USA* **84**, 1974– 1977.

Murphy, E. A. (1978) Genetics of longevity in man. In: *The Genetics of Aging* (ed. Schneider, E. L.). New York: Plenum Press, pp. 261–301.

Naeye, R. L. (1983) Maternal age, obstetric complications, and the outcome of pregnancy. *Obstetrics and Gynecology* **61**, 210–216.

Nahoul, K. and Roger, M. (1990) Age-related decline of plasma bioavailable testosterone in adult men. *Journal of Steroid Biochemistry* **35**, 293–299.

Navot, D., Bergh, P. A., Williams, M. A., Garrisi, G. J., Guzman, I., Sandler, B. and Grunfeld, L. (1991) Poor oocyte quality rather than implantation failure as a cause of age-related decline in female fertility. *Lancet* **337**, 1375–1377.

Naylor, A. F. (1974) Sequential aspects of spontaneous abortion: maternal age, parity, and pregnancy compensation artifact. *Social Biology* **21**, 195–204.

Neaves, W. B., Johnson, L., Porter, J. C., Parker, C. R. and Petty, C. S. (1984) Leydig cell numbers, daily sperm production, and serum gonadotropin levels in aging men. *Journal of Clinical Endocrinology and Metabolism* **59**, 756–763.

Nicosia, S. V. (1986) Ovarian changes during the climacteric. In: *Aging, Reproduction, and the Climacteric* (eds Mastroianni, L. and Paulsen, C. A.). New York: Plenum Press, pp. 179–199.

Nicosia, S. V. (1987) The aging ovary. *Medical Clinics of North America* **71**, 1–9.

Nieschlag, E. and Michel, E. (1986) Reproductive functions in grandfathers. In: *Aging, Reproduction, and the Climacteric* (eds Mastroianni, L. and Paulsen, C. A.). New York: Plenum Press, pp. 59–71.

Nieschlag, E., Lommers, V., Freischem, C. W., Langer, K. and Wickings, E. J. (1982) Reproductive function in young fathers and grandfathers. *Journal of Clinical Endocrinology and Metabolism* **55**, 676–681.

Nordling, C. O. (1953) A new theory on the cancer inducing mechanism. *British Journal of Cancer* **7**, 68–72.

Olshansky, S. J., Carnes, B. A. and Cassel, C. (1990) In search of Methuselah: estimating the upper limits to human longevity. *Science* **250**, 634–640.

Palloni, A. and Tienda, M. (1986) The effects breastfeeding and pace of childbearing on mortality at early ages. *Demography* **23**, 31–52.

Peters, R. H. (1983) *The Ecological Implications of Body Size*. Cambridge: Cambridge University Press.

Pirke, K. M. and Doerr, P. (1973) Age related changes and interrelationships between plasma testosterone, oestradiol, and testosterone-binding globulin in normal adult males. *Acta Endocrinologica* **74**, 792–800.

Pirke, K. M., Sintermann, R. and Vogt, H. J. (1980) Testosterone and testosterone precursors in the spermatic vein and in the testicular tissues of old men. *Gerontology* **26**, 221.

Potter, R. G., Wyon, J. B., New, M. and Gordon, J. E. (1965) Fetal wastage in eleven Punjab villages. *Human Biology* **37**, 262–273.

Promislow, D. E. L. (1992) Senescence in natural populations of mammals: a comparative study. *Evolution* (in press).

Public Health Service (1991) *Vital Statistics of the United States*, 1988, Vol. III, Part A. PHS publication no. 91-1101. Hyattsville, MD: Public Health Service, US Department of Health and Human Services.

Purifoy, F. E., Koopmans, L. H. and Mayes, D. M. (1981) Age differences in serum androgen levels in adult males. *Human Biology* **53**, 499–511.

Reiss, M. J. (1989) *The Allometry of Growth and Reproduction*. Cambridge: Cambridge University Press.

Resseguie, L. J. (1974) Pregnancy wastage and age of mother among the Amish. *Human Biology* **46**, 633–639.

Reznick, D. N. (1985) Costs of reproduction: An evaluation of the empirical evidence. *Oikos* **44**, 257–267.

Reznick, D. N., Perry, E. and Travis, J. (1986) Measuring the cost of reproduction: A comment on papers by Bell. *Evolution* **40**, 1338–1344.

Richardson, S. J., Senikas, V. and Nelson, J. F. (1987) Follicular depletion during the menopausal transition: evidence for accelerated loss and ultimate exhaustion. *Journal of Clinical Endocrinology and Metabolism* **65**, 1231–1237.

Rodenheffer, R. J., Gerstenblith, G., Becker, L. C., Fleg, J. L., Weisfeldt, M. L. and Lakatta, E. G. (1984) Exercise cardiac output is maintained with advancing age in healthy human subjects: cardiac dilation and increased stroke volume compensate for a diminished heart rate. *Circulation* **69**, 203–213.

Romeu, A., Muasher, S. J. and Acosta, A. A. (1987) Results of in vitro fertilization attempts in women 40 years of age and older: the Norfolk experience. *Fertility and Sterility* **47**, 130–136.

Rose, M. R. (1984) Genetic covariation in *Drosophila* life history: untangling the data. *American Naturalist* **123**, 565–569.

Rose, M. R. (1991) Evolutionary Biology of Aging. New York: Oxford University Press.

Rose, M. R. and Charlesworth, B. (1980) A test of evolutionary theories of senescence. *Nature* **287**, 141–142.

Rose, M. R. and Charlesworth, B. (1981a) Genetics of life history in *Drosophila melanogaster*. I. Sib analysis of adult females. *Genetics* **97**, 173–186.

Rose, M. R. and Charlesworth, B. (1981b) Genetics of life history in *Drosophila melanogaster*. II. Exploratory selection experiments. *Genetics* **97**, 187–196.

Rose, M. R. and Service, P. M. (1985) Evolution of aging. *Reviews of Biological Research in Aging* **2**, 85–98.

Royer, G. L., Seckman, C. E., Schwartz, J. H., Bennett, K. P. and Hendrix, J. W. (1984) Relationship between age and levels of total, free, and bound testosterone in healthy subjects. *Current Therapy Research* **35**, 345–353.

Rubens, R., Dhont, M. and Vermeulen, A. (1974) Further studies on Leydig cell function in old age. *Journal of Clinical Endocrinology and Metabolism* **39**, 40–45.

Santow, G. and Bracher, M. (1989) Do gravidity and age affect pregnancy outcome. *Social Biology* **36**, 9–22.

Sauer, M. V., Paulson, R. J. and Lobo, R. A. (1990) A preliminary report on oocyte donation extending reproductive potential to women over 40. *New England Journal of Medicine* **323**, 1157–1160.

Scheiner, S. M., Caplan, R. L. and Lyman, R. F. (1989) A search for trade-offs among life history traits in *Drosophila melanogaster*. *Evolution and Ecology* **3**, 51–63.

Schwartz, D. and Mayaux, M. J. (1982) Female fecundity as a function of age. *New England Journal of Medicine* **306**, 404–406.

Selvin, S. and Garfinkel, J. (1976) Paternal age, maternal age and birth order and the risk of a fetal loss. *Human Biology* **48**, 223–230.

Service, P. M. and Rose, M. R. (1985) Genetic covariation among life-history components: the effect of novel environments. *Evolution* **39**, 943–945.

Service, P. M., Hutchinson, E. W. and Rose, M. R. (1988) Multiple genetic mechanisms for the evolution of senescence in *Drosophila melanogaster*. *Evolution* **42**, 708–716.

Seymour, F. I., Duffy, C. and Koernev, A. (1935) A case of authenticated fertility in a man of 94. *Journal of the American Medical Association* **105**, 1423–1424.

Shapiro, S., Levine, H. S. and Abramowicz, M. (1970) Factors associated with early and late fetal loss. *Advances in Planned Parenthood* **6**, 45–63.

Sherman, B. M. and Korenman, S. G. (1976) Hormonal characteristics of the human menstrual cycle throughout reproductive life. *Journal of Clinical Investigation* **55**, 699–706.

Sherman, B. M., West, J. H. and Korenman, S. C. (1976) The menopausal transition: analysis of LH, FSH, estradiol, and progesterone concentrations during menstrual cycles of older women. *Journal of Clinical Endocrinology and Metabolism* **42**, 629–636.

Shock, N. W. (1972) Energy metabolism intake and physical activity of the aging. In: *Nutrition in Old Age* (ed. Carlson, L. A.). Uppsala: Almquist and Wiksell.

Sing, C. F. and Boerwinkle, E. (1987) Genetic architecture of inter-individual variability in apolipoprotein, lipoprotein and lipid phenotypes. In: *Molecular Approaches to Human Polygenic Disease* (ed. Bock, G. and Collins, G. M.). CIBA Foundation Symposium 130. New York: Wiley, pp. 99–121.

Sniffen, R. C. (1950) The testis. I. The normal testis. *Archives of Pathology* **50**, 259–284.

Snowdon, D. A., Kane, R. L., Beeson, W. L., Burke, G. L., Sprafka, J. M., Potter, J., Iso, H., Jacobs, D. R. and Phillips, R. L. (1989) Is early natural menopause a biologic marker of health and aging? *American Journal of Public Health* **79**, 709–714.

Snyder, P. J., Reitano, J. F. and Utiger, R. D. (1975) Serum LH and FSH responses to synthetic gonadotropin-releasing hormone in normal men. *Journal of Clinical Endocrinology and Metabolism* **41**, 938–945.

Sokal, R. R. (1970) Senescence and genetic load: evidence from *Tribolium*. *Science* **167**, 1733–1734.

Sokal, Z. (1964) Morphology of the human testis in various periods of life. *Folia Morphologica* **23**, 102–111.

Sørensen, T. I. A., Nielsen, G. G., Andersen, P. K. and Teasdale, T. W. (1988) Genetic and environmental influences on premature death in adult adoptees. *New England Journal of Medicine* **12**, 727–732.

Sparrow, D., Basse, R. and Rowe, J. W. (1980) The influence of age, alcohol consumption and body build on gonadal function in man. *Journal of Clinical Endocrinology and Metabolism* **51**, 508–512.

Stevenson, A. C., Warnock, H. A., Dudgeon, M. Y. and McClure, J. H. (1958) Observations on the results of pregnancies in women resident in Belfast. *Annals of Human Genetics* **23**, 382–420.

Takahashi, J., Higashi, Y., LaNasa, A., Yoshida, K. I., Winters, S. J., Oshima, H. and Troen, P. (1983) Studies of the human testis. XVIII. Simultaneous measurement of nine intratesticular steroids: evidence for reduced mitochondrial function in testes of elderly men. *Journal of Clinical Endocrinology and Metabolism* **56**, 1178–1187.

Tataryn, I. V., Meldrum, D. R., Lu, K. H., Frumar, A. M. and Judd, H. L. (1979) LH, FSH, and skin temperature during the menopausal hot flash. *Journal of Clinical Endocrinology and Metabolism* **49**, 152–154.

Tenover, J. S., Matsumoto, A. M., Clifton, D. K. and Bremner, W. J. (1988) Age-related alterations in the circadian rhythms of pulsatile luteinizing hormone and testosterone secretion in healthy men. *Journal of Gerontology* **43**, M163–M169.

Tinkle, D. W. and Hadley, N. F. (1975) Lizard reproductive effort: caloric estimates and comments on its evolution. *Ecology* **56**, 427–434.

Tobin, J. D. (1981) Physiological indices of aging. In: *Aging: A Challenge to Science and Society*, Vol. 1. *Biology* (eds Danon, D., Shock, N. W. and Marois, M.). New York: Oxford University Press.

Treloar, A. R., Boynton, R. E., Behn, B. G. and Brown, B. W. (1967) Variation of the human menstrual cycle through reproductive life. *International Journal of Fertility* **12**, 77–126.

Treloar, S. A. and Martin, N. G. (1990) Age at menarche as a fitness trait: nonadditive genetic variance detected in a large twin sample. *American Journal of Human Genetics* **47**, 137–148.

Tsitouras, P. D., Martin, C. E. and Harman, S. M. (1982) Relationship of serum testosterone to sexual activity in healthy elderly men. *Journal of Gerontology* **37**, 288–293.

United Nations (1991) *Demographic Yearbook 1989*. New York: United Nations.

Urban, R. J., Veldhius, J. D., Blizzard, R. M. and Dufau, M. L. (1988) Attenuated release of biologically active luteinizing hormone in healthy aging men. *Journal of Clinical Investigation* **81**, 1020–1029.

van Dijk, T. (1979) On the relationship between reproduction, age, and survival in two carabid beetles: *Calathus melanocephalus* L. and *Pterostichus coerulescens* L. (Coleoptera, Carabidae). *Ecologia* **40**, 63–80.

van Look, P. F. A., Lothian, H., Hunter, W. M., Michie, E. A. and Baird, D. T. (1977) Hypothalamic–pituitary–ovarian function in perimenopausal women. *Clinical Endocrinology* **7**, 13–31.

van Noord-Zaadstra, B. M., Looman, C. W. N., Alsbach, H., Habbema, J. D. F., te Velde, E. R. and Karbaat, J. (1991) Delayed childbearing: effect of age on fecundity and outcome of pregnancy. *British Medical Journal* **302**, 1361–1365.

Vaupel, J. W. (1988) Inherited frailty and longevity. *Demography* **25**, 277–287.

Vermeulen, A., Rubens, R. and Verdonck, L. (1972) Testosterone secretion and metabolism in male senescence. *Journal of Clinical Endocrinology and Metabolism* **34**, 730–735.

Vermeulen, A., Deslypere, A. and de Meirleir, K. (1989) A new look to the andropause: altered function of the gonadotrophs. *Journal of Steroid Biochemistry* **32**, 163–165.

Verwoerdt, A., Pfeiffer, E. and Wang, H. S. (1969) Sexual behavior in senescence. II. Patterns of sexual activity and interest. *Geriatrics* **24**, 137–154.

Virro, M. R. and Shewchuk, A. B. (1984) Pregnancy outcome in 242 conceptions after artifical insemination with donor sperm and effects of maternal age on the prognosis for successful pregnancy. *American Journal of Obstetrics and Gynecology* **148**, 518–524.

vom Saal, F. S. and Finch, C. E. (1988) Reproductive senescence: phenomena and mechanisms in mammals and selected vertebrates. In: *The Physiology of Reproduction*. Vol. 2 (eds Knobil, E., Neill, J. D., Ewing, L. L., Greenwald, G. S., Markert, C. L. and Pfaff, C. L.). New York: Raven Press, pp. 2351–2413.

Wallinga, J. H. and Bakkar, H. (1978) Effect of longterm selection for litter size in mice on lifetime reproductive rate. *Journal of Animal Science* **46**, 1563–1571.

Warburton, D. and Fraser, F. C. (1964) Spontaneous abortion risks in man: data from reproductive histories collected in a medical genetics unit. *American Journal of Human Genetics* **16**, 1–25.

Waterhouse, J., Muir, C., Shanmugaratnam, K., Powell, J. (eds) (1982) *Cancer Incidence in Five Continents*, Vol. IV. Lyon: International Agency for Research on Cancer.

Wattiaux, J. M. (1968) Cumulative parental effects in *Drosophila subobscura*. *Evolution* **22**, 406–421.

Weiss, K. M. (1981) Evolutionary perspectives on human aging. In: *Other Ways of Growing Old* (eds Amoss, P. and Harrell, S). Stanford: Stanford University Press, pp. 25–51.

Weiss, K. M. (1985) The biology of aging, and the quality of later life. In: *Aging 2000: Our Health Care Destiny*, Vol. I: *Biomedical Issues* (eds Gaitz, C. and Samorazski, T.). New York: Springer, pp. 29–49.

Weiss, K. M. (1989a) Are the known chronic diseases related to the human lifespan and its evolution? *American Journal of Human Biology* **1**, 307–319.

Weiss, K. M. (1989b) A survey of human biodemography. *Journal of Quantitative Anthropology* **1**, 79–151.

Weiss, K. M. (1990) The biodemography of variation in human frailty. *Demography* **27**, 185–206.

Weiss, K. M. (1993) *Genetic Variation and Human Disease: Principles and Evolutionary Approaches*. Cambridge: Cambridge University Press.

Weiss, K. M. and Chakraborty, R. (1984) Multistage models and the age pattern of familial polyposis coli. *Cancer Investigation* **2**, 443–448.

Weiss, K. M. and Chakraborty, R. (1988) Multistage models and the age-patterns of cancer: does the statistical analogy imply genetic homology? In: *Familial Adenomatous Polyposis* (ed. Herrera, L.). New York: A. R. Liss, pp. 77–89.

Whittemore, A. and Keller, J. B. (1978) Quantitative theories of carcinogenesis. *SIAM Review* **20**, 1–30.

Wilcox, A. J. and Gladen, B. C. (1982) Spontaneous abortion: the role of heterogeneous risk and selective fertility. *Early Human Development* **7**, 165–178.

Wilcox, A. J., Weinberg, C. R., O'Connor, J. F., Baird, D. D., Schlatterer, J. P.,

Canfield, R. E., Armstrong, E. G. and Nisula, B. C. (1988) Incidence of early loss of pregnancy. *New England Journal of Medicine* **319**, 189–194.

Williams, G. C. (1957) Pleiotropy, natural selection, and the evolution of senescence. *Evolution* **11**, 398–411.

Williams, G. C. (1966) *Adaptation and Natural Selection: A Critique of Some Current Evolutionary Thought.* Princeton, NJ: Princeton University Press.

Winters, S. J. and Troen, P. (1982) Episodic luteinizing hormone (LH) secretion and response of LH and follicle-stimulating hormone to LH-releasing hormone in aged men: evidence for coexistent primary testicular insufficiency and an impairment in gonadotropin secretion. *Journal of Clinical Endocrinology and Metabolism* **55**, 560–565.

Winters, S. J., Sherins, R. J. and Troen, P. (1984) The gonadotropin suppressive activity of androgen is increased in elderly men. *Metabolism* **33**, 1052–1059.

Woessner, J. F. (1963) Age-related changes of the human uterus and its connective tissue framework. *Journal of Gerontology* **18**, 220.

Wood, J. W. (1987) The genetic demography of the Gainj of Papua New Guinea, 2. Determinants of effective population size. *American Naturalist* **129**, 165–187.

Wood, J. W. (1989) Fecundity and natural fetility in humans. In: *Oxford Reviews of Reproductive Biology* (ed. Milligan, S. R.). Oxford: Oxford University Press, pp. 61–109.

Wood, J. W. (1990) Fertility in anthropological populations. *Annual Review of Anthropology* **19**, 211–242.

Wood, J. W. (1994) *Dynamics of Human Reproduction: Biology, Biometry, Demography.* Hawthone, NY: Aldine de Gruyter Press.

Wood, J. W. and Weinstein, M. (1988) A model of age-specific fecundability. *Population Studies* **42**, 85–113.

Wood, J. W., Holman, D. J., Weiss, K. M., Buchanan, A. V. and LeFor, B. (1992a) Hazards models for human population biology. *Yearbook of Physical Anthropology* **35**, 43–87.

Wood, J. W., Weiss, K. M., Buchanan, A. V., Holman, D. J., Weinstein, M. and Chang, M.-C. (1992b) Joint estimation of effective fecundability and the proportion of couples sterile from censored waiting time data. (Submitted for publication.)

Yerushalmy, J., Bierman, J. M., Kemp, D. H., Conner, A. and French, F. E. (1956) Longitudinal studies of pregnancies on the island of Kauai, Territory of Hawaii: analysis of previous reproductive histories. *American Journal of Obstetrics and Gynecology* **71**, 80–96.

Zumoff, B., Strain, G. W., Kream, J., O'Connor, J., Rosenfeld, R. S., Levin, J. and Fukushima, D. K. (1982) Age variation of the 24-hour mean plasma concentrations of androgens, estrogens, and gonadotropins in normal adult men. *Journal of Clinical Endocrinology and Metabolism* **54**, 534–538.

# 3

# The Genetics of Longevity in Humans

TRUDY R. TURNER AND MARK L. WEISS

## INTRODUCTION

Few topics of human biology attract more general attention than "aging." Yet knowledge of the determinants and variability in aging parameters are severely limited. In large part this deficiency results because we lack a clear picture as to what constitutes "aging," why it occurs and why individuals age at different rates. In this paper we review some of the theories concerning the genetics of aging. Additionally, we review the limited literature on the anthropological genetics of aging. For this purpose, we define anthropological genetics as aspects of heredity which are of anthropological significance. This is a much broader definition than the generally accepted restriction to the genetics of small populations, associated aspects of demography, and an emphasis on within and between population variability. This extended definition is largely a result of the minimal literature on anthropological genetics of aging in any narrower sense. Of prime interest in this regard are questions as to why some individuals or populations live longer than others.

Besides surveying the limited information on conventional topics such as population variability in genetics of human aging, we will briefly review developments in the molecular genetics of aging. Many of the newest developments in aging research come from work using invertebrate models, e.g., *Caenorhabditis elegans*, a free-living nematode, and the fruit fly, *Drosophila melanogaster*. While much recent work has focused on such models, it is debatable as to the appropriateness of extrapolating from data gathered on invertebrates to vertebrates, particularly mammals and humans. Thus, we also review data on the primary vertebrate model, inbred strains of mice.

## BIOMARKERS OF AGING

To track the aging process in individuals and populations, it is necessary to have appropriate biomarkers by which to judge its progress. In evaluating and choosing these markers it is important to note the difference between biological alterations which are secondary to aging processes *per se* and disease states which are associated with aging or are simply age-related.

Biomarkers of aging can be defined as age-dependent changes correlated with chronological aging (Johnson, 1990). These changes range from visible phenotypic changes to subtle biochemical changes. In humans a senescent phenotype can be recognized by common observations such as the thinning and loss of hair, wrinkling of skin, loss of visual and auditory acuity, ocular cataracts, muscular weakness, hardening of the arteries, varicose veins, menopause in females, some increased propensity to fall and some loss of short-term memory (Martin, 1988: 262).

Other changes during aging occur in nutritional requirements and diet, hormone resting levels and inductions, tissue responses to hormonal stimuli, immune response potentials and autoimmune titers, activity levels, obesity, and accumulation of lipofuscins (Shmookler Reis, 1988: 272). The effects of aging on enzyme levels of animals at various ages and other physiological changes of aging are well documented [see the *CRC Handbook of Biochemistry in Aging* (Florini, 1981), the *CRC Handbook of Physiology in Aging* (Masaro, 1981), and *Biological Markers of Aging* (Reff and Schneider, 1982)].

Much of the work on biomarkers has been done on mice and rats. Harrison and Archer (1988) examined a series of biological systems including those that measure underlying malfunctions affecting health such as open-field activity and tight-wire performance; those that directly affect health such as wound healing and hemoglobin concentration; those that measure the aging of cellular macromolecules due to glycosylation such as tail collagen; those that measure organ function such as urine concentration; and those that measure re-growth rate such as hair growth. Different genotypes of inbred mice showed different aging patterns. The authors suggest that while some of these changes in biological systems may predict longevity, they function as independent time clocks in different inbred strains of mice. The expression of an androgen responsive gene, $\alpha$-2 globin, is independent of changes in serum androgen levels and is an additional biomarker of aging in rodents (Mooradian, 1990). Russell and Seppa (1990) in their study of single gene effects on aging in the nematode *C. elegans* have five biomarkers of aging: survival, movement rate, lipofuscin level, $\beta$-glucosidase activity and $\beta$-*N*-acetyl-glucosaminidase activity. One of the biomarkers of aging, signaling the onset of senescence in *Drosophila*, is reduced fertility and fecundity of females (Arking, 1987a, b).

Mooradian (1990) suggests that while biomarkers demonstrate a quantitative correlation between a biological parameter and the age of the subject, the biological parameter must also not be altered by disease or nutritional state. He uses age-related changes in the replicative capacity of fibroblasts, glycation of collagen, and alkali-induced DNA unwinding rate as biomarkers.

Martin (1988) makes a distinction between public and private markers of aging. Public markers are common to a species while private markers are responsible for intraspecific genetic variation in aging and can be classified as either polymorphisms or mutations. However, most of the private markers Martin studied are responsible for disease states that decrease the life span of the individual possessing the variant. Tully (1988) and Mooradian (1990) suggest that studying age-related diseases will not contribute significantly to the understanding of the normal processes of aging.

However, the distinction blurs as one considers the ramifications and implications of specific changes, e.g., loss of skin elasticity is an indication of a loss of the ability to maintain a steady state, a loss which can have severe consequences in many organ systems. In fact many biomarkers of aging include some reference to functional decline. As disease generally involves a loss of function, one can see the dilemma of trying to separate "normal" loss of function from disease-related losses.

One of the biomarkers of aging in human females is menopause. Snowdon *et al.* (1989) compared 5,287 naturally postmenopausal and 3,166 surgically postmenopausal white female Seventh Day Adventists between the ages of 55 and 100. Results indicated that the likelihood of premature death decreased with increasing age at natural menopause until the age of 55. Early menopause was associated with substantial excess mortality. Age at menopause may then be considered a predictor of longevity. A decline in fertility and female sexual behavior are also biomarkers in *Macaca mulatta* (Short *et al.*, 1989; Bowden *et al.*, 1990).

Smith (see Holden, 1987), studying four generations of an Amish family, found that those males with a deletion in the arm of the Y-chromosome lived substantially longer than males who did not have this deletion. However, males generally appear to be more vulnerable than females to infant mortality, while X-linked immunoregulatory genes appear to contribute to a greater resistance to infectious disease.

Recombinant DNA techniques have been used in the nematode to look for biochemical biomarkers of aging. To date, none of the three chromosomal regions examined by Johnson *et al.* (1987) contains the major locus, age-1, that specifies a long life span in certain inbred strains. Two-dimensional gel electrophoresis also failed to reveal any qualitative changes in proteins that would signal senescence.

The only biochemical biomarker that has shown a consistent association with aging is in the HLA system. This is true for the H-2 region in mice (see "Mice: A Vertebrate Model," pp. 86–88). Takata *et al.* (1987) have observed a low phenotype frequency of HLA-DRw9 in 82 centenarians and 20 nonagenarians in Okinawa, Japan. Among the Japanese, HLA-DRw9 is related to most autoimmune diseases. There is also a high frequency of DR-1. An absence of DR-1 is also associated with autoimmune disease in this population. The authors suggest that DRw9 is a risk factor and DR-1 is a favorable factor for longevity in these populations.

Most of the studies on phenotypic biomarkers have been conducted to track the course of the aging process and are not predictive of length of life. Studies concerned with genetic biomarkers, however, attempt to be predictive. The only study with some marginal success is the HLA system in humans. The histocompatibility system seems to be predictive in mice as well. While some authors have attempted to use biomarkers as a means for testing various theories of aging, perhaps the only conclusion that can be reached is that a genetic predisposition for long life is simply not having genes that will cause death at an early age. This idea corresponds to Vaupel's (1988) idea of inherited frailty and further studies of aged individuals may confirm the role of the HLA system in longevity.

## THEORIES OF AGING

There are several theoretical models to account for the aging process at the cellular level. These fall into two categories which have been called programmed and stochastic. The program models ascribe aging to phenomena which are built into the cells' genome, while stochastic models attribute aging to accumulations of random decrements over time.

### Programmed Aging

Many of the program theories flow from the demonstration by Hayflick and Moorhead (1961) and Hayflick (1965) that in cell culture human diploid fibroblasts have a limited life span which is related to the number of elapsed cell divisions rather than to the passage of time *per se*. In this view, senescence is the last stage in an aging process which starts at conception. As cells divide, genetic switches are turned on and off in a programmed fashion to account for the events we collectively describe as development and aging.

This view has the appealing feature of making senescence a part of a continuum of development. Certainly, there are regulatory switches known at the genetic level for aspects of early development. The mechanisms controlling the progression from embryonic to fetal to adult hemoglobins in higher primates are becoming quite well documented at the molecular level (Stamatoyannopoulos, 1991). There is even some evidence for regulatory gene involvement in aging in *Drosophila melanogaster* (Shepard *et al.*, 1989).

Three lines of evidence in particular have provided support for the programmed theory of aging. First, there is Hayflick's observation and its implicit program. Human diploid fibroblast behavior can be further investigated by inducing the cells to enter a quiescent stage during which division ceases. This is accomplished through manipulation of the culture media. Proliferation can be induced by introduction of the missing growth factors. This provides a reversible loss of growth for comparison with senescence.

In the 1970s, Martin *et al.* (1974), Bell *et al.* (1978) and others suggested that fibroblasts in cell culture become terminally differentiated and thus cease dividing. Were this the case one might well expect to find synthesis of comparable arrays of molecules in differentiated cells and senescent ones. Recently, in reviewing the use of human diploid fibroblasts in aging research, Goldstein (1990), noted that there are some protein and mRNA similarities between terminally differentiated and senescent cells. He suggests common, or at least analogous pathways involving the repression of growth-stimulating genes and the expression of growth-inhibitory genes, but there are also significant differences. If a battery of proteins or mRNA could be identified, they would be important biomarkers of the aging process.

In searching for genetic programming of senescence, one process that has been proposed is the production of DNA synthesis inhibitors. Smith (1990) reviews information on a number of inhibitors isolated from cultured cells; as yet such inhibitors have been hinted at (Stein et al., 1990), but have not been identified in senescent cells. While favoring the view that cellular aging is a process caused by the active inhibition of DNA synthesis, Smith (1990) acknowledges that there is no reason to rule out the possibility that the loss of function is secondary to other, possibly stochastic, alterations of cell function. The general uncertainty about the applicability of results gathered on human diploid fibroblast cultures has prompted some to advocate utilization of cells of the immune system for research into cellular aging (Miller, 1989).

Additional data that have led some to propose a strict genetic program for aging comes from the study of pathologies causing "accelerated aging." Progeria is a term applied to two very rare disorders which cause phenotypes reminiscent of rapid aging and which are under relatively simple genetic control: Hutchinson–Gilford syndrome or progeria of youth (sometimes referred to simply as "progeria") and Werner's syndrome or progeria of the adult. In the former, the affected individual suffers from retarded growth, loss of hair, thin skin, and a very low weight to height ratio. The median age at death is 12 years and death usually occurs due to congestive heart failure or myocardial infarcts. While the syndromes are reminiscent of old age, other characteristics of normal aging, such as cataracts and osteoporosis, are not present. Progeria is strongly suspected of being caused by an autosomal dominant allele. Werner's syndrome is clearly caused by an autosomal recessive and differs from progeria in several ways. Yet, the fact that both mirror aspects of what one would expect of "premature aging," implies to some that the normal aging process is under strong genetic control, and a small number of genetic loci at that (Hayflick, 1987). It has been hypothesized by Goldstein et al. (1990) that Werner's syndrome results from an inability to repress a locus which produces an inhibitor of DNA synthesis; again looking to an internal programmed senescence.

Thirdly, at the organismal level, the life histories of semelparous species provide support to those who argue for programmed senescence. Semelparous species, such as the salmon, exhibit high fecundity for a short period after maturity, followed by rapid aging and death. The constancy of this process within species is taken as strong evidence for genetic "programming" (Kirkwood, 1989). Evidence indicates that the transition into "old age" is mediated by hormonal changes. In salmon, for instance, castration can delay death for several years (Russell, 1987). The female octopus (Octopus hummelincki) drastically reduces food intake after laying her eggs and normally dies within days of their hatching. Surgical removal of her optic nerve after egg laying results in resumption of eating and a significantly extended life span (Kirkwood, 1985).

Iteroparous species, such as humans, also evidence hormonally conditioned age changes which are taken to reflect genetic programs. Menopause clearly is one such, as is greying of the hair. Involution of the thymus can be reversed by hormonal manipulation (Kelly *et al.*, 1987). Genetically influenced programs occur in iteroparous species; but it is not clear that they cause aging.


## Stochastic Aging

For some time, stochastic processes have been favored in attempting to account for the aging process. Here, the decline in function, at least at a cellular level, is ascribed to the accumulation of errors in one or more molecular species. Again, a variety of permutations on the basic concept have been offered; one which has received much support is the "free radical theory."


### *Free Radical Theory*

Normally, organic molecules are held together by chemical bonds which consist of two electrons. In organic molecules, these bonds may unite a hydrogen atom and part of the molecule, generically known as a "radical." Each electron involved in a bond has a "spin" and the two electrons spin in opposite directions to form a bond with no net spin; an energetically favorable state. When a chemical bond is broken, the resulting species may each retain one unpaired electron and hence have a net spin. Radicals with an odd electron are known as "free radicals," and most are quite reactive as they attempt to find an electron with which to pair. When a free radical reacts so as to capture an electron, the donor in turn becomes a free radical; reactions involving free radicals involve the propagation of more free radicals. This situation continues until two free radicals react and form a stable bond involving two electrons.

Free radicals are constantly being formed *in vivo* as a consequence of a variety of phenomena. Radiation sources may split bonds and generate free radicals and enzyme-catalyzed reactions may do the same. Depending on their reactivity, free radicals have differing half-lives; a hydroxyl radical's is $7 \times 10^{-10}$ s, while others may live for days. As a consequence, different radicals can diffuse greater or lesser distances from their site of origin and this affects their biological consequences (Pryor, 1984).

In 1956, Denham Harman first proposed that the progressive accumulation of somatic deterioration which we call "aging," might result from damage induced by free radicals. Random deleterious chemical changes accumulate in systems throughout the body and lead to progressive loss in the ability to maintain homeostasis. According to this theory, damage is done to somatic DNA which, in turn, leads to defective proteins and/or reduced ability to replicate accurately. In fact this is a modification of the earlier "wear and tear" theory of aging.

There is a wealth of evidence that various free radicals are capable of interacting with and altering DNA. Hydroxyl radicals are known to cause chemical changes in all components of the DNA, though not with equal efficiencies. The altered DNA moieties can then undergo a wide variety of further reactions. The chemistry of these reactions is further complicated by differential changes to native double-stranded DNA, as opposed to the individual constituents of the DNA.

Various lines of evidence support this general theory but some data remain to be explained. The effects of ionizing radiation are mediated through the formation of free radicals and in a number of ways radiation damage mimics aging effects (Pryor, 1987). Free radicals are known to be, or suspected to be, involved in the etiology of a number of diseases associated with old age. This list includes many forms of cancer and atherosclerosis. To many, the most compelling evidence for a role for free radicals in aging is the inverse relationship between the metabolic rate of a mammalian species, a key aspect in the rate of production of free radicals, and the species' average life span (Harman, 1983). However, one might expect that antioxidants, such as vitamin E, which retard the rate of free radical oxidative damage could thus increase species' *maximum* life span. To date this has not been demonstrated. However, some mammals fed a diet high in antioxidants do have a greater *mean* life span (Harman, 1984). This would imply that free radicals do not set the upper bound of species-specific life spans; but that their suppression allows a greater percentage of the species to approach this boundary. The inability of free radical inhibitors to elongate the life span is currently taken to be one of the strongest arguments against the free radical theory of aging.

Organisms have evolved mechanisms to prevent the damage free radicals are capable of causing. Enzymes, such as superoxide dismutase (SOD) and catalase, serve as capable free-radical scavengers or inhibitors of free-radical reactions. Most free radicals are produced in the mitochondria as a result of aerobic metabolism and in fact the mitochondrial DNA codes for the enzyme SOD-2. As virtually nothing is known about population variability for free-radical-inhibiting enzymes in humans, their investigation could have great potential in clarifying variability in phenomena related to aging.

## DNA Repair

A number of the theories of aging which have been advanced are not mutually exclusive, but rather reflect modifications or elaborations which develop with increasing data and understanding. Along these lines, some ascribe the maximum achievable life span of an organism to the evolved efficiency of mechanisms to repair damage done to the DNA—whether it be the result of free radicals or other agents. Various DNA repair mechanisms exist. Damaged oligonucleotides can be excised by exonucleases and the complementary strand used as a template for the construction of a corrected copy. Ames and colleagues (1985) described an enzyme, a DNA glycosylase, which recognizes and excises thymine glycol, a derivative of thymine known to be produced by free radical damage. The damaged bases are excreted in the urine, providing a marker for tracking oxidative damage to the DNA. In fact, Saul *et al.* (1987) find for three species that the higher the metabolic rate the higher the excretion of damaged bases and the shorter the life span. On the other hand, they did not find a relationship between age and levels of damaged bases in the urine of humans. Again, there are no data on population variability in this marker.

In the context of rates of evolution in the order Primates, Goodman (e.g., Czelusniak *et al.*, 1982) has long maintained that the higher primates have evidenced a decreasing rate of change at the molecular level. Proponents of this view have discussed a number of mechanisms which might account for a slowdown in hominoid evolution including more efficient DNA repair mechanisms (Koop *et al.*, 1989). If in fact there are more efficient repair mechanisms in the higher primates, they may exist because of evolutionary pressures related to extension of the life span.

## Error Catastrophe

While Denham linked the aging process to the accumulation of somatic mutations, Orgel (1963) proposed an alternative molecular mechanism. In Orgel's view, aging was a function of accumulated errors in the translation and transcription of proteins. Any one of these errors would likely have negligible effects but their accretion would lead to a threshold at which the metabolic machinery develops catastrophic malfunctions. The error catastrophe theory pictures a cascade of effects as the faulty proteins precipitate further errors in protein synthesis and functioning.

This theory provides a number of testable hypotheses. If random errors are introduced into amino-acid sequences with age, molecular forms should become increasingly heterogeneous over time. While studies in the early 1970s seemed to indicate that this was indeed the case, at least for some proteins, these results have since proven to be largely artifactual or the result of slowing of protein turnover, which in turn can lead to the intracellular accumulation of denatured proteins. It is a change in the conformation of the molecules which leads to a loss of fidelity, not errors in synthesis. Other proteins were shown not to exhibit any structural alterations in aged cells (Rothstein, 1987).

As many of the molecules involved in DNA repair are proteins, it is theoretically possible to combine aspects of both the error catastrophe and free radical theories. Might errors in the synthesis of enzymes which interact with DNA lead to inaccuracies in replication or DNA repair processes? Again, there is no experimental evidence to support this view. DNA polymerases from young and old humans are equally faithful in DNA replication, and the DNA repair enzymes from young and old cells are equally efficient (Rothstein, 1987). While now even Orgel agrees that the error catastrophe theory is untenable, it is still potentially interesting to investigate the conformational changes which aging proteins exhibit.

## Advanced Glycosylated End-Products

Evidence of complex conformational changes in a variety of proteins has been accumulating due to an overlap in research on diabetes and aging. This is not entirely unexpected as several aging processes appear to be accelerated in diabetics. Additionally, diabetics have long been known to have high levels of a minor component of hemoglobin known as $HbA_{1C}$. It has been demonstrated that this component is a glycated hemoglobin formed by the nonenzymatic glycosylation of the protein (Koenig *et al.*, 1976; Bunn and Higgins, 1981; Cerami *et al.*, 1987). If hemoglobin structure can be altered by long-term exposure to high levels of sugar, might not that of other proteins?

Through the Maillard reaction, which is also responsible for "browning" of foods, proteins can be irreversibly modified to form advanced glycosylated end-products (AGE). Cross-links between collagen molecules, for instance, can be formed by AGEs and it is suspected that such cross-linkages might account for some of the phenotypic characteristics of aging. Most intriguingly, collagen linked with AGEs on arterial walls has been shown to trap proteins including low-density lipoproteins (Cerami *et al.*, 1987) and thus may contribute to the formation of atherosclerotic plaques. When incubated with glucose, solutions of other proteins will also form AGEs. Lens crystallins appear to become cross-linked under long-term high glucose conditions and refract light in a cataract-like fashion. Additionally, AGEs are known to interact with DNA and may interfere with DNA repair mechanisms as demonstrated *in vitro* by Bucala *et al.* (1985).

## Other Models

A variety of other permutations have been offered over the years. One model attributed senescence to simple wear and tear (Weisman, 1891). The minor insults and detriments an organism encounters each day simply wear it out. However, raising organisms in protected environments neither prevents aging nor extends the maximum life span. If the wear and tear model is a stochastic model, then the programmed counterpart is the rate of living model and dates back even further (Buffon, 1749) with Pearl (1928) as a later proponent. Basically this holds that a species' metabolic rate is the cause of organismal wear and tear. However, Arking *et al.* (1988) demonstrated that different strains of *Drosophila melanogaster*, with equivalent metabolic profiles, could have significantly different maximum life spans. Numerous other models have been advanced with greater or lesser experimental support. One relates the effect of dietary restriction to the intracellular replacement of macromolecules. Another attributes aging to damage of the mitochondria. A number of additional models can be parceled into either the programmed senescence or the stochastic aging camps.

The apparent dichotomy between active, programmed determinants of aging and stochastic causes has been much discussed in the literature (Holliday, 1986; Arking, 1988; Lints, 1989; Rose, 1989). For a number of the protagonists the discussion is framed against a backdrop of evolutionary "necessity." Evolution is taken as the ultimate cause of aging (e.g., Rose and Graves, 1989); senescence is then a direct consequence of the decline in the force of selection with age. As Rose and Graves state ". . . as natural selection fades out (in the life of an organism with separate soma and germ lines), it is inevitable . . . that the functional performance of the adult body should deteriorate with age. This, for evolutionary biologists, is the sole and sufficient cause of senescence (p. B27)." Two genetic mechanisms are put forward to account for the evolution of aging: antagonistic pleiotropy and age-specific selection effects. Alleles which exhibit antagonistic pleiotropy evidence opposite effects on fitness at different times in the life cycle. Some increase reproductive potential early in life while reducing reproductive abilities later in life (see Crews and Gerber, this volume). While alleles which exhibit such antagonistic pleiotropy are subject to strong control by selection, alleles with age-specific effects evidenced in the postreproductive period are relatively invisible to selection. Age-specific effects can thus lead to increased genetic variability. These mechanisms are not mutually exclusive. Under either or both regimes one can imagine that senescence could result from different alleles in different populations. It may be that there is no universal physiological mechanism underlying aging (see Wood *et al.*, this volume).

Many of those embroiled in the programmed versus stochastic causation debate invoke evolution as the ultimate arbiter; each position being defended via recourse to the action of evolutionary forces, particularly selection. For the programmed camp, the genetic program exists because it is adaptive and that requires natural selection. To some who favor stochastic explanations the evolutionary question becomes "how did longevity evolve?"—senescence being the "easily" explained decay of homeostasis. Analogies can be drawn between this view and the "probable mutation effect" by which Brace (1963) explained the loss of anatomical structures over evolutionary time.

All of these sometimes competing theories and processes are leading to a picture of complex gene–environment interactions at the cellular and molecular levels; a situation which makes population genetic studies very difficult. These complexities are further demonstrated by invertebrate studies.

## GENETICS AT THE ORGANISMAL LEVEL

### Invertebrate Models

A number of factors are making use of invertebrate models of aging increasingly attractive and two in particular are being used extensively, *D. melanogaster* and *C. elegans*. Much is already known about the genetics of each species and *C. elegans* offers a distinct advantage in that the developmental fate of every cell has been mapped. Of course, one can manipulate these organisms with minimal cost and legislative regulation and they have short generations. Molecular tools also allow manipulations and investigations which were previously impossible. The applicability of this information to humans or other primates is not always immediately apparent, however.

Possibly the most important demonstration using invertebrates is that one can select for increased life span. This was accomplished in both *D. melanogaster* (Rose and Charlesworth, 1981; Luckinbill *et al.*, 1984) and *C. elegans* (Johnson and Wood, 1982; Friedman and Johnson, 1988). Luckinbill and co-workers selected for female fruit flies that reproduced late in life (the "long-lived" strain) and for those that reproduced early in life (the "short-lived" strain). This selective regime had much greater effect on longevity when an environmental component was introduced. When the "long-lived" strain was reared under high larval density, selection increased their mean life span significantly: the mean female life span for the Oregon R wild type strain is $51 \pm 20$ days; the comparable statistic for the long-lived strain (L) is $77 \pm 14$ days (Arking, 1987b). However, the strain selected for earlier reproduction was not significantly different from the control strain. The ability to achieve dramatic increases in life span implies a significant genetic variance at high rearing-densities. *C. elegans* strains have been bred with maximum life spans as much as 70% greater than that of the wild type (Johnson, 1987). And, unlike most other models, *C. elegans* strains bred for life traits do not evidence inbreeding depression (Johnson and Wood, 1982). Invertebrate models have demonstrated a number of important points. First, that life span is a variable, heritable trait. Secondly, the life span seen in wild populations is not necessarily the maximum life span for that species (Johnson *et al.*, 1988). At least in *C. elegans*, selection has not favored longevity. The locus responsible for the extended life span, *age-1*, also reduces fertility, a case of antagonistic pleiotropy.

The genes that control longevity it would seem are not the genes affecting the rate of development. In *D. melanogaster*, Arking *et al.* (1988) find that extension of the postreproductive period almost completely accounts for the increases noted in life span.

These studies also indicate that the number of loci involved in aging is not a very large number. Arking and Dudas (1989) speculate that there might be "several genes localized on the third chromosome" of *D. melanogaster* responsible for the regulation of longevity. And as noted in *C. elegans*, mutants at one locus are responsible for a 70% increase in longevity. These results are in line with earlier estimates by Cutler (1975) that a small number of regulatory changes may have been responsible for significant shifts in the maximum life span of hominids over geological time.

Does the demonstration of genetic variation necessarily rule out an important role for stochastic processes in senescence? Arking does not tie the extended life phenotype to a rejection of the free-radical or other stochastic processes. In fact, he determined that the antioxidant defenses of the L-strain were significantly higher than those of the controls. Null mutants for SOD and catalases have also been identified in *D. melanogaster* (Bewley *et al.*, 1986; Campbell *et al.*, 1986) and as the free-radical theory predicts, the mutants die young. Tomalsoff (in Arking, 1988) found similar results in primates.

## Mice: A Vertebrate Model

Mice are frequently chosen as models in genetic studies because of several features of their life histories; short life span, rapid development, small size, fecundity, and the fact that there are several inbred strains where genotypes can be compared, hybridized and backcrossed (Ingram, 1990). The National Institute on Aging has a registry describing the various stocks of mice, appropriate uses, biological characteristics, known age-dependent physiological and behavioral changes, and husbandry techniques (Sprott, 1983). Mice are especially useful for studies of genetics and aging since there are large differences in life span of different strains. The strains can differ by only a few loci, making it possible to study the role of individual loci in determining life span (Russell, 1966). Four kinds of genetically defined stocks of mice are commonly used in aging studies. Inbred lines are used for strain comparisons, especially in examination of the effects of specific loci on functional systems, such as the immune system. Single gene mutants are used to determine the role of discrete metabolic or biochemical alterations in the aging process. Genetically selected stocks are used to study the existence of genetic contributions to age-related changes and F1 hybrids are used to examine hybrid vigor (Sprott, 1983).

Mice have been used experimentally to test various hypotheses about aging. To test the antioxidant/free-radical hypothesis of aging, Reynolds (see Sprott, 1987) attempted to correlate the amount of serum uric acid, an antioxidant, with locomotor activity and life span. The correlations were very weak and not consistent with the hypothesis of free radical formation and aging. Schneider and Reed (1985) discuss other experiments where different strains of mice were given SOD and other antioxidants in an attempt to extend life span. In humans SOD declines with age. In mice additional SOD functioned only to extend life span in strains that had a genetic predisposition to life shortening diseases (Schneider and Reed, 1985: 55).

To test the hypothesis that aging results from DNA damage, Su and colleagues (1984), compared *Mus musculus* to *Peromyscus leucopus* which has a life span 2.5 times longer than *Mus*. They found that the shorter-lived species had a faster rate of DNA damage accumulation and tolerated a lower maximum extent of damage than the longer-lived species. Considerable work has been done on sister chromatid exchange (SCE) and aging. SCE formation is a measure of DNA repair capacity. A decrease of SCE formation with age would favor the DNA repair theory of aging. There is some age-dependent SCE formation. However, strain differences weaken the support for this hypothesis (Sprott and Combs, 1990). Some work has also been done on the relationship between DNA transcription and aging. Age-related changes were found in histone H1 subtypes, which inhibit DNA transcription (Sprott, 1987).

Studies on aging in mice have demonstrated that individual life spans in certain inbred lines can be extended by diet restriction. Harrison and Archer (1987) were able to increase longevity in all strains they examined except B6. There have been several reports of hybrid vigor when inbred strains of mice are crossed (Russell, 1966; Ingram and Reynolds, 1982; Sprott, 1983, 1985). This probably results from the elimination of deleterious recessives from each inbred strain. Several authors have correlated sex differences with life-span differences (Waldron, 1983; Meyer *et al.*, 1989; Smith and Warner, 1989). Smith and Warner (1989) discuss the advantages of a female genotype. DNA polymerase alpha, the principal enzyme of DNA replication, maps to the X-chromosome. There is X-reactivation with age in mice, thus allowing for an extra locus for this enzyme. Meyer *et al.* (1989) found some correlation of sex and effects of H-2 haplotype.

One of the most active research areas in aging and mice is the genetic analysis of the decline of immune function and the increase in autoimmune phenomena with age (Sprott, 1983, 1985, 1987; Sprott and Combs, 1990). Meredith and Walford (1977) found that longer-lived strains of mice usually maintained T-cell function longer than other strains. Sprott (1983) summarized the work of several other researchers who have found that the major histocompatibility complex (MHC) plays a significant role in immunological age changes. Some of these studies are of congenic mice (strains identical at all loci except the one of interest) differing only in the H-2 haplotype. The MHC genes control the immune system of which H-2 is a part. Studies of the H-2 region of chromosome 17 indicate that changes here can lead to significant changes in life span. Several other studies confirm the involvement of the H-2 histocompatibility group in longevity (see Sprott, 1987, and Sprott and Combs, 1990, for discussion).

## Heritability and Longevity in Humans

The relative contributions to human longevity of individual genotypes and the environment have continued to interest researchers. Since the early 1900s there have been several studies that have estimated heritability ($H^2$) for longevity in humans as between 0.00 and 0.49. These studies can be divided into two groups: those that have examined genealogical records over a long period of time; and those that have sampled from a special subgroup of the population, such as twins, the insured, or working class families from Baltimore (Cohen, 1964). However, there are serious methodological problems, especially with the older studies, which raise questions about the validity of their conclusions.

The earliest genealogical studies were based on published collections of records of many families. Beeton and Pearson (1899) used old English genealogical records including Foster's *Peerage of Great Britain and Ireland*, Burke's *Landed Gentry of the British Empire* and the *Society of Friends Records*. These records indicated a positive correlation between the length of life of parents and offspring. However, there are several aspects of the records that challenge these conclusions. Only males are included since pedigrees were traced only through the male line. There was a tendency to omit individuals who died before the age of 21. These early deaths probably accounted for about 30% of all deaths during the time period covered by these records. Late adult deaths are also omitted (Cohen, 1964; Rose and Bell, 1971). These same problems are seen in later studies using collections of genealogies for data. Holmes (1928), using Allstrom's *Dictionary of Royal Lineage*, and Stoessiger (1932), using Pearson's *Family Data*, both found a correlation between parents and offspring for longevity. Jalavisto (1951), using the *Genealogical Records of Finnish and Swedish Middle Class and Nobility* extending from 1500 to the early 20th century, found that both maternal and paternal longevity was associated with the longevity of the offspring. However, the effect of maternal longevity was greater. Besides having all the problems associated with old genealogical records, this study also failed to control for any social class differentials.

A. G. Bell (1918) initiated an alternative way of using genealogical records to determine the heritability of longevity. He studied a single family, the Hydes, who were all descended from William Hyde, who died in 1681 in Norwich, Connecticut. He found an almost direct relationship between the life span of parents and offspring (Cohen, 1964). However, only about one-third of the individuals in the genealogy are included in his analysis. There is also an over-representation of early adult deaths. In 1864, the date the records end, several of the older members of the lineage were still alive and thus excluded from the analysis. Wilson and Doering (1926) attempted to correct this problem in their analysis of the Elder Peirces, descendants of John Pars Weaver of Watertown, Massachusetts, who lived around 1640. They included in their analysis only those individuals who had a chance to reach age 95 by the cut-off date of 1880. However, they also restricted their data to males and to fathers of sons who themselves were fathers. This introduced another source of sampling error and confounded fertility with the analysis of longevity. Pearl (1931) conducted one study using genealogical information from five long-lived American families and found no correlation between longevity of parents and offspring. Yuan (1931, 1932) conducted a landmark study of longevity on a five century (1365–1914) Chinese genealogy. This was the first time that life-table techniques were used to correlate parental and offspring longevity. He found that parental life expectancy was greater among long-lived sons and sons' life expectancy was greater if parents were long lived. However, differences of correlations between the life tables of the short and long lived were small.

All of these studies suffer from the same flaws that are inherent in the use of old genealogies. The data are often incomplete and inaccurate, especially with the age of death of females, if they are even included. In addition there may be secular trends in mortality over several centuries. Individuals may have died of causes that have little to do with a genetic predisposition to longevity.

The second group of studies differs from the first in that instead of relying on historical data, investigators collected data from sample populations. This approach was pioneered by Pearl and Pearl (1934). Extensive histories of families of working men in the Baltimore area were collected by a staff of field workers. These records include more than 100,000 individuals. Additionally, studies were conducted on the families of extremely longevous individuals, those living past 90 years. In his analysis Pearl introduces the TIAL (total immediate ancestral longevity) index. The ages at death of an individual's six immediate ancestors are summed. The TIAL for the longevous group seems to be fairly homogeneous and higher in nonagenarians. However, there is some bias in the selection of a sample group, since all six ancestors must be dead at the time of sampling. The conclusions are also based on incomplete and unverified data, and the final analysis was based on only a fraction of the available sample (Cohen, 1964; Rose and Bell, 1971). Preas (1945) used data collected for a morbidity study of Cattaraugus County in upstate New York. Mortality rates were lowest for offspring with both parents surviving to age 70 and highest with both parents dead under the age of 70 (Cohen, 1964). In Preas' study, more fertile parents were over-represented in the sample and there was large attrition due to missing observations. Zonneveld and Polman (1957) surveyed 3,000 people over the age of 65 and found that a larger percentage of parents of 80-year-olds had reached that age than parents of people in the younger age groups. However, age at death was not included and about one-quarter of the sample was not used because of lack of information. The same problems of incompleteness of data, selection bias and the use of unverified data appear in this series of studies, as well as in the studies using historical records of genealogy.

During the 1960s and 1970s Pearl's original data were reanalyzed (Murphy, 1978). Abbott *et al.* (1978) have tried to correct for some of the problems in the original data set, but still face the problems of missing information. They conclude that the additive genetic component of the variance in longevity is less than 10% of the total phenotypic variance (Abbott *et al.*, 1978: 105). Recently, Philippe (1978) studied the population of Isle-aux-Coudres, Quebec, Canada. This population is relatively uniform in socioeconomic and medicosocial characteristics. Philippe suggests that differences in age at time of death in this genetically homogeneous population are due to the effect of the environment. He suggests that the heritability of survival is nearly zero (Philippe, 1978: 128). In the most recent study of longevity, Bocquet-Appel and Jakobi (1990) used path analysis to distinguish transmissible and non-transmissible components of longevity in genealogies from the village of Arthez d'Asson (Pyreneés Atlantiques, France) from the 18th century onwards. They estimated the heritability of longevity at 0.16.

Cohen (1964), in the most comprehensive review of studies of the heritability of aging, discusses another class of studies, those conducted by insurance companies or actuarial societies. She reviews nine studies conducted between 1903 and 1942. Most of these studies indicate a positive correlation between age at death of parents and age at death of offspring. Early insurance applications asked the age and cause of death of the parents of the insured. Investigators used this as a source of data and had very large sample sizes. However, it is not certain whether these individuals represent a homogeneous population, as was claimed by some of the investigators. Also the data upon which these studies are based have numerous defects, especially in validity and in the selection of applicants for inclusion. There seems to be considerable misstatement of ages and causes of death of parents and sibs on the forms. Family history may also be a factor in choosing the applicants to be insurees. Inferences from these data are fairly limited (Cohen, 1964: 162).

Two final special sample groups of the population have been used to determine the heritability of longevity: twins and adopted children. The initial work on senescent twins was reported in 1949 by Kallman and Sander. Their data is from over 2,000 twins participating in the New York State Psychiatric Institute Study of Aging Twins. Data analysis was limited, however, to a much smaller number of individuals who had reached 60 years of age, lived in or around New York, and spoke English (Bank and Jarvik, 1978: 304). The longitudinal study of these twins extended over three decades.

The total mean interpair life-span differences were consistently smaller in monozygotic than in dizygotic twins. This was especially true for females. For monozygotic twins the differences average 44.7 months, for dizygotic 66.5 months. The differences between monozygotic and dizygotic twins decreased with length of life, so that they nearly disappeared in male twins over the age of 80. This is because there may be less variability near the upper limit of the human life span (Cohen, 1964). One of the problems with an interpretation of the Kallman and Sander (1949) data is that only averages are given. There is no information on how many twin pairs were included in the comparisons. Hauge and Harvald (1961) derived their sample of twins from a compete registration of twins born in Denmark between 1870 and 1910. Questionnaires were sent to all twins and their near relatives. Inter-pair differences in the age of death of monozygotic twins were significantly less than in dizygotic twins (Cohen, 1964). One of the difficulties in the interpretation of the twin material is in how zygosity was determined. This is not made clear. Additionally, there may be some link between twinning and life span, so that twins are not a random sample of the population. Correlative to twin studies are studies on adoptive children. Wright (1988) reports on a study by Sørenson, who looked at the histories of 1,000 adoptive Danish children born between 1924 and 1926 and found that premature death, under the age of 50, may have a significant genetic component. This seems to agree with Abbott *et al.* (1978: 119) who suggest that long life may not be the result of non-specific genes for longevity but the absence of deleterious genes leading to premature death.

All of the studies described in this section had their root in the assumption that the children of long-lived parents were also long lived. While there may be corroborating evidence for this, the degree to which longevity is genetically controlled is questionable. Early estimates of heritability are much higher than more recent estimates. The data used for all of these studies are questionable at best. The only conclusion at this point is that if longevity in humans has any inherited component, it is very small.

## ANTHROPOLOGICAL GENETICS OF LONG-LIVED HUMAN POPULATIONS

There are three populations that have been thought to contain particularly long-lived individuals: the Hunzas of Pakistan, inhabitants of Vilcabamba in Ecuador, and inhabitants of the Caucasus in the Soviet Union. There are anecdotal accounts of the advanced ages attained by individuals of these groups in early reports of travelers to these regions. Leaf (1973, 1975) is, however, primarily responsible for describing and popularizing these groups as particularly longevous. Subsequent work, however, has failed to substantiate the extreme longevity of members of these communities. Social factors which invest aged individuals with increased status and misidentification are responsible for age exaggeration in these populations.

Hunza is located in the Karakoran Mountains in western Pakistan bordering on Afghanistan and China. This is an extremely isolated mountainous area with little contact with the rest of the world. Travelers to the area, particularly a British doctor, Sir Robert McCarrison, did much to popularize knowledge of the health, diet, and longevity of the people in the area. Leaf (1975) recounts meeting several nonagenarians and centenarians on his visit to the area. These physically active individuals continued to work in the fields and existed on a

Spartan diet. There are apparently no subsequent re-evaluations of this community and no documentation exists to substantiate the reports of extreme old age of some of the individuals in the community.

Better known and somewhat more accessible is the area around Vilcabamba in Ecuador. Captain George Coggeshall in 1825 claimed that individuals in the area were particularly healthy and described several people who were more than 90 and 100 years old. In 1959 an American physician, Dr Eugene Paine, described the area as remarkably free of heart disease. The government of Ecuador subsequently sent Dr Miguel Salvador, a cardiologist, to the area. He and his team conducted two surveys of the area in 1969 and 1970, and found the area had a low incidence of heart disease and a high proportion of longevous individuals. Leaf visited the area first the following year.

Vilcabamba is situated in the Andes mountains near the Peruvian border and about 100 miles from the Pacific. The area, like the Hunza area in Pakistan, is an isolated mountainous region. A census taken in 1971 recorded nine individuals out of 819 that were over the age of 100. If this number is normalized it would indicate 1,100 centenarians per 100,000 people in Vilcabamba. This contrasts with 63 per 100,000 in Azerbaijan, 39 for Georgia and three for the United States (Leaf, 1975: 47). Very old people remain active, farming and existing on about a 1,200 calorie diet that is very low in protein and fat. There are some written records, primarily baptismal records, for this area and they have been reanalyzed (Mazess and Forman, 1979).

Unlike the other two areas, the Caucasus are not remote or isolated. It is a mountainous area that stretches across a land bridge from the Black Sea to the Caspian Sea. Georgia, Azerbaijan, and Armenia are the three republics that make up the Caucasus. The first scientific expedition to study longevity and the physiological and health conditions in the Abkhasian part of Georgia was in 1937. Case reports were published on longevous individuals. However, there were no reliable documents establishing the ages of these people. Beginning in 1944 several additional expeditions under the direction of the Institute of Ethnography of the Academy of Science were conducted and a permanent medical research unit was established in the area. Well over 100 publications have dealt with longevity in the area (Medvedev, 1974). The Caucasus are less isolated than Vilcabamba and the Hunza. In addition, the climate and the altitude vary over the region and there is a much better level of nutrition. It was the bacteriologist Metchnikoff who first hypothesized that the fermenting agent of yogurt was responsible for the unusually long-lived individuals in the area (Leaf, 1975). The 1970 census lists between 4,500 and 5,000 centenarians in the Caucasus, making up 12% of the population. Two thirds of the centenarians are female. There have been several cases reported in the Soviet press of extreme old age, the oldest age reported being 168 years. However, this is an undocumented case. Recently another 5-year multi-disciplinary study of longevity was conducted in the Caucasus (Lelashvili and Dalakishvili, 1984) which included data on morphology, physiology, health, demography, and genetics.

Attempts to document extreme longevity indicate that most of the reported cases are the results of exaggeration of age by individuals. Age exaggeration seems to be common among the extremely elderly, especially where there is illiteracy and an absence of documentation (Mazess and Forman, 1979). Medvedev (1974) and Myers (1965) described this exaggeration of age and underestimation of mortality in the Soviet Union. Individuals exaggerate their age by about 20 years, especially since the long lived are highly esteemed and are heads of patriarchal families. Additionally, the Soviet Union used these supposedly long-lived individuals for propaganda. Some people claiming to be over 100 had deserted from the army during the First and Second World Wars and were using forged documents. Biological tests on individuals claiming to be over 100 also did not indicate extreme longevity. Mazess and Forman (1979) evaluated the age exaggeration in Vilcabamba by comparing the reported age of individuals with birth records and other collateral records of these individuals when they were between 20 and 50 years of age. They found cases of misidentification or sloppiness of identification of individuals. It was common to find individuals with the same surname and given name and in one case a niece was mistaken for her aunt. None of the 23 supposed centenarians in the area at the time was actually over 100. All were between 80 and 90. Additionally none of the "nonagenarians" was over 90. They did find that there was a high percentage of individuals over the age of 60 but concluded that this might reflect migration patterns more than any increased longevity in the area. Age exaggeration began at about 70 years of age, both for the ages of the living and the reported ages at death.

There is very little classical genetics information available on individuals or populations that evidence extreme longevity. Most comes from the multidisciplinary study of the populations in the Caucasus. Kipshidze et al. (1987) found that most longevous individuals in this area were blood group O and genotype MN. They suggest some form of selection for these genotypes but do not discuss the mechanism by which selection would operate to increase these genotypes. Jorgensen has also noted some age-related increase in O in populations in Germany and suggested that individuals with this genotype are less likely to get certain diseases and are a "little more fit" than the rest of the population (Jorgensen, 1977: 743). Lelashvili and Dalakishvili (1984) examined 11 red cell and three serum protein loci by electrophoresis in a population of 585 individuals from Abkhasian and Imeretian in Georgia. They found considerable polymorphism at these loci; only two loci were monomorphic. The two populations are in Hardy–Weinberg equilibrium, and do not differ significantly from neighboring populations. There is also no relationship between heterozygosity and age. Although there were some fluctuations in frequencies in various age groups, these were considered to be random events. Kuznetsova (1987) has examined chromosome polymorphisms in the C heterochromatin region in two populations from Abhasia and the Ukraine. Long-lived males were characterized by a large C segment on the Y-chromosome and a long Y-chromosome, while long-lived females have a relatively small-sized C segment on chromosome 9. Buckton et al. (1976), sampling individuals in Edinburgh, and Tsoneva et al. (1980, see Kuznetsova, 1987), sampling individuals from Bulgaria, have also found large C blocks on the Y-chromosome in aged individuals.

Smith (cited in Holden, 1987), working on chromosome polymorphism in another area of the world, found a deletion in the arm of the Y-chromosome in long-lived males in an Amish family. Sturgeon *et al.* (1969), in an examination of a population in southeastern Turkey, found an increased frequency of type P and Le(a−b−) in senescent individuals. Takata *et al.* (1987) also found a high incidence of DR-1 and a low incidence of DRw9 in the HLA system in Japanese centenarians (see "Biomarkers," pp. 76–79).

A multi-disciplinary study of aging and longevity in a Mennonite community in Kansas and Nebraska was conducted by Crawford and Rogers (1982). Community records date from its founding in the early 1600s to the population's emigration to the United States in 1874, and continue to the present. Blood samples were taken from 652 individuals, 360 females and 292 males, typed for red blood cell antigens. Heterozygosity levels for eight loci are high, 0.44–0.48, but these levels are independent of age. There are no significant statistical differences in frequencies between young and old groups of people.

Thus, there do not seem to be any populations where individuals routinely live longer than the proposed 100 year maximum and as yet there do not appear to be any easily discernible genetic markers in longevous humans.


## CONCLUSIONS

We have presented several theories of aging and the very limited information on genetics and aging in human populations. Regardless of the molecular mechanisms underlying aging, humans do have a maximum life span. The likelihood of reaching this maximum is dependent on genetic factors such as susceptibility to diseases and environmental stresses. The genetic predisposition for long life thus seems to depend on not having genes that will cause an early death. However, to date, the population perspective of anthropology and the fact that anthropology considers intra- and inter-population variability has not been applied to any significant degree. Opportunities to do so abound, in terms of allelic variability in allozymes such as SOD, histocompatibility loci, and oncogenes or in polygenic systems such as those that define susceptibility to arteriosclerosis or diabetes.


## REFERENCES

Abbott, M. H., Abbey, H., Bolling, D. R. and Murphy, E. A. (1978) The familial component in longevity—A study of offspring of nonagenarians: III Intrafamilial studies. *American Journal of Medical Genetics* 2, 105–120.

Ames, B. N., Saul, R. L., Schwiers, E., Adelman, R. and Cathcart, R. (1985) Oxidative DNA damage as related to cancer and aging: assay of thymine glycol, thymidine glycol, and, hydroxymethyluracil in human and rat urine. In: *Molecular Biology of Aging: Gene Stability and Gene Expression* (eds Sohal, R. S., Birnhaum, L. S. and Cutler, R. G.). New York: Raven Press, pp. 137–144.

Arking, R. (1987a) Genetic and environmental determinants of longevity in *Drosophila*. *Basic Life Sciences* **42**, 1–22.

Arking, R. (1987b) Successful selection for increased longevity in *Drosophila*: analysis of the survival data and presentation of a hypothesis of the genetic regulation of longevity. *Experimental Gerontology* **22**, 199–220.

Arking, R. (1988) Genetic analyses of aging processes in *Drosophila*. *Experimental Aging Research* **14**, 125–135.

Arking, R. and Dudas, S. P. (1989) Review of genetic investigations into the aging processes of *Drosophila*. *Journal of the American Geriatrics Society* **37**, 757–773.

Arking, R., Buck, S., Wells, R. A. and Pretzlaff, R. (1988) Metabolic rates in genetically based long lived strains of *Drosophila*. *Experimental Gerontology* **23**, 59–76.

Bank, L. and Jarvik, L. F. (1978) A longitudinal study of aging human twins. In: *The Genetics of Aging* (ed. Schneider, E. L.). New York: Plenum Press, pp. 303–333.

Beeton, M. and Pearson, K. (1899) Data for the problem of evolution in man. II. A first study of the inheritance of longevity and the selective death-rate in man. *Proceedings of the Royal Society London* **65**, 290–305.

Bell, A. G. (1918) *The Duration of Life and Conditions Associated with Longevity. A Study of the Hyde Genealogy*. Washington, DC: Genealogical Record Office.

Bell, E., Marek, L. F., Levinstone, D. S., Merrill, C., Sher, S., Young, I. T. and Eden, M. (1978) Loss of division potential *in vitro*: aging or differentiation. *Science* **202**, 1158–1163.

Bewley, G. C., Mackay, W. J. and Cook, J. L. (1986) Temporal variation for the expression of catalase in *Drosophila melanogaster*: correlations between rates of enzyme synthesis and levels of translatable catalase messenger RNA. *Genetics* **113**, 919–938.

Bocquet-Appel, J.-P. and Jakobi, L. (1990) Familial transmission of longevity. *Annals of Human Biology* **17**, 81–95.

Bowden, D. M., Short, R. and Williams, D. D. (1990) Constructing an instrument to measure the rate of aging in female pigtailed macaques (*Macaca nemestrina*). *Journal of Gerontology* **45**, 59–66.

Brace, C. L. (1963) Structural reduction in evolution. *American Naturalist* **97**, 39–50.

Bucala, R., Model, P., Russel, M. and Cerami, A. (1985) Modification of DNA by glucose-6-phosphate induces DNA rearrangements in a *E. coli* plasmid. *Proceedings of the National Academy of Sciences USA* **82**, 8439–8442.

Buckton, K. E., O'Riordan, M. L., Jacobs, P. A., Robinson, J. A., Hill, R. and Evans, H. J. (1976) C- and Q-band polymorphisms in the chromosomes of three human populations. *Annals of Human Genetics* **40**, 99–112.

Buffon (Leclerc, G. L., comte de) (1749) *Histoire naturelle, generale et particuliere*. Paris: Imprimerie Royale.

Bunn, H. and Higgins, P. J. (1981) Reaction of monosaccharides with proteins: possible evolutionary significance. *Science* **213**, 222–224.

Campbell, S. D., Hilliker, A. J. and Phillips, J. P. (1986) Cytogenetic analysis of the cSOD microregion in *Drosophila melanogaster*. *Genetics* **112**, 205–215.

Cerami, A., Vlassara, H. and Brownlee, M. (1987) Glucose and aging. *Scientific American* **256**, 90–96.

Cohen, B. H. (1964) Family patterns of mortality and life span. *Quarterly Review of Biology* **39**, 130–181.

Crawford, M. H. and Rogers, L. (1982) Population genetic models in the study of aging and longevity in a Mennonite community. *Social Science and Medicine* **16**, 149–153.

Cutler, R. G. (1975) Evolution of human longevity and the genetic complexity governing aging rate. *Proceedings of the National Academy of Sciences USA* **72**, 4664–4668.

Czelusniak, J., Goodman, M., Hewett-Emmett, D., Weiss, M. L., Venta, P. J. and Tashian, R. E. (1982) Phylogenetic origins and adaptive evolution of avian and mammalian haemoglobin genes. *Nature* **298**, 297–300.

Florini, J. R. (1981) *CRC Handbook of Biochemistry in Aging*. Boca Raton, FL: CRC Press.

Friedman, D. B. and Johnson, T. E. (1988) A mutation in the *age-1* gene in *Caenorhabditis elegans* lengthens life and reduces hermaphrodite fertility. *Genetics* **118**, 75–86.

Goldstein, S. (1990) Replicative senescence: the human fibroblast comes of age. *Science* **249**, 1129–1133.

Goldstein, S., Murano, S. and Shmookler Reis, R. J. (1990) Werner syndrome: a molecular genetic hypothesis. *Journal of Gerontology: Biological Sciences* **45**, B3–B8.

Harman, D. (1956) Aging: a theory based on free radical and radiation chemistry. *Journal of Gerontology* **11**, 298–300.

Harman, D. (1983) Free radical theory of aging: consequences of mitochondrial aging. *Age* **6**, 86–94.

Harman, D. (1984) Free radicals and the origination and, evolution, and present status of the free radical theory of aging. In: *Free Radicals in Molecular Biology, Aging, and Disease* (eds Armstrong, D., Sohal, R. S., Cutler, R. G. and Slater, T. F.). New York: Raven Press, pp. 1–12.

Harrison, D. E. and Archer, J. R. (1987) Genetic effects on responses to food restriction in aging mice. *Journal of Nutrition* **117**, 376–382.

Harrison, D. E. and Archer, J. R. (1988) Biomarkers of aging: tissue markers, future research needs, strategies, directions and priorities. *Experimental Gerontology* **23**, 309–321.

Hauge, M. and Harvald, B. (1961) Malignant growths in twins. *Acta Genetica et Statistica Medica* **11**, 372–378.

Hayflick, L. (1965) The limited *in vitro* lifetime of human diploid cell strains. *Experimental Cell Research* **37**, 614–636.

Hayflick, L. (1987) Origins of longevity. In: *Modern Biological Theories of Aging* (eds Warner, H. R., Butler, R. N., Sprott, R. L. and Schneider, E. L.). New York: Raven Press, pp. 21–34.

Hayflick, L. and Morehead, P. S. (1961) The serial cultivation of human diploid cell strains. *Experimental Cell Research* **25**, 585–621.

Holden, C. (1987) Why do women live longer than men? *Science* **238**, 158–160.

Holliday, R. (1986) Testing molecular theories of cellular aging. In: *Dimensions in Aging* (eds Bergener, M., Ermini, M. and Stahelin, H. B.). New York: Academic Press, pp. 21–34.

Holmes, S. J. (1928) Age at parenthood, order of birth, and parental longevity in relation to the longevity of offspring. *University of California Publications in Zoology* **31**, 359–375.

Ingram, D. K. (1990) Perspectives of genetic variability in behavioral aging of mice. In: *Genetic Effects on Aging II* (ed. Harrison, D. E.), W. Caldwell, NJ: Telford, pp. 205–231.

Ingram, D. K. and Reynolds, M. A. (1982) The relationship of genotype, sex, body weight, and growth parameters to lifespan in inbred and hybrid mice. *Mechanisms of Ageing and Development* **20**, 253–266.

Jalavisto, E. (1951) Inheritance of longevity according to Finnish and Swedish genealogies. *Annales Medicae Internae Fenniae* **40**, 263–274.

Johnson, T. E. (1987) Aging can be genetically dissected into component processes using long-lived lines of *Caenorhabditis elegans*. *Proceedings of the National Academy of Sciences USA* **84**, 3777–3781.

Johnson, T. E. (1990) Increased life-span of age-1 mutants in *Caenorhabditis elegans* and lower Gompertz rate of aging. *Science* **249**, 908–912.

Johnson, T. E. and Wood, W. B. (1982) Genetic analysis of life-span in *Caenorhabditis elegans*. *Proceedings of the National Academy of Sciences USA* **79**, 6603–6607.

Johnson, T. E., Friedman, D. B., Fitzpatrick, P. A. and Conley, W. L. (1987) Mutant genes that extend life span. *Basic Life Sciences* **42**, 91–100.

Johnson, T. E., Conley, W. L. and Keller, M. L. (1988) Long-lived lines of *Caenorhabditis elegans* can be used to establish predictive biomarkers of aging. *Experimental Gerontology* **23**, 281–295.

Jorgensen, G. (1977) A contribution to the hypothesis of a "little more fitness" of blood group O. *Journal of Human Evolution* **6**, 741–743.

Kallman, F. J. and Sander, G. (1949) Twin studies on senescence. *American Journal of Psychiatry* **106**, 29–36.

Kelly, K. W., Brief, S., Westly, H. J., Novakofski, J., Bechtel, P. J., Simon, J. and Walker, E. R. (1987) Hormonal regulation of the age-associated decline in immune function. *Annals of the New York Academy of Sciences* **496**, 91–97.

Kipshidze, N. N., Pivovarova, I. P., Dzorbenadze, D. A., Agadzanov, A. S. and Shavgulidze, N. A. (1987) The longevous people of Soviet Georgia. In: *Realistic Expectations for Long Life* (ed. Lesnoff-Caravaglia, G.). New York: Human Sciences Press, pp. 83–110.

Kirkwood, J. L. (1985) Comparative and evolutionary aspects of longevity. In: *Handbook of the Biology of Aging, 2nd edn* (eds Finch, C. E. and Schneider, E. L.). New York: Van Nostrand Reinhold, pp. 27–42.

Kirkwood, J. L. (1989) Evolution and aging. *Genome* **31**, 398–405.

Koenig, R. J., Peterson, C. M., Kilo, C. and Cerami, A. (1976) Hemoglobin $A_{IC}$ as an indicator of the degree of glucose intolerance in diabetes. *Diabetes* **31** (Suppl.) 47–51.

Koop, B. F., Tagle, D. A., Goodman, M. and Slightom, J. L. (1989) A molecular view of primate phylogeny and important systematic and evolutionary questions. *Molecular Biology and Evolution* **6**, 580–612.

Kuznetsova, S. M. (1987) Polymorphism of heterochromatin areas on chromosomes 1, 9, 16, and Y in long lived subjects and persons of different ages in two regions of the Soviet Union. *Archives of Gerontology and Geriatrics* **6**, 177–186.

Leaf, A. (1973) Getting old. *Scientific American* **229**, 45–52.

Leaf, A. (1975) *Youth in Old Age*. New York: McGraw-Hill.

Lelashvili, N. G. and Dalakishvili, S. M. (1984) Genetic study of high longevity index populations. *Mechanisms of Ageing and Development* **28**, 261–271.

Lints, F. A. (1989) The rate of living theory revisited. *Gerontology* **35**, 36–57.

Luckinbill, L. S., Arking, R., Clare, M. J., Cirocco, W. C. and Buck, S. (1984) Selection for delayed senescence in *Drosophila melanogaster*. *Evolution* **38**, 996–1003.

Martin, G. M. (1988) Constitutional genetic markers of aging. *Experimental Gerontology* **23**, 257–267.

Martin, G. M., Sprague, C. A., Norwood, T. H. and Pendergrass, W. R. (1974) Clonal selection, attenuation and differentiation in an *in vitro* model of hyperplasia. *American Journal of Pathology* **74**, 137–154.

Masaro, J. (1981) *CRC Handbook of Physiology in Aging.* Boca Raton, FL: CRC Press.

Mazess, R. B. and Forman, S. H. (1979) Longevity and age exaggeration in Vilcabamba, Ecuador. *Journal of Gerontology* **34**, 94–98.

Medvedev, Z. A. (1974) Caucasus and Altay longevity: a biological or social problem. *The Gerontologist* **14**, 381–387.

Meredith, P. J. and Walford, R. L. (1977) Effect of age on response to T- and B-cell mitogens in mice congenic at the H-2 locus. *Immunogenetics* **5**, 109.

Meyer, T. E., Armstrong, M. J. and Warner, C. M. (1989) Effects of H-2 haplotype and gender on the lifespan of A and C57BL/6 mice and their F1, F2, and backcross offspring. *Growth, Development and Aging* **53**, 175–183.

Miller, R. A. (1989) The cell biology of aging: immunological models. *Journal of Gerontology: Biological Sciences* **44**, B4–B8.

Mooradian, A. D. (1990) Biomarkers of aging: do we know what to look for? *Journal of Gerontology* **45**, 183–186.

Murphy, E. A. (1978) Genetics of longevity in man. In: *The Genetics of Aging* (ed. Schneider, E. L.). New York; Plenum Press, pp. 261–301.

Myers, R. J. (1965) Analysis of mortality in the Soviet Union according to 1958–59 life tables. *Transactions of Society of Actuaries* **16**, 309–317.

Orgel, L. E. (1963) The maintenance of the accuracy of protein synthesis and its relevance to ageing. *Proceedings of the National Academy of Sciences USA* **67**, 517–521.

Pearl, R. (1928) *The Rate of Living.* London: University of London Press.

Pearl, R. (1931) Longevity: a pedigree. *Human Biology* **3**, 133–137.

Pearl, R. and Pearl, R. D. (1934). *The Ancestry of the Long-Lived.* Baltimore: Johns Hopkins Press.

Phillipe, P. (1978) Familial correlation of longevity: an isolate based study. *American Journal of Medical Genetics* **2**, 121–129.

Preas, S. (1945) Length of life of parents and offspring in a rural community. *Milbank Memorial Fund Quarterly* **23**, 180–196.

Pryor, W. A. (1984) Free radicals in autoxidation and in aging. In: *Free Radicals in Molecular Biology, Aging and Disease* (eds Armstrong, D., Sohal, R. S., Cutler, R. G. and Slater, T. F.). New York: Raven Press, pp. 13–35.

Pryor, W. A. (1987) The free-radical theory of aging revisited: a critique and a suggested disease-specific theory. In: *Modern Biological Theories of Aging* (eds Warner, H. R., Butler, R. N., Sprott, R. L. and Schneider, E. L.). New York: Raven Press, pp. 89–112.

Reff, M. E. and Schneider, E. L. (1982) *Biological Markers of Aging.* US Health and Human Services publication no. 82-2221, Washington, DC.

Rose, C. L. and Bell, B. (1971) *Predicting Longevity.* Lexington, MA: Heath Lexington Books.

Rose, M. R. (1989) Genetics of increased lifespan in *Drosophila. BioEssays* **11**, 132–135.

Rose, M. R. and Charlesworth, B. (1981) Genetics of life history in *Drosophila melanogaster* II. Exploratory selection experiments. *Genetics* **97**, 187–196.

Rose, M. R. and Graves, J. L., Jr (1989) What evolutionary biology can do for gerontology. *Journal of Gerontology: Biological Sciences* **44**, B27–29.

Rothstein, M. (1987) Evidence for and against the error catastrophe hypothesis. In: *Modern Biological Theories of Aging* (eds Warner, H. R., Butler, R. N., Sprott, R. L. and Schneider, E. L.). New York: Raven Press, pp. 139–154.

Russell, E. S. (1966) Lifespan and aging patterns. In: *Biology of the Laboratory Mouse* (ed. Green, E. L.). New York: McGraw-Hill, pp. 511–519.

Russell, R. L. (1987) Evidence for and against the theory of developmentally programmed aging. In: *Modern Biological Theories of Aging* (eds Warner, H. R., Butler, R. N., Sprott, R. L. and Schneider, E. L.). New York: Raven Press, pp. 35–61.

Russell, R. L. and Seppa, R. I. (1990) Effects of single-gene mutations on aging, as measured with biomarkers. In: *Genetic Effects on Aging II* (ed. Harrison, D. E.). W. Caldwell, NJ: Telford Press, pp. 129–152.

Saul, R. L., Gee, P. and Ames, B. N. (1987) Free radicals, DNA damage, and aging. In: *Modern Biological Theories of Aging* (eds Warner, H. R., Butler, R. N., Sprott, R. L. and Schneider, E. L.). New York: Raven Press, pp. 113–129.

Schneider, E. L. and Reed, J. D. (1985) Modulations of aging processes. In: *Handbook of the Biology of Aging*, 2nd edn (ed. Finch, C. E. and Schneider, E. L.). New York: Van Nostrand Reinhold, pp. 45–76.

Shepard, J. C. W., Walldorf, U., Hug, P. and Gehring, W. J. (1989) Fruit flies with additional expression of the elongation factor EF-1alpha live longer. *Proceedings of the National Academy of Sciences USA* **86**, 7520–7521.

Shmookler Reis, R. J. (1988) Strategies and criteria for the development of molecular biomarkers of senescence. *Experimental Gerontology* **23**, 271–280.

Short, R., England, N., Bridson, W. E. and Bowden, D. M. (1989) Ovarian cyclicity, hormones, and behavior as markers of aging in female pigtailed macaques (*Macaca nemestrina*). *Journal of Gerontology* **44**, B131–138.

Smith, D. W. E. and Warner, H. R. (1989) Does genotypic sex have a direct effect on longevity? *Experimental Gerontology* **24**, 277–288.

Smith, J. R. (1990) DNA synthesis inhibitors in cellular senescence. *Journal of Gerontology: Biological Sciences* **45**, B32–B35.

Snowdon, D. A., Kane, R. L., Beeson, L., Burker, G. L., Sprafka, M., Potter, J., Iso, H., Jacobs, D. R. and Phillips, R. L. (1989) Is early natural menopause a biologic marker of health and aging? *American Journal of Public Health* **79**, 709–714.

Sprott, R. L. (1983) Genetic aspects of aging in *Mus musculus*: January 1981–February, 1982. In: *Review of Biological Research in Aging*, Vol. 1 (ed. Rothstein, M.). New York: Alan R. Liss, pp. 73–80.

Sprott, R. L. (1985) Genetic aspects of aging in *Mus musculus*. In: *Review of Biological Research in Aging*, Vol. 2 (ed. Rothstein, M.). New York: Alan R. Liss, pp. 99–104.

Sprott, R. L. (1987) Genetic aspects of aging in *Mus musculus*. In: *Review of Biological Research in Aging*, Vol. 3 (ed. Rothstein, M.). New York: Alan R. Liss, pp. 71–76.

Sprott, R. L. and Combs, C. A. (1990) Genetic aspects of aging in *Mus musculus*. In: *Review of Biological Research in Aging*, Vol. 4 (ed. Rothstein, M.). New York: Wiley–Liss, pp. 73–80.

Stamatoyannopoulos, G. (1991) Human hemoglobin switching. *Science* **252**, 383.

Stein, G. H., Beeson, M. and Gordon, L. (1990) Failure to phosphorylate the retinoblastoma gene product in senescent human fibroblasts. *Science* **249**, 666–669.

Stoessiger, B. (1932) On the inheritance and duration of life and cause of death. *Annals of Eugenics* **5**, 105–178.

Sturgeon, P., Beller, S. and Bates, E. (1969) Study of blood group factors in longevity. *Journal of Gerontology* **24**, 90–95.

Su, C. M., Brash, D. E., Turturro, A. and Hart, R. W. (1984) Longevity-dependent organ-specific accumulation of DNA damage in two closely related murine species. *Mechanisms of Ageing and Development* **27**, 239–247.

Takata, H., Suzuki, M., Ishii, T., Sekiguchi, S. and Iri, H. (1987) Influence of major histocompatibility complex region genes on human longevity among Okinawan-Japanese centenarians and nonagenarians. *Lancet* **2** (8563), 824–826.

Tully, T. (1988) Response to Dr George Martin. *Experimental Gerontology* **23**, 269–270.

Vaupel, J. W. (1988) Inherited frailty and longevity. *Demography* **25**, 277–287.

Waldron, I. (1983) Sex differences in human mortality: the role of genetic factors. *Social Science and Medicine* **17**, 321–333.

Weisman, A. (1891) *Essays upon Heredity and Kindred Biological Problems*, 2nd edn, Vol. 1. Oxford: Clarendon Press.

Wilson, E. B. and Doering, C. R. (1926) The elder Pierces. *Proceedings of the National Academy of Sciences USA* **12**, 424–432.

Wright, K. (1988) Nature, nurture and death. *Scientific American* **258**, 34–38.

Yuan, I. C. (1931) Life tables for a southern Chinese family from 1365 to 1849. *Human Biology* **3**, 157–159.

Yuan, I. C. (1932) The influence of heredity upon the duration of life in man based on a Chinese genealogy from 1365 to 1914. *Human Biology* **4**, 41–68.

Zonneveld, R. J., van and Polman, A. (1957) Hereditary factors in longevity. *Acta Genetica et Statistica Medica* **7**, 160–162.

# 4

# Cousin Marriage and the X-Chromosome: Evolution of Longevity and Language

## SOLOMON H. KATZ AND DAVID F. ARMSTRONG

### INTRODUCTION

One of the most important and consistent findings concerning the human life cycle is the presence of an extended period of postreproductive longevity. Evidence for the universality and antiquity of this phenomenon includes the following: a nearly universal cross-cultural distribution of terms for grandparents, widespread potential for the significant expression of postreproductive longevity in modern societies lacking medical care, and fossil evidence for postreproductive longevity in prehistoric societies. However, the evolutionary basis for this human biological phenomenon continues to be debated.

Although random mating is a major feature of evolutionary models, its role in human evolutionary population genetics has always been in question because of evidence from contemporary hunters and gatherers suggesting that most of human evolution took place under conditions of restricted population size in association with processes of random drift and socially defined inbreeding. Random drift and inbreeding have a long and well-developed literature, beginning with the earlier works of Sewall Wright and Haldane. However, it was not until the initial insights of Hamilton (1964), the further refinements of Trivers (1971), and the application of their theories to humans that the concept of kin selection was successfully applied to the evaluation of selective advantages accruing to various kinds of social relations among humans.

Evolutionary theory generally suggests that, within a population, gene frequency changes due to selection are always large when compared with chance. However, in order for this statement to be true, the population must be large, the selection must not be weak, and the alleles in question must not be rare. In human populations, dispersal and geographic isolation often limit an individual's choice of mates to a small group of related neighbors within the surrounding locality. Thus, instead of natural selection, the potential effects of inbreeding and random drift may become the major sources of genetic variation. Hence, in accounting for population shifts under these conditions, a larger role for neutral or chance changes in gene frequencies is favored over natural selection. (This is not to say that natural selection is an unimportant source of change in human populations, but that the frequency with which genetic change can be explained as a direct consequence of natural selection is less common than was previously believed.)

While non-random mating is one of the hallmarks of human populations, it is usually complicated by various social rules and customs regulating marriage. The widespread distribution of kinship systems that prescribe and proscribe marriage patterns has been a major topic of study throughout the history of anthropology (see Lévi-Strauss, 1969). Moreover, universalities of kinship ordinarily relate closely to the structure of social and economic obligation, and to cooperation between relatives, often resulting in care of relatives that is translatable in evolutionary terms to differential survival rates of descendants. Within the context of natural selection and random drift as important mechanisms for promoting genetic variation, the combination of prescribed and proscribed patterns of mating plays an enormous role in accounting for the distribution of genes within a population. To summarize, in human populations mating is not always random; it often operates within small isolated groups; it is often directed by proscriptive or prescriptive social conditions; these conditions often involve uneven distribution of care to specified descendants.

Moreover, selection can act on groups rather than individuals. Trivers (1971) has proposed the term "reciprocal altruism" to denote the component of enhanced fitness that emerges from behavioral interaction among cooperating related individuals. Empirical approaches such as the hypothetical "prisoner's dilemma" illustrate the potential effects of group selection. The relationship between the concepts of group selection and kin selection is clear. "Inclusive fitness" as proposed by Hamilton defines the condition that occurs when the survival of an offspring produced by one individual is enhanced by the behavior of its close genetic relatives—that is, finite numbers define the probabilities that offspring will be carrying copies of the particular chromosomes of those relatives.

This concept can be applied to the effects of X-chromosome inheritance, in which there are both male haploids and female diploids. X-expression in the next generation is equal in both sexes; because, although an X-linked gene in a female is transmitted to only half of her offspring and a gene in a male is transmitted to all of his daughters (but none of his sons), the female has twice as many offspring who can carry her chromosome as does the male.

However, when we consider the situation one generation removed (i.e., the grandparental generation), this equality among females no longer holds. In societies where grandmothers play a substantial role in the rearing of granddaughters and where through social prescription they live with their sons, it becomes significant that the son's daughter has a 100% chance of having at least one of the grandmother's X-chromosomes, while the daughter's daughter has only a 50% such chance. In cases where the grandmother lives with the son and cares for his children, there is an obvious advantage accruing to traits carried on her X-chromosomes. This suggests a conceptual framework for generating and testing hypotheses about the evolutionary effects of a grandmother's care, and hence the factors that might extend her lifespan, especially if any of those can be shown to be determined by alleles carried on the X-chromosome.

This latter point, in turn, suggests a variety of questions that we address in this paper: How large are these effects and what are their implications for the co-evolution of kinship systems and enhanced longevity? Are there other features of human behavior—the capacity for language, for example—that might have evolved simultaneously and that might involve similar genetic mechanisms? How could such systems have begun during the course of human evolution? What are the implications of these questions for established theories of social organization, predicated as they are upon the separation of human society from human biology? Finally, are there X-linked candidate genes with a potential for supporting this entire complex?


## METHODS OF CONSIDERATION

In order to investigate the degree to which the distribution of X-chromosomes between grandmothers and subsequent generations of their descendants might be influenced by kinship practices, we evaluated the genetic structures implied by several forms of prescribed or preferred cousin marriage that have been documented in the anthropological literature. Cousin marriage has been widely practiced among contemporary societies. Murdock's (1967) ethnographic atlas contains data on a stratified sample of societies that are described in the world ethnographic literature, and some form of cousin marriage is reported for nearly one half of these societies.

In particular, we have developed statistical models for analyzing the probabilistic effects of various patterns of cousin marriage with respect to the transmission of the X-chromosome and, implicitly, the likelihood that individual females will be able to make social investments in descendants who possess their X-chromosomes. These socially prescribed or preferred marriage patterns, particularly those involving the marriage of cross-cousins, are shown to have a significant impact on the ability of women to influence the transmission of their X-chromosomes in the grandchildren's generation and beyond. This effect has profound implications for the rate and direction of evolution of traits determined by X-chromosome loci.

There have been numerous interpretations of cousin marriage, from both sociological (e.g., Lévi-Strauss, 1969) and sociobiological (e.g., Alexander, 1979) points of view. We believe that our findings will add substantially to the understanding of this phenomenon as well as to the understanding of the evolution of the X-chromosome. We will show, in turn, that the evolution of the X-chromosome is related to the evolution of two uniquely human traits, postreproductive longevity and language, through the mediation of X-chromosome loci. More specifically, we will show that the selective advantages conferred by the capacity for language and longevity are mutually reinforcing through a positive feedback mechanism that involves cousin marriage.

In the discussion that follows, we will develop further the argument that systems of kinship and preferential marriage can act as mechanisms for influencing the genetic structures of small-scale social groups. This is clearly true in the case of incest avoidance within the nuclear family, but we argue that it may also be true of systems that favor marriage with certain relatives outside the nuclear family, particularly with respect to patterns of transmission of the sex chromosomes. Because of their asymmetrical distribution between males and females, it is possible to trace the inheritance of the X- and Y-chromosomes in ways that are not possible with the autosomal chromosomes.

Many previous interpretations of the genetic consequences of cousin marriage and inheritance patterns have tended to focus on the point of view of males and their probabilities of enhancing their selective fitness (e.g., Alexander, 1979). It has more recently been suggested that it may be productive to analyze such systems from the female point of view, particularly from the point of view of grandmothers. Hartung (1985: 666) has made this point succinctly: "The advantage of matrilineal inheritance is especially important to women because female mammals attain exceptional reproductive success primarily through their male offspring . . . [E]very mother with extraordinary sons has an extraordinary number of grandchildren." It is also worth noting that grandmothers are evolutionary veterans and are not species specific—there is abundant evidence of multi-generational matrilines among non-human primates (Cheney and Seyfarth, 1990: 25). We will analyze the effects of various patterns of cousin marriage from the multi-generational perspective of grandmothers and greatgrandmothers with respect to the transmission of their X-chromosomes.

To support our principal hypothesis, we will consider a particular X-linked locus involved in the action of the adrenal androgen dehydroepiandrosterone sulfate (DHEAS).

## STEROID SULFATASE AND THE TRANSMISSION OF THE X-CHROMOSOME

Katz *et al.* (1985) have proposed that DHEAS has a significant impact on the timing of gonadarche and apparently also on the maturation of the Central Nervous System during language acquisition and, finally, on the maintenance of postreproductive life span. Aside from its apparent importance in the development and maintenance of the human life cycle, DHEAS is also highly significant to our argument because the gene for steroid sulfatase, the enzyme controlling the conversion of DHEAS to the more active form DHEA, is on a very recently evolved portion of the X-chromosome.

Because of its location of the X-chromosome, DHEA's importance in the development and maintenance of the human life cycle will vary noticeably between the sexes—females of a population (who have twice as many X-chromosomes as males) control the evolution of X-linked traits but exhibit only partial (they may be heterozygous for the trait) or no (if it is inactivated or Lyonnized) X-chromosome expression. Males, on the other hand, have full expression of the traits on their single X-chromosome. As we suggested above, X-linkage is also highly significant in that its unique hemizygous mechanism of transmission to males may allow females in the grandparental and great grandparental generations to maximize their selective fitness with respect to traits carried on the X-chromosome through specific systems of kinship and marriage.

The possibility that grandparents could control the transmission of their X-chromosomes through systems of kinship and marriage acquires added significance when we note that the X and Y chromosomes of humans and chimpanzees have undergone rapid evolution (Yen *et al.*, 1988). In particular, the locus controlling steroid sulfatase activity is on the part of the X-chromosome that seems to have undergone the most radical evolutionary changes. In humans and chimps (but not other mammals) the gene controlling sulfatase activity is on the non-pseudoautosomal region of the X-chromosome and is not subject to the Lyon effect. Therefore, differences will automatically be expressed in males but, if recessive, must be in double dose to be expressed in females. Furthermore, among males there can be no crossing over of this segment of the X-chromosome with loci on the Y chromosome, since there is no homologous segment on the Y. Therefore, in males, the X-linked gene products from this region that are transmitted to the daughter must be the same as those that the father obtained from his mother.

Given the species specificity of the secretion of DHEAS, its important physiological correlates, and the unique evolutionary history of the X-linked steroid sulfatase locus, we have begun to study the (at least theoretical) effects that would be produced on the transmission of X-chromosomes in various forms of preferential marriage—in particular, those systems favoring matri-lateral or patrilateral cross-cousin marriage. These marriage systems are highly significant because they have been widely practiced in small-scale societies. We take our cue here from Lévi-Strauss (1969: 108), who points out, in a remarkable passage, that the human genome, in the causation of sex differences by the X- and Y-chromosomes, has a dual structure that mirrors in some ways the dual organizations of many human societies.

However, in developing the idea that an explanation of cross-cousin marriage might be used to form the cornerstone of a theory of human social structure, he goes on to assert that any explanation of this phenomenon must be purely sociological, because the degrees of kinship involved in any possible union of first cousins "are equivalent from a biological point of view." We will show that this assumption with respect to the X-chromosome is incorrect from the point of view of women, especially grandmothers.

## THE ELEMENTARY STRUCTURES OF KINSHIP

Central to Lévi-Strauss's sociological theory is the isolation of patterns of prescriptive or preferential (he makes no distinction between the two) cross-cousin marriage that can be described as atomic or elementary. These systems may be viewed as threefold: matrilateral, patrilateral, or bilateral. In addition, cousins may be classified as matri- or patrilateral parallel cousins. Figure 4-1 illustrates the types of first cousins. Note that parallel cousins are those descended from same-sex siblings and cross-cousins are those descended

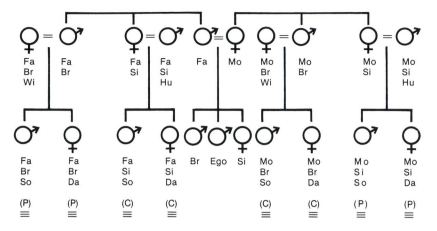

**Figure 4-1**   First cousin taxonomy. P = parallel; C = cross. From Honigman (1959: 386). Reprinted by permission of HarperCollins Publishers, Inc.

from opposite-sex siblings. From male ego's point of view, his matrilateral cousins are those related to him through his mother, and his relationships to his patrilateral cousins are through his father. In Figure 4-2, we illustrate a bilateral cross-cousin marriage system—the classic Kariera type—in which the matri- and patrilateral cross-cousins would structurally be the same person.

Lévi-Strauss states that these cousins are equivalent from a biological point of view, meaning that any pair of first cousins, whether matrilateral, patrilateral, cross or parallel, has the same coefficient of relationship, $\frac{1}{16}$ or 0.0625. This means, in turn, that with respect to any particular chromosome, first cousins have a probability of 0.0625 of being identical by descent (Haldane and Jayakar, 1962). However, this assumption is only correct from the point of view of the cousins themselves and with respect only to the autosomal chromosomes. We will take the point of view of women with respect to the probability that various of their descendants will have at least one of their X-chromosomes.

As we pointed out above, the sex chromosomes in the male are hemizygous. Therefore, it is critically important to know the location of males in the chain of offspring leading from a female to a particular descendant. The reason for this is simple: males cannot transmit X-chromosomes to their sons and they have only one X-chromosome to transmit to their daughters—that which they received from their mothers. Therefore, males act as gateways in the transmission of X-chromosomes (Figure 4-3).

It has long been known that the coefficient of inbreeding has to be calculated differently for the sex chromosomes than for the autosomal chromosomes, for the reasons outlined above (Haldane and Moshinsky, 1939; Haldane and Jayakar, 1962). In particular, Haldane and Moshinsky (1939; Haldane and Jayakar, 1962) have calculated coefficients of inbreeding with respect to the X-chromosome for the female offspring of cousins involved in various types of cousin marriage (this coefficient has the same value as the

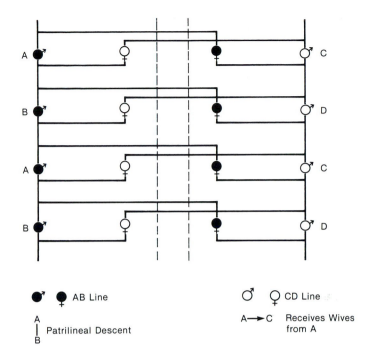

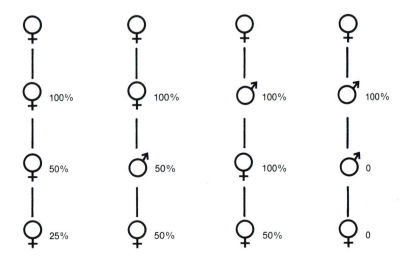

**Figure 4-2** Idealized bilateral marriage system: the Kariera System. From Livingstone (1959: 363). Reprinted by permission of the *Journal of Anthropological Research* and Dr Frank Livingstone.

**Figure 4-3** Possible pathways of transmission of X-chromosomes: great-grandmother to great-granddaughter (probabilities of inheriting at least one of GGM's X-chromosomes).

**Table 4-1**  X-linked coefficients of relationship[a] (=X-linked inbreeding coefficients for female offspring).

|                              |         |
| ---------------------------- | ------- |
| Bilateral cross-cousins      | 18.75%  |
| Matrilateral parallel cousins | 18.75% |
| Matrilateral cross-cousins   | 12.50%  |
| Patrilateral parallel cousins | 0.00%  |
| Patrilateral cross-cousins   | 0.00%   |

[a]This terminology has been used in a variety of ways.
We follow the usage in Haldane and Jayakar (1962).

coefficient of relationship for the parents and is undefined for males, as males have only one X-chromosome) (see Table 4-1). We have added a coefficient for "bilateral cross-cousins," calculated according to the Kariera-type model and assuming the genetic relatedness of the founding sibships (see footnote 1, Table 4-4). Under the given assumptions, the value of this coefficient is the same as that for matrilateral parallel cousins. In all of these cases, the coefficient of inbreeding depends critically upon the numbers of males and females in each pathway of descent leading from the common ancestor.

Coefficients of inbreeding have to do with the increased probability that an inbred marriage will produce offspring who are homozygous at particular loci. We take a different perspective—one that considers the probability that a particular woman's X-chromosomes will be present in various of her descendants. The method of calculating this probability is conceptually similar to the method of calculating inbreeding coefficients for the X-chromosome.

Consider a matrilateral cross-cousin marriage. In general, the probability that a child will inherit one of his or her ancestor's chromosomes is halved for each generation the child is removed from the ancestor. As we explained above, this is not the case with the sex chromosomes. The possible pathways of descent of the X-chromosome and the associated probabilities of inheriting at least one of the founding woman's X-chromosomes are presented in Figure 4-4. Note that the probabilities associated with the various pathways are radically different depending upon whether the donor and the recipient are male or female. Note also that these pathways assume no inbreeding, that is, they assume random mating at the outset. The situation becomes more complicated at the point where the marriage partners are inbred—in Figure 4-4, the point at which the cousins marry.

In general, we need to have more detailed knowledge concerning the possible sex-chromosome combinations for each of the people, in each of the pathways. Starting with the founding couple, the female's X-chromosomes are labeled $X_1$ and $X_2$, and the male's X-chromosome is labeled X. The possible combinations of X-chromosomes in their offspring are as shown in Figure 4-4 (in this and succeeding generations, any X-chromosome not from the founding female is labeled simply X). The probabilities that each descendant will have at least one of the founding woman's X-chromosomes are given as percentages. These individuals produce the matrilateral cross-cousins in the third tier of Figure 4-4. Finally, the offspring of the matrilateral cross-cousins have the possible combinations of X-chromosomes shown in the bottom tier of the

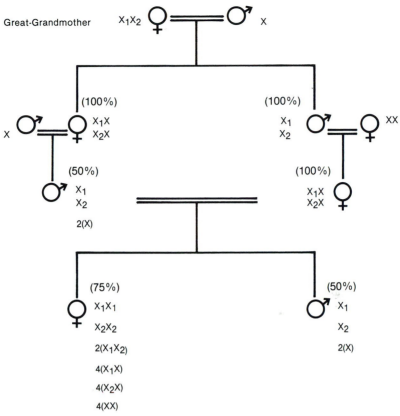

**Figure 4-4**  Transmission of the X-chromosome: matrilateral cross-cousin marriage (probability of inheriting one of founding woman's X-chromosomes).

figure. The probability that a female produced by this union will have at least one of the great-grandmother's X-chromosomes is thus $12/16$ or 0.75 and the probability that she will actually be identical (share the same two chromosomes) with her great-grandmother ($X_1X_2$) is $2/16$ or 0.125.

We have also calculated these probabilities for the patrilateral cross-cousin pattern. Compared to the patrilateral pattern, the probability is greatly increased for a woman's great-granddaughters, in the ideal situation, by rules favoring matrilateral cross-cousin marriage. In fact, the probability of inheriting one of great-grandmother's X chromosomes is three times higher in the matrilateral (0.75) than in the patrilateral pattern (0.25—Figure 4-5).

In cases where there is no inbreeding prior to the marriage of the first cousins, these probabilities can be calculated according to simple formulas. As we show in Figure 4-3, there are simple rules for calculating the decreasing probability of having the founding woman's X-chromosome among the various possible non-inbred lines of descent. At the point where the first cousins marry, the following rules apply for calculating the probabilities that their male and female offspring will have one of the great-grandmother's X-chromosomes. Male offspring cannot inherit X-chromosomes from their fathers, so their

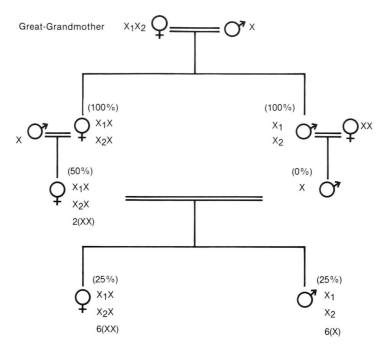

**Figure 4-5**   Transmission of the X-chromosome: patrilateral cross-cousin marriage (probability of inheriting one of founding woman's X-chromosomes).

probability is simply the female cousin's probability reduced by one half, or $P_{GGS} = 1/2P_{FC}$, where $P_{GGS}$ is the probability that the great-grandson will have one of the founding woman's X-chromosomes and $P_{FC}$ is the same probability for his mother, the female cousin. The situation for the great-granddaughters is more complicated. In general, their probability is the sum of the probabilities associated with inheritance from their mothers and fathers, i.e., ½ from their mothers, and 1 from their fathers. However, this must be reduced by the probability of inheriting one of the founding woman's X-chromosomes from both parents. The overall formula can be written as follows: $P_{GGD} = (P_{MC} + \frac{1}{2}P_{FC}) - \frac{1}{2}P_{MC}P_{FC}$, where MC = male cousin.

We have also examined the probabilities that would be produced by a bilateral cross-cousin marriage rule in its simplest, or Kariera-type, form, in which the matri- and patrilateral cross-cousins are structurally the same person. In this last analysis, we have employed the formal model of Livingstone (1959). Note that in this pattern, the probabilities are slightly enhanced over those produced by the matrilateral situation (Table 4-2). This is true because we must assume that a woman's brother may have one of her X-chromosomes (see above concerning calculation of the inbreeding coefficient).

It is important also to discuss the probabilities of inheritance of X-chromosomes under various pathways that would be encountered under conditions of random assortment. In Figure 4-6, we outline the separate pathways that make up the matri- and patrilateral cross-cousin marriage

**Table 4-2** Probabilities that great-grandchildren will have at least one of great-grandmother's X-chromosomes.

|  | Female (%) | Male (%) | Average (%) |
|---|---|---|---|
| Bilateral cross-cousins | 81.25 | 62.50 | 71.88 |
| Matrilateral cross-cousins | 75.00 | 50.00 | 62.50 |
| Patrilateral parallel cousins | 50.00 | 50.00 | 50.00 |
| Matrilateral parallel cousins | 62.50 | 25.00 | 43.75 |
| Patrilateral cross-cousins | 25.00 | 25.00 | 25.00 |

patterns. The probability of appearance of at least one of the founding grandmother's X-chromosomes in each of the descendants is that which would occur under strict patterns of random mating. Note that the average of the probabilities under these pathways is always less than that which would occur if marriage had been with the particular cross-cousin. Note also that the average for the random mating pathways in the matrilateral pattern is greater than the probabilities inherent in the *actual* patrilateral cross-cousin marriage system.

There is a complicating factor that we have not considered here—the possible effect on these probabilities that would result from the presence of general inbreeding within small-scale populations. We have not considered this

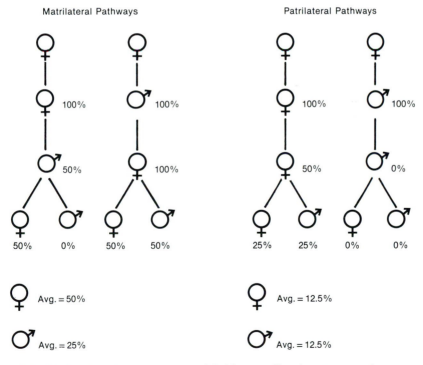

**Figure 4-6** Probability that great-grandchildren will inherit one of a woman's X-chromosomes with random mating and assuming separate pathways involved in matrilateral and patrilateral cross-cousin marriage.

effect, because our purpose here is to discuss the formal properties of these systems and to view them as reproductive strategies for females, with respect to their own chromosomes.

There is another genetic question that needs to be discussed—under any of the systems of marriage that we have discussed, women may have great-grandchildren other than those that result from the cousin pairs we have been considering. For example, note (Figure 4-5) that, in the patrilateral cross-cousin pattern, the founding woman's son's daughter has a 100% probability of having one of her X-chromosomes. However, she might choose to marry another one of her grandmother's grandchildren; and, even if she marries an unrelated man, her children will still have a 50% probability of having one of the great-grandmother's X-chromosomes. The advantage to her grandmother that the matrilateral pattern conveys is the increased chance that she will marry her cross-cousin and that their daughter's probability of having one of the grandmother's X-chromosomes will increase to 75%. This underscores the importance of patrilocality and the son's daughter in enhancing the effectiveness of kin investment for the grandmother. With patrilocal residence, the founding woman has an increased chance of making a social investment in her son's daughter, who *must* have one of her X-chromosomes. Matrilateral cross-cousin marriage further enhances any such investment by the grandmother, because her son's daughter marries a man who has a 50% chance of having one of her X-chromosomes.

We have also calculated these probabilities for matri- and patrilateral parallel cousins, possible marriage patterns that do not figure in Lévi-Strauss's analysis, for reasons that will become apparent below. (Table 4-2 summarizes data for all of the possible patterns.)

In the next stage of this analysis, we construct what we are calling, with apologies to Lévi-Strauss, a great-grandmother's elementary structures cost–benefit analysis. The idea here is to reduce the relative genetic advantage of each possible marriage pattern by the relative risk of inbreeding at the X-chromosome. The result is what we have called "net advantage." According to the ancient conventions of double-entry bookkeeping, we have entered the benefits on the right as credits and the relative risks on the left as debits. Note that costs and benefits here have been given equal numerical weights, a convention that we have adopted for conceptual simplicity only, and, thus, "net advantage" has relative value only and only given the stated assumptions. The last line in the chart contains the average values for these metrics under conditions of random assortment, the baseline condition. The "benefit ratio" is simply the net advantage for each case divided by the advantage in the baseline condition (Table 4-3).

To this point we have not discussed the prevalence of the various forms of preferential marriage in the ethnographic record, leaving our discussion at a formal level. We feel that it is very important to consider this distribution, however, employing the *Ethnographic Atlas* (Murdock, 1967) as a base. Table 4-4 displays the rank ordering of the rates of occurrence of the possible preferential marriage patterns against the rank orderings of the benefit ratios. There is remarkable correspondence between these two rank orderings, a

**Table 4-3** Great-grandmother's elementary structures: cost–benefit analysis.

| Cousin marriage pattern | Genetic cost (inbreeding) (%) | Genetic benefit (probability of inheriting X-chromosome (%) | Net advantage (%) | Benefit ratio |
|---|---|---|---|---|
| Bilateral cross-cousin | −18.75 | 71.88 | 53.13 | 2.125 |
| Matrilateral cross-cousin | −12.50 | 62.50 | 50.00 | 2.000 |
| Patrilateral parallel cousin | 0.00 | 50.00 | 50.00 | 2.000 |
| Matrilateral parallel cousin | −18.75 | 43.75 | 25.00 | 1.000 |
| Patrilateral cross-cousin | 0.00 | 25.00 | 25.00 | 1.000 |
| Random assortment | 0.00 | 25.00 | 25.00 | 1.000 |

**Table 4-4** Cousin marriage rules compared to net advantages to great-grandmother.

| Rank order of frequencies of first cousin preference rules | Rank order of net advantages to great-grandmother |
|---|---|
| Multilateral first cousin marriage with predominantly cross-cousin preference<br>24% | Bilateral (Kariera) cross-cousin marriage pattern<br>53% |
| Matrilateral first cross-cousin preference<br>9% | Matrilateral cross-cousin marriage pattern<br>50% |
| Patrilateral parallel cousin preference<br>3% | Patrilateral parallel cousin marriage pattern<br>50% |
| Patrilateral cross-cousin preference<br>2% | Patrilateral cross-cousin marriage pattern<br>25% |
| Matrilateral parallel cousin preference<br>0% | Matrilateral parallel cousin marriage pattern<br>25% |
| *First cousin marriage not allowed/second or other cousin preference*<br>*62%* | *Average of descent pathways under random assortment*<br>*25%* |

1. The categories of cousin marriage included are groupings of categories from the Murdock (1967) *Ethnographic Atlas*. These groupings include Murdock categories as follows:

   Multilateral first cousin marriage with predominantly cross-cousin preference (Cc, C, Q, Qc, Tc, T).
   Matrilateral first cross-cousin preference (Cm, Mm, M, Em, Fm, Qm, Tm, E, F).
   Patrilateral first cross-cousin preference (Cp, Pp, P, Gp, Qp, Tp, G, Dp, D).
   Patrilateral parallel cousin preference (Qa, Da, Fa).
   Second or other cousin or cousin marriage not practiced (N, O, R, S).

2. The calculations of coefficients of inbreeding and estimates of great-grandmother's expectations concerning her X-chromosomes for "bilateral cross-cousins" are based on the idealized Kariera system. The method of calculation assumes that in the founding sibships, one of the sister's X-chromosomes may be shared by her brother and the other may not be. Our calculation represents the averages of the situations for matrilateral cross-cousins without inbreeding and with maximal inbreeding, i.e., where the brother in the founding sibship has one of his sister's X-chromosomes. These estimates are intended to show that there should be a small increment in the net advantage to the great-grandmother over the simple matrilateral cross-cousin situation.

correspondence that appears even more remarkable when we consider that societies with some form of preferential marriage rules make up almost half of those (47%) in the *Ethnographic Atlas*. Clearly, preferential cousin marriage is quite widespread, especially in preindustrial societies, and it is distributed in much the way we would predict from our analysis of genetic advantages to females, if we were to consider it as a reproductive strategy for maximizing fitness.

However, as Lévi-Strauss (1969: 30) and others have indicated, preferential marriage rules do not always or even often result in marriages between the preferred relatives. Moreover, people practicing these forms of marriage have no knowledge of the chromosomal theory of inheritance. Nevertheless, practiced continuously over long periods of time, these marriage patterns should produce statistical effects, depending on the degree to which the idealized situation is realized, in the directions we have indicated. Furthermore, as we discuss in the next section, in societies where cousin marriage is practiced, there are demographic factors that will automatically tilt mate selection in the direction of the matrilateral cross-cousin.

## DEMOGRAPHIC FACTORS IN SYSTEMS OF COUSIN MARRIAGE

It can be demonstrated that in social groups where cousin marriage is practiced, age differences between spouses will automatically tip the system in the direction of matrilateral cross-cousin marriage. On average boys reach puberty, hence marriageable age, about 2 years later than girls. This means that, again on average, a man's father's sisters will marry before the man's father does. This means, in turn that his father's sister's daughters will, again on average, be older than he is and will tend to reach marriageable age well before he does. Exactly the opposite will be true of his mother's brother's daughters. Thus, in societies where cousin marriage is practiced there will be, in general, for each man, a larger pool of marriageable mother's brother's daughters than of father's sister's daughters (Figure 4-7). It is suggested that in societies where marriage with mother's brother's daughter is "preferred," this preference may represent little more than recognition of reality. It is easy to show that matrilateral cross-cousin marriage is also more likely than either form of parallel cousin marriage, but to a lesser degree.

This reinforces our argument concerning the likely effects of cousin marriage on the transmission of the X-chromosome. That is, in any society where cross-cousin marriage is practiced, it is likely that the preponderant marriage pattern will be matrilateral, and the posited effects of matrilateral cross-cousin marriage on transmission of the X-chromosome will naturally follow.

## LONGEVITY AS AN EVOLUTIONARY PROBLEM

Next, we will consider the evolution of two uniquely human traits and show how they are related through the evolution of the X-chromosome. We stated

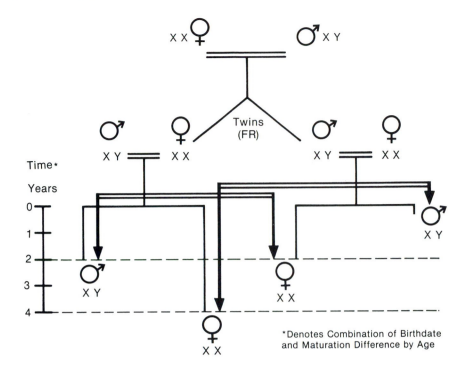

Males reach sexual maturity two years later than females. Assuming that reproductive capacity is attained two years earlier in females, the following are true:

1. On average, the male twin reproduces two years later than the female twin. The probable matings follow a matrilateral cross-cousin marriage pattern since both progeny reach sexual maturity at the same time.

2. Patrilateral cross-cousin marriage is improbable. Because the female is born two years before the male and also matures two years earlier, there would be a four-year difference between the male and female in attainment of sexual maturity.

**Figure 4-7** Sex differences in maturation rate favor matrilateral over patrilateral cross-cousin marriage.

above that there is substantial evidence that a gene, that for DHEA, on the X-chromosome is substantially implicated in development of the biological substrates of longevity and language. Longevity well past the end of reproductive capacity is a relatively rare phenomenon among mammals, and occurs among humans but to a much smaller degree among other primates (see Figure 4-8). Longevity is a problem for traditional evolutionary theory, because the mechanism of natural selection can only with great difficulty deal with the existence of large numbers of non-reproductive individuals. Modern sociobiological concepts, such as kin selection, can be invoked to deal with this phenomenon, but we will not dwell on those in detail here.

We argue that among humans longevity can be partly explained by a combination of increases in the reproductive success of social groups that have

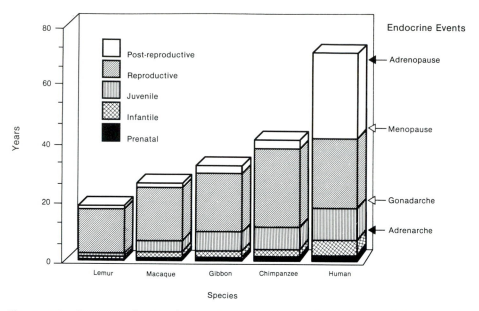

**Figure 4-8** Postreproductive longevity in primates. Adapted from Schultz (1969: 149).

elders who can act as the repositories of collective transgenerational knowledge about the social group and its environment and, in addition, by the effect of individual elders who enhance their fitness by promoting the survival of their direct descendants identified through the maintenance of kinship systems. In either case, language is the key to maintenance of knowledge (especially historical knowledge) about the social group (kinship system) and the survival of its members within the natural environment.

What we are arguing is a variant of what has come to be known as the "grandmother hypothesis," an evolutionary argument for the development of postmenopausal life span in women. The "grandmother hypothesis" invokes the concept of kin investment. According to Hill (1991: 4): "That hypothesis assumes that there are greater fitness pay-offs, at some age, to investment in grandchildren (and possibly other kin) than can be obtained by continued direct reproduction. . . (e.g., Williams 1957; Hamilton, 1966; Trivers, 1972; Alexander, 1974; Gaulin, 1980; Hawkes *et al.*, 1989)." In contradiction to this model, it has been suggested that postmenopausal life span is not a special trait at all, but is simply an artifact of recent improvements in living conditions. Hill (1991) argues convincingly that postmenopausal longevity must be a special trait (see Wood *et al.*, this volume, for a different argument).

In its most general form, the "grandmother hypothesis" is relatively non-specific with respect to the mechanics of kin investment, but, as we suggested above, storage of knowledge is clearly a key attribute that would facilitate the process. The effectiveness of elders as repositories of this knowledge is greatly enhanced by the symbol-encoding capacity of human languages. Recent models for the evolution of language and for the first appearance of languages recognizably like modern ones have tended to suggest that their beginnings are linked to the development of complex technology in the Upper Paleolithic (see e.g., Davidson and Noble, 1989). Models such as these appear to be out of synchrony with paleoanatomic, especially paleoneurological, evidence that suggests an early beginning of the path toward language (e.g., Falk, 1987, discusses the continuing controversy concerning the antiquity of human cerebral reorganization. Accumulating evidence suggests that this had begun at least by the appearance of *Homo habilis*).

Our model suggests that it was the *information storage* function of language, relating to knowledge about the social structure and environment of the social group, rather than support of technology, that was the key selective factor in its evolution. Note that the archaeological record cannot support or falsify this hypothesis, as kinship systems do not leave a direct material residue and that our main purpose here is not to argue for a particular age for either language or longevity (for a very recent and comprehensive review of the evidence relevant to the antiquity of language see Dibble, 1989).

## LANGUAGE AS AN EVOLUTIONARY PROBLEM

The model we are promoting is compatible with those that support a relatively early beginning of language evolution (Armstrong, 1989), and it avoids the problem posed by Premack (1986: 133) that language is "an embarrassment for evolutionary theory because it is vastly more powerful than one can account for in terms of selective fitness." It is true that it is more powerful than it needs to be to support relatively simple technologies, the production techniques for which can be learned by observation and imitation. However, it may be just powerful enough to support complex social systems and to store transgenerational knowledge about the environment (Armstrong, 1989; Pinker and Bloom, 1990).

We also propose a model for the evolution of language and longevity that relies on the mechanism of natural selection, and that is explicitly "adaptationist." The notion, introduced above, that natural selection, adaptationism in general, is insufficient to explain the power and complexity of human language is not new and is traceable at least to the early writings of Chomsky (see Piattelli-Palmarini, 1989, for a recent review). Piattelli-Palmarini (1989) has recently introduced an argument invoking the Edelman (1987) "neural Darwinism" model to support the Chomskyan, non-adaptationist notion of fixed neural structures underlying language and language evolution through random "macro" mutation processes. We will not discuss this argument at length here, but will observe that the same "neural Darwinism" argument has recently been used to argue *against* the Chomskyan model of language development (Rosenfield, 1988: 156–159). We point out simply that the issue is far from settled, but that we believe adaptationist arguments can be supported in the evolution of human language, and our purpose is to present such an argument here. In particular, we will argue that it is possible to identify positive feedback systems involving neural, genetic, demographic, and social and linguistic factors, all contributing to the propagation of the biological substrates of language and longevity.

Given our previous arguments concerning the value of elders, we suggest therefore, that language co-evolves with longevity in females. Language clearly has primacy within this theoretical model. At least rudimentary forms of language enhance the selective advantage of longevity, but the converse of this may not be true. We observe also that evidence for the antiquity of longevity will be very difficult to evaluate (see, e.g., Trinkaus, 1985, and Trinkaus and Tompkins, 1990, on age at death of Neandertals; Hill, 1991), as the fossilization process would have been sampling from a very constricted segment of a steeply sloping population pyramid (see, Hill, 1991). We propose also that the evolution of longevity would be on an exponential track, with very slight increments at first and larger increments as the positive feedback progresses, up to a limit dictated by the kinship system itself, if the enhancement is through kin investment.

In support of the notion that the development of kinship systems has primacy as a selective factor in the evolution of the biological substrates of language and longevity is the accumulating evidence concerning kin recognition and incest avoidance in non-human primates (Gouzoules, 1984; Cheney and Seyfarth, 1990). This suggests a firm biological foundation for the substrates of family life and their presence prior to the hominid split from the other primates.

## THE EVOLUTION OF X-LINKED TRAITS

In the case of societies practicing preferential matrilateral or bilateral cross-cousin marriage we would expect, as we have shown above, to find that the evolution of X-linked traits is promoted through the social and genetic investment of grandmothers in their granddaughters, the genetic pay-off coming in the great-grandchildren's generation. This relationship between social and genetic investment would reinforce the selective advantage of longevity in females (the female must live long enough to make the investment in the descending generations) and possibly passively enhance the evolution of longevity in males.

A specific positive feedback mechanism would have the following character-istics. First, a female would have to have a mutation at the steroid sulfatase locus that enhanced her capacity for longevity. This would increase her likelihood of living long enough to make a social investment in her grandchil-dren and great-grandchildren. Second she would have to live in a society practicing matrilateral or biateral cross-cousin marriage, preferably with patrilocal residence—this would increase the probability that the grandchildren and great-grandchildren in whom she made the social investment would have her X-chromosome and, hence, her steroid sulfatase gene.

The importance of viewing the potential genetic effects of cousin marriage from a statistical point of view cannot be overemphasized. We have shown that these marriage rules existed in at least ideal form in a very high proportion of the ethnographic universe. We suggest that their practice in even a fraction of the world's social groups could produce, given gene flow between social groups, a profound effect on the evolution of the X-chromosome species wide. This effect, again, would be realized through a positive feedback process.

## IMPLICATIONS FOR BIOCULTURAL EVOLUTIONARY THEORY

We have chosen to examine the inter-relationships among these phenomena, because they are central to the development of human social life, and because we believe that an understanding of their inter-relatedness will move us toward an understanding of the biocultural nature of hominid evolution. At first glance, these phenomena appear to stand along a continuum of biological determination. Starting with the capacity for longevity, we have a phenomenon among humans that appears to be entirely under biological or genetic control (although its expression would depend very much upon social factors, such as medical care). Second, language would appear to be a cultural phenomenon that is closely correlated with genetically based developmental and anatomic features unique to the hominids. Third, systems of kinship and marriage, with the possible exception of the universal avoidance of incest within the nuclear family, would appear to be entirely culturally based.

This final point has been most persuasively and strikingly argued by Lévi-Strauss. While recognizing the possibility that incest avoidance may have a biological component, he establishes the adoption of prescriptive marriage systems involving cousins as the key step in the movement from a biological to a sociological level of determinism. He asserts that it is "the prohibition of incest, which presents, without the slightest ambiguity, and inseparably combines, the two characteristics in which we recognize the conflicting features of two mutually exclusive orders. . . . Here therefore is a phenomenon which has the distinctive characteristics both of nature and of its theoretical contradiction, culture (Lévi-Strauss, 1969: 8–10)."

Lévi-Strauss is not the first to point out the importance of the incest taboo in the evolution of family life and, hence, human social organization—Freud (1950) is a notable forerunner, and it is not our purpose to review this literature here. We are more interested in Lévi-Strauss's inference from this idea, namely that it is the appearance of *prescriptive* marriage systems, the so-called elementary structures of kinship, that demonstrates humankind's crossing of the cultural Rubicon, out of the realm of the biological.

The general principle cannot be more clearly and forcefully stated than this:

> It is precisely because cross-cousin marriage disregards the biological factor that it should be able to establish that the origin of the incest prohibition is purely social, and furthermore to reveal what its real nature is. It is not enough to repeat that the prohibition of incest is not based on biological grounds. What then is its basis? This is the real question, and while it remains unanswered the problem cannot be said to have been resolved. For the most part, an answer to this is very difficult to give because the prohibited degrees of kinship, taken as a whole, are biologically

closer than the permitted degrees. Consequently, there is always a doubt as to whether it is the biological degree, or the social degree, which is the basis of the institution. The difficulty is completely eliminated only in the case of cross-cousin marriage, for if we can understand why degrees of kinship which are equivalent from a biological point of view are nevertheless considered completely dissimilar from the social point of view, we can claim to have discovered the principle, not only of cross-cousin marriage, but of the incest prohibition itself (Lévi-Strauss, 1969: 122).

We have shown, on the contrary, that the cross-cousins Lévi-Strauss discusses are not equivalent from a biological point of view, and that it makes a great deal of difference genetically whether a society prescribes marriage with the matrilateral or the patrilateral cross-cousin. We have also shown that there are complex evolutionary relationships of positive feedback among the phenomena of language, longevity and prescriptive or preferential marriage systems, and that these positive feedback relationships may have profound effects on the evolution of particular loci on the X-chromosome.

Human sociobiologists have taken up the issue of human mating patterns, especially cousin marriage (Alexander, 1979; Hartung, 1985). Their arguments have centered on the question of uncertain paternity and lineage extinction as biological explanations for matrilineal inheritance and matrilateral cross-cousin marriage. We do not dispute this suggestion, but have approached the genetic and evolutionary impact of cousin marriage from a different perspective. There is nothing contradictory in these approaches—they merely highlight the possibility that there may be multiple causes and effects with respect to phenomena as complicated as these.

With regard to this final point, there is more general relevance to our argument from developments in sociobiology, or more recently, human behavioral ecology (see, e.g., Irons, 1991). According to Irons (1991: 60), human behavioral ecology has had as its central assumption "that the evolution of the human capacity and propensity to absorb a culture was accompanied by the evolution of psychological mechanisms that tended, at least in the environments of evolution, to keep culturally influenced behavior directed toward reproductive goals." That is, in essence, that human culture was adaptive, in the sense of increasing the reproductive fitness of the populations that possessed it, "at least in the environments of evolution." The final phrase here is critical to our acceptance of this notion. Irons is not completely clear as to what is meant by "the environments of evolution," but it seems to mean something like "probably preneolithic, certainly preindustrial." This qualification is necessary, because it is relatively easy to point out recent culturally defined behaviors that are clearly nonadaptive in the sense of adaptation given above.

We have suggested above that our approach is "coevolutionary." Irons (1991: 60) has succinctly summarized the difference between theories based in human behavioral ecology and those based on co-evolutionary principles:

> However, in contrast to some of the co-evolutionary theories . . ., it is not assumed that culture itself consistently leads people away from their reproductive goals. Rather culture is something individuals use and manipulate in pursuit of the

proximate goals that, in the environments of human evolution, were reproductively advantageous.

This approach has certainly been productive when applied to simple societies, but, as Irons suggests, it breaks down when applied to more complex, more highly *structured* social groups. Having said this, however, we note that we have explicated an example of a social structure which, in fact, appears to further the "reproductive goals" of women in simple, as well as some highly complex societies.

Moreover, we do not believe that it is necessary always to invoke unknown biologically based "psychological" mechanisms to explain the existence of social phenomena with biological or genetic implications. It is difficult to imagine a genetic mechanism that would cause people to choose to marry their matrilateral cross-cousins. We believe that a more plausible and parsimonious explanation in this case involves demographic factors and group survivability and competitiveness.

## CONCLUSION

In conclusion, we note that it is language, and only language, that makes possible the maintenance of complex systems of kinship, marriage, and inheritance. The sociostructural advantages of the systems of kinship and marriage that we have discussed here have been analyzed by Lévi-Strauss and many others, and it is not our purpose to review those here. These sociostructural effects have to do with the establishment of inter-family relationships, the formation of alliances and the management of politics in small-scale societies. We do not dispute the importance of these sociostructural factors. We propose that, in addition, systems of preferential marriage, coupled with incest avoidance, provided these social groups with a powerful mechanism for managing genetic structures as well as social systems. Incest avoidance clearly has the effect of minimizing the deleterious effects of inbreeding in social groups where potential marriage partners are likely to be close relatives. We suggest, following Lévi-Strauss, that preferential marriage becomes the obverse of incest avoidance, but from a biological as well as a sociostructural point of view, by optimizing the genetic effects of the marriage patterns of these relatives.

From an evolutionary point of view, we note that there appears to be a reciprocal relationship between these purely behavioral factors and genetic factors involving the X-chromosome, tending to promote evolution of a vitally important set of loci within social groups that have the particular social structures. These behavioral systems, then, can be seen as co-evolutionary with genetically based developmental systems that promote the development of longer life spans and complex languages, which in turn could enhance the social effectiveness of commonly practiced marriage patterns. We cannot evaluate the extent to which such practices may have existed prehistorically. We do know, however, that extremely complex systems of kinship and marriage co-existed, in modern times, with the simplest of technologies, and that these would have been impossible to practice in the absence of well-developed languages or people who had lived long enough to store extensive knowledge about the social group and the inter-relatedness of its members. We note also that patterns of preferential cousin marriage existed at the geographic poles of the enthnographic world, namely in Australia, South America, and Africa. Barring independent invention or diffusion, an early origin for these practices is suggested by the historical distribution. We believe that these factors taken together reinforce the need for increasing attention to be paid not only to the purely social consequences of various types of social structures, but also to their potential genetic effects as well.

We have shown that genetic, demographic, and social factors can interact to establish a mutually reinforcing positive-feedback system which should have the effect of enhancing the effects of selection for loci on the X-chromosome. We believe that this demonstration promotes the theoretical notion of gene-culture co-evolution.

# REFERENCES

Alexander, R. D. (1974) The evolution of social behavior. *Annual Review of Ecology and Systematics* **5**, 325–383.

Alexander, R. D. (1979) *Darwinism and Human Affairs*. Seattle: University of Washington Press.

Armstrong, D. F. (1989) Comments on Davidson and Noble, The archaeology of perception: traces of depiction and language. *Current Anthropology* **30**, 137–138.

Cheney, D. L. and Seyfarth, R. M. (1990) *How Monkeys See the World*. Chicago: University of Chicago Press.

Davidson, I. and Noble, W. (1989) The archaeology of perception: traces of depiction and language. *Current Anthropology* **30**, 125–156.

Dibble, H. (1989) The implications of stone tool types for the presence of language during the Lower and Middle Palaeolithic. In: *The Human Revolution: Behavioural and Biological Perspectives on the Origins of Modern Humans* (eds Mellars, P. and Stringer, C.). Edinburgh: Edinburgh University Press, pp. 415–432.

Edelman, G. M. (1987) *Neural Darwinism: The Theory of Neuronal Group Selection*. New York: Basic Books.

Falk, D. (1987) Brain lateralization in primates and its evolution in hominids. *Yearbook of Physical Anthropology* **30**, 107–126.

Freud, S. (1950) *Totem and Taboo*. New York: W. W. Norton. Originally published in 1913.

Gaulin, S. J. (1980) Sexual dimorphism in the human post-reproductive lifespan: Possible causes. *Journal of Human Evolution* **9**, 227–232.

Gouzoules, S. (1984) Primate mating systems, kin associations, and cooperative behavior: evidence of kin recognition? *Yearbook of Physical Anthropology* **27**, 99–134.

Haldane, J. B. S. and Jayakar, S. D. (1962) An enumeration of some human relationships. *Journal of Genetics* **58**, 81–107.

Haldane, J. B. S. and Moshinsky, P. (1939) Inbreeding in Mendelian populations with special reference to human cousin marriage. *Annals of Eugenics* **9**, 321–340.

Hamilton, W. D. (1964) The genetical evolution of social behavior. *Journal of Theoretical Biology* **7**, 1–52.

Hamilton, W. D. (1966) The moulding of senescence by natural selection. *Journal of Theoretical Biology* **12**, 12–45.

Hartung, J. (1985) Matrilineal inheritance: new theory and analysis. *Behavioral and Brain Sciences* **8**, 661–688.

Hawkes, K., Connell, J. F. and Blurton Jones, N. G. (1989) Hardworking Hadza grandmothers. In: *Comparative Socioecology: The Behavioural Ecology of Humans and Other Mammals* (eds Standen, V. and Foley, R. A.). Oxford: Blackwell Scientific Publications.

Hill, K. (1991) The evolution of premature reproductive senescence and menopause in human females: an evaluation of the "grandmother hypothesis" (Manuscript).

Honigman, J. J. (1959) *The World of Man*. New York: Harper and Row.

Irons, W. (1991) How did morality evolve? *Zygon* 26.1.79–89.

Katz, S. H., Hediger, M. L., Zemel, B. S. and Parks, J. S. (1985) Adrenal androgens, body fat and advanced skeletal age in puberty: new evidence for the relations of adrenarche and gonadarche in males. *Human Biology* **57**, 401–413.

Lévi-Strauss, C. (1969) *The Elementary Structures of Kinship*. Boston: Beacon Press.

Livingstone, F. B. (1959) A formal analysis of prescriptive marriage systems among the Australian aborigines. *Southwestern Journal of Anthropology* **15**, 361–372.

Murdock, P. (1967) *Ethnographic Atlas*. Pittsburgh: University of Pittsburgh Press.

Piattelli-Palmarini, M. (1989) Evolution, selection and cognition: from "learning" to parameter setting in biology and in the study of language. *Cognition* **31**, 1–44.

Pinker, S. and Bloom, P. (1990) Natural language and natural selection. *Behavioral and Brain Sciences* **13**, 4. 707–65.

Premack, D. (1986) *Gavagai! or the Future History of the Animal Language Controversy*. Cambridge, MA: The MIT Press.

Rosenfield, I. (1988) *The Invention of Memory*. New York: Basic Books.

Schultz, A. H. (1969) *The Life of Primates*. New York: Universe Books.

Trinkaus, E. (1985) Pathology and the posture of the La Chapelle-aux-Saints Neandertal. *American Journal of Physical Anthropology* **67**, 19–42.

Trinkaus, E. and Tompkins, R. L. (1990) The neandertal life cycle: the possibility, probability, and perceptibility of contrasts with recent humans. In: *Primate Life History and Evolution* (ed. C. J. Rousseau). New York: Wiley-Liss.

Trivers, R. L. (1971) The evolution of reciprocal altruism. *Quarterly Review of Biology* **46**, 35–57.

Trivers, R. L. (1972) Parental investment and sexual selection. In: *Sexual Selection and the Descent of Man* (ed. Campbell, B.). Chicago: Aldine.

Williams, G. C. (1957) Pleiotropy, natural selection, and the evolution of senescence. *Evolution* **11**, 398–411.

Yen, P. H., Marsh, B., Allen, E., Tsai, S. P., Ellison, J., Connolly, L., Nelswanger, K. and Shapiro, L. J. (1988) The human X-linked steroid sulfatase gene and a Y-encoded pseudogene: evidence for an inversion of the Y chromosome during primvate evolution. *Cell* **56**, 1123–1135.

# III
## POPULATIONS, ENVIRONMENT, AND MORBIDITY

# 5

# Primate Gerontology: An Emerging Discipline

## C. JEAN DeROUSSEAU

## INTRODUCTION

The field of primate aging is in its infancy, although there have been several reviews and edited volumes describing age-related changes in old primates (Bowden, 1979; Davis and Leathers, 1985; Pavelka and Fedigan, 1991). The field has grown along with primatology in general from description through explanation to experimentation, but it still lacks a cohesive framework. In this paper I review the major sources of data on aging in non-human primates, and identify three themes within primatology with direct or indirect significance to human aging. These themes are also evolutionary in nature and may help to define a true "primate gerontology." They are: behavior and physiology; nutrition and aging; and life history.

To date, primate research on aging has been dominated by medical research with its emphasis on identifying animal models that mimic human aging disorders and then on finding treatments that halt or reverse those problems of aging. A wide variety of physiological age changes that have possible impacts on behavior have been noted in non-human primates. However, field studies in primatology present conflicting evidence about the impact of physiological aging on behavior, while there appears to be an inverse effect of behavior (social stress) on biology. The view of primates as individuals with mutually accommodating biological and behavioral systems is not only of import to the aging field but also a view that must be incorporated into anthropological models of non-human primate and human evolution.

Although many different age-related disorders have been documented in non-human primates (see Committee on Animal Models for Research on Aging, 1981; Cornelius and Simpson, 1984), those that are influenced by nutrition have come to the forefront. Diseases such as atherosclerosis and diabetes can be found or induced and manipulated in non-human primate models; their study has led scientists into areas, such as the impact of dietary restriction on aging, with theoretical importance to the understanding of human aging.

Primate life history, the third area I identify as significant to our understanding of aging, has been greatly facilitated by longitudinal field studies. As researchers accumulate more and more accurate information about the primate life cycle in nature, comparisons of patterns of growth, reproduction, and mortality are being made, and the relationships between these parameters of life history examined. Significantly, comparative work in this area is also contributing to a better theoretical understanding of the evolution of aging.

## A BRIEF HISTORY OF AGING STUDIES IN PRIMATOLOGY

Early observations of primates were concerned with description, particularly with collecting type specimens to catalog each new species that was discovered. Museums collected skins and skeletons, while zoos went after token live animals. Museum specimens offered the first evidence that age-related diseases occurred in wild populations, while animals in zoos and other institutions provided data on longevity and case histories of disorders that closely resembled those observed with human aging.

More recently, a true gerontology of non-human primates has become possible because of two research trends through the 20th century: (1) a recognition by medical researchers that non-human primates are valuable models for the study of human health; and (2) an understanding in primatology that long-term behavioral studies with identification of individual animals is an unusually productive approach to primate behavior.

First of all, as primates were increasingly used for medical purposes, breeding colonies were established to secure a steady supply of animals, and primates, especially rhesus monkeys, became a standard laboratory animal. Individual animals matured and aged in captivity, providing an intimate view of primate ontogeny in many biological systems. These colonies became opportunities not only for medical research in general, but also for gerontology to gather systematic data on longevity and age-related diseases.

Secondly, longitudinal studies following the health and behavioral histories of individual animals began to provide detailed information about growth, reproduction, and aging in different species of primates. These data have led to the study of patterns of reproduction and mortality, or life-history research in primates, as well as to the continuing appraisal of the role that older animals play in natural primate societies.

### Skeletal "Populations"

In the early half of this century large samples of non-human primates were shot for museums and other collectors, their skins and skeletons becoming a permanent catalog of primate species. Although the age of individual specimens was seldom known, the collections consisted of animals of all ages, and offered an early view of age-related disorders in non-human primates.

Studying these collections, Adolph Schultz, one of the first students of modern primate population biology, was able to say that "arthritis, sinus infections, dental decay and fractured bones have not appeared with civilization in modern man, but are just as prevalent in many kinds of other primates, living under natural conditions" (Schultz, 1969: 189–190). Other skeletal surveys before and after Schultz's have corroborated his finding that natural populations include individuals with age-related disorders (see Fox, 1939; DeRousseau, 1988; Lovell, 1990), although the frequency of disease is not always high (Rothschild and Woods, 1992). This is an important point because of notions that aging is unique to humans, whose culture protects the aged, and that in nature, animals that are not "fit," such as the aged, are weeded out by natural selection. Clearly, the early skeletal evidence and more recent field observations (see later section on behavior) belie these assumptions.

Certainly, museum populations of skeletons must be used for aging studies with caution. First of all, in many cases museum collections are not samples of populations in nature, but accumulations from many different populations. In addition, diseased specimens may reflect a bias in sampling (i.e., the most disabled individuals being the most likely to be caught or shot), while the chronological age of each specimen can only be estimated.

Despite these difficulties, such skeletal collections offer a cross-sectional view of some aging parameters that are difficult to obtain in living populations, e.g., the fine details of arthritic degeneration. With regard to the adequacy of the sampling, many museum collections include subsets derived from single localities that are more likely to truly represent natural populations. Among these are some parts of the gibbon collection at the Museum of Comparative Zoology at Harvard University, the ape collection at the Cleveland Museum of Natural History, the tamarin collection at the Museum at Michigan State University, and the Neil Tappen Collection at the University of Wisconsin at Milwaukee (some Old World monkeys; Albrecht, 1982).

With regard to age estimation, there are fairly reliable indicators of skeletal age in humans (see Stewart, 1979), and although forensic markers need further study in non-human primates, one can divide an unknown skeletal sample of primates into juvenile, young adult, adult, and old adult using stages of epiphyseal and pubic symphysis fusion (Rawlins, 1975; Cheverud, 1981).

One promising new development for skeletal studies of aging involves the establishment of skeletal collections associated with long-term breeding colonies of non-human primates. Among these are the Cayo Santiago rhesus monkey collection housed in the Department of Anatomy at the University of Puerto Rico (see DeRousseau, 1990), a collection of chimpanzees from the Gombe National Park in Kenya (see Zihlman et al., 1990), a collection of monkeys at the Primate Research Facility of the Bowman Gray School of Medicine (D. Weaver, personal communication), and a collection of Japanese macaques currently being assembled from the Arashiyama West colony in Texas (McDonald Pavelka, personal communication).

The value of these collections is that specimens come with a history, including in many cases dates of birth and death. Thus, chronological ages and other aspects of life history can be compared to parameters of biological aging.

The problem with these samples is, however, that with the exception of the Gombe chimpanzee skeletons, they are derived from captive populations. Although the colonies are captive to varying degrees (some are provisioned yet free-ranging), they do not necessarily age "naturally."

Interestingly, the contrast between captive and natural populations has become an important one with some significance for aging studies (Kessler *et al.*, 1986; DeRousseau, 1990; Rothschild and Woods, 1992). These studies and others on growth (discussed later) clearly show the importance of environment in the expression of the primate life cycle and age-related disease.

This is an important observation for several reasons. First of all, it suggests that age-related disorders in non-human primates are influenced by "life style" mimicking the human condition. Secondly, it demonstrates the adaptable nature of non-human primate, not just human, lives. This points the way toward the comparative study of adaptability, an approach that may clarify why aging does *not* occur (e.g., as fast in humans as it does in mice; see later discussion).

## The Elderly in Zoos and Research Laboratories

For over a century zoos have collected and exhibited non-human primates from all over the world. As replacement costs have risen, increasing effort has been made to enhance zoo environments and maintain animals in good health, and indeed many zoo primates do survive into old age. More recently, laboratories associated with universities, medical centers, and drug companies have established their own colonies of non-human primates for research (although this research direction is becoming less popular due to both rising costs and the animal rights movement). These animals too have often been maintained in captivity for a long time in an attempt to use them cost-effectively.

In both cases, animals were usually captured when they were juveniles, easily trapped, and manageable, so that their chronological ages were determinable based on maturational criteria such as tooth eruption and epiphyseal closure. As these animals aged and others were born in captivity, individual primates with ages that were accurate or well estimated accrued in zoos and research institutions.

### *Maximum Life Span*

Although the circumstances under which zoo and laboratory animals live are "artificial," they do in many cases act like human culture to favor survival. Food is usually abundant and medical care is usually prompt. Thus, captive animals may fulfill the potential of their species for longevity, and in doing so provide some of the best estimates for species' maximum life span. In addition, individual animals may live long enough to exhibit the same age-related diseases that are observed in humans.

Various compilations of ages at death in zoos and research facilities include those by Cutler (1976) and Harvey *et al.* (1987). Schultz (1969) presented these data in a classic figure showing the relationship of growth and reproductive periods to life span in five representative species of primates (see Figure 4-8,

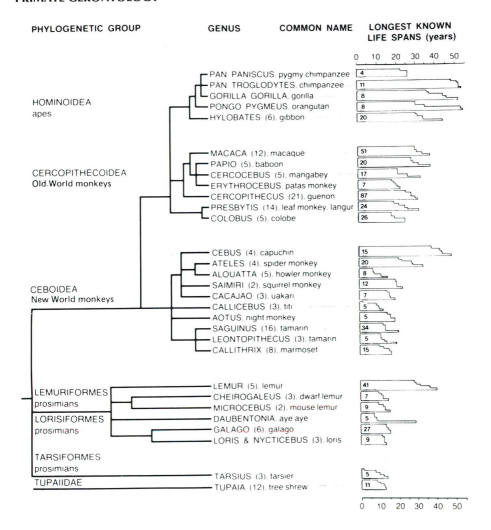

| PHYLOGENETIC GROUP | GENUS | COMMON NAME | LONGEST KNOWN LIFE SPANS (years) |

**Figure 5-1** The five maximum life spans recorded for each of 30 Primate genera. Numbers in parentheses are the number of species in each genus. Numbers in histograms are the number of old individuals noted for each genus. The figure is reproduced from Bowden and Williams (1984) and was constructed from records maintained by M. L. Jones of the San Diego Zoo.

Katz and Armstrong, this volume). He argued from these comparisons that life span has lengthened through primate evolution, and that only humans show a "postreproductive" phase of life (but see Watts, 1990; see also later section on menopause).

Bowden and Jones (1979) and Bowden and Williams (1984) present a more extensive taxonomy of longevities using data compiled by M. L. Jones since 1941 (Figure 5-1). These and other life-cycle estimates from captive animals supplement the data from natural populations on which life-history research is based (see later section on life history).

Maximum life spans derived from captive animals are, of course, not equivalent to maximum life spans in natural circumstances. In addition, maximum life span may not be the best variable to measure a species' longevity; life expectancy may be more meaningful biologically. In one sense, maximum life span derived from zoos and research institutions may be most significant as a measure of adaptability to captive conditions.

On the other hand, it may be argued that longevities derived from animals in captivity are most comparable precisely because they are *not* an expression of natural but varied habitats. They are instead the outcome of living in more or less similar contexts presented with more or less similar stressors, to which no one species should be particularly well adapted. Thus, species variation in longevity is less likely to be due to differences in environment, and more likely to be due to differences in genetic potential. This variation may, in turn, be most appropriate for comparisons to human longevity, since certain aspects of captivity, like relative social isolation, mimic conditions often associated with human aging.

Clearly, comparative work on longevities, taking into account differences between zoos and research facilities, is called for to justify this logic. It is probable that zoos vary considerably in animal husbandry and that longevities may reflect this variation. If this is so, the comparative use of zoo life spans would be questionable, but of great practical import for the understanding of human longevity and for primate conservation efforts. In other words, variation in animal management may be an opportunity to study the impact of environment on longevity in non-human primates.

### Spontaneous Age-related Disease

Age-related diseases that have occurred "spontaneously," i.e., were not induced experimentally, in captive non-human primates include rheumatoid arthritis (Brown *et al.*, 1974), atherosclerosis (Kaplan *et al.*, 1985), diabetes mellitus (Howard, 1983), osteoporosis (Sumner *et al.*, 1989), degenerative joint disease (DeRousseau, 1990), and a host of other degenerative conditions (Bowden, 1979; Davis and Leathers, 1985). What environmental stimuli might be involved in their expression, and whether such disorders are a problem for primates in nature or not, awaits further study. Similarly, their impact on longevity is unclear.

At present, the occurrence of these diseases means that non-human primates may act as experimental models for human disease. Since non-human primates are akin to humans both phylogenetically and in complexity of adaptation, they are particularly suited as models for age-related disorders, which are largely multivariate in etiology. The documentation of "stress" in free-ranging baboons (Sapolsky, 1990) and the impact of social stress on the cardiovascular, immune, and reproductive systems (see later section on social stress) suggests that even this seemingly human facet of disease causation is part of the disease process in non-human primates.

## Primate Research Centers

Over the course of this century, colonies of non-human primates were set up for various reasons, both in their native lands and in the industrialized countries of the world. Animals in some colonies ranged freely in native habitats (e.g., the howler monkeys on Barro Colorado Island off Panama); others were free-ranging, but displaced from their original locations and provisioned (e.g., the rhesus monkeys of Cayo Santiago off Puerto Rico); and others were held captive in enclosures ranging from corrals to individual cages (e.g., the Sukhumi Primate Research Station established by the Soviet Union in 1924). (See Haraway, 1989, for a recent review.)

In the United States, some colonies were dedicated to understanding primate behavior and biology, e.g., the Yale University Laboratories of Primate Biology founded by Robert Yerkes (apes), or to conservation, e.g., the Duke University Primate Center (prosimians). However, most were established to supply animals needed by medical research. These breeding colonies were also used for research, much of it focusing on the reproductive system and tropical diseases, topics of obvious importance to the successful breeding of captive primates.

Although breeding animals was a high priority of many colonies, not many were successful, and in the 1950s and 1960s the National Institutes of Health provided the funds to set up seven Regional Primate Research Centers to address the increasing shortage of laboratory animals in the United States. These are located: in Atlanta affiliated with Emory University (the Yerkes Laboratories becoming one of the centers); in Beaverton, Oregon affiliated with the University of Oregon; near Boston affiliated with Harvard University; in Davis, California; in Madison, Wisconsin affiliated with the University of Wisconsin; in New Orleans; and in Seattle affiliated with the University of Washington. By 1980 these centers housed 12,000 animals (Haraway, 1989: 122).

Over the years several of the centers sponsored by the National Institutes of Health have amassed a considerable number of aged animals, providing a major resource for primate gerontology. Like the smaller samples of old animals in zoos and other institutions, center animals provide data on longevity and age-related diseases, and anatomical specimens for study.

The research centers are unique, however, as a resource for the systematic study of primate aging. This is not only because relatively large numbers of old animals may be easily accessed, but also because detailed medical, genealogical, and sometimes behavioral histories are available on many animals. It is the use of animals in primate centers which has boosted primate aging studies beyond the anecdotal phase (see, e.g., Bowden, 1979).

Also important to the development of a primate gerontology has been the bibliographic service maintained by the Primate Information Center, of the Regional Primate Research Center in Seattle.[1] This service has generated

[1]Address: Primate Information Center, SJ-50, University of Washington, Seattle, WA 98195, USA. Telephone: 206-543-4376.

several bibliographies on aging in primates listing 148 references in 1978 (Caminiti, 1978) and 460 references in later updates (Williams, 1984; Caminiti, 1985).

From one vantage point, it is those primate colonies that are semi-naturalistic, and not the Research Centers, that offer the best resource for aging studies. They are after all more representative of natural behavior and physiology. These include: Cayo Santiago, Arashiyama West, and Morgan Island. Several of these have set the standard for longitudinal behavioral studies, but include some degree of handling for medical examination and treatment.

On the other hand, the variety of circumstances under which animals are maintained offers an excellent opportunity to explore aspects of aging associated with life style. For example, initial comparisons of the Cayo Santiago colony and the Wisconsin Regional Primate Center show that some aging changes seem to be consistent between free-ranging and caged animals while others vary considerably (DeRousseau, 1984, 1990).

## Longitudinal Field Studies

Following the collecting phase of primatology when specimens were brought home to the laboratory or compound, the field approach brought the researcher to the home territories of the different primate species (see DeVore, 1965). It rapidly became apparent that the longer a primate group was observed in its natural habitat, the more complete was the understanding of social organization and behavior. An observer could learn to recognize individual animals, note kin relationships, even construct family trees if the observation period was long enough. Today field studies of 12 months or longer are commonplace (see Smuts et al., 1987), and longitudinal fieldwork has become one of the most productive research trends in primate behavior.

To the study of aging, this has meant: (1) an improvement in the age estimations of free-ranging animals, and thus, in species estimates of life span; and (2) the possibility of studying the biology and behavior of animals with known or well-estimated chronological ages in nature. The range of possible studies is extended when behavioral observations are combined with trapping procedures for marking and examining individual animals, as is increasingly the case. In particular, documentation of the relationship between chronological and biological age in natural settings is increasingly possible.

Among the earliest and most long-lived programs to date are those established at Cayo Santiago, Puerto Rico (rhesus monkeys; Carpenter, 1972; Rawlins, 1979), at Arashiyama and several other sites in Japan (Japanese macaques; Huffman, 1991) with one derivative site in Texas (Fedigan, 1991), and at the Gombe National Park in Kenya (chimpanzees; Goodall, 1983, 1986). All of these programs employed provisioning to some extent to cluster animals for study[2] (Asquith, 1989). They all identified, aged, and sexed

---

[2]The Japanese and Kenyan study sites are within the natural habitats of the animals. Cayo Santiago, on the other hand, was established in 1938 with animals from India, and provisioning there is not simply an observational tool. Although Cayo Santiago animals are free-ranging, they cannot leave the island and cannot survive on its natural vegetation alone.

individual animals, censused animals regularly, and determined genealogical relationships when possible.

This baseline data on age and kinship provided important clarifications of primate behavior, such as the inverse relationship of age and dominance in sibling female macaques (Koyama, 1967; Sade, 1967) and the differences in dominance patterns with age observed between male and female chimpanzees (Bygott, 1979). In addition, it allowed the actual measurement of life-cycle variables in free-breeding populations, and spurred the rise of demographic and life-history study (described below). One measure of the productivity of longitudinal study is the current interest in actual measures of lifetime reproductive success in non-human primates (Fedigan *et al.*, 1986; Cheney *et al.*, 1988).

Because of their long-term nature, each of these sites has become a focus for the study of aging in non-human primates. At the Arashiyama sites both in Japan and Texas, special attention has been paid to the behavior of old animals (Nakamichi, 1984; McDonald Pavelka, 1990). At the Cayo Santiago site, physiological aspects of aging have been studied with data collected at the annual trapping to tattoo animals (Bito *et al.*, 1982; DeRousseau *et al.*, 1986; Turnquist, 1986). The skeletons of well-observed chimpanzees at Gombe have been collected at death and studied relative to their known life-history events (Jurmain, 1989; Zihlman *et al.*, 1990).

A considerable number of other longitudinal field programs have been conducted (see Richard, 1985; Smuts *et al.*, 1987) leading to other observations on aging. Of particular interest are those describing postmenopausal females in natural groups (see later section on menopause). Although these are still largely anecdotal, it seems clear that use of longitudinal data for aging studies will bring new insights to our understanding of human aging, both behavioral and physiological.

## NEW RESEARCH DIRECTIONS IN PRIMATE GERONTOLOGY

Studies relevant to our understanding of primate aging can be grouped by type of data available, as they were in the preceding sections. Age-related diseases of the skeleton (museum collections), longevity (zoo and primate facility records), primates as models for human physiological aging (medical research in zoos and primate facilities), life history and aging in primate societies (colony and field studies) emerge as major topics under current investigation.

In the following sections these studies are regrouped into three areas that I believe are particularly important for their relevance to human aging and for their evolutionary content. These are: behavior, nutrition, and life history. Studies in nutrition and behavior have practical significance, leading us to a better appreciation of what may modify the process and experience of human aging. Life history is a theoretical concept that emphasizes the inter-relatedness of life-cycle phases and the importance of context and feedback. In defining these areas, I draw upon complementary research that does not fall under the rubric of aging, but is important in a theoretical overview. For example, the impact of provisioning on maturation is not about aging *per se*, but the principle that life-cycle parameters may respond to diet is relevant to our understanding of aging.

Although each area of research stands alone for its contributions to the field of aging, the research discussed also works together as a framework for research in primate gerontology. It exemplifies "life-history thinking" (DeRousseau, 1990) in which the life cycle of the individual organism is examined at higher levels of organization. The study of behavior and aging examines the interaction of the individual life cycle with its larger social context. The impact of nutrition on aging is in some sense an examination of the individual life cycle in one aspect of its ecological context. Formal life-history study takes the life-cycle characteristics of the organism and compares them across species, a third level of organization.

## Social Behavior and Aging in Primates

### Physiological Aging and Behavior

The primate adaptation includes certain anatomical features that are linked to behavior and comprise the whole animal. Among these are convergent orbits for binocular vision, a tendency for uprightness and grasping hands for mobility with dexterity, a tendency for single offspring with long inter-birth intervals, and a large and complex brain that allows for differing degrees of inter-personal awareness, learning, and manipulation of the environment.

Variation in these traits is generally considered to be species specific. Yet, visual, musculoskeletal, reproductive, and cognitive processes also vary by age within primate species (see the following sections). We might expect that this variation, too, would be linked to behavior (see DeRousseau *et al.*, 1986).

On the other hand, Dolhinow (1984) suggests that loss of function with age is likely to predispose the older monkey to predation, accidents, etc., so that animals that are old physiologically and behaviorally are rare in nature. However, many age-related declines begin early in ontogeny (e.g., loss of accommodation, joint mobility) and may still exert an impact on behavioral capacities.

*The Senses: Presbyopia and Presbyacusis.* A survey of the Cayo Santiago rhesus macaques and the Wisconsin Regional Primate Research Center showed that an age-related decline in the ability to accommodate the eye to near objects was present in both colonies (Bito *et al.*, 1982). Behaviorally, this means that all fine discrimination of food objects and the ability to focus while grooming decline with age (Figure 5-2).

In addition, all animals over 15 years of age showed cataractous changes in their lens concomitant with decreased visual acuity (Kaufman and Bito, 1982). Although these changes have yet to be confirmed in feral populations, one might expect that an age-related loss of acuity might effect such behaviors as arboreal locomotion, foraging, and even recognition of conspecifics.

Other senses too show age-related declines in non-human primates similar

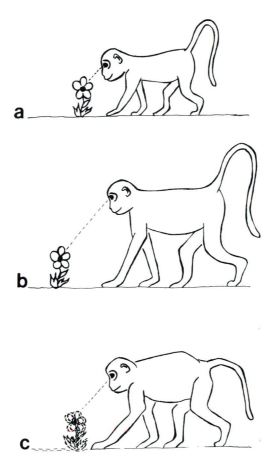

**Figure 5-2** Functional consequences of loss of accommodative amplitude in rhesus monkeys. (a) A young animal can focus at very short distances, a phenomena that is probably necessary for normal development, but that far exceeds the capability of an adult. This ability is consistent with the distances that are routine for a small animal, often clinging to its mother. (b) An animal at the beginning of the second decade of life has lost about half of its maximal accommodative amplitude, but can still function normally. Because of increases in body size due to growth, its accommodative ability is still consistent with distances characteristic of routine activities such as grooming and foraging. (c) An old animal with no ability to accommodate cannot bring objects at arm's length, or directly in front of its hand on the ground, into focus. Although it is physiologically handicapped, experience and social support may ameliorate its functional difficulties. Reproduced from DeRousseau *et al.* (1986).

to those found in humans. For example, there are neuronal losses (Hawkins *et al.*, 1985) and hearing deficits (Bennett *et al.*, 1983) in older monkeys. These too might compromise an older animal's social interactions.

*Locomotion: Osteoarthritis and Osteoporosis.* Both degenerative joint disease and osteoporosis occur in non-human primates (Fox, 1939; Schultz, 1969;

Bowden *et al.*, 1979). Osteoporosis appears to be responding to activity levels and reproductive stresses (DeRousseau, 1985a; Sumner *et al.*, 1989) while joint degeneration may be strongly influenced by biomechanical factors (DeRousseau, 1988). Whatever the etiology, both disorders can compromise the activity patterns and levels of older animals.

In my own studies of osteoarthritis in captive macaques, a significant portion of animals over 12 years of age showed joint degeneration concomitant with functional losses (DeRousseau, 1985b), and measurements of joint mobility in anesthetized animals showed loss of mobility well before the development of osteoarthritis (DeRousseau *et al.*, 1983). Recent work by Rothschild suggests that feral groups do not show the same frequencies of joint disease, but his samples are not of known age.

Several research groups have developed experimental monkey models of osteoporosis, and some cases of bone loss in older primates are known. The spinal kyphosis often observed in old animals may be partially due to loss of vertebral bone (Gorman, 1983), and thus also exemplify a physical constraint on behavior due to aging.

*Menopause and Age-related Changes in Reproduction.* Many studies have begun to document age-related variation in reproduction both in free-ranging and captive populations (Strum and Western, 1982; Paul and Kuester, 1988; Harley, 1990; Sade, 1990) and several describe postmenopausal females in nature (Waser, 1978; Nishida *et al.*, 1990; Borries *et al.*, 1991). In addition, various hormonal and anatomical changes similar to those observed in human menopause have been noted in non-human primates, including macaques and chimpanzees (Van Wagenen, 1972; Hodgen *et al.*, 1977; Graham *et al.*, 1979; Gould *et al.*, 1981). On the whole, the evidence for a menopause in non-human primates has been interpreted as support for the "grandmother hypothesis," that a period of postreproduction in females will be selected for because it contributes to the survival of grandchildren and latest offspring (Gaulin, 1980; Hrdy, 1981; Lancaster and King, 1985).

A recent review (Pavelka and Fedigan, 1991), however, suggests that although there may indeed be age-related decline in reproduction, the evidence for a true menopause is scarce (see also Small, 1984). On re-examination physiological studies show many more animals that continue to reproduce into old age than those that do not. In their survey Pavelka and Fedigan were able to identify only one monkey (Graham *et al.*, 1979) and one ape (Gould *et al.*, 1981) that show the oocyte depletion characteristic of human menopause (see Wood *et al.*, this volume). In addition, the authors argue that evidence for the cessation of ovarian cycles in behavioral studies is also rare. Importantly, of 11 aged female chimpanzees studied by Nishida *et al.* (1990), five of 11 ceased to show estrous swellings in the few years before their death; six of 11, however, *continued to cycle*.

By Pavelka and Fedigan's (1991) criteria for a human-like menopause, that (1) *all* females (2) cease to experience menstrual cycles (3) approximately *halfway* through the maximum life span, non-human primates do not show a true menopause. Interestingly, chimpanzees continue to cycle until about 50 years of age (Graham, 1979) but do not live much longer than that. Pavelka and Fedigan suggest that an oocyte supply of 50 years may be characteristic of apes including humans, and the uniqueness of humans is therefore in the expansion of life span.

*Cognitive Function and Age-related Changes in the Brain.* There is an extensive body of literature on cognitive and neural aging in primates, particularly in macaques (see reviews by Bowden and Williams, 1984; Davis, 1985; Price *et al.*, 1985; Dean and Bartus, 1988; Moss *et al.*, 1988; Price *et al.*, 1990). Old monkeys often show age-related changes in both cognition, e.g., contraction of memory or increased behavioral stereotypy, and neural physiology, e.g., plaque formation, pigment accumulation, that are similar to human aging. In this respect they are a critical model for examining human disorders such as Alzheimer's Disease, as well as aging, although direct correspondences between cognitive decline and neural change remain tentative.

That such changes affect behavior in a normal social context seems likely, although Bowden and Williams (1984) suggest that at least some age-related changes that emerge in cognitive tests may actually be adaptive under natural conditions. For example, reduced curiosity and increased behavioral stereotypy may be useful conservative characteristics of the older experienced monkey, that result in avoidance of potentially risky situations.

### Behavioral Studies

There is evidence that rates of social behavior in Japanese macaques decline with age (Nakamichi, 1991). In other words, older animals tend to groom and interact with other monkeys less frequently than younger animals. This patterning has been interpreted as an isolation analogous to the one observed in elderly humans. Other studies, however, find no such effect and attribute a social bias to our willingness to find that old monkeys are also socially isolated (McDonald Pavelka, 1988, 1990, 1991). Dominance rank may complicate simple relationships between age and behavior (Borries *et al.*, 1991; McDonald Pavelka, 1991).

Other behaviors that have been associated with age in non-human primates include an unwillingness to accept innovation, leadership in times of hardship, etc. Borries (1988) has suggested that support of grandchildren may be part of the role of old females in langur society. Whether there is a unique role for the aged in monkey society remains controversial, and may depend on the species and social organization being studied.

Maxim (1979) has suggested that primates with social organizations built around female kinship and coalitions will tend to support females, while those societies that are organized around male–male relationships will support males. By this model, one would not expect females to become socially isolated with age in macaque society, while males might more easily become peripheral. Male rhesus macaques on Cayo Santiago, especially lower-ranking animals, do appear to become socially peripheral with age while females do not (personal observation). Female peripheralization may be characteristic of old langurs which are organized into one-male reproductive units (Borries *et al.*, 1991).

Clearly, more data on species with different social systems, and on both males and females, is necessary.

## Social Stress, Disease, and Immunity

While in many cases it is physiology that limits or changes behavior (see preceding sections), it is clear that behavior may in turn influence physiology. This is best exemplified in humans in the correlation between "stress" and disease (see Weiner, 1977), most likely due to the impact of psychosocial state on the neuroendocrine system and ultimately on the immune system (see Mayer, this volume).

Both the neuroendocrine effects of social stress (Sapolsky, 1990) and an age-related decline in immune function (Ershler *et al.*, 1988) have been documented in non-human primates, suggesting a basic similarity to the human systems. Recent experiments presenting captive cynomolgus monkeys with the stress of social reorganization also show that social context can modulate immune function (Cunnick *et al.*, 1991; Kaplan *et al.*, 1991b), as well as the expression of age-related diseases, such as atherosclerosis (Kaplan *et al.*, 1983), and even ovarian function (Kaplan *et al.*, 1984).

The effect of social state upon such variables that are directly related to survival and reproduction is one of the most exciting new directions in primatology. Its significance for the understanding of aging has yet to be explored.

## Nutrition and Aging in Non-human Primates

Many contemporary diseases of aging are related to diet. These range from arteriosclerosis which is so ubiquitous that some researchers consider it to be a true parameter of "aging" to diabetes which increases in frequency with age. Non-human primates develop some of these diseases spontaneously, while others can be induced with appropriate stimuli. Because of the multi-factorial life-style etiologies of most age-related diseases, non-human primates make valuable models for research into causes and treatments of such disorders.

Research into nutrition-related disorders that occur with advancing age in non-human primates has led several teams toward calorie-restriction studies. It has been known for some time that rodents fed low-calorie or low-protein diets live longer and show less loss of vitality with age (see Masoro, 1984; Merry, 1986). Research on non-human primates suggests that there may indeed be a relationship between diet, aging, and longevity in higher primates, and may eventually offer insights into basic mechanisms of human aging.

## Obesity and Diabetes

Spontaneous obesity is not infrequent in captive non-human primates from prosimians to apes, and can occur in natural populations as well (Kemnitz, 1984; Schwartz, 1987; Hansen, 1992). When a female is obese, her offspring may grow larger than normal (Kemnitz *et al.*, 1988), and presumably be subject to obesity in later life.

In many cases macaque obesity precedes a diabetic condition that is remarkably similar to Type 2 non-insulin-dependent diabetes in humans (Hansen *et al.*, 1993). This non-insulin-dependent diabetes in rhesus monkeys and a non-obesity-related diabetes in *Macaca nigra* (Howard, 1983; Howard and Yasuda, 1990) have become important models for the understanding of human diabetes.

The etiology of these conditions in non-human primates appears to be multi-factorial. Approximately 70% of all mature *M. nigra* show some carbohydrate impairment or overt diabetes (Howard, 1983: 10) which is not associated with obesity, implying that some, presumably genetic, species characteristic is predisposing these animals to disease. On the other hand, middle-aged rhesus monkeys often develop obesity in captivity, presumably related to the conditions of captivity; about 50% of obese monkeys develop diabetes (Kemnitz, personal communication). Undoubtedly dietary and social factors play a role in the expression of these disorders, among them the amount of fiber in the diet and relaxation of the social inhibitions associated with dominance rank (Kemnitz, 1984).

## Cardiovascular Disease

Similarities in the patterning of atherogenesis in monkeys and humans have stimulated much research on atherosclerosis in non-human primates, including squirrel monkeys, rhesus and cynomologus macaques, and baboons. While much of this work is aimed at using diet or drugs to regress lesions, some of it has focused on behavioral influences on atherogenesis, noting the role of social stability, dominance rank, and reproductive status on various measures of atherosclerosis (see reviews by Kaplan *et al.*, 1985, 1991a).

Results clearly indicate that non-human primates, especially macaques, are among the best animal models of atherosclerosis available. In addition to showing spontaneous age-related changes that are similar to the human condition, they approach the social complexity of humans, and show the same idiosyncranicity in the expression of the disease (Clarkson *et al.*, 1985).

## Variation in Provisioning

Current interest in so-called "provisioned" groups of primates has emphasized whether behavioral characteristics of natural and provisioned groups are similar (see Fa and Southwick, 1988; Asquith, 1989), with some concern over the reliability of data collected on provisioned populations. On the other hand, variation in provisioning is clearly an opportunity to explore the behavioral and physiological responses of a species to differing environments, and some work in this direction has begun.

In general, birthrates appear to rise while age at first reproduction and mortality decrease, with substantial provisioning (Loy, 1988; Lyles and Dobson, 1988). Alternatively, when conditions seem stressful, reproduction may be postponed (Kaplan *et al.*, 1984).

Growth also varies with the conditions of captivity (Watts, 1986; DeRousseau, 1990) as does the frequency of obesity (cf. Kemnitz, 1984; Schwartz *et al.*, 1993). Figure 5-3 presents data comparing growth and aging in two colonies of rhesus monkeys maintained under different conditions. Note that the colony

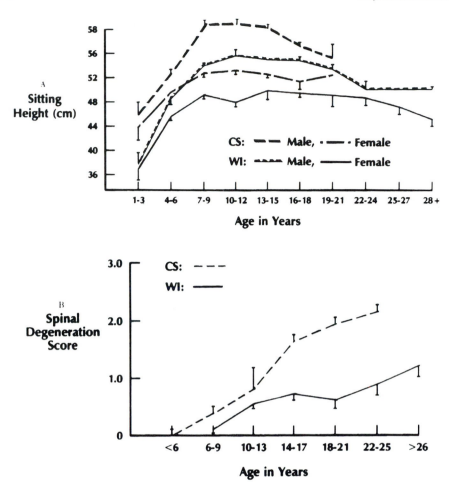

**Figure 5-3** Cross-sectional comparisons of growth and aging measures of the spine, in two colonies of rhesus monkeys. CS = Cayo Santiago, Caribbean Primate Research Center; WI = Wisconsin Regional Primate Research Center and University of Wisconsin Department of Psychology Laboratories. Lines connect mean values. Bars represent standard errors. (A) Mean sitting height by age. (B) Mean scores of osteoarthritic change in the lower spine by age: 0 = none; 4 = severe. Reproduced from DeRousseau (1990).

with delayed growth also shows a slower rate of osteoarthritic development and a longer life span. These results bring a new awareness of life-cycle plasticity to the study of aging.

### Calorie-Restriction Studies

Studies of diet and of nutritionally related disorders in primates have led several research teams to begin calorie-restriction projects in monkeys, whereby one experimental group is given a reduced ration and compared to a control group, both physiologically and behaviorally (Holden, 1990; Ingram *et al.*, 1990; Weindruch *et al.*, 1991; Kemnitz *et al.*, manuscript). Calorie restriction does, of course, result in less weight and body fat, but is also beginning to show some effect upon insulin levels (Kemnitz *et al.*, 1992). This research direction is important both practically and theoretically. It promises insights into age-related disorders tied to age, and into mechanisms of aging.

## Primate Life Histories and Demographics

The evolution of the primate life cycle has become a topic of interest to paleoanthropologists (Bromage, 1990; Stringer *et al.*, 1990; Trinkaus and Tompkins, 1990), primate biologists (Watts, 1990), and behaviorists (Hrdy, 1981), who are amassing more and more data on life-cycle variation both in fossil and contemporary species. These improved determinations of reproductive schedule and life span in non-human primates are valuable assets for understanding human aging and longevity.

### Life-History Theory and Research

In 1954 Cole drew a sharp distinction between life history and demographics in his article, "The population consequences of life-history phenomena." By life history he referred to the typical reproduction schedule of a species, including such characteristics as variation in clutch size, age at first reproduction, and life span. "Life-history tactics" have come to include such characteristics as body size, brain size, growth and mortality patterns, which although not related to reproduction, are related to the processes of maturation to reproductive age.[3] Demography referred to population size and composition.

Life-history theory then generally examines the consequences of certain aspects of the life cycle for population growth. Life-history study of non-human primate groups has examined both within- and between-species variation. Research within species is largely concerned with documenting determinants of reproduction and components of mortality, as well as with constructing life tables of age–sex-specific reproduction and mortality. Research across species is often correlative, asking what reproductive variables cluster with what mortality patterns and ecological contexts. Cross-species research must by definition summarize within-species variation, and in this sense information is lost.

Undoubtedly, one of the sources of variation within species is the ability of most organisms to adapt to their specific circumstances during growth. This phenotypic plasticity in maturation can be described mathematically as a species "norm of reaction" and shown to maximize fitness under varying conditions (e.g., Stearns and Koella, 1986). To my knowledge use of this model has not been applied to non-human primates.

---

[3]I have argued that instead of life history comprising a specific set of ontogenetic traits, it is more an approach whereby whatever is studied is considered in an ontogenetic framework (see DeRousseau, 1990: 1–3).

## Comparative Life Histories in Primates

The intensive study of both captive and feral primates has accumulated increasingly detailed information about both growth (Watts, 1985) and reproductive patterns (Dunbar, 1987, 1988). Although Schultz's early work (1969) suggested that some simple evolutionary trends seemed responsible for variation in the primate life cycle, Watts (1990) shows that data to date do not support this notion, and instead that different systems (reproductive, skeletal, dental) have evolved somewhat independently. In addition, individual non-human primates like individual humans seem capable of adjusting their maturation rates to accommodate circumstances (DeRousseau and Reichs, 1987; DeRousseau, 1990; see Figure 5-3).

Similarly, individual primates seem to show a variety of reproductive patterns, depending on dominance, age, food supply, etc. (see reviews by Jolly, 1985; Dunbar, 1988). One interesting reproductive variant within species is that infant survivorship can actually be better in older females who are more experienced at caring for their offspring (Dolhinow et al., 1979).

Although the relationship between reproduction and life span in individual primates in nature is still little studied, several studies have shown a positive relationship between age and reproductive success. Studying Amboseli baboons, Altmann et al. (1988) showed that the number of surviving offspring was highly correlated with the age of the mother. One study on the Arashiyama West colony (Fedigan et al., 1986) was able to show that "lifetime reproductive success" (total number of offspring living to age 5) in provisioned Japanese monkeys depended most strongly on reproductive life span. A follow-up study by Fedigan (1991) found that matrilines composed of long-lived individuals tended to weigh more as well as reproduce more than short-lived matrilines. Interestingly, the two most dominant lineages of five examined "were the lightest, shortest-lived, and least productive" (Fedigan, 1991: 150).

The impacts of various sources of mortality on life span are even less clear from field studies. Four main causes of mortality in free-ranging populations of non-human primates have been identified by Dunbar (1988): starvation, disease, temperature stress, and predation. Variation on how these stressors impact on a given individual may depend on reproductive condition, dominance rank, or proximity to predators (Altmann et al., 1988; Cheney et al., 1988). The standard model life table for Old World monkeys derived by Gage and Dyke (1988) suggests that various causes of death may be age dependent in some environments and age independent in others. In general, data on mortality does not clarify what selective pressures might be operating to effect life span.

There is some evidence that there may be a trade-off between reproductive effort and mortality. Fedigan et al. (1986) found an inverse relationship between fecundity per year (total number of births divided by reproductive life span) and infant survivorship in Japanese macaques, suggesting that reducing birth intervals increases the risk of infant mortality.

By far the most systematic examination of life-history variables relative to life span has been across species. From these studies it seems clear that the primate life cycle is not unusual among mammals and that many aspects of ontogeny in primates are highly correlated with one another at the species level (Harvey and Clutton-Brock, 1985; Harvey et al., 1987).

The most well-cited correlation of life-history traits in primates is the positive correlation of life span with brain weight independent of body weight (Sacher, 1959, 1975). Although Harvey et al. (1987) found the same result, he suggests that the finding could be an artifact of the greater individual variation in body than in brain weight.

Interestingly, there is a very high correlation between age at first reproduction and life expectancy in mammals, body weight held constant (Harvey and Zammuto, 1985). When both body weight and age at first reproduction are held constant, the correlation between life span and brain size in primates is negligible (Harvey et al., 1987). Thus, the more important relationship may be one that signals a trade-off between reproductive effort and mortality.

## Where Do We Go From Here?

There are many theories of how and why we age (see Finch, 1991; Rose, 1991), all of which have some empirical support. Although these ideas are generally perceived as competing theories, it may be useful to consider them instead as deriving from observations at different levels of organization, and thus representing differing perspective on the aging process.

For example, a focus on changes in macromolecules over time may lead to hypotheses about the role of cross-linking in aging, while a focus on patterns of reproduction and mortality in populations may lead to an evolutionary interpretation of aging. If these perspectives compete as models for why we age, information is lost. If, instead, we consider that each level of organization is part of the story, new questions arise about the interactions between those levels, and a synthesis may emerge (see Wood et al., this volume, for a discussion of the interaction between physiological and population characteristics of aging in humans).

In this paper, too, I have presented material on aging in non-human primates from several levels of organization. Each one shows exciting data that could be important to understanding mechanisms of primate aging. Behavioral studies are engaged in a debate over the role of the elderly in society, while physiological studies suggest both that aging may limit behavior, and that behavior may in turn affect aging. In particular, social stress may affect atherogenesis, ovulation, and immune function. The field of nutrition and aging has developed models for obesity, diabetes, and atherosclerosis, as well as long-term experiments examining the impact of dietary restrictions on aging. Life-history studies are amassing vast amounts of data describing patterns of reproduction and longevity both within and between species that suggest that a "trade-off" between reproduction and mortality may be both an individual and a species trait.

Taken together, the sum is more than its parts, however. Each of these areas of study includes some attention to interactions between the relevant levels of organization, e.g., diet or social stress affecting physiological aging, or aging affecting inter-birth intervals. Those interactions in a sense define the plasticity in the various systems of the organism, and direct our attention toward those processes by which the organism adjusts to its circumstances.

The notion of the "adaptable individual" will surely play a role in our understanding of aging. What mechanisms have evolved to negotiate the environment at all the various levels of organization? Are not these the true "traits" on which evolution has proceeded, and which offer the most hope for the modification of human aging? Ways in which the primates vary in such mechanisms will, I predict, be the most important contribution of primate gerontology in the next several decades.

## REFERENCES

Albrecht, G. H. (1982) Collections of nonhuman primate skeletal materials in the United States and Canada. *American Journal of Physical Anthropology* **57**, 77–97.

Altmann, J., Hausfater, G. and Altmann, S. A. (1988) Determinants of reproductive success in savannah baboons. *Papio cynocephalus*. In: *Reproductive Success* (ed. Clutton-Brock, T. H.). University of Chicago: Chicago, pp. 403–418.

Asquith, P. J. (1989) Provisioning and the study of free-ranging primates: history, effects, and prospects. *Yearbook of Physical Anthropology* **32**, 129–158.

Bennett, C. L., Davis, R. T. and Miller, J. M. (1983) Demonstration of presbycusis across repeated measures in a nonhuman primate species. *Behavioral Neuroscience* **97**, 602-607.

Bito, L. Z., DeRousseau, C. J., Kaufman, P. L. and Bito, J. W. (1982) *Investigative Ophthalmology and Visual Science* **23**, 23–31.

Borries, C. (1988) Patterns of grandmaternal behaviour in free-ranging Hanuman langurs (*Presbytis entellus*). *Human Evolution* **3**, 239–260.

Borries, C., Somner, V. and Srivastava, A. (1991) Dominance, age, and reproductive success in free-ranging female Hanuman langurs. *International Journal of Primatology* **12**, 231–257.

Bowden, D. M. (ed.) (1979) *Aging in Nonhuman Primates*. Van Nostrand Reinhold Co.: New York.

Bowden, D. M. and Jones, M. L. (1979) Aging research in nonhuman primates. In: *Aging in Nonhuman Primates* (ed. Bowden, D. M.). Van Nostrand Reinhold: New York, pp. 1–13.

Bowden, D. M. and Williams, D. D. (1984). Aging. In: *Advances in Veterinary Science and Comparative Medicine*, Vol. 28. Research on Nonhuman Primates (ed. Hendrickx, A. G.). Academic Press, Inc.: Orlando, FL, pp. 305–341.

Bowden, D. M., Teets, C., Witkin, J. and Young, D. M. (1979) Long bone calcification and morphology. In: *Aging in Nonhuman Primates* (ed. Bowden, D. M.). Van Nostrand Reinhold Company: New York, pp. 335–347.

Bromage, T. G. (1990) Early hominid development and life history. In: *Primate Life History and Evolution* (ed. DeRousseau, C. J.). Wiley–Liss: New York, pp. 105–114.

Brown, T. McP., Clark, H. W. and Bailey, J. S. (1974) Natural occurrence of rheumatoid arthritis in great apes—a new animal model. *Proceedings of the*

*Zoological Society of Philadelphia Centennial Symposium on Scientific Research*, pp. 43–79.

Bygott, J. D. (1979) Agonistic behavior, dominance, and social structure in wild chimpanzees of the Gombe National Park. In: *The Great Apes* (eds Hamburg, D. A. and McCown, E. R.). Benjamin/Cummings: Menlo Park, CA, pp. 405–428.

Caminiti, B. (1978) *The Aged Nonhuman Primate: A Bibliography*. Primate Information Center, Regional Primate Research Center, University of Washington, Seattle.

Caminiti, B. (1985) *The Aged Nonhuman Primate, 1976–1985*. Primate Information Center, Regional Primate Research Center, University of Washington, Seattle.

Carpenter, C. R. (1972) Breeding colonies of macaques and gibbons on Santiago Island, Puerto Rico. In: *International Symposium on Breeding Nonhuman Primates for Laboratory Use* (ed. Beveridge, W. I.). Karger: Basel, pp. 76–87.

Cheney, D. L., Seyfarth, R. M., Andelman, S. J. and Lee, P. C. (1988) *Reproductive Success* (ed. Clutton-Brock, T. H.). University of Chicago Press: Chicago, pp. 384–402.

Cheverud, J. M. (1981) Epiphyseal union and dental eruption in *Macaca mulatta*. *American Journal of Physical Anthropology* **56**, 157–167.

Clarkson, T. B., Kaplan, J. R. and Adams, M. R. (1985) The role of individual differences in lipoprotein, artery wall, gender, and behavioral responses in the development of atherosclerosis. *Annals of the New York Academy of Sciences* **454**, 28–45.

Committee on Animal Models for Research on Aging (1981) *Mammalian Models for Research on Aging*. National Academy Press: Washington, DC.

Cornelius, C. E. and Simpson, C. F. (eds) (1984) *Advances in Veterinary Science and Comparative Medicine*, Vol. 28. *Research on Nonhuman Primates*. Academic Press, Inc.: New York.

Cunnick, J. E., Cohen, S., Rabin, B. S., Carpenter, A. B., Manuck, S. B. and Kaplan, J. R. (1991) Alterations in specific antibody production due to rank and social instability. *Brain Behavior and Immunity* **5**, 357–369.

Cutler, R. G. (1976) Evolution of longevity in primates. *Journal of Human Evolution* **5**, 169–202.

Davis, R. T. (1985) The effects of aging on the behavior of rhesus monkeys. In: *Behavior and Pathology of Aging in Rhesus Monkeys* (eds Davis, R. T. and Leathers, C. W.) Alan R. Liss, Inc.: New York, pp. 57–82.

Davis, R. T. and Leathers, C. W. (eds) (1985) *Behavior and Pathology of Aging in Rhesus Monkeys*. Alan. R. Liss, Inc.: New York.

Dean, R. L. and Bartus, R. T. (1988) Behavioral models of aging in nonhuman primates. In: *Psychopharmacology of the Aging Nervous System* (eds Iversen, L. L., Iversen, S. D. and Snyder, S. H.). Plenum Press: New York, pp. 325–392.

DeRousseau, C. J. (1984) Variation in patterns of growth and aging in rhesus monkeys (abstract). *American Journal of Physical Anthropology* **63**, 151.

DeRousseau, C. J. (1985a) Aging in the musculoskeletal system of rhesus monkeys. III. Bone loss. *American Journal of Physical Anthropology* **68**, 157–167.

DeRousseau, C. J. (1985b) Aging in the musculoskeletal system of rhesus monkeys. II. Degenerative joint disease. *American Journal of Physical Anthropology* **67**, 177–184.

DeRousseau, C. J. (1988) *Osteoarthritis in Rhesus Monkeys and Gibbons. A Locomotor Model of Joint Degeneration*. S. Karger AG: Basel, Switzerland.

DeRousseau, C. J. (ed.) (1990) *Primate Life History and Evolution*. Wiley-Liss: New York.

DeRousseau, C. J. and Reichs, K. J. (1987) Ontogenetic plasticity in nonhuman primates. I. Secular trends in the Cayo Santiago macaques. *American Journal of Physical Anthropology* **73**, 279–287.

DeRousseau, C. J., Rawlins, R. G. and Denlinger, J. L. (1983) Aging in the musculoskeletal system of rhesus monkeys: I. Passive joint excursion. *American Journal of Physical Anthropology* **61**, 483–494.

DeRousseau, C. J., Bito, L. Z. and Kaufman, P. L. (1986) Age-dependent impairments of the rhesus monkey visual and musculoskeletal systems and apparent behavioral consequences. In: *The Cayo Santiago Macaques* (eds Rawlins, R. G. and Kessler, M. J.). State University of New York Press: Albany, pp. 232–251.

DeVore, I. (ed.) (1965) *Primate Behavior: Field Studies of Monkeys and Apes*. Holt, Rinehart and Winston: New York.

Dolhinow, P. (1984) The primates: age, behavior, and evolution. In: *Age and Anthropological Theory* (eds Kertzer, D. I. and Keith, J.). Cornell University Press: New York, pp. 65–81.

Dolhinow, P., McKenna, J. J. and Vonder Haar Laws, J. (1979) Rank and reproduction among female langur monkeys: Aging and improvement (They're not just getting older, they're getting better). *Aggressive Behavior* **5**, 19-30.

Dunbar, R. I. M. (1987) Demography and reproduction. In: *Primate Societies* (eds Smuts, B. B., Cheney, D. L., Seyfarth, R. M. Wrangham, R. W. and Struhsaker, T. T.). University of Chicago Press: Chicago, pp. 240–249.

Dunbar, R. I. M. (1988) *Primate Social Systems*. Cornell University Press: Ithaca, NY.

Ershler, W. B., Coe, C. L., Gravenstein, S., Schultz, K. T., Klopp, R. G., Meyer, M. and Houser, W. D. (1988) Aging and immunity in nonhuman primates: I. Effects of age and gender on cellular immune function in rhesus monkeys (*Macaca mulatta*). *American Journal of Primatology* **15**, 181–188.

Fa, J. E. and Southwick, C. H. (eds.) (1988) *Ecology and Behavior of Food-Enhanced Primate Groups*. Alan R. Liss, Inc.: New York.

Fedigan, L. M. (1991) History of the Arashiyama West Japanese macaques in Texas. In: *The Monkeys of Arashiyama* (eds Fedigan, L. M. and Asquith, P. J.). State University of New York Press: Albany, pp. 140–154.

Fedigan, L. M., Fedigan, L., Gouzoules, S., Gouzoules, H. and Koyama, N. (1986) Lifetime reproductive success in female Japanese macaques. *Folia primatologica* **47**, 143–157.

Finch, C. E. (1991) *Longevity, Senescence, and the Genome*. University of Chicago Press: Chicago.

Fox, H. (1939) Chronic arthritis in wild mammals. *Transactions of the American Philosophical Society n.s.* **31**, 71–149.

Gage, T. B. and Dyke, B. (1988) Model life tables for the larger Old World monkeys. *American Journal of Primatology* **16**, 305–320.

Gaulin, S. J. C. (1980) Sexual dimorphism in the human post-reproductive lifespan: Possible causes. *Journal of Human Evolution* **9**, 227–232.

Goodall, J. (1983) Population dynamics during a 15-year period in one community of free-living chimpanzees in the Gombe National Park, Tanzania. *Zeitschrift Tierpsychologie* **61**, 1-60.

Goodall, J. (1986) *The Chimpanzees of Gombe: Patterns of Behavior*. Harvard University Press: Cambridge, MA.

Gorman, L. (1983) Bone loss and osteoporosis in rhesus monkeys. *American Journal of Physical Anthropology* **60**, 200–201.

Gould, K. G., Flint, M. and Graham, C. E. (1981) Chimpanzee reproductive senescence: A possible model for evolution of the menopause. *Maturitas* **3**, 157–166.

Graham, C. E. (1979) Reproduction function in aged female chimpanzees. *American Journal of Physical Anthropology* **50**, 291–300.

Graham, C. E., Kling, O. R. and Steiner, R. A. (1979) Reproductive senescence in female nonhuman primates. In: *Aging in Nonhuman Primates* (ed. Bowden, D. M.). Van Nostrand Reinhold: New York, pp. 183–209.

Hannah, J. S., Verdery, R. B., Bodkin, N. L., Hansen, B. C., Le, N.-A. and Howard, B. V. (1991) Changes in lipoprotein concentrations during the development of noninsulin-dependent diabetes mellitus in obese rhesus monkeys (*Macaca mulatta*). *Journal of Clinical Endocrinology* **72**, 1067–1072.

Hansen, B. C. (1992) Obesity and diabetes in monkeys. In: *Obesity* (eds Bjorntorp, P. and Brodoff, B. M.). Lippincott: New York, pp. 256–265.

Hansen, B. C., Bodkin, N. L., Jen, K.-L. C. and Ortmeyer, H. K. (1993) Primate models of disease. In: *Proceedings of the International Diabetes Federation*. Elsevier Science Publishers, B.V.: Amsterdam, Netherlands.

Haraway, D. (1989) *Primate Visions*. Routledge: New York.

Harley, D. (1990) Aging and reproductive performance in langur monkeys (*Presbytis entellus*). *American Journal of Physical Anthropology* **83**, 253–261.

Harvey, P. H. and Clutton-Brock, T. H. (1985) Life history variation in primates. *Evolution* **39**, 559–581.

Harvey, P. H. and Zammuto, R. M. (1985) Patterns of mortality and age at first reproduction in natural populations of mammals. *Nature* **15**, 319–320.

Harvey, P. H., Martin, R. D. and Clutton-Brock, T. H. (1987) Life histories in comparative perspective. In: *Primate Societies* (eds Smuts, B. B., Cheney, D. L., Seyfarth, R. M., Wrangham, R. W. and Struhsaker, T. T.). University of Chicago Press: Chicago, pp. 181–196.

Hawkins, J. E., Jr, Miller, J. M., Rouse, R. C., Davis, J. A. and Rarey, K. (1985) Inner ear histopthology in aging rhesus monkeys (*Macaca mulatta*). In: *Behavior and Pathology of Aging in Rhesus Monkeys* (eds Davis, R. T. and Leathers, C. W.). Alan R. Liss, Inc.: New York, pp. 137–154.

Hodgen, G. D., Goodman, A. L., O'Connor, A. and Johnson, D. K. (1977) Menopause in rhesus monkeys: Model for study of disorders in the human climacteric. *Am. J. Obstet. Gynecol.* **127**, 581–584.

Holden, C. (1990) Primate secret to longevity. *Science* **250**, 1335.

Howard, C. F. (1983) Diabetes and carbohydrate impairment in nonhuman primates. In: *Nonhuman Primate Models for Human Diseases* (ed. Dukelow, W. R.). CRC Press, Inc.: Boca Raton, FL, pp. 1–36.

Howard, C. F., Jr and Yasuda, M. (1990) Diabetes mellitus in nonhuman primates: Recent research advances and current husbandry practices. *Journal of Medical Primatology* **19**, 609–625.

Hrdy, S. B. (1981) "Nepotists" and "altruists": the behavior of old females among macaques and langur monkeys. In: *Other Ways of Growing Old: Anthropological Perspectives* (eds Amoss, P. T. and Harrell, S.) Stanford University Press: Stanford, CA, pp. 59–76.

Huffman, M. A. (1991) History of the Arashiyama Japanese macaques in Kyoto, Japan. In: *The Monkeys of Arashiyama* (eds Fedigan, L. M. and Asquith, P. J.). State University of New York Press: Albany, pp. 21–53.

Ingram, D. K., Cutler, R. G., Weindruch, R., Renquist, D. M., Knapka, J. J., April, M., Belcher, C. T., Clark, M. A., Hatcherson, C. D., Marriott, B. and Roth, G. S. (1990) Dietary restriction and aging: The initiation of a primate study. *Journal of Gerontology* **45**, B148-B163.

Jolly, A. (1985) *The Evolution of Primate Behavior*. Macmillan Publishing Company: New York.

Jurmain, R. (1989) Trauma, degenerative disease, and other pathologies among the Gombe chimpanzees. *American Journal of Physical Anthropology* **80**, 229–237.

Kaplan, J. R., Manuck, S. B., Clarkson, T. B., Lusso, F. M., Taub, D. M. and Miller, E. W. (1983) Social stress and atherosclerosis in normocholesterolemic monkeys. *Science* **220**, 733–735.

Kaplan, J. R., Adams, M. R., Clarkson, T. B. and Koritnik, D. R. (1984) Psychosocial influences on female "protection" among cynomolgus macaques. *Atherosclerosis* **53**, 283–295.

Kaplan, J. R., Manuck, S. B., Clarkson, T. B. and Prichard, R. W. (1985) Animal models of behavioral influences on atherogenesis. *Advances in Behavioral Medicine* **1**, 115–163.

Kaplan, J. R., Adams, M. R., Clarkson, T. B., Manuck, S. B. and Shively, C. A. (1991a) Social behavior and gender in biomedical investigations using monkeys: studies in atherogenesis. *Laboratory Animal Science* **41**, 334–343.

Kaplan, J. R., Heise, E. R., Manuck, S. B., Shively, C. A., Cohen, S., Rabin, B. S. and Kasprowicz, A. L. (1991b) The relationship of agonistic and affiliative behavior patterns to cellular immune function among cynomolgus monkeys (*Macaca fascicularis*) living in unstable social groups. *American Journal of Primatology* **25**, 157–173.

Kaufman, P. L. and Bito, L. Z. (1982) The occurrence of senile cataracts, ocular hypertension and glaucoma in rhesus monkeys. *Experimental Eye Research* **34**, 287–291.

Kemnitz, J. W. (1984) Obesity in macaques: spontaneous and induced. In: *Advances in Veterinary Science and Comparative Medicine* Vol. 28 (eds Cornelius, C. E. and Simpson, C. F.). Academic Press, Inc.: Orlando, FL, pp. 81–114.

Kemnitz, J. W., Engle, M. J., Flitsch, T. J., Perelman, R. H. and Farrell, P. M. (1988) Obesity in pregnancy: Consequences for maternal glucoregulation and fetal growth. In: *Nonhuman Primates Studies on Diabetes, carbohydrate Intolerance, and Obesity*. (ed. Howard, C. F.). Alan. R. Liss, Inc.: New York, pp. 29–41.

Kemnitz, J., Baum, S., Elson, D., Roecker, E. Weindruch, R., Barden, H., Kaufman, P., Crawford, K. and Ershler, W. (1992) Caloric restriction and aging in rhesus macaques. Abstract of paper given at FASEB Annual Meetings.

Kemnitz, J. W., Weindruch, R., Roecher, E. B., Crawford, K., Kaufman, P. L. and Ershler, W. B. (n.d.) Dietary restriction of adult male rhesus monkeys: design, methodology and preliminary findings from the first year of study. (Manuscript, Wisconsin Regional Primate Research Center, Madison.

Kessler, M. J., Turnquist, J. E., Pritzker, K. P. H. and London, W. T. (1986) Reduction of passive extension and radiographic evidence of degenerative knee joint diseases in cage-raised and free-ranging aged rhesus monkeys (*Macaca mulatta*). *Journal of Medical Primatology* **15**, 1–9.

Koyama, N. (1967) On dominance rank and kinship of a wild Japanese monkey troop in Arashiyama. *Primates* **8**, 189–216.

Lancaster, J. B. and King, B. J. (1985) An evolutionary perspective on menopause. In: *In Her Prime: A New View of Middle-Aged Women* (eds Brown, J. K. and Kerns, V.). Bergin and Garvey: South Hadley, MA, pp. 13–20.

Lovell, N. C. (1990) *Patterns of Injury and Illness in Great Apes: A Skeletal Analysis*. Smithsonian Institution Press: Washington, DC.

Loy, J. (1988) Effects of supplementary feeding on maturation and fertility in primate groups. In: *Ecology and Behavior of Food-Enhanced Primate Groups* (eds Fa, J. E. and Southwick, C. H.). Alan R. Liss, Inc.: New York, pp. 153–166.

Lyles, A. M. and Dobson, A. P. (1988) Dynamics of provisioned and unprovisioned primate populations. In: *Ecology and Behavior of Food-Enhanced Primate Groups* (eds Fa, J. E. and Southwick, C. H.). Alan R. Liss, Inc.: New York, pp. 167–198.

Masoro, E. J. (1984) Food restriction and the aging process. *Journal of the American Geriatrics Society* **32**, 296–300.

Maxim, P. E. (1979) Social behavior. In: *Aging in Nonhuman Primates* (ed. Bowden, D. M.). Van Nostrand Reinhold Company: New York, pp. 56–70.

McDonald Pavelka, M. S. (1988) *Aging in Female Japanese Monkeys: Primatological Contributions to Gerontology*. Doctoral Thesis, Department of Anthropology, University of Alberta, Edmonton, Alberta, Canada.

McDonald Pavelka, M. S. (1990) Do old female monkeys have a specific social role? *Primates* **31**, 363–373.

McDonald Pavelka, M. S. (1991) Sociability in old female Japanese monkeys: human versus nonhuman primate aging. *American Anthropology* **93**, 588–598.

McDonald Pavelka, M. S., Gillespie, M. W. and Griffin, L. (1991) The interacting effect of age and rank on the sociability of adult female Japanese monkeys. In: *The Monkeys of Arashiyama* (eds Fedigan, L. M. and Asquith, P. J.). State University of New York Press: Albany, pp. 194–207.

Merry, B. J. (1986) Dietary manipulation of ageing: an animal model. In: *The Biology of Human Ageing* (eds Bittles, A. H. and Collins, K. J.). Cambridge University Press: Cambridge, pp. 225–242.

Moss, M. B., Rosene, D. L. and Peters, A. (1988) Effects of aging on visual recognition memory in the rhesus monkey. *Neurobiology of Aging* **9**, 495–502.

Nakamichi, M. (1984) Behavioral characteristics of old Japanese monkeys in a free-ranging group. *Primates* **25**, 192–203.

Nakamichi, M. (1991) Behavior of old females: comparisons of Japanese monkeys in the Arashiyama East and West groups. In: *The Monkeys of Arashiyama* (eds Fedigan, L. M. and Asquith, P. J., State University of New York Press: Albany, pp. 175–193.

Nishida, T., Takasaki, H. and Takahata, Y. (1990) Demography nd reproductive profiles. In: *The Chimpanzees of the Mahale Mountains: Sexual and Life History Strategies*. University of Tokyo Press: Tokyo, pp. 63–97.

Paul, A. and Kuester, J. (1988) Life-history patterns of Barbary macaques (*Macaca sylvanus*) at Affenberg Salem. In: *Ecology and Behavior of Food-Enhanced Primate Groups* (eds Fa, J. E. and Southwick, C. H.). Alan R. Liss, Inc.: New York, pp. 199–228.

Pavelka, M. S. M. and Fedigan, L. M. (1991) Menopause: a comparative life history perspective. *Yearbook of Physical Anthropology* **34**, 13–38.

Price, D. L., Cork, L. C., Struble, R. G., Kitt, C. A., Price, D. L., Jr, Lehmann, J. and Hedreen, J. C. (1985) Neuropathological, neurochemical, and behavioral studies of the aging nonhuman primate. In: *Behavior and Pathology of Aging in Rhesus Monkeys* (eds Davis, R. T. and Leathers, C. W.). Alan R. Liss, Inc.: New York, pp. 113–135.

Price, D. L., Koo, E. H., Wagster, M. V., Walker, L. C., Wenk, G. L., Applegate, M. D., Kitt, C. A. and Cork, L. C. (1990) Behavioral, cellular, and molecular biological studies of aged nonhuman primates. *Advances in Neurology* **51**, 83–89.

Rawlins, R. G. (1975) Age changes in the pubic symphysis of *Macaca mulatta*. *American Journal of Physical Anthropology* **42**, 477–487.

Rawlins, R. G. (1979) Forty years of rhesus research. *New Scientist* **82**, 108–110.

Richard, A. F. (1985) *Primates in Nature*. W. H. Freeman and Co.: New York.

Rose, M. R. (1991) *Evolutionary Biology of Aging*. Oxford University Press: New York.

Rothschild, B. M. and Woods, R. J. (1992) Osteorarthritis, calcium pyrophosphate deposition disease, and osseous infection in Old World primates. *American Journal of Physical Anthropology* **87**, 341–347.

Sacher, G. A. (1959) Relation of lifespan to brain weight and body weight in mammals. In: *Ciba Foundation Colloquia on Ageing*. Vol. 5. *The Lifespan of Animals* (eds Wolstenholme, G. E. W. and O'Connor, M.). Churchill: London.

Sacher, G. A. (1975) Maturation and longevity in relation to cranial capacity in hominid evolution. In: *Primate Functional Morphology and Evolution* (ed. Tuttle, R. H.). Mouton Publishers: The Hague, pp. 417–441.

Sade, D. S. (1967) A longitudinal study of social behavior of rhesus monkeys. In: *The Functional and Evolutionary Biology of Primates* (ed. Tuttle, R.). Aldine-Atherton: Chicago, pp. 378–398.

Sade, D. S. (1990) Intrapopulation variation in life-history parameters. In: *Primate Life History and Evolution* (ed. DeRousseau, C. J.). Wiley–Liss: New York, pp. 181–194.

Sapolsky, R. M. (1990) Stress in the wild. *Scientific American*, January issue.

Schultz, A. H. (1969) *The Life of Primates*. Universe Books: New York.

Schwartz, S. M. (1987) Spontaneous obesity in the Cayo Santiago macaque. *American Journal of Primatology* **12**, 370.

Schwartz, S. M., Kemnitz, J. W. and Howard, C. F. (1993) Obesity in free-ranging rhesus macaques. *International Journal of Obesity* **17**, 1–9.

Small, M. F. (1984) Aging and reproductive success in female *Macaca mulatta*. In: *Female Primates: Studies by Women Primatologists* (ed. Small, M. F.). Alan R. Liss, Inc.: New York, pp. 249–259.

Smuts, B. B., Cheney, D. L., Seyfarth, R. M., Wrangham, R. W. and Struhsaker, T. T. (eds) (1987) *Primate Societies*. University of Chicago Press: Chicago.

Stearns, S. C. and Koella, J. C. (1986) The evolution of phenotypic plasticity in life-history traits: Predictions of reaction norms for age and size at maturity. *Evolution* **40**, 893–913.

Stewart, T. D. (1979) *Essentials of Forensic Anthropology*. Charles C. Thomas: Springfield, IL.

Stringer, C. B., Dean, M. C. and Martin, R. D. (1990) A comparative study of cranial and dental development within a recent British sample and among Neandertals. In: *Primate Life History and Evolution* (ed. DeRousseau, C. J.). Wiley–Liss: New York, pp. 115–152.

Strum, S. C. and Western, J. D. (1982) Variations in fecundity with age and environment in olive baboons (*Papio anubis*). *American Journal of Primatology* **3**, 61–76.

Sumner, D. R., Morbeck, M. E. and Lobick, J. J. (1989) Apparent age-related bone loss among adult female Gombe chimpanzees. *American Journal of Physical Anthropology* **79**, 225–234.

Trinkaus, E. and Tompkins, R. L. (1990) The Neandertal life cycle: The possibility, probability, and perceptibility of contrasts with recent humans. In: *Primate Life History and Evolution* (ed. DeRousseau, C. J.). Wiley–Liss: New York, pp. 153–180.

Turnquist, J. E. (1986) Joint mobility as a function of age in free-ranging rhesus monkeys (*Macaca mulatta*). In: *The Cayo Santiago Macaques* (eds Rawlins, R. G. and Kessler, M. J.). State University of New York Press: Albany, pp. 253–262.

van Wagenen, G. (1972) Vital statistics from a breeding colony: Reproduction and pregnancy outcome in *Macaca mulatta*. *Journal of Medical Primatology* **1**, 3–28.

Waser, P. M. (1978) Postreproductive survival and behavior in a free-ranging female mangabey. *Folia Primatologica (Basel)* **29**, 142–160.

Watts, E. S. (ed.) (1985) *Nonhuman Primates Models for Human Growth and Development*. Alan R. Liss, Inc.: New York.

Watts, E. S. (1986) Skeletal development. In: *Comparative Primate Biology*, Vol. 3. *Reproduction and Development* (ed. Dukelow, W. R.). Alan R. Liss, Inc.: New York, pp. 415–439.

Watts, E. S. (1990) Evolutionary trends in primate growth and development. In: *Primate Life History and Evolution* (ed. DeRousseau, C. J.) Wiley–Liss: New York, pp. 89–104.

Weindruch, R. H., Kemnitz, J. W., Roecker, E. B., Kaufman, P. L. and Erchler, W. B. (1991) Dietary restriction of adult rhesus monkeys: findings from the first year of study. The *Gerontologist* **31** (Special Issue II), 78.

Weiner, H. (1977) *Psychobiology and Human Disease*. Elsevier: New York.

Williams, J. (1984) *Age Primate Learning and Behavior, 1940–1983*. Primate Information Center, Regional Primate Research Center, University of Washington, Seattle.

Zihlman, A. L., Morbeck, M. E. and Sumner, D. R., Jr (1989) Tales of Gombe chimps as told in their bones. *Anthroquest* **40**, 20–22.

Zihlman, A. L., Morbeck, M. E. and Goodall, J. (1990) Skeletal biology and individual life history of Gombe chimpanzees. *Journal of Zoology* **221**, 37–62.

# 6

# Chronic Degenerative Diseases and Aging

## DOUGLAS E. CREWS AND LINDA M. GERBER

## INTRODUCTION

One goal of biological anthropology is to explore and document human biological variation within and between populations. Longevity and patterns of chronic degenerative diseases vary across today's many populations and the likelihood is that they have varied throughout hominid evolution. Where life expectancy is low, the constellation of infectious, parasitic, and nutritional disease, poor maternal conditions, congenital childhood diseases, and accidents contribute overwhelmingly to morbidity and mortality. In contrast, where longevity extends to the seventh and eighth decades, a group of conditions, collectively identifiable as chronic degenerative diseases, lead morbidity and mortality statistics.

The purpose of this chapter is to explore the adaptive and evolutionary bases for the high frequency of chronic degenerative conditions among elderly individuals living in today's cosmopolitan societies. To accomplish this goal, we first articulate minimal conditions that may allow labeling any particular disorder as a chronic degenerative disease. Next, prehistorical evidence and historical reports are reviewed to document that an increase in such chronic degenerative conditions has accompanied the extension of human life expectancy into the seventh and eight decades. Demographic, sociocultural, and life-style changes that have combined to usher in today's "epidemic" of chronic degenerative diseases are examined in turn. Following this, a model, based on "thrifty genotypes" with pleiotropic effects that may be described as "antagonistic" interacting with changing sociocultural environments and ecological settings, is offered to help explain the present "epidemic" of chronic degenerative diseases. Possible examples of "thrifty-pleiotropic" phenotypes are explored to illustrate the model and several natural experimental settings that may be used to test predictions from the proposed model are detailed in a final section.

## VARIATION IN HUMAN CHRONIC DEGENERATIVE DISEASES: TRENDS AND CORRELATES

### Chronic Degenerative Diseases

A multitude of conditions may fall into the category chronic degenerative diseases. At minimum, chronic degenerative diseases may be defined as those conditions that lead to progressive deterioration in one or more clinical, metabolic, or physiological traits that can be measured on a continuous scale (Crews and James, 1991). Medically, chronic degenerative disease states are commonly diagnosed when a specific metabolic and/or physiological parameter falls above or below a particular critical value (Sing *et al.*, 1985). Examples of such parameters include blood glucose, serum cholesterol, body mass index, and blood pressure which are used to define diabetes, hypercholesterolemia, obesity, and hypertension, respectively. Critical values for diseases based on such parameters are often arbitrary, such as the point at which blood pressure is diagnostic of hypertension (Pickering, 1961) or at which blood glucose is diagnostic of diabetes mellitus (Harris, 1985; Foster, 1989). Frequently, such definitions have been based on retrospective or prospective population data showing that individuals with elevated or depressed values are at greater risk of morbidity and mortality. Additionally, some chronic diseases may be insidious in their onset and present only when symptoms are recognized clinically, for example, neoplastic diseases, slow virus infections, and human immunodeficiency viruses. Such diseases will not necessarily show progressive deterioration and continuous decline to a critical value.

Importantly, many disease cut-points change as diagnostic instrumentation and expertise improve, such as has occurred with cholesterol and blood pressure (American Heart Association, 1988). Whereas, in the case of cancer, an ongoing process of unregulated cell proliferation is not diagnosed until the resulting cell mass becomes sufficiently large to be identified by state-of-the-art diagnostic techniques, that are themselves continually improving. Indeed, the majority of present-day chronic noninfectious degenerative diseases are the end-product of complex and poorly defined series of events initiated at an unknown point and progressing over a good portion of an individual's life (see Hutt and Burkitt, 1986). The etiology and presentation of such conditions represent complex interactions among genes, environment, personal life history, and medical technology. Thus, etiologies are often difficult to establish, since most people with these disorders have sub-clinical diseases and many disease-free individuals share features, or risk factors, in common with those affected.

Among the most commonly recognized chronic degenerative diseases are those that are the leading killers of adults in 20th century cosmopolitan societies—coronary heart disease, cerebrovascular disease, cancer, and diabetes. Chronic infections, modern examples of which are acquired immune deficiency syndrome and kuru, also represent chronic degenerative diseases, although they commonly are not recognized as such. Still other conditions, such as osteoporosis, osteoarthritis, multiple sclerosis, amyotrophic lateral sclerosis, cystic fibrosis, and Alzeheimer's disease, that are less frequently cited as causes of death are obviously chronic degenerative diseases. Other conditions, such as sickle cell anemia, phenylketonuria, some psychiatric disorders, arthritis, epilepsy, and familial hypercholesterolemia also fit this minimal definition. Additionally, certain conditions that occur during infancy, childhood, or early adulthood and frequently cause premature death, for example, progeria and Werner's syndrome, which may, in some ways, resemble premature aging, or amyotrophic lateral sclerosis and Huntington's chorea, are also associated with progressive deterioration in multiple physiological parameters. (Several of these disorders are examined in more detail by Strong and Garruto, Plato et al., and Miles and Brody in this volume.) Such examples suggest that neither age nor eventual mortality are necessary or sufficient criteria for describing chronic degenerative diseases, which may strike at any age from birth through old age.

In this chapter, we focus on the chronic degenerative conditions that contribute to the majority of morbidity and mortality among members of late 20th century cosmopolitan populations who have survived past their prime reproductive years, and that will likely remain leading causes of morbidity and mortality through the next century. Trends in morbidity and mortality for these conditions with both time and age have been extensively documented for both "developing" and "cosmopolitan" populations (Preston, 1976, Gerber, 1980, 1984; Gerber and Madhavan, 1980; Crews and MacKeen, 1982; Eaton and Konner, 1985; Baker and Crews, 1986; Keith and Smith, 1988; Yamagishita and Guralnick, 1988; Cohen, 1989; Crews, 1989) and are not detailed here. Instead, prehistorical and historical evidence for several chronic degenerative conditions and their possible associations with human evolutionary trends are explored.

## Prehistorical and Historical Evidence

Prehistorical and historical evidence does not support the notion that populations ancestral to ours completely escaped chronic degenerative diseases. The Old Man of La'Chapelle aux Saints [circa 40,000 years before present (YBP)] suffered from osteoarthritis (Williams, 1973) and both Egyptian (circa 5,000 YBP) and New World (circa 8,500 YBP) mummies retain direct evidence of gallstones (Chakraborty, personal communication, 1991[1]; Hinkle, 1987). Additionally, the Egyptian mummies show evidence of osteoarthritis and atherosclerosis (Hinkle, 1987). Historically, early Asian, Greek, and Egyptian records vividly record both insulin-dependent (IDDM) and non-insulin-dependent diabetes mellitus (NIDDM) and hypertension (see Ruskin, 1956; Papaspyros, 1964). Although their prevalences may now be greater than at any earlier period in human history or prehistory, such chronic degenerative conditions likely have affected *Homo sapiens sapiens* throughout our species'

[1]Dr R. Chakraborty's recent investigation of 36 female Atacameño Indian mummies, aged 40 years and older from Chile, revealed definite evidence of gallstones in 75% (27/36) of these individuals.

evolutionary history (Hinkle, 1987) and even our pre-*Homo* ancestors, as they do modern non-human primates (see DeRousseau, 1989 and this volume).

Morbidity and mortality in the 18th and 19th centuries were generally consequences of infectious and nutritional diseases; at the same time, descriptions of the diseases of affluence and over-nutrition were increasing and the first consistent evidence of coronary heart disease, atherosclerosis, and NIDDM among well-to-do classes was beginning to accumulate (Cohen, 1989). Obesity-related diabetes and gout were recognized as diseases of wealth and affluence as early as the Greek and Roman eras and through the middle ages and later centuries (see Rushkin, 1956; Cohen, 1989). Many of the other chronic degenerative diseases common in 20th century societies, such as hypertension, cerebrovascular disease, neoplasms, digestive and renal pathologies, and the major neurological disorders, Alzheimer's and Parkinsonism, were not fully described until the 19th and 20th century.

As the major chronic degenerative conditions were being identified, described, and increasing in prevalence, median and average life expectancies at birth were increasing to levels above those that had ever been known (Deevey, 1950; Weiss, 1981, 1984, 1989). Prior to the modern era, few members of most populations probably survived beyond the fourth and fifth decades of life. Thus, chronic degenerative diseases that today generally make their first appearance around the sixth and later decades of life, would not have been exposed to the full force of natural selection since they would not have greatly influenced reproductive variation prior to the 19th and 20th centuries. Natural selection would of course have acted on any aged adults during earlier epochs, however, a relative decline in the potency of selection would be associated with age since few people survived or reproduced at later ages. Still, any individual who did survive and reproduce at an age beyond which few conspecifics lived could have a disproportionate impact on the evolving gene pool if they contributed disproportionately to future generations or increased their own inclusive fitness by continued parental and grandparental investment. Possible examples of these patterns may occur among the Ifaluk, residents of the North Pacific Island of Yap, where adults with living parents have more offspring than adults whose parents have died (Turke, 1988, 1991), or among the Yanomami, natives of the Amazonian basin tropical rain forest, where long-lived men tend to acquire more wives and have more offspring (Chagnon, 1974).

Based on such data, a proximate cause for recent increases in the incidence and prevalence of chronic degenerative conditions is that these diseases generally afflict people over 50 years old, an age group that has increased disproportionately in cosmopolitan industrialized populations as the median and mean ages of survivorship have been extended to seven decades and longer (Adams and Smouse, 1985; Stini, 1991; see Miles and Brody, this volume). However, the ultimate causes of these increases likely include numerous factors in addition to life extension and modern life styles. Among these causes are complex networks of gene–environment interactions that have evolved secondary to adaptive strategies that our species and its progenitors developed to survive in the variety of ecological settings they were exposed to during their evolution. Numerous findings support this assertion; for example, both free-ranging and captive non-human primates apparently show signs of atherosclerosis (McGill *et al.*, 1960, 1981) and osteoarthritis (DeRousseau, 1989 and this volume) with increasing age. Thus, genetic features predisposing to such chronic degenerative diseases may be secondary to selective pressures that acted on the hominid gene pool even prior to the appearance of modern humans (*Homo sapiens sapiens*) about 100,000–250,000 years ago (Hinkle, 1987; Eaton *et al.*, 1988).

The appearance of several chronic degenerative conditions at ages that likely were near the upper limit of human survival and reproduction through most of human evolution, along with their exponential increase thereafter, also suggest that natural selection has acted so as to retard disease progression during the period of maximum human reproductive potential (Williams, 1957; Hamilton, 1966; Alexander, 1990; Rose, 1991). Data showing that individual life spans are highly correlated within families, indicate a strong genetic component to longevity (Sørensen *et al.*, 1988), although these genetic factors likely interact with similarly strong environmental factors. It follows that any genetic predispositions which enhanced survival and reproduction, either directly or indirectly, would have been subject to positive selective pressures throughout evolutionary history. A number of genetic traits may have been selected simply because they masked the late-acting detrimental pleiotropic effects of other genes with early-acting positive effects (Williams, 1957; Wood *et al.*, this volume). Today, these late-acting detrimental effects, due to increased life expectancies, may be subject to stronger natural selection than they were during previous stages of human evolution.

## Sociocultural and Life-style Changes

Degenerative diseases occur most frequently in people who survive past the fourth decade of life, a segment of human populations that was very small even in European populations as recent as 300 years ago (Hinkle, 1987). Given the small group size of individuals at risk and the few cases that received available medical attention, it is not surprising that medical definitions and diagnoses for many of these diseases were not classified and described until the present century (Hinkle, 1987; Crews and James, 1991). However, the knowledge that demographic changes have occurred and biomedical knowledge has improved does not explain how these diseases evolved, why they perpetuate, and why they seem to mainly affect individuals over 40 years old.

Although available data are limited in numerous ways, extensive mortality statistics do document ages and causes of death in European and European-derived populations since the 17th century (see, for example, Preston, 1976). These data document declines in childhood and maternal mortality and increases in life expectancy that have accompanied improvements in sanitation, nutrition, and medical care in the general population. These developments have been associated with increased life expectancy at all ages, most significantly at birth, but no obvious extension in maximum life span. These sociodemographic trends have so profoundly influenced patterns of longevity and mortality that they are today incorporated into theories of demographic and epidemiological transitions (Teitlebaum, 1975; Omran, 1977; Baker and Garruto, 1992; Baker and Bindon, 1993).

After completing these transitions, populations include a large proportion of persons aged 50 years and older and have higher mortality rates from heart diseases, cancer, and diabetes than populations that have not experienced these transitions. Children generally mature earlier in such populations and menarche often occurs as early as 11 or 12 years, as compared to ages as old as 16 years in more isolated rural societies (Beall, 1983, 1986). For women, these changes are associated with earlier reproductive maturation and longer reproductive periods. However, ages at first pregnancy have shown a secular trend toward older ages in most cosmopolitan populations since the 19th century and remain well above those of women from more rural societies (Micozzi, 1987). Today, populations with such long female reproductive periods generally show mortality rates from breast and cervical cancer above those of populations where girls mature at later ages (see Hsieh et al., 1990). This may reflect a misfit between present sociocultural circumstances that dictate delayed reproduction and the early attainment of reproductive capacity that likely was the adaptive strategy among human females during earlier phases of human evolution.

On average, women in Westernized cosmopolitan societies are physiologically prepared for reproduction as early as 13–14 years of age (Beall, 1983). During earlier phases of human evolution, early attainment of reproductive potential was likely an evolutionary advantage. In such circumstances, as in modern gathering/hunting societies, most women likely remained pregnant and/or lactating from soon after puberty continuously until menopause (Lancaster and King, 1985). Thus, the hormonal context of most human females during most of human evolution was relatively high levels of circulating progesterone and lactating hormones, compared to continued high estrogen levels found among women in contemporary cosmopolitan societies (Lancaster and King, 1985). Interpretation of such data suggests that high rates of breast and cervical cancer observed in these societies may not necessarily be secondary to an aging population nor do they follow from a fundamental change in human reproductive physiology. Instead they appear to follow sociocultural changes related to improved nutrition during infancy, childhood, and adolescence leading to earlier sexual maturation, as well as cultural pressures to postpone first pregnancy, fewer births per woman, and longer reproductive and postreproductive life expectancies.

Complex social, cultural, demographic, and life-style changes have significantly altered the means of production, improved the availability of calorie- and fat-dense but fiber-poor foods, and increased exposure to pollution and other stressors of modern life such as noise and radiation (Schell, 1991). A number of these changes have been examined elsewhere (Eaton and Konner, 1985; Smyer and Crews, 1985; Eaton et al., 1988; McGarvey et al., 1989; Crews and James, 1991; Schell, 1991) and they appear to have direct and indirect influences on the incidence and prevalence of chronic degenerative diseases and human longevity.

Cardiovascular diseases, cancer, diabetes, osteoporosis, irritable bowel syndrome, hypertension, and obesity may closely follow "western-style" changes in diet and physical activity (Burkitt *et al.*, 1974; Trowell and Burkitt, 1981; Kritchevsky, 1986; McGarvey *et al.*, 1989). Evidence for this general proposition continues to accumulate. Diverticulosis and colorectal cancer, frequent digestive system disorders in many cosmopolitan societies, are likely, in part, traceable to their fiber-poor and fat-rich diets (Burkitt *et al.*, 1974). The "epidemic" of vascular diseases and NIDDM may similarly follow from diets high in calories and social changes predisposing to low levels of habitual physical activity, that lead to obesity, hypertension, and hypercholesterolemia. Obesity in many individuals likely results from life-long patterns of physical inactivity, ingestion of an overabundance of calorie-dense food, and genetic differences between individuals (see McGarvey *et al.*, 1989). In some individuals, hypertension may be positively related to sodium intake (INTERSALT, 1988, 1989); however, for most individuals, hypertension may be more related to obesity. In both cases, a genetic predisposition, to salt retention or efficient extraction and storage of calories, is likely. Similarly, ingestion of large amounts of animal products rich in saturated fats, by increasing the overall consumption of fat, may lead to hypercholesterolemia in some people, but not in others. Definite genetic factors (e.g., apolipoproteins, low-density lipoprotein receptor variants) have been documented to be associated with such interindividual variations in lipid metabolism. The accumulated evidence strongly suggests that genetic-based susceptibilities to each of these conditions are coded in the human gene pool. These may contribute to individual variability in the development of chronic degenerative diseases and their associated risk factors.

Clearly the etiology of the major chronic degenerative diseases is multi-factorial and, at least in part, secondary to susceptible genotypes participating in social and cultural traditions that help to maintain an environmental setting in which life may continue long after the attainment of maximum reproductive potential. Recent sociocultural developments apparently have exposed some aspects of this accumulated human genetic variation as detrimental to the survival of adults who live past their reproductive prime. Evolutionarily, any genetic characteristic that predisposed to conservation of scarce resources and nutrients likely had positive selective value. Today, deleterious consequences of these characteristics, predispositions to chronic degenerative processes in a species whose females live 30–50 years beyond their reproductive years and whose males live significantly beyond their peak reproductive years, have become apparent.

Currently, the epidemiological and clinical focus of chronic disease research is on identifying and preventing risk factors, e.g., elevated cholesterol, high blood pressure, elevated triglycerides, and impaired glucose metabolism. The hunt is on to find the molecular bases for these risk factors. However, the established risk factors for such multi-factorial chronic degenerative diseases are themselves likely to be of polygenic origin. That is, multiple genetic variants likely predispose individuals to very similar disease phenotypes (Sing *et al.*, 1985). Most research designs aggregate these phenotypes because understanding of the disease processes are not sufficiently sophisticated to detect their variable etiologies and determine associations with demographic, psychological, and physiological instruments that are themselves problematic (James and Baker, 1990). Each specific phenotype may be the result of gene–environment interactions at the individual level and each genotype may have evolved in response to different environmental pressures (see James and Baker, 1990).

## AN EVOLUTIONARY THEORY OF AGING AND CHRONIC DEGENERATIVE DISEASE

The combination of two well-developed genetic models, thrifty genes (Neel, 1962, 1982) and genes that show antagonistic pleiotropy (Williams, 1957), may help to explain many observations such as we have just detailed.

### Thrifty Genotypes and Human Evolution

The purpose of this section is to illustrate how extension of the thrifty gene model may help explain how various risk factors came to be associated with chronic degenerative diseases. The idea of a "thrifty genotype" was first proposed by J. V. Neel in 1962 to account for the high prevalence of diabetes in some populations. Neel (1962) suggested that through mutation and selection a variant "thrifty" genotype (or genotypes) was produced and increased in its relative representation in human populations exposed to fluctuating periods of scarcity and abundance in foodstuffs. In 1982, Neel restated this model and applied it only to NIDDM.

Hypothetically, when access to caloric resources was not constant, and consequently, there were periods of relative deprivation, individuals with "thrifty" genotypes would have had a selective advantage over individuals without these genes. For example, an enhanced phenotypic ability to process food efficiently into energy and store it as fat could be the result of genes that enhance metabolic extraction of energy or that allow more rapid sequestration of energy in adipose tissues. Such thrifty genotypes might code for proteins that lead to a greater insulin response (hyperinsulinemia) following the ingestion of food. The consequent phenotype would store more excess energy as adipose tissue. Muscle cell resistance to the action of insulin would enhance this storage activity. Neel suggested that when populations, including some members with such thrifty genotypes, were exposed to periods of food scarcity or starvation, that the thrifty phenotypes would be expected to outcompete "non-thrifty" phenotypes (Neel, 1962, 1982). In contrast, in modern-day high-calorie environments with little need for physical activity, these same phenotypes could face a mortality disadvantage in later life. They would continuously experience hyperinsulinemia, show peripheral muscle resistance to insulin, store more calories as adipose tissue, and become obese as is observed in many contemporary populations. Obesity-related NIDDM may thus be a disease of overabundance, exposed when genetically determined mechanisms for conservation of scarce calories continually encounter a surfeit of calories (Neel, 1962; McGarvey *et al.*, 1989). Importantly, these thrifty variants might continue to be associated with efficient or early sexual maturation and reproduction and be beneficial, rather than detrimental, during early life and the years of maximum reproductive effort to the extent that they are associated with a reproductive advantage.

Similar types of evolutionary processes may have led to a multiplicity of thrifty genotypes, suggesting that Neel's basic model may be applicable to several additional chronic degenerative diseases. Further elaboration of these concepts may help to explain associations between several such conditions that today generally appear among elderly members of cosmopolitan societies and appeared among well-to-do members of some societies during earlier centuries. Several essential elements of such evolutionary scenarios follow. (1) An established metabolic need for a resource that was either scarce or overly abundant during earlier periods of hominid and human evolution. (2) Selective pressures: (a) favoring reproduction and survival of individuals who were more adept at acquiring, extracting, utilizing, or recycling scarce resources; or (b) that did not favor increased frequencies of genes predisposing to efficient mechanisms for acquiring, extracting, utilizing, or recycling resources readily available in the environment. (3) Average and median life expectancies that, in general, did not extend greatly beyond the ages of maximum reproductive potential among early hominids and humans. (This is not to imply that comparatively long-lived individuals could not have been found during all evolutionary horizons, only that they would have been relatively rare.) (4) Genes having positive early-acting effects on the metabolism of such scarce resources, but detrimental late-acting pleiotropic effects, that could be incorporated into the hominid gene pool through the action of evolutionary forces.

Given the spectrum of chronic degenerative diseases and their associated risk factors, we may postulate several resources that likely were relatively scarce during most of our species' evolutionary history—highly concentrated energy and nutrient sources (particularly animal fats and calorie-dense items such as fruits and nuts), foods rich in sodium chloride, and cholesterol-rich foods. We may also postulate several resources that were likely abundant during human and much of primate evolution—calcium, ascorbic acid, iodine, and iron. Several mechanisms by which selection could act to favor acquisition or utilization of scarce resources include taste preferences, efficiency of extraction, retention/conservation mechanisms, and resorption/deposition cycles; conversely, selective pressures should not favor development of these mechanisms for resources abundant in the environment of evolving hominids. Thrifty individuals, that is, those more efficient at acquiring, utilizing, retaining, and ultimately producing any scarce resource(s), should have achieved survival and reproductive advantages during earlier phases of hominid evolution. They still may achieve such advantages in present-day populations, even in cosmopolitan settings, during early life stages.

## Pleiotropy and Human Evolution

Genetic traits which predispose to morbidity and mortality prior to or during the reproductive years encounter stronger selective pressures against them than do those with later-acting effects (Williams, 1957; Hamilton, 1966). Such selective pressures should have assured that most genes predisposing to the development of NIDDM, coronary heart disease (CHD), cancer, or other chronic degenerative conditions at relatively young ages were selected out of early *Homo* populations. This process likely allowed genes with little influence on individual development of chronic degenerative diseases or those that predisposed individuals to developing them at ages beyond those of maximum reproductive potential to remain in the gene pool. Genes predisposing to chronic degenerative conditions during late life may have also led to individual selective advantages during developmental, maturational, and/or reproductive years, but predisposed to deleterious effects at ages beyond the species' usual reproductive span; that is, they show antagonistic pleiotropy (Williams, 1957; Rose, 1991; Wood *et al.*, this volume).

With regard to specific examples, two are: (1) genes that were associated with more efficient extraction of dietary cholesterol or enhanced the endogeneous production of cholesterol for synthesis of hormones essential to development during early life stages; or (2) genes that predisposed to more efficient accumulation of fat reserves during adolescence might have had a positive selective value. Today, however, their late-acting pleiotropic effects predispose many members of our society to obesity, atherosclerosis, and coronary heart disease during their later years. This positive selection for genes with late-occurring pleiotropic degenerative effects likely has been an important, if not major trend, in the evolution of humans as well as most other species (Williams, 1957; Hamilton, 1966; Rose, 1991; see Wood *et al.*, this volume). Data supporting this model of senescence have been reported following analyses of life tables from a variety of wild-living animal populations (Nesse, 1988) and from examination of several human genetic diseases (Albin, 1988). These and additional data were recently reviewed in relationship to antagonistic pleiotrophy and aging (Rose, 1991).

By combining Neel's (1962, 1982) thrifty genotype hypothesis with Williams' (1957) concept of antagonistic pleiotropy, it is possible to articulate a theory that predicts specific types of chronic degenerative diseases in humans and other species. Chronic degenerative diseases to be expected in humans are those that occur secondary to excessive accumulations of once scarce but now abundant resources (e.g., energy, cholesterol, salt), or, alternatively, that are secondary to decreased availability of resources that were abundant in previous ecological circumstances, and may remain abundant in today's environment, but that due to sociocultural changes are less available for metabolism (e.g., calcium, iron, iodine, fiber). The pleiotropic effect in the first case is that the underlying genotypes are thrifty and beneficial during youth, generally improving metabolic extraction, endogenous production, or retention/conservation, but as these show continued efficiency during late- and postreproductive years, they lead to detrimental outcomes associated with chronic degenerative diseases. In the later case, due to the relative recency of sociocultural changes leading to a relative metabolic scarcity of nutrients that had been abundant in diets of earlier populations, evolutionary time has not as yet been sufficiently long for any genetic predispositions toward efficient usage or extraction of these resources to have developed. Based upon this suggestion, resorption processes related to calcium stores of the skeleton may have recently been enhanced in response to calcium-poor diets that have followed settled agriculture; this enhancement may now predispose some individuals to osteoporosis (see Eaton and Nelson, 1991).

Any hypotheses developed to test this proposed model must determine whether available data support the suggestion that "thrifty gene" processes underlie many of the major chronic degenerative diseases and their associated risk factors in modern societies. A related question is whether the major chronic degenerative diseases of aging appear to be secondary to risk factor profiles that result from the antagonistic pleiotropy of thrifty genotypes (phenotypes) that have selective value in development and reproduction, but are associated with debilitation during later decades of life. We interpret available data as supporting both suggestions, although the second question will not be completely answered without additional data. The remaining sections of this chapter are directed toward both illustrating how the thrifty-pleiotropic gene model fits several chronic degenerative diseases of aging and to suggesting situations that may generate some tests of these assumptions and hypotheses generated from them.


## Thrifty Genes, Pleiotropy, Age, and Chronic Degenerative Diseases

Many of the known risk factors for vascular diseases cluster in the elderly, including hypertension, hyperglycemia, hypercholesterolmenia, and obesity. A major problem in defining chronic diseases is differentiating such disease states from aging. If a condition occurs in all members of a population as they age it is commonly viewed as aging rather than disease; however, it is also possible that a particular chronic degenerative disease might affect all members of the population if a particularly advantageous gene with a late-acting detrimental effect has been fixed in our gene pool. A second and related problem is that many chronic degenerative diseases and their related risk factors occur simultaneously, such as NIDDM with obesity, hypertension with renal impairment, or atherosclerosis with hypertension and coronary heart disease (see Laragh and Brenner, 1990). When such simultaneity occurs, it is difficult to ascribe a particular pathology to any one precipitating factor, and the one cause–one disease model of traditional epidemiology breaks down. This suggests that a single gene or gene complex may affect several metabolic systems and thus cause multiple "diseases." An indication of antagonistic pleiotropy?

During the last 10,000 years, and particularly over the past several generations, the human environment has changed dramatically (Fenner, 1970; Stini, 1971; Harrison, 1973; Baker and Baker, 1977; Baker, 1984; Eaton et al., 1988). It is thus possible that some genes which conferred selective advantages in our scavanging, gathering, and hunting past may today put us at a disadvantage with respect to chronic diseases and longevity, although, possibly, not reducing our reproductive potential during earlier years (Levi and Anderson, 1975; Eaton *et al.*, 1988; James *et al.*, 1989; McGarvey *et al.*, 1989; Crews, 1990; Crews and James, 1991). Considering these concepts, it is reasonable to suggest that a contributor to the increased prevalence of chronic degenerative diseases in present-day cosmopolitan populations is a lack of fit between our genetic predispositions and modern environments (James and Baker, 1990). A particular focus of research in this area has been on changes in dietary factors (Stini, 1971; Eaton and Konner, 1985; Eaton and Nelson, 1991); however, social and physical environments are also drastically changed and changing (Baker, 1984). All of these alterations are significantly affecting our health, in part through their impact on the development of degenerative diseases. Thus, in addition to the life-style and demographic changes described earlier, there are likely significant genetic and environmental causes for the presence and persistence of chronic degenerative diseases in modern populations.

We are members of a species that is the product of millions of years of adaptation to a mobile life style with a diet rich in plant foods, supplemented with occasional animal products of generally low-fat content. This life style typified Australopithecines and early *Homo species* that existed between 7 to 0.5 million years ago, about 280,000–350,000 generations (using either 25 or 20 years as an average generation); these populations likely lived only 15–20 years on average (Cutler, 1976; Weiss, 1981, 1984, 1989). Although still the subject of much current debate, our direct ancestors likely spent about 0.5 million years, 20,000–25,000 generations, in a scavenging/gathering/hunting life style. The early settled agricultural and nomadic pastoral period of human social organization has lasted for about 10,000 years, or 400–500 generations, and Neolithic Agriculturalists averaged about 25 years of life as did Classic/Medieval Europeans (Weiss, 1981, 1984, 1989). For less than 200 years, 8–10 generations, human beings have been developing mechanized agriculture and a diet including heavy reliance on domesticated animal products. During this period, life expectancy at birth has increased from 43 to 75 years (see Deevey, 1950; Weiss, 1981, 1984, 1989). Thus, our gene pool is the product of evolution in a mobile, plant-eating, short life expectancy ecological niche, but we live today in a sedentary, fat-rich/fiber-poor ecological niche, with an extended life span, much of which has never been so strongly exposed to the sieve of natural selection.

## APPLICATIONS OF MODEL TO DISEASE ASSOCIATIONS IN SELECTED SETTINGS

To illustrate the proposed model, evaluate its applicability to chronic degenerative diseases, and develop theory-based hypotheses for future testing, several risk factor–disease associations are examined. The first, obesity-related hyperglycemia and NIDDM, has been widely cited as a "thrifty genotype" and may provide an ideal example of antagonistic pleiotropy. Two others, plasma lipids with coronary heart disease and salt/sodium intake with hypertension, do not provide such clear models of thrifty genes and their pleiotropic effects and their genetic bases remain largely unknown. In addition, two resources that presumably were not scarce during hominid evolution, ascorbic acid and calcium, are briefly examined.

## Obesity-related Hyperglycemia and Diabetes

The classical situation to best illustrate the value of the thrifty-pleiotropic model is likely to be the decreased ability to tolerate a glucose load and the increasing prevalence of NIDDM among middle-aged and elderly members of many cosmopolitan and developing populations. In brief, during earlier phases of evolution, humans and their predecessors may frequently have found themselves in ecological settings of nutrient and resource scarcity. If the available food supply were cyclical, waning from abundance to starvation, any enhanced ability to store energy as adipose tissue might carry a positive selective value. To the degree that such a "thrifty" gene predisposed individuals possessing it to achieve greater reproductive success, relative to their peers, the gene would increase in frequency in the population. Originally, such variant genes may have arisen in some isolated population through mutation. There they may have increased in frequency or even have become fixed in small populations by random genetic drift. Later, via migration and interbreeding, these genes may have entered other population groups, have eventually attained variable frequencies, and have been maintained at a range of frequencies due to variable degrees of selective advantage in different ecological settings. The late-acting effects of such genes—NIDDM, impaired glucose tolerance, and nonenzymatic glycation of macromolecules—may seldom have been observed prior to the development of ecological settings typified by nutrient and resource overabundance. These thrifty genes may have led to increased survival, improved growth and development, and/or enhanced reproductive ability in early and middle age, traits that would have been associated with large variations in reproductive success; their late-acting effects would include impaired glucose tolerance, NIDDM, nonenzymatic glycation, and mortality at ages that were not associated with large variations in reproductive success. Natural selection would not be an effective agent against any late effects that did not produce a negative effect on reproduction, but such genes might be fixed based on their early positive effects.

Glucose tolerance declines with age in the absence of overt diabetes (Andres, 1971; Orchard et al., 1982; Kreisberg, 1987; Shimokata et al., 1991). In both men and women this decline with age is independent of fatness, fat patterning, and physical fitness (Shimokata et al., 1991). This age-related increase in circulating glucose is associated with a number of phenotypic alterations that occur secondary to the nonenzymatic glycation of macromolecules and that appear to mimic age-related changes seen in older persons (Cerami, 1985, 1986, provide a complete description of these associations). Evidence that such alterations may be secondary to specific genes comes from data suggesting that the general impairment of carbohydrate metabolism with increasing age may be due to age-related declines in the induction of enzymes involved with carbohydrate metabolism (Tollefsbol, 1987); an impairment that in turn apparently plays a role in general cellular senescence. Nonenzymatic glycation, possibly secondary to such delays of enzyme induction, may promote the premature aging characteristic of persons with diabetes (Cerami, 1985, 1986).

Another major feature of NIDDM is peripheral insulin resistance of muscle and adipose cells (Reaven, 1984; DeFronzo, 1988). The resistance may be part of a thrifty genotype promoting maintenance of adequate blood glucose during periods of caloric deficit. During periods of severe starvation, individuals possessing genes predisposing to insulin resistance might outcompete other persons who could not maintain euglycemia. Such hypoglycemic persons would be at risk of death from wasting or brain damage, or might have their reproductive potential decreased by successive cycles of feast and famine. On the other hand, thrifty genotypes may have stored excess energy (i.e., glucose) in adipose and liver cells during times of feasting and hyperglycemia (see Wendorff and Goldfine, 1991, for a recent review). These thrifty genotypes remain useful for development, maturation, and maintenance of the body via euglycemia in the described ecological setting. However, when they encounter an ecological setting with a constant surfeit of calories, obesity, and secondary (i.e., obesity-induced) insulin resistance may occur. This may lead to continuous hyperglycemia, insulin resistance, decreased insulin responsiveness of pancreatic beta-cells, and, ultimately, to the expression of overt NIDDM.

During the preceding several million years of our species' evolutionary history, the late-acting detrimental effects of such thrifty genes were offset by beneficial early effects accruing to individuals who maintained euglycemia through their prime reproductive years. When food supplies are unstable, predispositions to metabolize and to efficiently store energy in times of abundance or retrieve previously stored energy during times of deprivation would be advantageous. Any gene-based trait that contributed to glucose homeostasis would have had a selective advantage, contributed to survival during extreme environmental stress, and affected reproductive variation.

These considerations suggest that efficient energy storage and some degree of overweight should have been adaptive at particular life stages and led to improved survival relative to age–sex-matched peers, even if this trait was associated with somewhat earlier mortality. Evolutionarily, traits that predisposed reproductive age females to maintain euglycemia during times of caloric stress, compared to conspecifics who tended toward hypoglycemia, might be associated with longer reproductive spans, more mature and less frail neonates, shorter birth intervals, shorter generation times, greater completed fertility, and more surviving offspring. If these traits were associated with a deficit in maximum attainable life span, this cost would be offset by higher fertility. Evidence that this may be an appropriate model for at least some stages of human evolution is available for modern populations. For example, infants with birth weights below 5 pounds are at increased risk of neonatal mortality compared to babies with higher birth weights. Furthermore, in modern low-calorie environments with ecologically scarce resources, sexual maturation, onset of fecundity, and childbearing are delayed and longer generation spans are observed than in more cosmopolitan populations. Longer maturational periods subject individuals to greater risks of death prior to mating and childbearing. Individuals with thrifty genes promoting euglycemia in such resource-poor environments would be at an advantage; diabetic pathologies would likely not be expressed in low-calorie environments; a longer reproductive span would be achieved by women with earlier maturation due to more efficient use of calories; and, earlier births relative to conspecifics would be advantageous. In such circumstances, women maintaining adequate glycemia, in the upper range of "normal," during gestation could produce larger and healthier neonates than their competitors who maintained euglycemia at levels minimally consistent with live birth. In addition, offspring of women expressing this trait might be more likely to survive and ultimately reproduce because of their more propitious birth weights, maturity at birth, and possession of thrifty genes. Such genotypes may predispose some women to gestational diabetes in cosmopolitan societies, while in earlier epochs, they allowed similar women to maintain adequate glycemia in the face of nutritional stress. Today, birth defects and oversized neonates may be associated with thrifty genotypes, but such outcomes may remain unlikely in situations of caloric stress.

Based on the thrifty-pleiotropic gene models of chronic disease a number of research questions may be asked. Do individuals who survive to reproductive age tend to be somewhat heavier than their peers who have died? Do overweight individuals generally leave more surviving offspring than their lower weight peers? Are there reproductive disadvantages associated with being underweight? Is gestational diabetes seen in low-calorie environments and are detrimental outcomes expressed as they are in high-calorie environments? Does the frequency of clinically diagnosed gestational diabetes increase with modernization and/or availability of a surfeit of calories? Do women who show gestational diabetes also show earlier ages at menarche? Partial answers to several of these questions are likely available in existing data sets; complete answers may need to await collection of additional data. Such research will improve our understanding of the possible association of thrifty-pleiotropic genes with health, survival, reproduction, and chronic degenerative diseases.

## Plasma Lipids and Coronary Heart Disease

A large number of gene products that participate in the metabolism of lipids and lipoproteins have been identified (Berg, 1987; Scott, 1987). Several variants may be associated with specific abnormalities of lipid metabolism (Kottke, 1986; Utermann et al., 1989); those identified thus far appear to be rare variants and may only represent extreme genotypes from a wide range of minor and major variants in receptors, enzymes, and co-enzymes associated with lipid metabolism. These variants may contribute to major differences in lipid levels, such as familial hypercholesterolemia, or produce only subtle differences such as are associated with some of the apolipoproteins. All variants are likely to be differentially distributed in various population groups, for example, the apolipoproteins (Kamboh and Ferrell, 1990). In general, about 30–40% of ingested cholesterol is absorbed from the diet; however, additional cholesterol is produced endogenously by the liver from available fatty acids (Linscheer and Vergroesen, 1988). Once cholesterol is available in the circulation, little is excreted since no efficient mechanism for cholesterol excretion is found in humans (Connor and Connor, 1985). Thrifty genes predisposing individuals to more efficient extraction, retention, storage, production, recycling, and conservation of cholesterol thus have a limited range of variation within which to affect cholesterol levels. To illustrate somewhat the range of possible phenotypes, two non-Western traditional living populations residing in rather unique ecological settings are reviewed in some detail, Greenland and Alaskan Eskimos and the African Maasai.

As early as 1914, a high dietary intake of fat (47% of calories) was reported among Greenland Eskimos (Bang *et al.*, 1976). Similarly, dietary records for inhabitants of two northern Alaska Eskimo villages, from the summer and the winter of 1971–1972, revealed that in one village, the diet consisted of caribou, seal, and beluga whale with lesser amounts of walrus, birds, and fish, and the percentage of calories from fat among adults was 43% (Bell and Heller, 1978). In the other village, native staples included baleen and beluga whale, seal, and fish, and calories from fat approximated 36%.

However, this high-fat diet does not translate into the chronic disease profile that one might expect based upon European experience. For example, despite diets with similar amounts of fat and cholesterol among Greenland Eskimos and Danes, among both men and women and at all ages, the former showed lower mortality rates from coronary heart disease (CHD) than the latter. The observed Eskimo-to-Dane ratio of mortality rates was 0.5 or below in most age groups (Kromann and Green, 1980; Bjerregaard and Dyerberg, 1988). Although total calories from fat and the quantity of cholesterol consumed were quite similar in these two populations, the Danish diet included twice as much saturated fat (Bang *et al.*, 1976). Furthermore, Eskimos consumed large amounts of omega-3 polyunsaturated fatty acids, the principal fatty acid in cold water marine animals that are the major contributors to the diet of Eskimos—seal, walrus, and whale (Leaf and Weber, 1988). Based upon these data, high dietary intake of omega-3 fatty acids has been postulated as a protective factor against CHD in Eskimos, and other populations (Bang *et al.*, 1972, 1976). However, among Greenland Eskimos living in Denmark, total lipid and cholesterol levels approximate those of native Danes and are a good deal above those of non-migrant Greenland Eskimos (Bang and Dyerberg, 1972). These data have been interpreted as suggesting that a change in ecological circumstances, to a diet with more saturated fat and cholesterol, rather than genetic factors, have led to a more atherogenic lipid profile of migrant Greenland Eskimos (Draper, 1980). Additional data supporting this view come from a study of two villages in southwest Alaska, where a gradient in average plasma cholesterol with degree of dietary acculturation was reported (Draper, 1976). In these villages, about 40% of the population showed hypercholesterolemia with an average plasma cholesterol level of 256 mg/dl.

These accumulated data suggest that, until recently, Eskimo populations were protected from possible deleterious sequela of their high cholesterol diet by their consumption of high levels of fat from marine sources or, perhaps, other factors that remain unidentified at present. Evidence for this suggestion includes that ingestion of fish oil and/or omega-3 fatty acids is associated with reduced triglycerides and very low density lipoproteins, suppression of hepatic triglyceride and apolipoprotein B production, increased removal of very low density lipoproteins from the circulation, an increase of bile in the feces, along with a blunted serum cholesterol increase following a meal rich in cholesterol (Leaf and Weber, 1988). In the presence of omega-3 fatty acids, cholesterol derived from marine sources would be less likely to lead to hypercholesterolemia, even in the presence of thrifty mechanisms for efficient extraction, retention, and conservation of cholesterol. However, dietary change to saturated non-marine fat sources has led Eskimos to express an atherogenic lipid profile and they therefore may now be at increased risk for CHD, as are most other human populations.

The thrifty-pleiotropic model of chronic degenerative diseases developed here suggests that genetic mechanisms should have evolved to enhance production of cholesterol in a fat- and cholesterol-poor environment from food resources generally available to evolving hominids, i.e., land animals and plant products. These thrifty traits may have been circumvented in the traditional ecological setting of Eskimos. In an ecological setting with high intakes of omega-3 fatty acids, hypercholesterolemia and CHD should not be significant problems, since populations subsisting in these settings will have their genetic propensity limited by the influence of these fatty acids. In such ecological settings, selection may even favor more efficient mechanisms to extract, retain, and/or utilize cholesterol and its precursors. When such populations encounter a surfeit of cholesterol and saturated fats from land mammals, they may be at increased risk of hypercholesterolemia and later CHD because of these enhanced abilities. Based on the thrifty-pleiotropic gene model, two testable hypotheses are suggested. On an isocaloric diet high in omega-3 fatty acids, but without other sources of fatty acids or cholesterol, Greenland Eskimos should show higher serum cholesterol levels than age–sex-matched Europeans on the same diet. Similarly, on an isocaloric diet high in fats and cholesterol from animal, but not fish, sources, Greenland Eskimos should also show higher serum cholesterol levels than age-sex-matched Europeans.

An additional "unique" population is the Masai of Kenya and Tanzania. The Masai subsist on a diet high in animal products, but are reported to have a low incidence of cardiovascular diseases (Mann et al., 1964; Scrimshaw and Guzman, 1968). As such, their ecological situation may allow additional tests of the thrifty-pleiotropic gene model of chronic degenerative diseases. One study among the Masai compared serum cholesterol values of men living in their usual rural environment to men who had lived for some time in urban areas and to a European control group (Day et al., 1976). Although the Masai diet of milk, supplemented with blood and meat, has a cholesterol content similar to European and Western diets, both Masai groups had cholesterol levels significantly lower than the European group. Furthermore, the rural Masai group had levels significantly lower than the urban group, despite a similar diet. The investigators found that obesity alone could not account for the increased cholesterol level of the urban sample and hypothesized that some change in life style (e.g., amount of exercise, physical fitness) was a factor causing this difference in cholesterol.

The data suggest that in the traditional setting, an ecological balance exists between diet, activity, and serum cholesterol. This balance may be dependent on a population-wide lowering of the efficiency of cholesterol extraction, reabsorption, or conservation, since it is an overly abundant resource for this population. In this situation, genetic mechanisms that predispose to less efficient extraction of dietary cholesterol or to low endogenous production would not be selected against and might increase in frequency in the population. When Masai move to different ecological settings these predispositions are retained and their cholesterol levels remain well below those of their European counterparts, although higher than traditional-living Masai, even on an altered diet. The thrifty-pleiotropic gene model suggests that the relaxed selection for thrifty extraction or metabolism of cholesterol would lead to an increase in genetic variation associated with these activities and perhaps positive selection to conserve energy by reducing unneeded expenditures to conserve already abundant amounts of cholesterol. In this case, the proposed hypothesis from the thrifty-pleiotropic model is almost the reverse of that applied to the Eskimos. On an isocaloric diet either high or low in animal fat and cholesterol, the Masai should show lower serum cholesterol levels than age–sex-matched Europeans because of relaxed selection for thrifty genes.

## Salt Intake and Blood Pressure

Data are now available exploring the relation of sodium intake to blood pressure both within populations and between various populations. The INTERSALT study (INTERSALT, 1988, 1989; Stamler, 1991) demonstrated that the tendency of blood pressure to increase with age was related to salt intake and that salt intake was related to blood pressure in normotensive as well as hypertensive persons within different populations. Although this relation has been found in many populations and ethnic groups, blacks, especially American blacks, have been found to be more "salt-sensitive" than American whites (Luft et al., 1991). A number of hypotheses have been presented to explain the responsiveness of blood pressure to salt.

Helmer (1967) speculated that African populations probably experienced high salt losses due to sweating and thus, adapted genetically to their environment by having an enhanced ability to conserve or retain salt. Gleiberman (1973), Wilson (1986), and Jackson (1991) added the influence of low dietary salt on the evolution of salt conservation. Grim (1988) also proposed the "slavery hypothesis of hypertension," suggesting that salt loss in diarrheal stools and vomit selected for enhanced ability to conserve or retain salt. A consolidation of these theories led Wilson and Grim (1991) to state a genetic–environmental interactive theory of the etiology of salt-sensitive high blood pressure in American blacks: "An enhanced genetic-based ability to retain or conserve salt would increase in populations in which reproductive success is decreased by high morbidity and/or mortality from Na+ losses in sweat, stools, or vomit" (p. I-123). They hypothesized that in American blacks, because of the high mortality they experienced as a result of the transatlantic slave trade (Middle Passage), caused largely by salt- and water-depletive diseases, any genes that predisposed to salt loss would have been strongly selected against. Thus, the founding population for African Americans would have included only individuals who survived this selective stress and should have included individuals with an enhanced ability to conserve salt. This ability, today, is of course detrimental, due to the abundance of dietary salt, and may explain in part the greater prevalence of sodium-sensitive high blood pressure in American blacks.

The transatlantic Middle Passage may have constricted genetic variability and magnified the potential for salt-sensitive hypertension in American blacks through genetic drift and selection. The general consensus is that this historical event was a selective pressure for an enhanced ability to conserve salt in American blacks (Grim, 1988; Jackson, 1991; Wilson and Grim, 1991). The finding that diuretics work better to control hypertension in black than in white Americans lends some support to their proposal. Today, this genetic capability serves as another example of a thrifty-pleiotropic genotype, the late-acting detrimental pleiotropic effect being an increased risk of salt-sensitive hypertension, whereas such salt retention was likely beneficial in previous periods. The thrifty-pleiotropic model suggests several questions for future testing. Do African Americans show a greater frequency of salt-sensitive hypertension than do European Americans? On a controlled low-salt diet, do African Americans show greater sodium retention than European Americans? During episodes of extreme heat stress, whether experimentally or environmentally induced, do African Americans show less fluid and electrolyte loss than age–sex-matched European Americans?

## Ascorbic Acid and Calcium

This discussion would not be complete without at least a brief review of some resources that likely have been readily available throughout the majority of human evolution. These may include at least ascorbic acid, calcium, iron, and iodine, each associated with a well-recognized deficiency disease, scurvy, osteoporosis, anemia, and goiter/cretinism, among others. Diets in many cosmopolitan societies are low in calcium and iron and these are associated with age-related increases in osteoporosis and anemia, respectively. The thrifty-pleiotropic model implies that since these resources have been abundant throughout the majority of human evolution, thrifty genes for their efficient extraction, utilization, and/or conservation have not been associated with selective advantages and should not be widely distributed in humans.

For instance, humans do not produce ascorbic acid endogenously. This suggests that vitamin C has been a readily available nutrient, rather than a scarce resource, for some large portion of hominid evolution and that loss of the metabolic pathway to its synthesis resulted from relaxed selection for this trait or, perhaps, positive selection to conserve energy by eliminating an unnecessary metabolic pathway. Based upon present data, modern humans do not appear to show an identifiable environmentally induced chronic degenerative disease related to excess or low vitamin C as they age. Formation of oxalate stones in the kidney has been suggested as an example of a condition related to excessive vitamin C intake, however, recent data do not support this association (Hornig *et al.*, 1988). Similarly, scurvy is not associated with aging, but occurs as a vitamin deficiency in very specific circumstances (Hornig *et al.*, 1988).

Unfortunately for the many sufferers from osteoporosis, humans do appear to show an environmentally-induced calcium-related chronic degenerative disease. Calcium is plentiful in the natural environment and in many foods available to gatherers/hunters who previously inhabited a variety of ecological zones, but today may be a scarce resource among most agricultural peoples, including our own United States population (Eaton and Nelson, 1991). The calcium resorption/deposition process that characterizes modern humans and is apparently associated with osteoporosis in later life, may have been amplified as genes promoting calcium scavanging have increased in response to this culturally determined change in human ecology. Perhaps genes controlling the deposition/resorption processes of skeletal calcium stores have recently been exposed to new selective pressures as agriculture has led to calcium-poor diets (see Eaton and Nelson, 1991). Furthermore, it may be that modern predispositions to osteoporosis are related to the recency of this change and the slow pace of evolution. Mechanisms for more efficient calcium absorption and metabolism may be developing; however, in the meantime, calcium remains a poorly absorbed and dietarily scarce nutrient.

## OVERVIEW AND FUTURE PERSPECTIVES

Based upon the review of data and theory presented here, longevity likely represents a suite of compromises between individual reproductive success and continued maintenance of the individual soma, such that a number of physiological systems become prone to breakdown at or about the same time (Hamilton, 1966; Williams, 1957; Rose, 1991). Several avenues for continued transdisciplinary human population biology research into the adaptive and evolutionary association of chronic degenerative diseases and aging in addition to those enumerated in preceding sections appear to be emerging. For example, heterozygosity may be associated with higher longevity and later onset of disease in humans (Johnson, 1988). Data supporting this hypothesis would support the thrifty-pleiotropic gene model of aging and chronic degenerative diseases proposed here. Heterozygosity could in part mask late-acting antagonistic pleiotropic effects of the homologous gene product. Production of two protein types and co-dominance would produce three phenotypes. Multiple loci involvement would produce a range of phenotypes and continuous variation. Partial tests of this effect may readily be made with any number of currently identifiable DNA, protein, and restriction fragment length polymorphisms. Long-lived individuals should show different genotypic frequencies than young and middle-aged conspecifics, as they do for the apolipoprotein E polymorphism (see Scott, 1987). This alone is circumstantial evidence of an association between such traits and variation in longevity. Traditionally, biological anthropologists and human population biologists have examined polymorphisms of blood proteins to establish population affinities. Although some differences between long-lived and short-lived persons may be encountered with such data, it is more likely that most genetic predispositions to longevity are dependent on thrifty-pleiotropic genes coding for regulatory, receptor, and repair proteins, rather than structural and metabolic proteins (see Turner and Weiss, this volume).

Another avenue for testing aspects of the thrifty-pleiotropic model of aging and chronic degenerative diseases is the large amount of variability in the amount and degree of disability and chronic degenerative disease observed in older men and women (Stout and Crawford, 1988; Guralnik et al., 1991). One implication of antagonistic pleiotropy identified by Williams (1957) is that the late-occurring detriment should be related to a number of different genes, some contributing to the early benefit, some contributing to the late detriment, and still others counteracting the late detriment. Another implication is that, at the population level, the frequency of pleiotropic genes may be relatively high throughout the gene pool; this should produce a strong correlation between disability and disease in any one system with that of all other systems (Williams, 1957). In such a situation, the degree of disability or chronic degenerative disease in a population should be normally distributed at any specific age. Furthermore, the age of the onset and degree of disability or chronic degenerative disease should be correlated in any population, although they need not be closely related for all individuals. Any one individual only has a certain probability of receiving any particular "thrifty-pleiotropic" gene at any particular locus. Therefore, only a limited number of persons will receive a full complement of the most detrimental late-acting deleterious effects, most of which should occur at about the same age, providing health care workers with a small percentage of patients who are 40–50 years old and die of chronic degenerative diseases. Conversely, an additional small percentage of individuals may receive few, if any, genes with detrimental effects and represent that small cadre of long-lived, cigarette-smoking, fat-eating, heavy drinking centenarians who are featured in media headlines. These also are the patterns that have recently been reported following research on elderly individuals in several cosmopolitan settings (Stout and Crawford, 1988; Olshansky et al., 1990; Guralnik et al., 1991). Although such data support a thrifty-pleiotropic model of aging and chronic disease, continued research is needed to document that age of onset of such conditions is positively skewed and that age of onset has increased during human evolution. This should be expected in a successful species because there is always positive selection for modifiers that will delay or lessen any detrimental pleiotropic effects of genes with early-acting positive effects when their deleterious late effects occur prior to cessation of reproduction and parental investment (Williams, 1957; Turke, 1991). However, the late effects will continue to be observed since some "thrifty-pleiotropic" games are expected to be fixed in the gene pool due to their early positive effect (see Williams, 1957).

It is not likely that any single disciplinary focus will be sufficient to unravel the complex web of causality that relates aging to morbidity and mortality due to chronic degenerative diseases. Biological anthropology and, specifically, human population biology, with its transdisciplinary approach to the study of human disease processes, may be in a unique position to contribute significantly to a broader understanding of the evolutionary and adaptive significance of the multi-factorial processes, represented by diseases such as NIDDM, CHD, cancer, osteoporosis, hypertension, hyperlipidemia, and hyperglycemia, which today account for over 70% of mortality and disability in technologically complex cosmopolitan societies, and to explain their apparent causal association with age (see Baker, 1982; Little and Haas, 1989). Advances in molecular biology are occurring rapidly; yet, their application to the study of chronic degenerative diseases remains in its nascence. As these techniques become more sophisticated, the need to interpret and integrate their results into an adaptive and evolutionary framework will increase. Pursuit of these molecular factors and an understanding of their genetic and evolutionary bases may best be achieved through collaborative efforts of biomedical anthropologists, epidemiologists, gerontologists, and molecular biologists.

## ACKNOWLEDGMENTS

We thank Paul W. Turke, Ph.D., for his useful comments on an earlier version of this manuscript and for sharing his unpublished manuscript "Evolution of the 100 Year Lifespan." We also wish to thank Bea DiFabio, M.S., R.D., for her insightful comments and suggestions on an earlier version along with our other colleagues who read various sections and added suggestions.

## REFERENCES

Adams, J. and Smouse, P. E. (1985) Genetic consequences of demographic changes in human populations. In: *Diseases of Complex Etiology in Small Populations* (eds, Chakraborty, R. and Szathmary, E. J. E.), New York: Alan R. Liss, pp. 147–178.

Albin, R. L. (1988) The pleiotropic gene theory of senescence: supportive evidence from human genetic disease. *Ethology and Sociobiology* 9, 371–382.

Alexander, R. D. (1990) *How Did Humans Evolve? Reflections on the Uniquely Unique Species*. The University of Michigan, special publication no. 1, Museum of Zoology. Ann Arbor, MI.

American Heart Association, The Joint National Committee on Detection, Evaluation, and Treatment of High Blood Pressure (1988) The 1988 Report. *Archives of Internal Medicine* 148, 1020–1038.

Andres, R. (1971) Aging and diabetes. *Medical Clinics of North America* 55, 835–845.

Baker, P. T. (1982) Human population biology: a viable transdisciplinary science. *Human Biology* **54**, 203–220.

Baker, P. T. (1984) The adaptive limits of human populations. *Man (NS)* **19**, 1–14.

Baker, P. T. and Baker, T. S. (1977) Biological adaptations to urbanization and industrialization: some research strategy considerations. In: *Colloquia in Anthropology*, Vol. I. (ed. Wetherington, R. K.). Fort Burgwin Research Center, Australia, pp. 107–118.

Baker, P. T. and Bindon, J. R. (1993) Health Transition in the Pacific Islands. *American Journal of Human Biology* **5**, 5–7.

Baker, P. T. and Crews, D. E. (1986) Mortality patterns and some biological predictors. In: *The Changing Samoans: Behavior and Health in Transition* (eds Baker, P. T., Hanna, J. M. and Baker, T. S.). Oxford University Press, Oxford: pp. 93–122.

Baker, P. T. and Garruto, R. M. (1992) Health transition: examples from the Western Pacific. *Human Biology* **64**, 785–789.

Bang, H. O. and Dyerberg, J. (1972) Plasma lipids and lipoproteins in Greenlandic west coast Eskimos. *Acta Medica Scandinavica (Stockholm)* **192**, 85–94.

Bang, H. O., Dyerberg, J. and Hjorne, N. (1976) The composition of food consumed by Greenland Eskimos. *Acta Medica Scandinavica (Stockholm)* **200**, 69–73.

Beall, C. M. (1983) Ages at menopause and menarche in a high altitude Himalayan population. *Annals of Human Biology* **10**, 365–370.

Beall, C. M. (1986) Factors associated with menopause status in a high altitude Tibetan population. *American Journal of Physical Anthropology* **69**, 174.

Bell, R. and Heller, C. A. (1978) Nutrition studies: an appraisal of the modern North Alaskan Eskimo diet. In: *Eskimos of Northwestern Alaska: A Biological Perspective* (eds Jamison, P. L., Zegura, S. L. and Milan, F. A.). Stroudsburg, PA: Dowden, Hutchinson & Ross, Inc., pp. 145–156.

Berg, K. (1987) Genetics of coronary heart disease and its risk factors. In: *Molecular Approaches to Human Polygenic Disease* (eds Bock, G. and Collins, G. M.). Chichester, UK: John Wiley & Sons Ltd, pp. 14–33.

Bjerregaard, P. and Dyerberg, J. (1988) Mortality from ischemic heart disease and cerebrovascular disease in Greenland. *International Journal of Epidemiology* **17**, 514–519.

Burkitt, D. P., Walker, A. R. P. and Painter, N. S. (1974) Dietary fiber and disease. *JAMA* **229**, 1069–1074.

Cerami, A. (1985) Hypothesis: glucose as a mediator of aging. *Journal of the American Geriatrics Society* **33**, 626–634.

Cerami, A. (1986) Aging of proteins and nucleic acids: what is the role of glucose. *Trends in Biochemical Sciences* **11**, 311–314.

Chagnon, N. A. (1974) *Studying The Yanomamo*. New York: Holt, Rinehart, and Winston.

Cohen, M. N. (1989) *Health and the Rise of Civilization*. New Haven, CT: Yale University Press.

Connor, W. E. and Connor, S. L. (1985) The dietary prevention and treatment of coronary heart disease. In: *Coronary Heart Disease: Prevention, Complications, and Treatment* (eds Connor, W. E. and Bristow, J. D.). Philadelphia: J. B. Lippincott, pp. 43–64.

Crews, D. E. (1989) Cause-specific mortality, life expectancy, and debilitation in aging Polynesians. *American Journal of Human Biology* **1**, 347–353.

Crews, D. E. (1990) Anthropological issues in biological gerontology. In: *Anthropology and Aging: Comprehensive Reviews* (ed. Rubinstein, R. L.). Boston, MA: Kluwer Academic Publishers, pp. 11–38.

Crews, D. E. and James, G. D. (1991) Human evolution and the genetic epidemiology of chronic degenerative diseases. In: *Applications of Biological Anthropology to Human Affairs* (eds. Lasker, G. W. and Mascie-Taylor, N.). Cambridge: Cambridge University Press, pp. 186–207.

Crews, D. E. and MacKeen, P. C. (1982) Mortality related to cardiovascular disease and diabetes mellitus in a modernizing population. *Social Sciences and Medicine* **16**, 175–181.

Cutler, R. G. (1976) Evolution of longevity in primates. *Journal of Human Evolution* **51**, 169–202.

Day, J., Carruthers, M., Bailey, A. and Robinson, D. (1976) Anthropometric, physiological and biochemical differences between urban and rural Masai. *Atherosclerosis* **23**, 357–361.

Deevery, E. S. (1950) The probability of death. *Scientific American* **182**, 58–60.

DeFronzo, R. A. (1988) The triumvirate: B-cell, muscle, liver: a collusion responsible for NIDDM. *Diabetes* **37**, 667–687.

DeRousseau, C. J. (1989) *Osteoarthritis in Rhesus Monkeys and Gibbons: A Locomotor Model of Joint Degeneration*. Contributions to Primatology, Vol. 25. New York: Karger.

Draper, H. H. (1976) A review of recent nutritional research in the Arctic. In: *Circumpolar Health* (eds Shephard, R. J. and Itoh, S.). Toronto: University of Toronto Press, pp. 120–129.

Draper, H. H. (1980) Nutrition. In: *The Human Biology of Circumpolar Populations* (ed. Milan, F. A.). Cambridge: Cambridge University Press, International Biological Programme, No. 21. pp. 257–284.

Eaton, S. B. and Konner, M. J. (1985) Paleolithic nutrition: a consideration of its nature and current implications. *New England Journal of Medicine* **312**, 283–289.

Eaton, S. B. and Nelson, D. A. (1991) Calcium in evolutionary perspective. *American Journal of Clinical Nutrition* **54**, 281S–287S.

Eaton, S. B., Konner, M. J. and Shostak, M. (1988) Stone agers in the fast lane: chronic diseases in evolutionary perspective. *American Journal of Medicine* **84**, 739–749.

Fenner, F. (1970) The effects of changing social organisation on the infectious diseases of man. In: *The Impact of Civilisation on the Biology of Man* (ed. Boyden, S. V.). Camberra: Australian University Press, pp. 48–68.

Foster, D. W. (1989) Diabetes mellitus. In: *The Metabolic Basis of Inherited Disease*, 6th edn (eds. Scriver, C. R., Beaudet, A. L., Sly, W. S. and Valle, D.). New York: McGraw-Hill, Inc:, pp. 375–397.

Gerber, L. M. (1980) The influence of environmental factors on mortality from coronary heart disease among Filipinos in Hawaii. *Human Biology* **52**, 269–278.

Gerber, L. M. (1984) Diabetes mortality among Chinese migrants to New York City. *Human Biology* **56**, 449–458.

Gerber, L. M. and Madhavan, S. (1980) Epidemiology of coronary heart disease in migrant Chinese populations. *Medical Anthropology* **4**, 307–320.

Gleiberman, L. (1973) Blood pressure and dietary salt in human populations. *Ecology of Food and Nutrition* **2**, 143–156.

Grim, C. E. (1988) On slavery, salt and the higher blood pressure in black Americans (abstract). *Clinical Research* **36**, 426A.

Guralnik, J. M., LaCroix, A. Z., Branch, L. G., Kasl, S. V. and Wallace, R. B. (1991) Morbidity and disability in older persons in the years prior to death. *American Journal of Public Health* **81**, 443–447.

Hamilton, W. D. (1966) The moulding of senescence by natural selection. *Journal of Theoretical Biology* **12**, 12–45.

Harris, M. (1985) *The Sacred Cow and the Abominable Pig: Riddles of Food and Culture*. New York: Simon and Schuster.

Harrison, G. A. (1973) The effects of modern living. *Journal of Biosocial Science* **5**, 217–228.

Helmer, O. M. (1967) Hormonal and biochemical factors controlling blood pressure. In: *Les Concepts de Claude Bernard sur le Milieu Interieur*. Paris: Masson & Cie, pp. 115–128.

Hinkle, L. E. (1987) Stress and disease: the concept after 50 years. *Social Science and Medicine* **25**, 561–566.

Hornig, D. H., Moser, U. and Glatthaar, B. E. (1988) Ascorbic acid. In: *Modern Nutrition in Health and Disease* (eds Shils, M. E. and Young, V. R.). Philadelphia: Lea & Febiger, pp. 417–435.

Hsieh, C. C., Trichopoulos, D., Katsouyanni, K. and Yuasa, S. (1990) Age at menarche, age at menopause, height and obesity as risk factors for breast cancer: associations and interactions in an international case-control study. *International Journal of Cancer* **15**, 796–800.

Hutt, M. S. and Burkitt, D. P. (1986) *The Geography of Non-Infectious Disease*. New York: Oxford University Press.

INTERSALT Cooperative Research Group (1988) INTERSALT: an international study of electrolyte excretion and blood pressure. Results for a 24 hour urinary sodium and potassium excretion. *British Medical Journal* **297**, 319–328.

INTERSALT Cooperative Research Group (1989) The INTERSALT Study. *Journal of Human Hypertension* **3**, 279–331.

Jackson, F. L. C. (1991) An evolutionary perspective on salt, hypertension, and human genetic variability. *Hypertension* **17**, (Suppl. I), I129–I132.

James, G. D. and Baker, P. T. (1990) Human population biology and hypertension: Evolutionary and ecological aspects of blood pressure. In: *Hypertension: Pathophysiology, Diagnosis, and Management* (eds Laragh, J. H. and Brenner, B. M.). New York: Raven Press, Ltd, pp. 137–145.

James, G. D., Crews, D. E. and Pearson, J. D. (1989) Catecholamines and stress. In: *Human Population Biology: A Transdisciplinary Science* (eds Little, M. A. and Haas, J. D.). New York: Oxford University Press. pp. 280–295.

Johnson, T. E. (1988) Genetic specification of life span: processes, problems, and potentials. *Journal of Gerontology: Biological Sciences* **43**, B87–B92.

Kamboh, M. I. and Ferrell, R. E. (1990) Genetic studies of human apolipoproteins XV: an overview of IEF immunoblotting methods to screen apolipoprotein polymorphisms. *Human Heredity* **40**, 193–207.

Keith, V. M. and Smith, D. P. (1988) The current differential in black and white life expectancy. *Demography* **25**, 625–632.

Kottke, B. A. (1986) Lipid markers for atherosclerosis. *American Journal of Cardiology* **57**, 11C–17C.

Kreisberg, R. A. (1987) Aging, glucose metabolism, and diabetes: current concepts. *Geriatrics* **42**, 67–72.

Kritchevsky, D. (1986). Geriatric diabetes: latest research on the role of dietary fiber. *Geriatrics* **41**, 117–122.

Kromann, N. and Green, A. (1980). Epidemiological studies in the Upernavik district, Greenland: incidence of some chronic diseases 1950–1974. *Acta Medica Scandinavica (Stockholm)* **208**, 401–406.

Lancaster, J. B. and King, B. J. (1985) An evolutionary perspective on menopause. In:

*In Her Prime: A New View of the Middle-Aged Women* (eds Brown, J. K. and Kerns, V). South Hadley, MA: Bergin & Garvey Publishers, pp. 13–20.

Laragh, J. H. and Brenner, B. M. (eds) (1990) *Hypertension: Pathophysiology, Diagnosis, and Management.* New York: Raven Press, Ltd.

Leaf, A. and Weber, P. C. (1988) Cardiovascular effects of omega-3 fatty acids. *New England Journal of Medicine* **318**, 549–557.

Levi, L. and Anderson, L. (1975) *Psychosocial Stress*, New York: Spectrum Publications.

Linscheer, W. G. and Vergroesen, A. J. (1988). Lipids. In: *Modern Nutrition in Health and Disease* (eds Shils, M. E. and Young, V. R.), Philadelphia: Lea & Febiger, pp. 71–107.

Little, M. A. and Haas, J. D. (eds) (1989) *Human Population Biology: A Transdisciplinary Science.* New York: Oxford University Press.

Luft, F. C., Miller, J. Z. and Grim, C. E. (1991) Salt sensitivity and resistance of blood pressure: age and race as factors in physiological responses. *Hypertension* **17**, (Suppl I), I102–I108.

Mann, G. V., Schaffer, R. D., Anderson, R. S. and Sandstead, H. H. (1964) Cardiovascular disease in the Masai. *Journal of Atherosclerosis Research* **4**, 289.

McGarvey, S. T., Bindon, J. R., Crews, D. E. and Schendel, D. E. (1989) Modernization and adiposity: causes and consequences. In: *Human Population Biology: A Transdisciplinary Science* (eds Little, M. A. and Haas, J. D.), New York: Oxford University Press, pp. 263–279.

McGill, H. C., Strong, J. P., Holman, R. L. and Werthessen, N. T. (1960) Arterial lesions in the Kenya Baboon. *Circulation Research* **8**, 670–679.

McGill, H. C., McMahan, C. A., Krushi, A. W. and Mott, G. E. (1981) Relationship of lipoprotein cholesterol concentrations to experimental atherosclerosis in baboons. *Atherosclerosis* **1**, 3–12.

Micozzi, M. (1987) Cross-cultural correlations of childhood growth and adult breast cancer. *American Journal of Physical Anthropology* **73**, 525–537.

Neel, J. V. (1962) Diabetes mellitus: a "thrifty genotype" rendered detrimental by progress? *American Journal of Human Genetics* **14**, 353–362.

Neel, J. V. (1982). The thrifty genotype revisited. In: *The Genetics of Diabetes Mellitus* (eds Kobberling, J. and Tattersall, R. B.). New York: Academic Press. pp. 283–293.

Nesse, R. M. (1988) Life table tests of evolutionary theories of senescence. *Experimental Gerontology* **23**, 445–453.

Olshansky, S. J., Carnes, B. A. and Cassel, C. (1990) In search of Methuselah: estimating the upper limits to human longevity. *Science* **250**, 634–640.

Omran, A. R. (1977) The epidemiological transition: a theory of the epidemiology of population change. *Milbank Memorial Fund Quarterly* **49**, 509–538.

Orchard, T. J., Becker, D. J., Kuller, L. H., Wagener, D. K., LaPorte, R. E. and Drash, A. L. (1982) Age and sex variation in glucose tolerance and insulin responses: parallels with cardiovascular risk. *Journal of Chronic Disease* **35**, 123–132.

Papaspyros, N. S. (1964) *The History of Diabetes, 2nd edn.* Stuttgart: Georg Thieme Verlag.

Pickering, G. W. (1961) *The Nature of Essential Hypertension.* New York: Grune and Stratton.

Preston, S. H. (1976) *Mortality Patterns in National Populations: With Special Reference to Causes of Death.* New York: Academic Press, Inc.

Reaven, G. M. (ed.) (1984) *International Diabetes Conference on Etiopathogenesis and Metabolic Aspects of Diabetes Mellitus*. Basel: Karger.

Rose, M. R. (1991) *Evolutionary Biology of Aging*. New York: Oxford University Press.

Ruskin, A. (1956) *Classics in Arterial Hypertension*. Springfield, IL: Charles C. Thomas.

Schell, L. M. (1991) Pollution and human growth: lead, noise, polychlorobiphenyl compounds and toxic wastes. In: *Applications of Biological Anthropology to Human Affairs* (eds. Lasker, G. W. and Mascie-Taylor, N.). Cambridge: Cambridge University Press, pp. 83–116.

Scott, J. (1987) Molecular genetics of common diseases. *British Medical Journal* **295**, 769–771.

Scrimshaw, N. S. and Guzman, M. A. (1968) Diet and atherosclerosis. *Laboratory Investigations* **18**, 623.

Shimokata, H., Muller, D. C., Fleg, J. L., Sorkin, J., Ziemba, A. W. and Andres, R. (1991) Age as an independent determinant of glucose tolerance. *Diabetes Care* **40**, 44–51.

Sing, C. F., Boerwinkle, E. and Moll, P. P. (1985) Strategies for elucidating the phenotypic and genetic heterogeneity of a chronic disease with a complex etiology. In: *Diseases of Complex Etiology in Small Populations* (eds Chakraborty, R. and Szathmary, E. J. E.). New York: Alan R. Liss, pp. 39–66.

Smyer, M. A. and Crews, D. E. (1985) "Developmental" intervention and aging: demographic and economic changes as a context for intervention. In: Advances in Motivation and Achievement (eds Kleiber, D. A. and Maehr, M. L.). Greenwich, CN: JAI Press Inc., pp. 189–215.

Sørensen, T. I. A., Nielsen, G. G., Andersen, P. K. and Teasdale, T. W. (1988) Genetic and environmental influences on premature death in adult adoptees. *New England Journal of Medicine* **12**, 727–732.

Stamler, R. (1991) Implications of the INTERSALT Study. *Hypertension* **17**, (Suppl. I), I16–I20.

Stini, W. A. (1971) Evolutionary implications of changing nutritional patterns in human populations. *American Anthropologist* **73**, 1019–1030.

Stini, W. A. (1991) The biology of human aging. In: *Applications of Biological Anthropology to Human Affairs* (eds Lasker, G. W. and Mascie-Taylor, N.) Cambridge: Cambridge University Press, pp. 208–236.

Stout, R. W. and Crawford, V. (1988) Active life expectancy and terminal dependency. Trends in long-term geriatric care over 33 years. *The Lancet* **6**, 281-283.

Teitlebaum, M. S. (1975) Relevance of demographic transition theory for developing countries. *Science* **188**, 420–425.

Tollefsbol, T. O. (1987) Gene expression of carbohydrate metabolism in cellular senescence and aging. *Molecular Biology and Medicine* **4**, 251–263.

Trowell, H. and Burkitt, D. P. (eds) (1981) *Western Diseases: Their Emergence and Prevention*. Cambridge, MA: Harvard University Press.

Turke, P. W. (1988) Helpers at the nest: child care networks on Ifaluk. In: *Human Reproductive Behavior* (eds Betzig, L., Borgerhoff Mulder, M. and Turke, P. W.), London: Cambridge University Press, pp. 173–188.

Turke, P. W. (1991) The pleiotrophic gene theory of senescence. *Association for Anthropology and Gerontology Newsletter* **12**, 5–7.

Utermann, G., Hoppichler, F., Dieplinger, H., Seed, M., Thompson, G. and Boerwinkle, E. (1989) Defects in low density lipoprotein receptor gene affect lipoprotein(a) levels: multiple interaction of two gene loci associated with premature atherosclerosis. *Proceedings of the National Academy of Sciences USA* **86**, 4171–4174.

Weiss, K. M. (1981) Evolutionary perspectives on human aging. In: *Other Ways of Growing Old: Anthropological Perspectives* (eds Amoss, P. T. and Harrell, S.). Stanford, CA: Stanford University Press, pp. 25–58.

Weiss, K. M. (1984) On the number of members of genus *Homo* who have ever lived, and some evolutionary interpretations. *Human Biology* **56**, 637–649.

Weiss, K. M. (1989) Are known chronic diseases related to the human lifespan and its evolution? *American Journal of Human Biology* **1**, 307–319.

Wendorff, M. and Goldfine, I. D. (1991) Archaeology of NIDDM: excavation of the "thrifty" genotype. *Diabetes* **40**, 161–165.

Williams, B. J. (1973) *Evolution and Human Origins*. New York: Harper and Row, Publishers.

Williams, G. C. (1957) Pleiotropy, natural selection, and the evolution of senescence. *Evolution* **11**, 398–411.

Wilson, T. W. (1986) Africa, Afro-Americans, and hypertension: An hypothesis. *Social Science History* **10**, 489–500.

Wilson, T. W. and Grim, C. E. (1991) Biohistory of slavery and blood pressure differences in blacks today: A hypothesis. *Hypertension* **17** (Suppl. I), I122–I128.

Yamagishita, M. and Guralnik, J. M. (1988) Changing mortality patterns that led life expectancy in Japan to surpass Sweden's: 1972–1982. *Demography* **25**, 611–624.

# 7

# Human Immune System Aging: Approaches, Examples, and Ideas

PETER J. MAYER

## INTRODUCTION

This chapter is intended to be a prelude to future studies and not a comprehensive review of the extensive literature in human immune system aging. The next section on the background to human immune system aging provides a brief summary of information relevant to the ideas and examples which follow. More detailed and thorough reviews of the subject are available (e.g., Goidl, 1987; Miller, 1989, 1991a; Schwab *et al.*, 1989; Segre *et al.*, 1989). (In reading these, and other, reviews one must be cautious about whether data refer to human or rodent studies; the distinction is not always made explicit.) The third section, biological anthropological perspectives on human immune system aging, is divided into the following conceptual areas explored in biological anthropology: (1) human biological diversity (population and sub-group variations in immune system aging); (2) biocultural perspectives (the interaction of biological and cultural influences on immune system aging); (3) ontogeny and gerontology (the continuum between development of the immune system, on the one hand, and its aging, on the other); and (4) evolutionary models of human immunosenescence. The concluding section suggests general applications of the concepts previously discussed and reflects the distinction made throughout the chapter between immune system aging, which refers to universal, progressive, cumulative, irreversible processes, and immunosenescence, which comprises that subset of processes which are pathogenic, dysfunctional, or detrimental.

This chapter is intended to be suggestive and not exhaustive, to highlight areas of mutual interest to biological anthropology and biological gerontology in the hope that cross-fertilization between the two might generate a kind of intellectual hybrid vigor. Despite the wealth of information gained from immunological experiments with rodents, reference in this chapter to these data is minimal because anthropologists focus their efforts on primates. Moreover, significant differences exist between rodent and human immune system aging (Ligthart and Hijmans, 1986, cf. Wade *et al.*, 1988), and one cannot simply assume that extrapolation across phylogenetic orders will be valid. Reference to non-human primate data is also infrequent, but this is due to a lack of such immunogerontological studies (see DeRousseau, this volume).


## BACKGROUND OF HUMAN IMMUNE SYSTEM AGING

The immune system consists primarily of peripheral tissues (spleen, lymph nodes, thymus) and central tissue (bone marrow). Pluripotent stem cells within the bone marrow act as a reservoir for renewing populations of other, more differentiated precursor cells. Bone marrow also harbors maturation factors for macrophages and B lymphocytes (B cells). While there have been a few studies with mice which seem to indicate little or no age-related change in bone marrow functions (Siskind, 1987), information about aging of this compartment of the human immune system is lacking. In contrast, much has been learned about human peripheral lymphoid system aging.

The immunologic theory of aging (Walford, 1969, 1974) focused attention on the centrality of thymic involution to immunosenescence and on the potential cascade of deteriorative effects due to loss of biological self-recognition (increased autoimmunity) with aging. Textbooks typically state that involution of the thymus gland is a morphological change—decrease in tissue mass and infiltration by fat cells—which begins around the time of puberty and accelerates thereafter with age. However, recent evidence suggests a more complicated situation: the thymus attains it maximal size soon after birth and does not change with age in healthy persons, although the volume of lymphatic tissue declines with age (Steinman, 1986); thymic involution accelerates after ca. age 30 (Tosi et al., 1982); the coefficient of variation in thymic wet weight is large (42–54%) and does not vary with age beyond age 10, although mean wet weight decreases by 62% (calculated from Kendall, 1981); and thymic tissue appears significantly disorganized in the oldest (63–91 years) age group studied to date (Kraft et al., 1988). While there appears to be consensus regarding an age-related increase in the proportion of fatty tissue (and a corresponding decrease in lymphatic tissue), postmortem studies that reported this conclusion are necessarily cross-sectional; definitive evidence for thymic involution awaits in vivo collection of longitudinal data, e.g., by computed tomography.

The thymus is the site of lymphocyte "education" (cellular differentiation) where pre-T-cells mature into regulatory and effector cells which have presumably "learned" to distinguish self from non-self as a consequence of the thymic microenvironment. This "educational" process presumably occurs by exposure of maturing T-cells to antigens of the major histocompatibility complex (MHC). Thymic involution correlates with a wide range of immune functional declines which diminish with age to levels of 5–30% of their peak youth values (Walford, 1982; cf. Twomey et al., 1982). What "triggers" thymic involution is unknown, although the following attributes suggest a significant role for genetic control: ubiquity among mammals studied, apparent universality among human beings, initiation of the involution process around the time of birth, and regularity/continuity of the process.

**Table 7-1**   A summary of reported findings in human immune system aging.

*Molecular and biochemical*
0        Complement function and levels
0        Interleukin-1 (IL-1) production
0        Prostaglandin production
0        B-cell growth factor production by T-cells
−        Interleukin-2 (IL-2) production
−        Number of chromosomes (especially X and Y) per cell
−        Induction of IL-2 and IL-2 receptor mRNA by PHA activation
−        Production of immunoglobins by T-cell-independent stimuli
+        Autoanti-idiotypes (not necessarily associated with disease)
+        Synthesis of prostaglandin
0/−     Antibody production
0/−     IL-2 receptor expression (− high affinity receptor)
0/−/+  $\gamma$-Interferon production
0/−/+  Serum levels of immunoglobins (IgA, IgG, IgM)

*Cellular*
0        Number of monocytes, macrophages, neutrophils
0        Number of pluripotent hematopetic stem cells
0        Antigen-processing by macrophages
0        Phagocytosis
0        B-cell function (0/− in very old >90 years)
+        Number of "uninducible" null (non-T, non-B) cells in bone marrow
+        Sensitivity to prostaglandin inhibition of lymphocyte stimulation (age >70 years)
+        Lymphocyte membrane rigidity (= −membrane fluidity)
+        Percentage of resting T-cells in the circulation
+        Suppressor activity of monocytes/macrophages
+        Helper T-cell stimulation of B-cell immunoglobin production
−        Migration ability of neutrophils
−        Suppressor T-cell suppression of B-cell immunoglobin production
−        Activity of cytotoxic T-cells
−        Number of oligopotent stem cells (precursors to T-cell subsets)
−        Proliferation and differentiation of B-cells to plasma cells
−        Oxidative burst in macrophage host defense response (neutrophils)
−        Protein synthesis following mitogenesis or activation
0/−     Proliferative response of T-cells to mitogens, antigens, lectins (e.g., phytohemagglutinin, PHA)
        −    Number of stimulatable cells
        −    Rate of entry into DNA synthesis phase of cell cycle
        −    Number of times stimulated cells will divide
        −    Total number of cell divisions *in vitro* (Hayflick limit)
        0/+  Time needed for cells to enter DNA synthesis phase
        0/+  Duration of cell cycle
0/−     Number and proportion of T-cells
0/−     Number of B-cells (−/+ in very old >90 years)
0/+     Number of natural killer (NK) cells (non-T-, non-B-cells)
0/+     Number of peripheral immature T-cells
−/+     Number of T-suppressor/cytotoxic cells (CD8+)
0/−/+  Number of T-helper/inducer cells (CD4+)
0/−/+  Ratio of CD4+/CD8+ cells
0/−/+  Platelet function
0/−/+  Cytotoxicity of NK cells

**Table 7-1** (cont)

*Physiological*

| | |
|---|---|
| + | Incidence and severity of infections |
| + | Autoimmunity (but not autoimmune disease) |
| + | Benign monoclonal gammopathies (homogeneous immunoglobins) |
| − | Thymic function (i.e., involution) |
| | 0/−    Levels of thymic hormones |
| | −     Hormone activity |
| − | Response to immunization (− response duration, − antibody levels) |
| − | Cell-mediated immunity (+ reactivation of shingles, tuberculosis) |
| − | Primary antibody response (T-cell dependent) |
| 0 | Secondary antibody response |
| 0/− | Inflammatory response |
| 0/− | Vigor of delayed-type hypersensitivity skin reaction |

0 = no change with age; − = decrease with age; + = increase with age.

Age-related changes in the immune systems of healthy adults can be documented at molecular, cellular, and physiological levels. Table 7-1 represents a compilation of such data from more than 200 reports. Some aspects of human immune system aging do not change with age or are the subject of conflicting reports, and some of these are also listed in Table 7-1. Aside from differences in study samples and disparities in technique, discrepant results are commonly due to simple comparisons between younger and older groups which ignore the likelihood that quantitative change in function is not linearly related to age. Age-related functional change typically assumes some peak value which differs in timing according to the parameter studied. In this context another important point is that mean differences between younger and older individuals may be observed even though substantial percentages of subjects in the old group outperform younger "control" subjects (e.g., in T-cell proliferation; Murasko *et al.*, 1991).

Many of the variables appearing in Table 7-1 are highly interrelated because cell-to-cell communication is required to initiate immune responses and to effect clonal expansion of immune system cells, and because soluble factors produced by organs and tissues (e.g., cytokines, hormones, neurotransmitters, thymic peptides) also influence the response of many cell types and subtypes. Thus, for example, decreased responsiveness of macrophages to mitogenic or antigenic stimulation (e.g., from fungi or bacteria) results in decreased production of interleukin-1 (IL-1); decreased levels of IL-1, or diminished responsiveness of post-thymic precursor T-cells to IL-1, results in decreased IL-2 production (with diminished autocrine effects, i.e., a dampening of positive feedback); decreased IL-2 results in a decreased number of activated helper/inducer T-cells ($T_h$-cells which carry the surface marker CD4), decreased microbiocidal activity of macrophages, and decreased natural killer (NK) cell activity. $T_h$-cells (CD4+), in turn, induce proliferation and clonal expansion of effector cells such as cytotoxic T-cells which kill, for example, virus-infected cells. $T_h$-cells, in concert with antigen-processing macrophages, also induce B-lymphocytes to differentiate into immunoglobin-producing plasma cells. This (oversimplified) cascade of events illustrates how age-related decreases in responsiveness or metabolism of a range of immune cells contribute to diminished efficacy of many T-cell-mediated responses, including host defense mechanisms such as cell- and humoral-mediated immunity. Consequently, the general consensus is that immunosenescence primarily emanates from T-cell functional declines. However, it is not known if all age-related T-cell dysfunction is intrinsically driven, caused by extrinsic changes, or some combination of both.

In general, then, immunogerontologists are struggling with the same issues that face all biological gerontologists: are the aging-related systemic changes which predispose to weaker immune responses genetically programmed? If so, are the initiating events intracellular or organ-specific? Or is the weakened response due to loss of "reserve capacity" or "maximum function" such that under challenge the ability to return the system to its normal range is comprised because each part of the complex system operates less than optimally over time? A corollary of the latter proposition, but a process which may reflect genetic control, is that elements of the regulatory system become imbalanced with aging. Examples of this include age-related increased T-cell suppressor activity and decreased helper/inducer activity.

## BIOLOGICAL ANTHROPOLOGICAL PERSPECTIVES ON HUMAN IMMUNE SYSTEM AGING

Immunogerontology is likely to be of continually increasing interest to biological anthropologists for at least four reasons. A primary interest of biological anthropologists, investigation of human biological diversity, finds evidence in the phenomenon that human beings become more varied, more different from one another, with age (Norris and Shock, 1966; Borkan, 1983; Rowe and Kahn, 1987; Chandra, 1989; Nelson and Dannefer, 1992; cf. Bornstein and Smircina, 1982; see also Wood et al., this volume) Longitudinal studies of immune function demonstrate increased variability in, for example, serum levels of IgA with increased age (Buckley et al., 1974). Moreover, intraindividual variability also increases with age, introducing a kind of immunological "mosaicism" (Miller, 1989, 1991b) in which some cells lose function whereas others of the same type do not. A second attribute of biological anthropology is elaboration of a biocultural perspective on human biological diversity, meaning that social, cultural, ecological, and historic factors help to co-determine biological differences. The role of nutrition in human immunosenescence, and the socioeconomic influences and cultural practices which affect what, how, and when people eat, illustrates this idea. A third focus of biological anthropologists has been human (and non-human primate) growth and development which, if individuals are followed long enough, becomes maturation and aging. In this regard the immune system may be especially valuable because so much is known of its genesis and because aspects of its age-related decline begin at puberty, where much of what is studied as growth and development continues as the study of maturation. A fourth area explored by biological anthropologists, human evolution, is relevant to immunogerontology with regard to possible consequences of natural selection.

A distinctive contribution of biological anthropology to gerontology in general may be to help distinguish between those human phenomena which are universal and species-specific and those aspects of aging which are idiosyncratic and environmental- or group-specific. The former type of data are likely to lead more directly to valid inferences about basic processes and mechanisms of biological aging, whereas the latter more likely reflect local or historical circumstances and may indicate pathophysiological conditions. Studies of the immune system, in particular, would benefit from cross-cultural and geographic comparisons since antigenic exposure (via infectious agents, food antigens, pollen) varies so greatly around the world that common responses likely reflect common processes. Conversely, heterogeneous responses could be due to genetic, ontogenetic, ecological, or cultural differences.

## Human Biological Diversity

Comparing biological variables between populations, or among sub-groups within one population, is conceptually simple and procedurally complex. The greatest difficulties entail defining group membership by means of valid scientific criteria and obtaining a representative sample of each group. Populations isolated by geography (e.g., island inhabitants; Friedlaender and Page, 1989) or social customs (e.g., Hutterites in Canada; Morgan, 1983) provide a way biological anthropologists have successfully resolved such difficulties. However, people living in developed and especially urbanized societies are heterogeneous, and admixture between previously separated populations compounds the complexities of validly defining biological groups and sampling their members. This may account for the scarcity of studies of biological diversity in immune system aging, although obviously such an explanation can not apply to the relative paucity of investigations of sexual dimorphism in immune system functioning.

### HLA and Disease Incidence

The major histocompatibility complex (MHC) refers to a unique collection of genes which, in human beings, code for the cell-surface glycoproteins known as human leukocyte antigens (HLAs). The immune system uses these determinants, one class of which appear on all somatic cells, to distinguish self from non-self. For instance, immune host defenses like cytotoxic T-cells must be able to determine whether a potential target is "friend or foe" by "reading" its HLA markers or detecting their absence. The antigens coded by the MHC genes help regulate immune response and thus there are good reasons to investigate this "supergene" complex for its potential role in immunological aging. For example, it has been shown that the MHC directly influences murine life span (Smith and Walford, 1978), and it may similarly affect human life span insofar as, for example, susceptibility to autoimmune diseases such as insulin-dependent diabetes and systemic lupus erythematosus correlates with specific MHC alleles (Walford, 1982).

Evolutionary significance of the HLA system may reside in the observed levels of polymorphism which could have arisen by natural selection acting on disease resistance or susceptibility, on maternal–fetal (in)compatibility, or on development of a cell-to-cell recognition system for differentiation and morphogenesis (Bodmer, 1972). Assuming that HLA phenotypes are stable during an individual's lifetime, one obvious question about this polymorphic system in relation to aging is: does the distribution of HLA antigens differ among different age cohorts in a population? The question does not appear to have been systematically investigated by, for example, looking specifically at societies with different adult age structures or at populations inhabiting different ecological niches. However, as was previously done for red blood cell markers and immunoglobins, population and group comparisons of HLA phenotypic frequencies have been compiled (e.g., Tsuji et al., 1986).

In support of a role for the MHC in immune system aging, there is evidence of substantial associations between HLA markers and disease, e.g., in addition to those listed above, ankylosing spondylitis, subacute thyroiditis, tuberculosis, multiple sclerosis, myasthenia gravis, and various arthritic conditions (reviewed in Yunis and Watson, 1982). Moreover, extremely long-lived Japanese Okinawans (nonagenarians and centenarians) appear to demonstrate a distinctive pattern of HLA-DR antigens (Takata et al., 1987; cf. Wainscoat et al., 1987) as do French Caucasians aged $\geq 90$ years, in a gender-specific pattern of HLA-C phenotypes (Proust et al., 1982). [HLA-A, -B, -C and -DR are the four loci which code for antigens of the human MHC; each locus is polymorphic, i.e., has multiple alleles.] Additionally, there are scattered reports of HLA frequency differences between younger and older healthy individuals (Macurova et al., 1975; Hansen et al., 1977; Batory et al., 1983). In contrast, others report no age-related trend in HLA markers (e.g., Yarnell et al., 1979; Blackwelder et al., 1982; Batory et al., 1983). Furthermore, the degree of heterozygosity at the MHC loci has also been investigated and found both to increase with age (e.g., Yasuda et al., 1980; Batory et al., 1983) and not to change with age (e.g., Yarnell et al., 1979; Blackwelder et al., 1982). Anthropologically interesting comparisons between Caucasians and Japanese, and among three Caucasian ethnic subgroups, all healthy persons aged $\geq 90$ years, revealed enigmatic shifts in zygosity for HLA-A, -B, -C, -DR (Hodge and Walford, 1980). In the Tuaregs, an inbred South Saharan population isolate, an unexpectedly low incidence of HLA-A and -B homozygotes may be an example of a selective advantage for HLA polymorphism that acts to maintain heterozygosity (Degos et al., 1974). However, the underlying biological mechanism and its possible relevance to immunosenescence are unknown.

In summary, then, insufficient consistent evidence exists to establish an association between HLA markers or heterozygosity and superior survival. This could be due to a true lack of relationship between the MHC and aging, to the insensitivity of current HLA-typing procedures, to co-variation between other genetic complexes and life span, to the balanced effects of competing selective pressures, to subtle, cumulative effects revealed only in the extremely old, or to the overwhelming influence of cohort (or period, i.e., historical) effects which mask biological aging effects. Additionally, given the known associations between HLA markers and diseases, there is the conceptual difficulty of disentangling pathophysiological effects associated with MHC genes from biological aging effects inferred to be influenced by MHC genes. In this regard it is interesting that in a study of 172 Hungarians aged 13–84 years the rate of age-related decline in T-cell function (stimulation by the plant lectin phytohemagglutinin, PHA) correlated significantly ($r = 0.55$–$0.84$) with HLA haplotypes (Batory et al., 1983).[1] Some haplotypes (combinations of HLA markers at different genetic loci) exhibit linkage disequilibrium among healthy "survivors," and this disequilibrium is associated with different rates of immune system aging (assessed by PHA stimulation). Hence it might be worthwhile to seek similar associations with other measures of immune function.

One can hypothesize that if the MHC influences longevity by means of the immune system, then some haplotypes will have a selective advantage within a particular environment (as evidenced by their over-representation among healthy elderly) and bearers of these haplotypes will exhibit immune function which is better than average for their age-matched cohort and similar to that of younger healthy individuals. A recent study of 17 "healthy" Kentucky centenarians supports this hypothesis with respect to HLA-A29/B7/B35 (Thompson et al., 1984). Observations of an association between particular haplotypes and reduced or enhanced gender-specific survival (e.g., Greenberg and Yunis, 1978; Proust et al., 1982) indicate that ontogenetic processes (i.e., sexual maturation) and sexual dimorphism also affect the possible influence of the MHC on longevity. (See also section on MHC regulation of biological aging, p. 201.)

Variation in a second polymorphic immune cell surface marker, the T-cell receptor, is reported to be associated with autoimmune diseases (Hoover and Capra, 1987). Age-related patterns of T-cell-receptor polymorphisms (comparable to those of the HLA system) are unknown.

### Sexual Dimorphism

The question as to why, on average, women outlive men in most countries has yet to be fully resolved (recently reviewed in Hazzard, 1989; Smith, 1989; Ory and Warner, 1990). A major issue is whether the phenomenon directly reflects underlying biological sexual dimorphism which is relatively insensitive to environmental variation (e.g., as seen in body size or secondary sexual characteristics such as body hair), or, instead, is a manifestation of gender

---

[1]While PHA stimulation is an admittedly limited measure, the percentage of activated cells correlated with survival in a 3-year follow-up study of 31 healthy elderly aged >80 years (Butenko, 1983) Moreover, among 403 elderly individuals aged 70–106 observed over a 25-month period, higher mortality was associated with very low lymphoproliferative response to three mitogens including PHA (Murasko et al., 1988). In addition, cross-sectional studies of both baboons (*Papio Cynocephalus*) (Eichberg et al., 1981) and rhesus macaques (Ershler et al., 1988a,b) report age-related decreases in PHA stimulation.

differences in exposure and susceptibility to disease and disability. Gender comparisons of life expectancy at various ages and life span in different populations, both contemporaneous and historical, will help to clarify the issue. Directly related to this issue is the focus on mechanisms which might mediate gender differences in survival, be they physiological or behavioral. The primary example of the former comprises hormones (e.g., the protective effects of estrogen to prevent coronary artery disease) and the latter includes differences in occupation or in life style, e.g., cigarette smoking. In addition, there is evidence to suggest an immunological basis to superior female survival (summarized in Purtilo and Sullivan, 1979). And while gender differences in exposure to stress have also been invoked, they have yet to be systematically investigated. (The possible role of stress in immunosenescence is discussed in the section on psychoneuroendocrinology and immune system aging, p. 193).

By virtue of possessing two X-chromosomes, females have a lower risk of expressing X-linked recessive mutations which might produce defective immune system components, either effectors or regulators. There are at least five X-linked recessive immunodeficient human syndromes (Horowitz and Hong, 1977), although their prevalence is low. Epidemiologic evidence indicates that males are more susceptible to lethal effects of infectious and parasitic diseases. For example, in the USA in 1980, the male/female ratio for incidence of acute infective and parasitic diseases per 100 persons per year was 0.88 (Verbrugge and Wingard, 1987), whereas the male/female ratio of age-adjusted mortality from pneumonia and influenza was 1.77 (Hazard, 1989). Moreover males have a higher incidence of cancer, especially lymphoma and leukemia (Hazard, 1989) and of two virus-associated neoplasms, Burkitt's lymphoma and nasopharyngeal carcinoma (Purtilo and Sullivan, 1979). Epidemiological studies also indicate that females suffer both higher incidence of autoimmune disorders (Purtilo and Sullivan, 1979; Hazzard, 1989) and greater severity since androgens suppress and estrogens accelerate autoimmune disease (Talal *et al.*, 1984). However, autoimmune diseases tend to be associated more with morbidity than with mortality. In general, for all diseases, women have higher rates of *morbidity* whereas men have higher rates of *mortality* (Verbrugge and Wingard, 1987).

Investigation of the basic mechanism(s) which contribute to sexual dimorphism in immunosenescence is at an early stage (Hazzard, 1990) even though observations of physiological and molecular differences have been made. For example:

1. There may be gender-specific age-related patterns of thymic involution (Simpson *et al.*, 1975; cf. Tosi *et al.*, 1982) possibly related to thymic–endocrine interaction (Rebar, 1984).
2. The age-related decline in mitogenic stimulation of T-cells occurs earlier in females (Delespesse *et al.*, 1974; cf. Yamakido *et al.*, 1985b), a difference which is reported to disappear after age 70 years (Mascart-Lemone *et al.*, 1982; Murasko *et al.*, 1988).
3. The number of circulating T-cells is reported to decrease in older men but not in older women (Mascart-Lemone *et al.*, 1982; cf. Goto and Nishioka, 1989).

4. Levels of total sum IgE (immunoglobin E) and of specific IgE antibody progressively decline in aging women but not in men (Delespesse et al., 1977; Hanneuse and Delespesse, 1978).

5. Females have higher levels of circulating immunoglobins than males (Grossman, 1990).

6. Older men may have reduced levels of $T_h$-cells (CD4+) and increased levels of suppressor T-cells (CD8+), compared to younger men, whereas women may demonstrate no change in these parameters with age (Mascart-Lemone et al., 1982; cf. Traill et al., 1985; Dworsky et al., 1989).

7. There are reports of decreased numbers and proportions of T-cell subsets in aging females (Hallgren et al., 1983; Nagel et al., 1983; Deviere et al., 1986).

8. Higher incidence of autoantibodies, especially non-organ-specific (Crespi et al., 1986) in aging females than in aging males (e.g., Traill et al., 1985) appears to be a consistent finding and has been reported for North American Blacks (Ockhuizen et al., 1982) and Caucasians (Cammarata et al., 1967) as well as Australian Caucasians (Mackay, 1971).

9. No sex or age difference in monocyte phagocytosis of yeast cells is reported (Sondell et al., 1990) although age-related decline in phagocytosis of antigen-coated red blood cells appears to be male-specific (Fulop et al., 1984).

10. The percentages of experimentally activated T cells and NK-cells increase more rapidly with advancing age in females than in males (Goto and Nishioka, 1989).

The many contradictory data may result from real population differences (e.g., Japanese versus Western European), from real biological aging differences (e.g., due to study sample differences in subjects' age range or "health"), from heterogeneity among the elderly, or from technical artifacts.

Sexual dimorphism in immune responses, with females producing a more active response than males, generally appears after sexual maturation, which strongly suggests an influential role for gonadal steroids (Grossman, 1990). Basic mechanisms which link the age-related immune phenomena listed above with biological gender differences most likely reside in interactions between sex hormones and cellular processes of proliferation and differentiation (e.g., T-cell; Holdstock et al., 1982; B-cell; Sthoeger et al., 1988), especially at the molecular genetic level. Suggested mechanisms may be related to impaired nuclear responsiveness to cytoplasmic signals (gender of subjects not reported: Gutowski et al., 1986) or gender-specific differences in chromatin structure as revealed by studies of DNA damage and repair (Stephens and Lipetz, 1983; Harris et al., 1985; Mayer et al., 1991).

### Blood Group Antigens and a Model of Restricted Idiotypic Repertoire with Aging

Biological anthropologists have traditionally investigated the worldwide distribution of blood group antigens (e.g., ABO alleles) in order to map population differences. The inference from allelic maps to mechanism often requires detailed ecological and biomedical knowledge. The classic example of this approach is the discovery of the co-distribution of the allele for sickle cell hemoglobin (heterozygosity protects against malaria, homozygosity causes disease), the incidence of *Anopheles gambiae* mosquitos infected by *Plasmodium falciparum*, the pathogen responsible for holoendemic malaria in Western Africa, and the historically recent adoption of slash and burn agriculture (Livingston, 1958). As illustrated by sickle cell disease, one goal of biological anthropology is to examine how cultural practices and evolutionary forces influence observed allelic distributions; in this regard the following model is of interest.

In response to presentation of antigens, B-cells from older individuals exhibit "profound diminution in medium- to high-affinity antibody" (Goidl *et al.*, 1990: 413) which has been interpreted to reflect a "restricted idiotypic repertoire." (An idiotype is an antigenic determinant located in or near the antigen-binding site of an antibody.) This loss of strongly binding antibody may be significant for morbidity and mortality since it could explain decreased resistance to infection in the elderly (Gardner, 1980; Phair *et al.*, 1988). Interest in the model for a restricted range of antibody response derives from the suggestion that older individuals who have shared an "ecological niche" throughout their lifetimes might also share patterns of reduced idiotypic expression as they age (Goidl *et al.*, 1990). The idea is that antigenic stimulation during one's lifetime—e.g., by infectious agents, antigens in food or the environment—eventually "depletes" idiotypic (antibody) diversity in the aged and that therefore antigenic stimulation common to a shared environment will lead to a shared pattern of restricted expression of idiotypes among the aged.

## Biocultural Perspective

Human survival in any environment necessitates internal adjustment to external circumstances (i.e., biological adaptation) as well as modification of external circumstances to internal requirements (i.e., cultural adaptation). In the context of human aging this type of approach has recently been referred to as "the interaction between psychosocial and physiologic variables" (Rowe and Kahn, 1987). However, what anthropologists cite as their biocultural approach has a slightly broader scope because it encompasses ecological variables as well, and these are particularly important in immunology since the immune system evolved to protect against external agents of potential morbidity and mortality which vary ecologically.

### Exposure to Immunological Stimuli

Infectious diseases represent the second most frequent cause of death in the elderly of developed countries (Bush and Kaye, 1990). Among the elderly morbidity and mortality from infections are due to interactions between endogenous immunosenescent processes and other factors such as malnutrition, decreased physical activity, increased therapeutic drug use, and exposure to pathogens. These other factors largely reflect cultural expectations, institutions, and behaviors which vary from group to group (e.g., Garruto and Gajdusek, 1975). For example, nosocomial infections (e.g., pneumonia), prevalent in Westernized societies where nursing homes and other group-living arrangements are utilized by the elderly, obviously could not occur in societies which lack such facilities. More generally, the segregation of age groups by residence, occupation, or social intercourse may affect exposure to immunologic stimuli. Similarly dietary customs, healing traditions, and what we have come to call life-style choices which are differentiated by age will influence what pathogens, antigens, allergens, etc. the immune systems of people of different ages contact. Consideration of these variables is likely to be intuitive or "common sense" for many health-care practitioners, but their systematic investigation within a cross-cultural biomedical framework might reveal substantial variation in patterns of human immune aging which suggest a wider range of adaptability and diversity than previously recognized. The formulation of an ecologically oriented hypothesis concerning antibody diversity and aging (see section on blood group antigens and a model of restricted idiotypic repertoire with aging, p. 191) represents another example of this approach.

### Psychoneuroendocrinology and Immune System Aging

One aspect of the biocultural perspective on human aging concerns "the mind-body problem," viz., how do non-biological factors processed by individuals influence their biological aging? Keeping in mind dangers of oversimplification and biological determinism, we can approach this question by looking to the relatively new field of psychoneuroimmunology (Solomon, 1985, 1990) (also known as neuroimmunomodulation and behavioral immunology) which is concerned with bidirectional interactions between the nervous system (psychic and somatic components) and the immune system. (For recent reviews, see Solomon, 1987; Freier, 1990). Observations which support the existence of such interactions include: presence of receptors for neurotransmitters and neuropeptides on lymphocytes and monocytes; innervation by the automatic nervous system of thymus, lymph nodes, spleen and bone marrow; experiments (not in human beings) in which manipulation of the hypothalamic–pituitary axis can stimulate or suppress immune function; evidence that thymic hormones (peptides) can affect neurotransmission (Lloyd, 1984); and the growing number of peptide messengers synthesized by elements of the neural, endocrine, and immune systems, e.g., somatostatin, $\beta$-endorphin, adrenocorticotrophic hormone, and IL-1 (Freier, 1990).

This explicitly reductionist approach examines possible mediators between psychosocial status, on the one hand, and functional changes in physiological (specifically immunological) parameters, on the other (e.g., Jemmott and Locke, 1984). The best studied of these potential mediating mechanisms comprise neuroendocrine aspects of the processing of "stressful" events. One general idea is that, under conditions of "stress," individuals with less "hardy" psychological states will be more vulnerable to morbidity and mortality associated with, if not causally related to, impaired immune function. Hence, depending upon individual differences in psychological and social circumstances, as people age, "stress" may exacerbate decreases in host defenses and in immune surveillance due to pre-existing immunosenescence.

Interest in the significance of the neuroendocrine–immune axis for biological aging is not new (recently reviewed in Meites *et al.*, 1987). However, application of social and behavioral data to biological studies of human aging, i.e., adoption of a biocultural approach, is recent. Within psychoneuroimmunology researchers have looked at cancer incidence and progression with age, and at loss and bereavement in the elderly. A recent conference on "neuroimmunomodulation" included reports which discussed these topics (Pierpaoli and Spector, 1988) and should be consulted for further references and details. A slightly older compendium offers a broader perspective on stress, immunity and aging (Cooper, 1984).

Endogenous opioids (endorphins) are released by the hypothalamic–pituitary axis in response to stress and directly affect the immune system by, among other things, increasing NK-cell activity, enhancing $\alpha$-interferon and IL-2 production, and influencing proliferation of mitogen-stimulated T-lymphocytes (Solomon *et al.*, 1988). An example of an aging-related change is the inhibition by $\alpha$-endorphin of T-cell proliferation in the mixed lymphocyte reaction (an *in vitro* analogue of graft rejection), which is present in younger healthy donors but is absent in older healthy donors (Barabino *et al.*, 1986).

Data on depression and bereavement support the idea that emotional state or major changes in one's life are associated with increased likelihood of morbidity and mortality (Bowling, 1987), and that mind and somatic health may be linked by neuroendocrine–immune interactions. For example, among recently widowed or divorced individuals: NK-cell activity is reduced, mitogenic stimulation of lymphocytes (both T and B) is reduced, there are fewer suppressor/cytotoxic T-cells (and an increase in the ratio of T-helper to T-suppressor/cytotoxic cells), and there are higher antibody titers to Epstein–Barr virus (Irwin *et al.*, 1987; Kiecolt-Glaser *et al.*, 1987; Baltrusch *et al.*, 1988). Specifically with regard to aging, one study found that otherwise healthy elderly subjects (aged > 65 years) who scored high on scales of psychological depression showed immune system impairments (e.g., decreased levels of IL-2, IL-4, NK-cell activity, mitogenic stimulation of lymphocytes) relative to non-depressed elderly (Guidi *et al.*, 1991). However, other reports are inconsistent (Monjan, 1984; Thomas *et al.*, 1985; Chandra, 1989) and more studies are needed.

The central role of "stress" in these examples highlights the significance of cultural systems in defining what is "stressful" and in helping to buffer against some of the dysphoric—and potentially physiologically dysfunctional—consequences of distressing states such as helplessness, anxiety, depression, and anomie. Medical anthropologists (and others) are actively investigating the role of social support systems in determining the course of individual aging. Early evidence from a study of 256 healthy, community living adults (aged 61–89 years) suggests that, in fact, stronger social support correlates with higher immune functioning (Thomas *et al.*, 1985). This example illustrates how biological and non-biological factors influence aging of the immune system.

## Nutrition and Immune System Aging

While nutrition and aging is detailed in Chapter 9, specific studies of the effects of nutrition on human immune system aging suggest how culturally influenced behavior (diet) can affect immunosenescence. (A recent review of this topic can be found in Chandra, 1985). In general, elderly are at risk for reduced consumption and absorption of micronutrients due to economic, psychosocial, sensory, dental, physiological, and pharmacological circumstances (Meydani, 1990). Studies of the relationship between nutritional status and aging immune function, many of which assay elderly subjects before and after nutritional supplementation, report the following results (references in Meydani, 1990). Vitamin C improves proliferative response of lympocytes to mitogens as well as delayed-type hypersensitivity skin response and levels of IgG, IgM, and complement C3 in healthy elderly; however, no difference in mitogenic response was reported between healthy elderly with unsupplemented high or low levels of vitamin C. Vitamin E improves proliferative response of lympocytes to mitogens as well as delayed-type hypersensitivity skin response and IL-2 production, and reduces prostaglandin production; moreover, higher (unsupplemented) levels of vitamin E correlate with stronger delayed-type hypersensitivity skin response and higher ratios of helper-inducer/cytotoxic-suppressor T-cells; however, vitamin E supplementation of chronic care patients did not improve antibody response to influenza vaccination. Vitamin $B_6$ improves mitogenic and antigenic responses of lymphocytes and their production of IL-2 as well as the percentage of helper-inducer (but not cytotoxic-suppressor) T-cells. Zinc improves delayed-type hypersensitivity skin reactions and increases anti-tetanus toxoid antibody formation and the percentage of circulating T-cells, but does not affect lymphocyte proliferation. Plasma levels of zinc are reduced in elderly humans, probably through a combination of reduced intake and reduced absorption (but not increased excretion) (Fabris *et al.*, 1990). Low levels of zinc may exacerbate independently arising effects of thymic involution inasmuch as thymulin, a thymic hormone, requires zinc to be activated.

The beneficial results on immune function of micronutrient supplementation in the elderly could be due to amelioration of malnutrition, non-specific immunostimulation, induction of non-immune systems (e.g., endocrine) or some combination of these. A partial answer to this question is provided by studies of older subjects in which correcting nutritional imbalance enhanced immune functioning (Chandra *et al.*, 1982; Chandra, 1989). These results support the idea that optimal nutritional status contributes to counteracting immunosenescence. However, the correlation is not perfect, indicating that other factors influence immunosenescence and that individuals differ in their response to nutrient supplementation. Moreover, two large recent studies of "healthy" elderly report no correlation between measures of nutritional status and immunological function (e.g., mitogenic stimulation, delayed-type hypersensitivity skin response, antibody and circulating immune complex levels; Chavance *et al.*, 1986; Goodwin and Garry, 1988).

## Ontogeny and Gerontology

The idea of a biological continuum between development and aging is well illustrated by the immune system, especially by the regular pattern of growth and involution of the thymus and its central role in T-lymphopoiesis. Disturbance of thymic physiology is thus likely to alter immune function significantly, whether it be through disruption during growth and development or as a consequence of post-maturational age-related changes. Examples of the former are considered in the section on early childhood malnutrition (p. 197) and can be contrasted with the beneficial interference of dietary restriction discussed in the section on dietary restriction and immune system aging (p. 198). As an example of the latter, recent studies demonstrate that thymic hormone supplementation in the elderly improves a range of immune responses (Jankovic et al., 1988; Ershler, 1990; Meroni et al., 1990).

Recent reinterpretation of a developmental shift in T-cell subsets suggests a cellular parallel with thymic growth and involution which may turn out to be causally related to it. Specifically the idea is that helper cells (CD4+) and suppressor cells (CD8+) represent different maturational stages of the same lineage (rather than members of separate lineages), with the former being so-called "memory" cells (CD29+), which have been previously activated, and the latter being "naive" (or "virgin") cells (CD45+), which have yet to be primed by antigen (Sanders et al., 1988). Evidence in support of the proposed developmental sequence is that less than 5% of T-cells from neonates are "memory" cells whereas adult T-cells comprise approximately 40% "memory" cells. [A similar developmental sequence has been observed in pigtailed macaques, although the actual cell surface markers and the magnitude of the shift in subset populations differ between the two species (Terao et al., 1988).] Beginning after birth, the accumulation of "memory" T-cells with age represents the cellular basis of protective immunity acquired via exposure to infectious agents. It is therefore of selective advantage to maintain a large diverse repertoire of these "memory" cells and that they be relatively long-lived (i.e., circulate for years rather than days or weeks). The relevance of this to aging was recently suggested by a model (Miller, 1991b) which hypothesizes, in part, that with age "memory" T-cells form an ever-increasing proportion of cells which are hyporesponsive and that therefore the proposed ontogenetic "conversion of virgin to memory T-cells" would be a primary element of immunosenescence. Partial support of the model derives from one cross-sectional human study which reported the predicted age-related decrease in CD45+ cells ("naive") but only a slight increase in CD29+ ("memory") cells (de Paoli et al., 1988).

### Growth Disruption and Adult Immune Dysfunction

*Vertebral Canal Size.* The hypothesis has been advanced that early poor growth may lead to reduced life span by perturbing neuroimmune function (Clark et al., 1986, 1989). The initial observation was a positive correlation between vertebral canal size and age at death in a skeletal collection of American Indian adults who lived 950–1300 A.D. Human vertebral canals reportedly cease growth by about age 4, when stable size and shape are attained; stunted vertebral canals may reflect malnutrition occurring either *in utero* or post-natally. Data collected from a living sample of English adults suggest that smaller canal size correlates with greater incidence of infection, whereas larger canal size correlates with greater incidence of autoimmune disease (Porter *et al.*, 1987). Data collected from 13 participants in the longitudinal Normative Aging Study (Boston) demonstrate moderate positive correlations between canal size and levels of thymosin-$\alpha_1$ (a thymic hormone), IL-2, mitogenic response of lymphocytes, NK-cell activity, and a significant negative correlation with thymosin-$B_4$ (another thymic hormone). However, multiple regression indicated that the best predictor of thymosin-$\alpha_1$ level was sitting height (not canal size), with which it was inversely correlated. A follow-up study 2.5 years later revealed the same pattern, with sitting height explaining 45% of the variation in thymosin-$\alpha_1$ level and vertebral canal size explaining an additional 12%. These results suggest that comparisons of thymosin-$\alpha_1$ between individuals should control for adult body size and that whatever aspect of neuroimmune development vertebral canal size measures, it is independent of body size. In sum, these preliminary results illustrate that early growth disturbance might predispose to later (adult) immune system dysfunction, possibly increasing morbidity and mortality. However, mechanism(s) linking neurological development and adult immune function, and the biological significance of vertebral canal size, remain unknown.

*Early Childhood Malnutrition.* The inter-relationships between nutritional status and immune function are complex and far from fully understood (recently reviewed in Chandra, 1988; Bendich, and Chandra, 1990), whether viewed alone or in the context of aging. Perhaps the best understood is zinc deficiency, the immunological consequences of which seem to share many similarities with protein-energy malnutrition and aging (Thompson *et al.*, 1984). Zinc deficiency in childhood can produce atrophy of lymphoid tissues including the thymus, resulting in a kind of accelerated or premature thymic involution. Later life consequences for immune function are unknown, although any adult sequelae of pre-adult zinc deficiency are likely to be related to the role of thymulin, a zinc-requiring thymic hormone, in regulating lymphocyte function. Zinc deficiency in the elderly has been correlated with immune incompetence, and its correction has yielded improved immune function (see section on nutrition and immune system aging, p. 195). But the time-scale involved is years, not decades, and thus far any long-term consequences of childhood zinc deficiency have not been reported. It is also unknown if zinc supplementation during growth and development can reverse thymic atrophy due to earlier zinc deficiency and thereby restore normal adult immune function.

Parallels between nutritional status and immunocompetence in infants and the elderly suggest commonalities of inadequacy shared by ontogeny and gerontology (Chandra, 1984). In addition to zinc deficiency just discussed, protein-energy malnutrition in the young, due to insufficient intake, premature birth, or both, results in thymic atrophy and cellular immune dysfunction.

These disruptions of normal growth and development seem to be quite similar to immunosenescence exacerbated by malnutrition (see section on nutrition and immune system aging, p. 195). Hence comparing the two extremes of the life span may be useful in that: (1) studies of the effects of nutritional supplementation on immune function (at any age) will yield insights about common underlying mechanisms; and (2) the application of dietary restriction techniques (see section on dietary restriction and immune system aging, p. 198) to human beings will benefit from understanding the effects of malnutrition on immune function.

## Dietary Restriction and Immune System Aging

Caloric restriction using a complete diet (e.g., feeding every other day) in rodents, usually initiated before sexual maturity, consistently extends mean and maximum life span by 25–40%. It is the only known intervention which reproducibly increases mammalian longevity. Among the effects assessed in rodents are the following immunological improvements: mitogenic response of lymphocytes, production of IL-2 and expression of IL-2 receptors, retarded thymic involution, increased numbers of helper T-cells, increased antibody production, increased T-cell cytolysis, increased induction of NK-cell activity, and, in stimulated lymphocytes, delayed age-related decreases in protein synthesis, in IL-2 activity and in mRNA level (Weindruch and Walford, 1988; Pahlavani et al., 1990). In contrast to these improvements, dietary restriction is also reported to: not affect serum thymic hormone levels; reduce numbers of lymphocytes and thymocytes; and decrease NK-cell cytolysis. On balance it appears that dietary restriction not only "retarded immune system maturation but also kept it younger longer" (Weindruch and Walford, 1988: 190). Age-associated pathology such as neoplasia and autoimmune disorders are also either delayed in appearance, decreased in incidence, or diminished in morbidity. (For recent review, see Weindruch and Walford, 1988.)

The relevance of these results for human and non-human primates has yet to be determined. In theory one can argue that "growth, development, and aging probably proceed by similar or identical mechanisms in most mammals, and nutritional modulation of these can be classified as a large-scale phenomenon. As such, one would expect the effects of dietary restriction to be translatable" from rodents to human beings (Weindruch and Walford, 1988: 301). In fact, empirical answers will be forthcoming as new studies in non-human primates report preliminary results (e.g., Weindruch et al., 1991). A cryptic note concerning clinical results in the former USSR refers to improved immunological parameters in rodents and states that "similar results were observed in obese patients administered a low-calorie diet" (Revskoy et al., 1985; citing an unreferenced study by Zalevskaya and Blagosklonnaya, 1981), but its significance cannot be judged.

## Evolutionary Models for Human Immunosenescence

Three major assumptions underlie any argument for evolution of a trait or complex of characteristics: (1) that the trait is genetically determined, at least in part; (2) that the trait ultimately (if indirectly) affects individual reproduction; and (3) that there is a biological mechanism which links genetic differences in the trait to individual reproductive success. While natural selection operates directly on variation in reproductive success, decreased morbidity or increased survival are clearly related to reproductive success and often substitute for it in evolutionary discussions. In the first two examples which follow, assumptions (2) and (3) translate into questions of diminished disease and mortality. Evidence which links aspects of immunosenescence to mortality comes from studies which demonstrate decreased survival over 1–3 years in elderly subjects with: milder delayed-type hypersensitivity skin reactions (Roberts–Thomson et al., 1974; Chandra, 1989), higher levels of autoantibodies (Mackay, 1972), lower levels of IgG (Buckley et al., 1974; cf. Lehtonen et al., 1990), fewer circulating lymphocytes (Chandra, 1989), or weaker response of lymphocytes to stimulation (Hallgren and Yunis, 1981; Murasko et al., 1988; cf. Lehtonen et al., 1990). In contrast to the limitations in the human data, all three assumptions are met by congenic mice (Lerner et al., 1988; Walford, 1990) in the third example below, MHC regulation of biological aging.

### Early Antigenic Exposure and Later Immune Response

Human beings (or any mammal) subject to immunosenescence and adapting to an environment relatively constant (predictable) in its distribution of pathogens would be at a selective advantage in mounting immune responses at younger rather than older ages. This holds because a more vigorous response (more rapid, of shorter duration), due to greater reserve capacity in youth, lessens the likelihood of morbidity or mortality (due to fewer complications) and increases chances of survival (due to quicker resumption of normal activity). Assuming that the immune system possesses some capacity for "memory" (e.g., see section on ontogeny and gerontology, p. 196), subsequent exposure to the same (or an antigenically similar) pathogen would elicit protective immunity. Hence, selection acting to decrease morbidity or mortality due to infectious disease at older ages would favor development of a long-term antigenic memory, especially in organisms with reduced immunocompetence due to senescence. Relaxing the assumption of relatively predictable pathogenic exposure during a person's lifetime—due, for example, to geographic mobility, exposure to inhabitants of other environments, changes in diet—would increase selective pressure against the specificity of an immune response in favor of a broadened repertoire. Long-term antigenic memory would continue to be advantageous.

This speculative scenario puts into an evolutionary context the recent suggestion as to why otherwise healthy elderly mount a decreased immune response to infection and yet avoid becoming ill. Namely, "because they have previously produced antibodies reactive with a sufficiently broad range of environmental pathogens to provide them with protection despite their reduced response to a new antigen" (Siskind, 1987: 238). In effect, pre-existing antibodies—and long-lived peripheral T-cells which "remember" previous antigenic exposures—effectively limit proliferation of the invading organism without inducing the immune response cascade elicited upon initial exposure (i.e. the "conventional" immune response). In short, "the distribution of idiotypes is established early in life," remains stable during an individual's lifetime, and may be "maintained by idiotype–anti-idiotype interactions with information stored in the population of long-lived peripheral T cells" (Siskind, 1987: 239–240). To test this hypothesis longitudinal data, perhaps from non-human primates, are required. [A prediction of this hypothesis, no change in antibody diversity after an (undefined) period of early exposure, contradicts a prediction of the "restricted idiotypic repertoire" model outlined above (see section on blood group antigens and a model of restricted idiotypic repertoire with aging, p. 191).]

### Immunosenescence as Protection Against Age-related Autoimmunity or Neoplasia

The recently raised "possibility that immune senescence might also convey benefits to the elderly organism" (Weksler et al., 1990: 402) presumes that selection acts to favor increased life span (or against increased morbidity and mortality) in older organisms by protecting against autoimmunity or neoplasia. On the assumption that an age-related increase in autoantibodies is inevitable, selection might favor the development of counteracting immunomodulatory processes which would act to limit immune response to autologous cells. Such downregulating mechanisms might include increases in suppressor T cell activity and in auto-antiidiotype antibody production (Weksler 1981). An unavoidable side effect of these processes of downregulation would be, specifically, decreased surveillance against foreign antigens and, in general, immunosenescence. In this scenario the genesis of autoantibodies is ultimately linked to thymic involution, or, possibly, to "prolonged exposure to autologous antigens" (Weksler, 1981). However, it is unclear how high levels of autoantibodies would exert a sufficiently strong selective pressure inasmuch as they are present in apparently otherwise healthy adults, and autoimmune disease is generally not fatal and occurs at relatively low prevalence (in recent times, anyway). Nevertheless the trade-off between relaxed tolerance of anti-self antibodies (i.e., increase autoimmunity) and heightened non-self tolerance (e.g., decreased infections) may reflect a balancing of selective pressures which influenced evolution of the immune system.

But what might cause age-related increased autoantibodies? Since normal pregnancy induces transient maternal immunodepression (presumably to minimize maternal–fetal incompatibility), it can be argued that higher levels of autoantibodies is the "cost" to females of child-bearing (Purtilo and Sullivan, 1979). Greater tolerance of "foreign" tissue (i.e., gestating offspring), perhaps by intermittent downregulation of normal non-self recognition/elimination processes [as hypothesized, for example, by the "alloantigenic challenge model of pregnancy" (Hoff et al., 1989: 75–77)], may result in greater autoantibody accumulation with age. This idea is testable since, if valid, one would expect a positive correlation between parity and levels of autoantibodies in otherwise similar women of the same age; conversely, comparing autoantibody levels among nulliparous women of different ages would reveal the extent to which autoantibody accumulation is independent of pregnancy and gestation.

While pregnancy results in significant depression of cellular but not humoral immune responses (Grossman, 1990), there may nevertheless be indirect long-term effects via, e.g., helper/inducer T-cells. Such a mechanism could be a pleiotropic byproduct of selection (Williams, 1957) for increased gestational time. (For a fuller discussion of pleiotropy see Wood *et al.*, this volume.) The apparent paradox that females have higher resistance to infection than males but also higher levels of circulating autoantibodies may reflect an evolutionarily selected compensatory mechanism (Grossman, 1990) in a system (female) subject to greater antigenic (self plus non-self) challenge.

With respect to age-related neoplasia, age-specific incidence of all cancers in the USA increases slowly from *ca.* age 20–40 years, rises more steeply until age 80, and then drops for survivors beyond age 80 years (Piantanelli, 1988). In apparent paradox, comparable tumors grow more slowly in elderly patients and metastasize less frequently than in younger patients (Ershler, 1986, 1987). Ignoring for the moment the apparent drop in cancer incidence beyond age 80, one might try to explain the paradox by postulating an age-related shift in the balance between "tumor-boosting" and "tumor-busting" capacities. Since most human tumors are only weakly antigenic (Ershler, 1986), direct anti-tumor immune system attack will not be effective and therefore immunosenescent weakening of tumor suppression can not explain the age-related cancer increase. Instead, as outlined by the immunofacilitation hypothesis (Kaesberg and Ershler, 1989), there may exist immune mechanisms which enhance tumor growth (e.g., a lymphokine with angiogenic properties) and which, during aging, senesce in the manner of other (documented) T-cell capacities. This hypothesis is being tested in a mouse model system (Weksler *et al.*, 1990).

The immunofacilitation hypothesis can not explain the decrease in age-related cancer incidence observed in people older than 80 years. However, this is not a major criticism since this segment of the population obviously includes an elite group of survivors who, by their very longevity and lack of morbidity, represent exceptional phenotypes [e.g., are less immune deficient than "younger elderly" (Murasko *et al.*, 1986)]. A greater difficulty arises from the recent suggestion that by decreasing tumor growth immunosenescence might benefit the host organism (Weksler *et al.*, 1990). According to evolutionary theory, selection is stronger at younger ages (where reproductive value is higher) and weaker at older ages. Hence, if neoplasia represented a potent source of morbidity or mortality, and if organisms were capable of counteracting such neoplastic growth, these counteractive measures would be under strong selective pressure to act at earlier ages. It may be, of course, that cancer-caused morbidity and mortality are only of recent historical significance for human beings, and thus there has not been sufficient evolutionary time to generate selective pressure.

### MHC Regulation of Biological Aging

The possible relationship between MHC gene products, the HLA system, and disease susceptibility was outlined above, as was evidence that HLA haplotypes are non-randomly represented among elderly "survivors." Walford (1987) has enlarged upon the suggestion that MHC modifies immunosenescence to propose that it regulates much of biological aging by influencing DNA repair, free-radical scavengers, mixed-function oxidases, neuroendocrine regulation, and certain developmental processes. He cites similarities among rodent, non-human primate, and human genomes to support the idea that the "entire MHC chromosomal region can be regarded as an interactive antibiosenescent system of ancient lineage" (Walford, 1987: 251). The obvious direct testable prediction of this hypothesis is a positive correlation between variability at the MHC locus (or HLA haplotypes) and variability in longevity. However, the difficulty of distinguishing aging from cohort and period effects without longitudinal data, plus the inherent "noise" in highly polymorphic outbred industrialized populations (Walford, 1987) make such a test potentially unrewarding. [Investigation of anthropological populations (Weiss, 1973) would reduce the noise attributable to an exceedingly heterogeneous gene pool.] Nevertheless, indirect predictions may be worth assessing, such as testing associations between MHC allelic variation or HLA haplotype variation and age-related rates of change in: efficacy of DNA repair, free radical scavenging, or mixed-function oxidase detoxification; immune responses, especially T-cell-dependent functions; and neuroendocrine–immune system interactions (see section on psychoneuroendocrinology and immune system aging, p. 193). A recent brief report of variation within promotor regions of the HLA system (Nepom et al., 1990), suggesting that such polymorphism may contribute to alterations in gene expression and regulation, is consistent with Walford's idea of a regulatory "supergene complex."

## CONCLUDING REMARKS AND PROSPECTS

In his presentation of the "extended" immunologic theory of aging, Walford (1987) makes the important point that in gerontological research discovering what *does not change with age* is perhaps equally important as investigating what does. This perspective promotes the establishment of age- and population-appropriate norms (variance as well as means) of immune function following thymic involution in "healthy" individuals. [Defining the latter is difficult, but rigorous attempts are being made, e.g., in Europe (Traill et al., 1985).] Aside from the clinical utility of age-appropriate and population-specific baselines, understanding fundamental aging processes requires that models of "successful" aging (Rowe and Kahn, 1987) be developed and tested. Comparisons across populations and environments may be especially valuable in this regard, as a means of testing hypotheses of immune function change or stasis among elderly "survivors" who a priori represent groups genetically and ontogenetically different from non-survivors. Immune system (and other) components that do not change with age among such individuals might be considered "biomarkers of surviving" in contrast to biomarkers of aging which are chosen precisely because they *do* change with age (see, e.g., Reff and Schneider, 1982; Mooradian, 1990). Both measures must be used to evaluate interventions designed to retard rates of aging: treatments which alter in a detrimental way processes observed to be unchanged in healthy elderly survivors are surely to be as avoided as treatments which accelerate other processes observed normally to decline with age.

Since aging is a phenomenon of individual organisms, it is important to at least be aware of, if not actively to investigate, genetic, ontogenetic, psychological, cultural, and ecological influences on human biological aging. The human immune system is an integrated part of a complex homeostatic hierarchy of systems which has been selected by the processes of evolution to function for more than 100 years. And while evolutionary change occurs at the level of the gene, natural selection acts at the level of the individual, operating on differential survival and reproduction of whole individuals, not separate parts. Moreover, since the immune system continually contacts most, if not all, cells, tissues, and organs, it can be expected to influence all other organismal systems (Cinader and Kay, 1986) and thus be more directly "exposed" to effects of natural selection. Adoption of this holistic perspective not only reminds us that neural, endocrine, and immune systems have co-evolved to interact reciprocally, but also warns us that elegant *in vitro* analyses may not translate into valid *in vivo* effects.

An evolutionary perspective cautions us against facile extrapolation across species, especially leaping from rodent to human without assessing mechanisms or processes in phylogenetically intermediate non-human primates. Ecologically, as well as biologically, our ancestral immunological stimuli and responses are shared with Old World monkeys and apes who live in social groups, enjoy omnivorous diets, and inhabit large and varied habitats. Hence, any human divergence from rodent models of the immune system is highly likely to be detected by cercopithecoid or hominoid animal models. Recently initiated investigation of the phenomenon of dietary restriction in non-human primates (e.g., Weindruch *et al.*, 1991) presents a prime example of the potential value of these animal models. (See also DeRousseau, this volume.)

Explanatory models of human immunosenescence can be divided into three types: active suppression, immunodeficiency, and dysregulation. Active suppression refers not only to the inhibitory effects of suppressor T-cells and antiidiotypic antibodies but also to downregulation of any immune function (e.g., IL-2 receptor expression), processes which may prove to involve fundamental epigenetic changes. Immunodeficiency pertains to loss of cellular function which may be due to decreased cell number, decreased metabolic activity (e.g., antibody production), structural change (e.g., increased membrane rigidity), or decreased biochemical activity (e.g., thymic hormones). Dysregulation concerns imbalance in finely orchestrated immune responses such that homeostatic norms are not maintained (e.g., increased benign monoclonal gammopathies, altered ratios of suppressor/inducer T-cells). Since examples of all three types of explanations can be found (see Table 7-1), no one model has come to predominate. Moreover, some observations invoke more than one model, e.g., increased prostaglandin production combined with increased sensitivity to prostaglandin inhibition of lymphocyte stimulation. In short, diverse decreases in immune system function with increasing age do not appear to be readily explained by a common mechanism. In addition there are equally diverse phenomena which increase with age or which do not change and therefore do not contribute to immunosenescence. Taking this broad view of human immune system aging illuminates how a wide variety of approaches, examples, and ideas proffered by biological anthropology can benefit immunogerontology.

## ACKNOWLEDGMENTS

I appreciate the helpful comments of Roy Walford and Rita Effros. Part of this work was supported by Biomedical Research Support Grant #2S07RR0540128.

## REFERENCES

References not cited refer to entries in Table 7-1.

Arlett, C. F. (1986) Human DNA repair defects. *Journal of Inherited Metabolic Disease* **1**(Suppl.), 69–84.
Baltrusch, H.-J. F., Seidel, J., Stangel, W. and Waltz, M. E. (1988) Psychosocial stress, aging and cancer. *Annals of the New York Academy of Sciences* **521**, 1–15.
Barabino, A., Morgano, A., Pierri, I., Rogna, S., Lotti, G. and Francesco, I. (1986) Effect of alpha-endorphin on mixed lympocyte reaction in young and aged healthy donors. In: *Immunoregulation in Aging* (eds Facchini, A., Haaijman, J. J. and Labo, G.). Rijswijk: EURAGE, pp. 143–149.
Batory, G., Onody, C., Gyodi, E., Nemeskeri, J. and Petrany, G. G. (1983) HLA and T-lymphocyte function in old age. *Human Immunology* **7**, 187–203.
Bender, K., Ruter, G., Mayerova, A. and Hiller, Ch. (1973) Studies on the heterozygosity at the Hl-A gene loci in children and old people. *Symposia Series in Immunobiological Standardization* **18**, 287–290.
Bender, K., Mayerova, A., Klotzbucher, B., Burckhardt, K. and Hiller, Ch. (1976) No indication of postnatal selection at the Hl-A loci. *Tissue Antigens* **7**, 118–121.
Bendich, A. and Chandra, R. K. (eds) (1990) *Micronutrients and Immune Functions.* New York: New York Academy of Sciences.
Blackwelder, W. C., Mittal, K. K., McNamara, P. M. and Payne, F. J. (1982) Lack of association between HLA and age in an aging population. *Tissue Antigens* **20**, 188–192.
Bodmer, W. F. (1972) Evolutionary significance of the HL-A system. *Nature* **237**, 139–145.
Borkan, G. A. (1983) Factors in clinical aging: variation in rates of aging. In: *Intervention in the Aging Process, Part A: Quantitation, Epidemiology, and Clinical Research* (eds Regelson, W. and Sinex, F. M.). New York: Alan R. Liss, pp. 99–111.
Bornstein, R. and Smircina, M. T. (1982) The status of the empirical support for the hypothesis of increased variablity in aging populations. *The Gerontologist* **22**, 258–260.
Bowling, A. (1987) Mortality and bereavement: a review of the literature on survival periods and factors affecting survival. *Social Science and Medicine* **24**, 117–124.
Brody, J. A. (1990) Chronic diseases and disorders: a hypothesis suggesting an

age-dependent versus an age-related class. In: *Biomedical Advances in Aging* (ed. Goldstein, A. L.). New York: Plenum, pp. 137–142.

Buckley, C. E., III, Buckley, E. G. and Dorsey, F. C. (1974) Longitudinal changes in serum immunoglobin levels in older humans. *Federation Proceedings* **33**, 2036–2039.

Bush, L. M. and Kaye, D. (1990) Epidemiology and pathogenesis of infectious diseases. *The Merck Manual of Geriatrics*. West Point, PA: Merck, Sharp & Dohme Research Laboratories.

Butenko, G. M. (1983) Ageing of the immune system and diseases. In: *Age-Related Factors in Carcinogenesis* (eds Likhachev, A., Anisimov, V. and Montesano, R.). Lyon: International Agency for Research on Cancer Publication no. 58, pp. 71–83.

Cammarata, R. J., Rodnan, G. P. and Fennell, R. H. (1967) Serum anti-gamma globulin and antinuclear factors in the aged. *Journal of the American Medical Association* **199**, 455–458.

Chandra, R. K. (1984) Nutritional regulation of immune function at the extremes of life: in infants and in the elderly. In: *Malnutrition: Determinants and Consequences* (eds White, P. L. and Selvey, N.). New York: Alan R. Liss, pp. 245–251.

Chandra, R. K. (1985) (ed.) *Nutrition, Immunity and Illness in The Elderly*. New York: Pergamon.

Chandra, R. K. (1988) (ed.) *Nutrition and Immunology*. New York: Alan R. Liss.

Chandra, R. K. (1989) Nutritional regulation of immunity and risk of infection in old age. *Immunology* **67**, 141–147.

Chandra, R. K., Joshi, P., Au, B., Woodford, G. and Chandra, S. (1982) Nutrition and immunocompetence of the elderly: effect of short-term nutritional supplementation on cell-mediated immunity and lymphocyte subsets. *Nutrition Research* **2**, 223–232.

Chavance, M., Herbeth, B., Janot, C., Vernhes, G. and Genetet, N. (1986) Effect of age and vitamin status on the mitogenic responses to PHA and anti-CD3 monoclonal antibody. In: *Immunoregulation in Aging* (eds Facchini, A., Haaijman, J. J. and Labo, G.). Rijswijk: EURAGE, pp. 177–183.

Cinader, B. and Kay, M. M. (1986) Differentiation of regulatory cell interactions in aging. *Gerontology* **32**, 340–348.

Clark, G. A., Hall, N. R., Aldwin, C. M., Armelagos, G. J., Borkan, G. A., Panjabi, M. M. and Wetzel, R. T. (1986) Poor growth prior to early childhood: Decreased health and life-span in the adult. *American Journal of Physical Anthropology* **70**, 145–160.

Clark, G. A., Aldwin, C. M., Hall, N. R., Spiro, A. and Goldstein, A. (1989) Is poor early growth related to adult immune aging? A follow-up study. *American Journal of Human Biology* **1**, 331–337.

Clark, G. A., Hall, N. R., Aldwin, C. M., Goldstein, A. L. and Steiner, R. C. (1990) Poor early growth and adult mental and somatic health. In: *Biomedical Advances in Aging* (ed. Goldstein, A. L.). New York: Plenum, pp. 331–346.

Converse, P. J. and Williams, D. R. R. (1978) Increased HLA-B heterozygosity with age. *Tissue Antigens* **12**, 275–278.

Cooper, E. L. (ed.) (1984) *Stress, Immunity, and Aging*. New York: Marcel Dekker.

Crespi, C., Zauli, D., Cometti, G., Bonavita, E., Bianchi, F. B. and Pisi, E. (1986) Spectrum of autoimmunity in aged individuals. In: *Immunoregulation in Aging* (eds Facchini, A., Haaijman, J. J. and Labo, G.). Rijswijk: EURAGE, pp. 331–336.

Degos, L., Colombani, J., Chaventre, A., Bengtson, B. and Jacquard, A. (1974) Selective pressure on HL-A polymorphism. *Nature* **249**, 62–63.

Delespesse, G., Duchateau, J., Bastenie, P. A., Lauvaux, J. P., Collet, H. and Govaerts, A. (1974) Cell-mediated immunity in diabetes mellitus. *Clinical and Experimental Immunology* **18**, 461–467.

Delespesse, G., De Maubeuge, J., Kennes, B., Nicaise, R. and Govaerts, A. (1977) IgE-mediated hypersensitivity in aging. *Clinics in Allergy* **7**, 155–160.

De Paoli, P., Battistin, S. and Santini, G. F. (1988) Age-related changes in human lymphocyte subsets: progressive reduction in the CD4 CD45R (suppressor inducer) population. *Clinical Immunology and Immunopathology* **48**, 290–296.

Deviere, J., Kennes, B., Closset, J., De Martelaer, V. and Neve, P. (1986) Effect of age, sex and health state on lymphocyte function. In: *Immunoregulation in Aging* (eds Facchini, A., Haaijman, J. J. and Labo, G.). Rijswijk: EURAGE, pp. 165–172.

Dworsky, R., Paganini-Hill, A., Ducey, B., Hechinger, M. and Parker, J. W. (1989) Lymphocyte immunophenotyping in an elderly population: age, sex and medication effects—a flow cytometry study. *Mechanisms of Ageing and Development* **48**, 255–266.

Eichberg, J. W., Heberling, R. L., Kalter, S. S., Morrison, J. D. and Lawlor, D. A., (1981) The influence of age and pregnancy on immune responses of baboons to mitogens and the baboon endogenous virus. *Developmental and Comparative Immunology* **4**, 135–144.

Ershler, W. B. (1986) Why tumors grow more slowly in old people. *Journal of the National Cancer Institute* **77**, 837–839.

Ershler, W. B. (1987) The change in aggressiveness of neoplasms with age. *Geriatrics* **42**, 99–104.

Ershler, W. B. (1990) Influenza and aging: immunological methods of enhancing influenza vaccine response in elderly people. In: *Biomedical Advances in Aging* (ed. Goldstein, A. L.). New York: Plenum, pp. 513–521.

Ershler, W. B., Coe, C. L., Gravenstein, S., Schultz, K. T., Klopp, R. G., Meyer, M. and Houser, W. D. (1988a) Aging and immunity in nonhuman primates: 1. Effects of age and gender on cellular immune function in rhesus monkeys (*Macaca mulatta*). *American Journal of Primatology* **15**, 181–188.

Ershler, W. B., Coe, C. L., Laughlin, N., Klopp, R. G., Gravenstein, S., Roecker, E. B. and Schultz, K. T. (1988b). Aging and immunity in non-human primates II. Lymphocyte response in thymosin-treated middle-aged monkeys. *Journal of Gerontology* **43**, B142–146.

Fabris, N., Mocchegiani, E., Muzzioli, M. and Provinciali, M. (1988) Neuroendocrine–thymus interactions: perspectives for intervention in aging. In: *Neuroimmunomodulation: Interventions in Aging and Cancer* (eds Pierpaoli, W. and Spector, N. H.). Annals of The New York Academy of Sciences, Vol. 521, pp. 72–87.

Fabris, N., Mocchegiani, E., Muzzioli, M. and Provinciali, M. (1990) Zinc, immunity, and aging. In: *Biomedical Advances in Aging* (ed. Goldstein, A. L.). New York: Plenum, pp. 271–282.

Freier, S. (1990) (ed.) *The Neuroendocrine–Immune Network*. Boca Raton, FL: CRC Press.

Friedlaender, J. S. and Page, L. B. (1989) Population biology and aging: the example of blood pressure. *American Journal of Human Biology* **1**, 355–366.

Fulop, T., Foris, G., Worum, I. and Leovey, A. (1984) Age-dependent changes of the Fc[gamma]-receptor-mediated functions of human monocytes. *International Archives of Allergy and Applied Immunology* **74**, 76–79.

Gardner, I. D. (1980) Aging and susceptibility to infections. *Reviews of Infectious Diseases* **2**, 801–810.

Garruto, R. M. and Gajdusek, D. C. (1975) Unusual progression and shifting clinical severity, morbidity and mortality in the 1969 Hong Kong (A/New Guinea/1/69 $H_3N_2$) influenza epidemic in New Guinea. *American Journal of Physical Anthropology* **42**, 302–303.

Gerkins, V. R., Ting, A., Menck, H. T., Casagrande, J. T., Terasaki, P. I., Pike, M. C. and Henderson, B. E. (1974) HL-A heterozygosity as a genetic marker of long-term survival. *Journal of the National Cancer Institute* **52**, 1909–1911.

Goidl, E. A. (ed.) (1987) *Aging and the Immune Response. Cellular and Humoral Aspects* New York: Marcel Dekker.

Goidl, E. A., Martin McEvoy, S. J., Bonilla, F. A., Kaushik, A. and Bona, C. A. (1990) Regulation of the expressed idiotypic repertoire in the normal immune response of the aged. In: *Biomedical Advances in Aging* (ed. Goldstein, A. L.). New York: Plenum, pp. 413–424.

Goodwin, J. S. and Garry, P. J. (1983) Relationship between megadose vitamin supplementation and immunological function in a healthy elderly population. *Clinical and Experimental Immunology* **51**, 647–653.

Goodwin, J. S. and Garry, P. J. (1988) Lack of correlation between indices of nutritional status and immunological function in elderly humans. *Journal of Gerontology* **43**, M46–49.

Goto, M. and Nishioka, K. (1989) Age- and sex-related changes of the lymphocyte subsets in healthy individuals: an analysis by two-dimensional flow cytometry. *Journal of Gerontology* **44**, M51–56.

Greenberg, L. J. and Yunis, E. J. (1978) Genetic control of autoimmune disease and immune responsiveness and the relationship to aging. *Birth Defects: Original Article Series* **XIV**, 249–260.

Grossman, C. J. (1990) Immunoendocrinology. In: *Basic and Clinical Endocrinology* (ed. Greenspan, F. S.). San Mateo, CA, Appleton and Lange, pp. 40–52.

Guidi, L., Bartoloni, C., Frasca, D., Antico, L., Pili, R., Cursi, F., Tempesta, E., Rumi, C., Menini, E., Carbonin, P., Doria, G. and Cambassi, G. (1991) Impairment of lymphocyte activities in depressed aged subjects. *Mechanisms of Ageing and Development* **60**, 13–24.

Gutowski, J. K., Innes, J. B., Weksler, M. E. and Cohen, S. (1986) Impaired nuclear responsiveness to cytoplasmic signals in lymphocytes from elderly humans with depressed proliferative responses. *Journal of Clinical Investigation* **78**, 40–43.

Haaijman, J. J. (1986) Perspectives in immunogerontology. In: *Immunoregulation in Aging* (eds Facchini, A., Haaijman, J. J. and Labo, G.). Rijswijk: EURAGE, pp. xi–xxix.

Hallgren, H. M. and Yunis, E. J. (1981) Immune function, immune regulation, and survival in an aging human population. In: *Immunological Aspects of Aging* (eds Segre, D. and Smith, L.). New York: Marcel Dekker, pp. 281–293.

Hallgren, H. M., Jackola, D. R. and O'Leary, J. J. (1983) Unusual pattern of surface marker expression on peripheral lymphocytes from aged humans suggestive of a population of less differentiated cells. *Journal of Immunology* **131**, 191–194.

Hanneuse, Y. and Delespesse, G. (1978) Influence of aging on IgE-reactions in allergic patients. *Clinics in Allergy* **8**, 165–174.

Hansen, H. E., Sparck, J. V. and Larsen, S. O. (1977) An examination of HLA frequencies in three age groups. *Tissue Antigens* **10**, 49–55.

Harris, G., Cramp, W. A., Edwards, J. C., George, A. M., Sabovljev, S. A., Hart, L., Hughes, G. R. V., Denman, A. M. and Yatvin, M. B. (1985) Radiosensitivity of peripheral blood lymphocytes in autoimmune disease. *International Journal of Radiation Biology* **47**, 689–699.

Hazzard, W. R. (1989) Why do women live longer than men? *Postgraduate Medicine* **85**, 271–284.

Hazzard, W. R. (1990) The sex differential in longevity. *Principles of Geriatric Medicine and Gerontology* (eds Hazzard, W. R., Andres, R., Bierman, E. L. and Blass, J. P.). New York: McGraw-Hill, pp. 37–47.

Hodge, S. E. and Walford, R. L. (1980) HLA distribution in aged normals. In: *Histocompatibility Testing 1980* (ed. Terasaki, P. I.). Los Angeles: UCLA Tissue Typing Laboratory, pp. 722–726.

Hoff, C., Garruto, R. M. and Durham, N. M. (1989) Human adaptability and medical genetics. In: *Human Population Biology. A Transdisciplinary Science* (eds Little, M. A. and Haas, J. D.). New York: Oxford University Press, pp. 69–81.

Holdstock, G., Chastenay, B. F. and Krawitt, E. L. (1982) Effects of testosterone, oestradiol and progesterone on immune regulation. *Clinical and Experimental Immunology* **47**, 449–456.

Hoover, M. L. and Capra, J. D. (1987) The T cells receptor and autoimmune disease. *Molecular Biology in Medicine* **4**, 123–132.

Horowitz, S. D. and Hong, R. (1977) The pathogenesis and treatment of immunodeficiency. *Monographs in Allergy* **10**, 1–198.

Irwin, M., Daniels, M., Bloom, E. T., Smith, T. L. and Weiner, H. (1987) Life events, depressive symptoms, and immune function. *American Journal of Psychiatry* **144**, 437–441.

Jankovic, B. D., Korolija, P., Isakovic, K., Popeskovic, L. J., Pesic, M. C., Horvat, J., Jeremic, D. and Vajs, V. (1988) Immunorestorative effects in elderly humans of lipid and protein fractions from the calf thymus: a double-blind study. In: *Neuroimmunomodulation: Interventions in Aging and Cancer* (eds Pierpaoli, W. and Spector, N. H.). Annals of The New York Academy of Sciences, Vol. 521, pp. 247–259.

Jemmott, J. B., III and Locke, S. E. (1984) Psychosocial factors, immunologic mediation, and human susceptibility to infectious diseases: how much do we know? *Psychological Bulletin* **95**, 78–108.

Kaesberg, P. R. and Ershler, W. B. (1989) The importance of immunosenescence in the incidence and malignant properties of cancer in hosts of advanced age. *Journal of Gerontology* **44**, 63–66.

Kelley, K. W., Davila, D. R., Brief, S., Simon, J. and Arkins, S. (1988) A pituitary-thymus connection during aging. In: *Neuroimmunomodulation: Interventions in Aging and Cancer* (eds, Pierpaoli, W. and Spector, N. H.). Annals of the New York Academy of Sciences, Vol. 521, pp. 88–98.

Kendall, M. D. (1981). Introduction. In: *The Thymus Gland* (ed. Kendall, M. D.). London: Academic Press, pp. 1–6.

Kiecolt-Glaser, J. K., Stephens, R. E., Lipetz, P. D., Speicher, C. E. and Glaser, R. (1985) Distress and DNA repair in human lymphocytes. *Journal of Behavioral Medicine* **8**, 311–320.

Kiecolt-Glaser, J. K., Fisher, L. D., Ogrocki, P., Stout, J. C., Speicher, C. E. and Glaser, R. (1987) Marital quality, marital disruption, and immune function. *Psychosomatic Medicine* **49**, 13–32.

Kraft, R., Fankhauser, G., Gerber, H., Hess, M. W. and Cottier, H. (1988) Age-related involution and terminal disorganization of the human thymus. *International Journal of Radiation Biology* **53**, 169–176.

Lehtonen, L., Eskola, J., Vainio, O. and Lehtonen, A (1990) Changes in lymphocyte subsets and immune competence in very advanced age. *Journal of Gerontology* **45**, M108–112.

Lerner, S. P., Anderson, C. P., Walford, R. L. and Finch, C. E. (1988) Genotype and reproductive aging of inbred female mice: effect of H-2 alleles. *Biology of Reproduction* **38**, 1035–1043.

Lewis, V. M., Twomey, J. J., Bealmear, P., Goldstein, G. and Good, R. A. (1978) Age, thymic involution, and circulating thymic hormone activity. *Journal of Clinical Endocrinology and Metabolism* **47**, 145–149.

Ligthart, G. J. and Hijmans, W. (1986) Ageing and the immune system in humans. In: *Immunoregulation in Aging* (eds Facchini, A., Haaijman, J. J. and Labo, G.). Rijswijk: EURAGE, pp. 157–164.

Livingston, F. B. (1958) Anthropological implications of sickle cell gene distribution in West Africa. *American Anthropologist* **60**, 533–562.

Lloyd, R. (1984) Possible mechanisms of psychoneuroimmunological interaction. *Advances* **1**, 42–51.

Mackay, I. R. (1972) Ageing and immunological function in man. *Gerontologia* **18**, 285–304.

Macurova, H., Ivanyi, P., Sajdlova, H. and Trojan, J. (1975) HL-A antigens in aged persons. *Tissue Antigens* **6**, 269–271.

Mascart-Lemone, F., Delespesse, G., Servais, G. and Kuntsler, M. (1982) Characterization of immunoregulatory T lymphocytes during ageing by monoclonal antibodies. *Clinical and Experimental Immunology* **48**, 148–154.

Mayer, P. J., Lange, C. S., Bradley, M. O. and Nichols, W. W. (1991) Gender differences in age-related decline in DNA double-strand break damage and repair in lymphocytes. *Annals of Human Biology* **18**, 405–415.

Meites, J., Goya, R. and Takahashi, S. (1987) Why the neuroendocrine system is important in aging processes. *Experimental Gerontology* **22**, 1–15.

Meroni, P. L., Barcellini, W., Borghi, M. O., Frasca, D., Vismara, A., Bamberga, P., Ferraro, G., Doria, G. and Zanussi, C. (1990) Immunopotentiating activity of thymopentin treatment in elderly subjects. In: *Biomedical Advances in Aging* (ed. Goldstein, A. L.). New York: Plenum, pp. 537–550.

Meydani, S. N. (1990) Micronutrients and immune function in the elderly. *Annals of The New York Academy of Sciences* **587**, 196–207.

Michael, S. D. and Chapman, J. C. (1990) The influence of the endocrine system on the immune system. *Immunology and Allergy Clinics of North America* **10**, 215–233.

Miller, R. A. (1989) The cell biology of aging: immunological models. *Journal of Gerontology* **44**, B4–8.

Miller, R. A. (1991a) Aging and immune function. *International Review of Cytology* **124**, 187–215.

Miller, R. A. (1991b) Accumulation of hyporesponsive, calcium extruding memory T cells as a key feature of age-dependent immune dysfunction. *Clinical Immunology and Immunopathology* **58**, 305–317.

Monjan, A. A. (1984) Effects of acute and chronic stress upon lymphocyte blastogenesis in mice and humans. In: *Stress, Immunity, and Aging* (ed. Cooper, E. L.). New York: Marcel Dekker, pp. 81–108.

Mooradian, A. D. (1990) Biomarkers of aging: do we know what to look for? *Journal of Gerontology* **45**, B183–186.

Morgan, K. (1983) Mortality changes in the Hutterite Brethren of Alberta and Saskatchewan, Canada. *Human Biology* **55**, 89–99.

Murasko, D. M., Nelson, B. J., Silver, R., Matour, D. and Kaye, D. (1986) Immunologic response in an elderly population with a mean age of 85. *American Journal of Medicine* **81**, 612–618.

Murasko, D. M., Weiner, P. and Kaye, D. (1988) Association of lack of mitogen-induced lymphocyte proliferation with increased mortality in the elderly. *Aging: Immunology and Infectious Disease* **1**, 1–6.

Murasko, D. M., Nelson, B. J., Matour, D., Goonewardene, I. M. and Kaye, D. (1991) Heterogeneity of changes in lymphoproliferative ability with increasing age. *Experimental Gerontology* **26**, 269–279.

Nagel, J. E., Chrest, F. J., Pyle, R. S. and Adler, W. H. (1983) Monoclonal antibody analysis of T-lymphocyte subsets in young and aged adults. *Immunological Communications* **12**, 223–237.

Nelson, E. A. and Dannefer, D. (1992) Aged heterogeneity: fact or fiction? The fate of diversity in gerontological research. *The Gerontologist* **32**, 17–23.

Nepom, B. S., Beatty, J., Nettles, J. and Nepom, G. T. (1990) Allelic polymorphisms among the regulatory regions of HLA class II genes. *Arthritis and Rheumatism* **33**, S31 (abstract #131).

Norris, A. H. and Shock, N. W. (1966) Aging and variability. *Annals of the New York Academy of Sciences* **134**, 591–601.

Ockhuizen, Th., Pandey, J. P., Galbraith, G. M. P., Fudenberg, H. H. and Hames, C. G. (1982) Autoantibodies and immunoglobin allotypes in healthy North American blacks of different age groups. *Mechanism of Ageing and Development* **19**, 103–111.

Ory, M. G. and Warner, H. R. (eds) (1990) *Gender, Health, and Longevity*. New York: Springer.

Pahlavani, M. A., Cheung, H. T., Cai, N.-S. and Richardson, A. (1990) Influence of dietary restriction and aging on gene expression in the immune system of rats. In: *Biomedical Advances in Aging* (ed. Goldstein, A. L.). New York: Plenum, pp. 259–270.

Phair, J. P., Hsu, C. S. and Hsu, Y. L. (1988) Ageing and infection. In: *Research and the Ageing Population* (eds Evered, D. and Whelan, J.). Chichester: Wiley, pp. 143–154.

Piantanelli, L. (1988) Cancer and aging: from the kinetics of biological parameters to the kinetics of cancer incidence and mortality. *Annals of the New York Academy of Sciences* **521**, 99–109.

Pierpaoli, W. and Spectro, N. H. (eds) (1988) *Neuroimmunomodulation: Interventions in Aging and Cancer*. Annals of the New York Academy of Sciences, **521**.

Porter, R. W., Drinkall, J. N., Porter, D. E. and Thorp, L. (1987) The vertebral canal. II. Health and academic status. A clinical study. *Spine* **12**, 907–911.

Proust, J., Moulias, R., Fumeron, F., Bekhoucha, F., Busson, M., Schmid, M. and Hors, J. (1982) HLA and longevity. *Tissue Antigens* **19**, 168–173.

Purtilo, D. T. and Sullivan, J. L. (1979) Immunological bases for superior survival of females. *American Journal of Diseases of Childhood* **133**, 1251–1253.

Rebar, R. W. (1984) Interaction between thymic hormones and other endocrine products. In: *Stress, Immunity, and Aging* (ed. Cooper, E. L.). New York: Marcel Dekker, pp. 173–186.

Reff, M. E. and Schneider, E. L. (eds) (1982) *Biological Markers of Aging*. United States Department of Health and Human Services, NIH Publication #82-2221, Bethesda, MD.

Revskoy, S. Yu, Poroshina, T. E., Kovaleva, I. G., Berstein, L. M., Ostroumova, M. N. and Dilman, V. M. (1985) Age-dependent metabolic immunodepression and cancer. In: *Age-Related Factors in Carcinogenesis* (eds. Likhachev, A., Anisimov, V. and Montesano, R.). Lyon: International Agency for Research of Cancer publication no. 58, pp. 253–259.

Roberts-Thomson, I. C., Whittingham, S., Youngchaiyud, U. and Mackay, I. R. (1974) Ageing, immune response, and mortality. *Lancet* **1**, 368–370.

Rowe, J. W. and Kahn, R. L. (1987) Human aging: usual and successful. *Science* **237**, 143–149.

Sanders, M. E., Makgoba, M. W. and Shaw, S. (1988) Human naive and memory T cells: reinterpretation of helper-inducer and suppressor-inducer subsets. *Immunology Today* **9**, 195–199.

Schaie, K. W. (1965) A general model for the study of developmental problems. *Psychological Bulletin* **64**, 92–107.

Schwab, R., Walters, C. A. and Weksler, M. E. (1989) Host defense mechanisms and aging. *Seminars in Oncology* **16**, 20–27.

Segre, D., Miller, R. A., Abraham, G. N., Weigle, W. O. and Warner, H. R. (1989) Workshop report. Aging and the immune system. *Journal of Gerontology* **44**, B164–168.

Shen, S. Y., Corteza, Q. B., Josselson, J., Gravenstein, S., Ershler, W. B., Sadler, J. H. and Chretien, P. B. (1990) Age-dependent enhancement of influenza vaccine responses by thymosin in chronic hemodialysis patients. In: *Biomedical Advances in Aging* (ed. Goldstein, A. L.). New York: Plenum, pp. 523–530.

Simpson, J. G., Gray, E. S. and Beck, J. S. (1975) Age involution in the normal human adult thymus. *Clinical and Experimental Immunology* **19**, 261–266.

Siskind, G. W. (1987) Aging and the immune system. In: *Modern Biological Theories of Aging* (eds Warner, H. R., Butler, R. N., Sprott, R. L. and Schneider, E. L.), New York: Raven, pp. 235–242.

Smith, D. W. E. (1989) Is greater female longevity a general finding among animals? *Biological Reviews* **64**, 1–12.

Smith, G. S. and Walford, R. L. (1978) Influence of the H-2 and H-1 histocompatibility systems upon life span and spontaneous cancer incidence in congenic mice. *Birth Defects Original Articles Series* **281**, 281–312.

Solomon, G. F. (1985) The emerging field of psychoneuroimmunology, with a special note on AIDS. *Advances* **2**, 6–19.

Solomon, G. F. (1987) Psychoneuroendocrinology: interactions between central nervous system and immune system. *Journal of Neuroscience Research* **18**, 1–9.

Solomon, G. F. (1990) Emotions, stress, and immunity. In: *The Healing Brain. A Scientific Reader* (eds Ornstein, R. and Swencionis, C.). New York: Guilford Press, pp. 174–181.

Solomon, G. F., Fiatarone, M. A., Benton, D., Morley, J. E., Bloom, E. and Makinodan, T. (1988) Psychoimmunologic and endorphin function in the aged. *Annals on the New York Academy of Sciences* **521**, 43–58.

Sondell, K., Athlin, L., Bjermer, L., Eriksson, S. and Norberg, B. (1990) The role of sex and age in yeast cell phagocytosis by monoctyes from healthy blood donors. *Mechanisms of Ageing and Development* **51**, 55–61.

Steinmann, G. G. (1986) Changes in the human thymus during aging. In: *The Human Thymus. Histophysiology and Pathology* (ed. Muller-Hermelink, H. K.). Current Topics in Pathology, Vol. 75, pp. 43–88. Berlin, New York: Springer-Verlag.

Stephens, R. E. and Lipetz, P. D. (1983) Higher order DNA repair in human peripheral leukocytes: a factor in aging and cancer? In: *Intervention in the Aging Process, Part B: Basic Research and Preclinical Screening* (eds Regelson, W. and Sinex, F. M.). New York: Alan R. Liss, pp. 155–173.

Sthoeger, Z. M., Chiorazzi, N. and Lahita, R. G. (1988) Regulation of the immune response by sex hormones 1. *In vitro* effects of estradiol and testosterone on pokeweed mitogen-induced human B cell differentiation. *Journal of Immunology* **141**, 91–98.

Takata, H., Suzuki, M., Ishii, T., Sekiguchi, S. and Iri, H. (1987) Influence of major histocompatibility complex region genes on human longevity among Okinawan-Japanese centenarians and nonagenarians. *Lancet* **ii**, 824–826.

Talal, N., Dauphinee, M. J. and Christadoss, P. (1984) Immune and endocrine factors in autoimmune disease. In: *Stress, Immunity, and Aging* (ed. Cooper, E. L.). New York: Marcel Dekker, pp. 187–193.

Terao, K., Rose, L. M., Sackett, G. P. and Clark, E. A. (1988) Development of lymphocyte subsets in pigtailed macaques. *Human Immunology* **21**, 33–48.

Thomas, P. D., Goodwin, J. M. and Goodwin, J. S. (1985) Effect of social support on stress-related changes in cholesterol level, uric acid level, and immune function in an elderly sample. *American Journal of Psychiatry* **142**, 735–737.

Thompson, J. S., Wekstein, D. R., Rhoades, J. L., Kirkpatrick, C., Brown, S. A., Roszman, T., Straus, R. and Tietz, N. (1984) The immune status of healthy centenarians. *Journal of the American Geriatrics Society* **32**, 274–281.

Tosi, P., Kraft, R., Luzi, P., Cintorino, M., Fankhauser, G., Hess, M. W. and Cottier, H. (1982) Involution of the human thymus. I. Size of the cortical area as a function of age. *Clinical and Experimental Immunology* **47**, 497–504.

Traill, K. N., Schonitzer, D., Jurgens, G., Bock, J., Pfeilschifter, R., Hilchenback, M., Holasek, A., Forster, O. and Wick, G. (1985) Age-related changes in lympho-cyte subset proportions, surface differentiation antigen density and plasma membrane fluidity: application of the EURAGE SENIEUR PROTOCOL admission criteria. *Mechanisms of Ageing and Development* **33**, 39–66.

Tsuji, K., Sato, K., Nose, Y., Inoku, H., Nakatsuji, T., Ando, A. and Ikewaki, N. (1986) Human class II antigens in different ethnic groups. In: *HLA Class II Antigens* (eds Solheim, B. G., Moller, E. and Ferrone, S.). Berlin: Springer-Verlag, pp. 154–168.

Twomey, J. J., Luchi, R. J. and Kouttab, N. M. (1982) Null cell senescence and its potential significance to the immunobiology of aging. *Journal of Clinical Investigation* **70**, 201–204.

Verbrugge, L. M. and Wingard, D. L. (1987) Sex differentials in health and mortality. *Women and Health* **12**, 103–145.

Wade, A. W., Green-Johnson, J. and Szewczuk, M. R. (1988) Functional changes in systemic and mucosal lymphocyte repertoirs with age: an updated review. *AGING: Immunology and Infectious Disease* **1**, 65–97.

Wainscoat, J. S., Peto, T. E. A. and Waswo, A. (1987) HLA genes and longevity. *Lancet* **ii**, 1399.

Walford, R. L. (1969) *The Immunologic Theory of Aging* Copenhagen: Munksgaard.

Walford, R. L. (1974) Immunologic theory of aging: current status. *Federation Proceedings* **33**, 2020–2027.

Walford, R. L. (1982) Studies in immunogerontology. *Journal of the American Geriatrics Society* **30**, 617–625.

Walford, R. L. (1987) MHC regulation of aging: an extension of the immunologic theory of aging. In: *Modern Biological Theories of Aging* (eds Warner, H. R., Butler, R. N., Sprott, R. L. and Schneider, E. L.). New York: Raven, pp. 243–260.

Walford, R. L. (1990) The major histocompatibility complex and aging in mammals. In:

*Molecular Biology of Aging* (eds. Finch, C. E. and Johnson, T. E.). New York: Alan R. Liss, pp. 31–41.

Weindruch, R. and Walford, R. L. (1988) *The Retardation of Aging and Disease by Dietary Restriction*. Springfield, IL: Charles C. Thomas.

Weindruch, R. H., Kemnitz, J. W., Roecker, E. B., Kaufman, P. L. and Erler, W. B. (1991) Dietary restriction of adult male rhesus monkeys: findings from the first year of study. *The Gerontologist* **31**, (Special Issue II), 78.

Weiss, K. M. (1973) Demographic models for anthropology. *Memoirs of the Society for American Archeology*, **27**.

Weksler, M. E. (1981) The senescence of the immune system. *Hospital Practice* October, 53–64.

Weksler, M. E., Kim, Y. T., Siskind, G. W. and Schwab, R. (1990) The clinical significance of immune senescence: Advantages and disadvantages. In: *Biomedical Advances in Aging* (ed. Goldstein, A. L.). New York: Plenum, pp. 401–404.

Williams, G. C. (1957) Pleiotropy, selection and the evolution of senescence. *Evolution* **11**, 398–411.

Yamakido, M., Yanagida, J., Ishioka, S., Matsuzaka, S., Hozawa, S., Akiyama, M., Kobuke, K., Inmizu, T. and Nishimoto, Y. (1985a) Detection of lymphocyte subsets by monoclonal antibodies in aged and young humans. *Hiroshima Journal of Medical Sciences* **34**, 87–94.

Yamakido, M., Yanagida, J., Ishioka, S., Matsuzaka, S., Hozawa, S., Akiyama, M., Kobuke, K., Inmizu, T. and Nishimoto, Y. (1985b) Interleukin-2 production and lymphocyte proliferation in aged and young humans. *Hiroshima Journal of Medical Sciences* **34**, 95–99.

Yarnell, J. W. G., St. Leger, A. S., Balfour, I. C. and Russell, R. B. (1979) The distribution, age effects and disease associations of HLA antigens and other blood group markers in a random sample of an elderly population. *Journal of Chronic Diseases* **32**, 555–561.

Yasuda, N., Tsuji, K. and Itakura, K. (1980) HLA heterozygosity in children and old people. *Tokai Journal of Experimental and Clinical Medicine* **5**, 165–169.

Yunis, E. J. and Watson, A. L. M. (1982) Histocompatibility, disease and aging. In: *Animal Models of Inherited Metabolic Diseases* (eds Desnick, R. J., Patterson, D. F. and Scarpelli, D. G.). New York: Alan R. Liss, pp. 327–349.

# 8

# Neuronal Aging and Age-related Disorders of the Human Nervous System

## MICHAEL J. STRONG AND RALPH M. GARRUTO

## INTRODUCTION

As different populations worldwide age *en block* and average life expectancy increases, dramatic increases in the prevalence of age-related neurodegenerative disorders can be expected, and with it massive social and economic burdens to society (Eveleth, this volume; Miles and Brody, this volume). This is true not only for Western cosmopolitan populations but also for many third world populations and many semi-isolated populations undergoing a "health transition" as they move into the modern world (Baker and Garruto, 1992; Miles and Brody, this volume). Among those who do develop a late onset neurodegenerative disorder, the majority will develop one or more of the dementias (Alzheimer's disease being the most predominant), parkinsonism or amyotrophic lateral sclerosis (Pfeffer *et al.*, 1987; Schoenberg *et al.*, 1987; Evans *et al.*, 1989). Additionally, increasing incidence rates independent of the aging of human populations have been described for several of these disorders, suggesting an increasing involvement of environmental factors in their etiology (Durrleman and Alperovitch, 1989; Lilienfeld *et al.*, 1989; Gunnarsson *et al.*, 1990). By understanding the normal mechanisms by which the human nervous system regulates neuronal populations, and how these cell populations undergo age-related attrition, the biological anthropologist, gerontologist and epidemiologist are provided with a link from cellular populations to human populations. It is this link that is likely to provide insight into the mechanisms by which the human nervous system ages in a disease state and allow the fruitful application of these concepts to the fields of human population biology and epidemiology.

The human nervous system is a dynamic structure capable of considerable plasticity throughout a human life span. By parcelling this plasticity into aging or non-aging phenomena, the nature of this process which encompasses not only neuronal senescence, but also neuronal proliferation and regression during development, is obscured. Indeed, the basic biological principals underlying the development of mature neuronal populations, with little intraspecies variability, often from neuronal pools twice exceeding the final neuronal requirements, may apply directly to our understanding of human neurodegeneration in which select neuronal populations degenerate to levels inadequate to maintain normal function.

Thus, we begin this chapter by looking at the process of neuronal proliferation and regression pre- and post-natally and examine how this process forms a continuum with "normal age-related" neuronal regression. Thereafter, we will review specific processes of adult-onset neurodegeneration in which this normal age-related neuronal regression is accelerated. In the final sections, we will discuss the concept of age-related disease syndromes and offer certain theoretical constructs and research perspectives on the aging nervous system. For the reader interested in pure and applied neurobiology, the scope of this chapter will be limited. Rather than provide an exhaustive review of the literature pertaining to each section, we have chosen to present a more concise conceptual overview with specific illustrative examples. This has, however, been supplemented by references to current and authoritative reviews of the relevant material.

## NEURONAL PROLIFERATION AND REGRESSION DURING PRENATAL DEVELOPMENT

In virtually every neural cell population studied, the process of cell death during neurogenesis is a normal phenomenon (extensively reviewed in Coleman and Flood, 1987). The initial process of cellular proliferation and differentiation is constant for each population of neurons and dependent on both intrinsic neuronal and regionally specific extrinsic factors. The process of selective neuronal death appears thereafter to 'prune' the neuronal populations to levels appropriate to the requirements of the target organ (Vogt and Vogt, 1946; Glücksmann, 1951; Oppenheim, 1975; Cunningham, 1982; Cowan et al., 1984).

The processes of neuronal proliferation and differentiation can be modulated by a variety of factors, both positive and negative. Positive modulating factors consist of hormonal influences (i.e., thyroid hormone, growth hormone), neurotrophic factors (endogenous, freely diffusible molecules which promote survival, growth and function of developing or adult neurons, i.e., nerve growth factor) (Hefti et al., 1989) and local mitogenic effects (i.e., notochord derived) (Williams and Herrup, 1988; Van Stratten et al., 1990). Negative modulating factors consist of local inhibitory effects upon the undifferentiated precursor cells, possibly mediated by matrix-specific proteins or adjacent cellular trophic factors. The extent of neuronal death is not only dependent upon the embryonic environment, but also on the size of the target field (Hamburger and Levi-Montalcini, 1949) and availability of synaptic contact target sites (Oppenheim, 1989). Rohrer (1990) has recently published a detailed review of this area of developmental neurobiology.

The process of proliferation and regression in neurogenesis has been extensively studied in the chick embryo lateral motor column innervation of the developing limb bud and will be briefly described here. The principles underlying this process have, however, been replicated in other developing neuronal populations (Hamburger and Levi-Montalcini, 1949; Lumsden, 1990). Within the developing lateral motor column, the initial neuronal proliferation is region-specific (Oppenheim *et al.*, 1989), occurs maximally by day 5 to 6.5 post-incubation (Hamburger, 1975) and demonstrates differences in the numbers of dividing cells between brachial and non-brachial spinal segments (Oppenheim *et al.*, 1989). The subsequent occurrence of cell death in the motor neuron population is related to specific interactions between these neurons, their target tissue (skeletal muscle) and primary sensory afferents (Okado and Oppenheim, 1984). As many as 50–53% of motor neurons in the lateral cell column are lost between days 5.5 and 9 of incubation, with little overlap between the period of proliferation and regression. This regression is accompanied by a concomitant loss of axons, ultimately resulting in a 1:1 pairing of motor neurons and projecting axons (Chu-Wang and Oppenheim, 1978b). This process can be inhibited by the presence of homogenates of embryonic hindlimb tissue (Oppenheim *et al.*, 1988), or by the transplantation of a supernumerary limb bud (Hamburger, 1939). It can be induced by the removal of the limb bud prior to the onset of naturally occurring cell death (Chu-Wang and Oppenheim, 1978a). In the majority of degenerating neurons, axons are present prior to the onset of degeneration, although it is not clear that all axons have formed functional connections with other neurons (Prestige and Wilson, 1972; Lamb, 1974). The signal for the induction of the degeneration appears synchronous with the contact of a population of neurons with a target tissue (e.g., when the peripheral areas become functionally innervated), suggesting a mechanism, in part, related to a target-derived trophic factor (Hughes, 1968).

Similar observations have been made for the induction of ventral horn motor neurons in the fetal mouse (Harris-Flanagan, 1969), *Xenopus laevis*, the South African clawed toad (Prestige, 1967; Lamb, 1974, 1977) and rat (Tada *et al.*, 1979). In the latter, neuronal regression has been observed to continue post-natally—a point relevant to our subsequent discussions (Rootman *et al.*, 1981). The ubiquitous nature of this neuronal proliferation and regression in vertebrate embryogenesis has been extensively reviewed elsewhere (Glück-smann, 1951).

## AGE-RELATED NEURONAL REGRESSION POST-NATALLY

As alluded to in the previous section, there is continued post-natal neuronal regression in the human nervous system. This process gives rise to certain characteristic morphological features, including: (1) a maximum size of the human brain which is attained by the age of 20–25 years, thereafter linearly regressing by 7–11% by the ages of 20–96; (2) a regionally specific neuronal loss; and (3) an increase in glial elements (Brody, 1955, 1970).

This observation of declining total brain weight with age during adulthood has been repeatedly confirmed in cross-sectional studies. Miller and colleagues

(1980) observed a constant mean brain weight between the ages of 20 and 50 in men and women with otherwise normal hemispheres, thereafter falling at a rate of approximately 2% per decade. The decline in brain weight was slightly greater in males than females. Similar data was obtained by Hubbard and Anderson (1981) studying brain weight as a function of cranial volume.

Numerous attempts through postmortem morphometric analyses have been made to correlate regional losses of defined neuronal populations with age. However, age-related neuronal attrition does not occur equally or at the same rate in all neuronal populations. Many fail to show significant age-related declines in number (Monagle and Brody, 1974; Konigsmark and Murphy, 1972), while others demonstrate significant differences in rates of attrition (Gowers, 1902). However, the process of age-related attrition does occur in the hippocampus, and because of the importance of this region to the neuropathological process in Alzheimer's disease, it has been extensively studied (Figure 8-1). Ball (1977) observed a negative correlation between nerve cell density and age in the hippocampus, with a much more precipitous drop for demented patients. Miller et al. (1984), in an analysis of the CA1 region of the hippocampus using an image analyzer in neurologically intact individuals (age range 15–96 years), observed a 3.6% decline in the absolute number of neurons per decade. This was accompanied by a 3.3% decrease per decade in hemisphere volume, a trend similar to that described by Mann et al. (1985). In a study of the neocortex and medial hippocampus, Anderson and colleagues (1983) studying patients from age 69 to 95 years, observed a 1% per annum loss of neurons, accompanied by a reduction in the volume of white matter but with a change in the actual cortical volume. Dam (1979), studying patients with age ranges between 21 and 91 years, observed an approximate 20% reduction in pyramidal and granular cell numbers in the hippocampus with age, a reduction that became significant only after the age of 68. Similar findings have been demonstrated in the amygdala (Herzog and Kemper, 1980) and subiculum (Shefer, 1972) (Figure 8-1).

The process of age-dependent neuronal drop-out is not restricted to the hippocampus. The cerebellum, in particular the Purkinje cell layer, is particularly vulnerable (Hall et al., 1975) (Figure 8-2). Torvik et al. (1986), in a postmortem analysis of men with an age range of 36 to 94 years, observed a significant decline in Purkinje cell numbers in all regions of the cerebellar vermis, but predominantly in the superior vermis. This decline began at approximately 60 years of age and was most profound by age 75. Similar findings were reported earlier in this century by Ellis (1919, 1920), although he observed that Purkinje cell numbers appeared stable until the third or fourth decade and thereafter declined. Ellis (1920) also observed a disappearance of the external granular cell layer from birth through age 12 months. Similar losses of neurons with age were observed in multiple pre- and post-rolandic samplings from healthy individuals age 18 through 95 (Henderson et al., 1980). In an analysis of the neurons in the locus ceruleus, Mann (1983) observed a 25% reduction in this neuronal population between the third and tenth decades of life while Vijayashankar and Brody (1979) found that the greatest reduction in these neurons occurred after age 63. While there are differences amongst

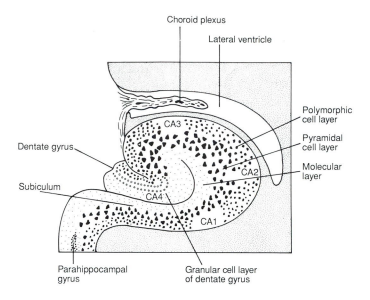

**Figure 8-1** Schematic diagram of the human hippocampal formation showing the cell layers and major anatomic sub-regions. Coronal section with medial surface at the left. Modified from Barr and Kiernan (1983) and reproduced with permission.

these studies, the observations clearly demonstrate neuronal attrition in both the cerebellum and hippocampus with age.

In the spinal cord, losses of ventral (anterior) horn motor neurons innervating skeletal muscle have also been observed with increasing age (Figure 8-3). Tomlinson and Irving (1977), studying the lumbosacral segments of spinal cords from neurologically intact individuals aged 13–95 years, observed no significant change in absolute neuronal numbers prior to age 60, but thereafter observed a mean loss of 24% by the age of 95, ranging from 5 to 50%. These losses were not accompanied by pathologic features of neurodegeneration in the anterior horn region. These changes have been verified in studies of spinal cord segments at lumbar levels L3, L4 and L5 in individuals ranging in age from 17 to 82 years, where a linear decline of 170–260 neurons per decade per segment was observed (Kawamura *et al.*, 1977). Similar reductions in spinal motor neurons at cervical levels C6 and C8 have been observed (Tsukagoshi *et al.*, 1979, 1980), and have been correlated with normal motor unit losses in the peripheral nervous system, specifically innervation to biceps brachii and brachialis muscles (Brown *et al.*, 1988).

The above studies illustrate several principles of age-dependent neuronal regression in healthy individuals. First, the weight of evidence suggests that the process of age-related neuronal loss is not linear throughout the human lifespan. For the majority of nuclear (neuronal population) regions, no significant decline appears to occur until around the sixth decade of life. Thereafter, significant loss of neurons (quantitatively measured by morphometric techniques) occurs and is associated with a reduction in mean brain

(a)

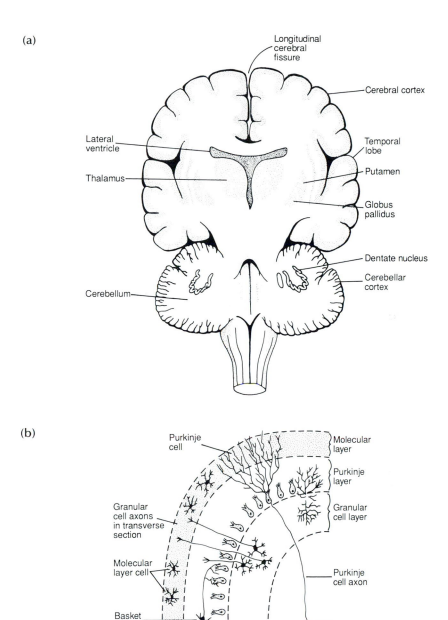

Longitudinal cerebral fissure

Cerebral cortex

Lateral ventricle

Temporal lobe

Putamen

Thalamus

Globus pallidus

Dentate nucleus

Cerebellar cortex

Cerebellum

(b)

Purkinje cell

Molecular layer

Purkinje layer

Granular cell axons in transverse section

Granular cell layer

Molecular layer cell

Purkinje cell axon

Basket cell

White matter

Golgi cell

**Figure 8-2** (a) Schematic anatomy of the cerebellum showing its juxtaposition to other brain landmarks. (b) Diagrammatic representation of a transverse section through the cerebellum showing various cell layers and cell types. (a) Modified from Carpenter and Sutin (1983) and reproduced with permission. (b) Modified from Gross (1959) and reproduced with permission.

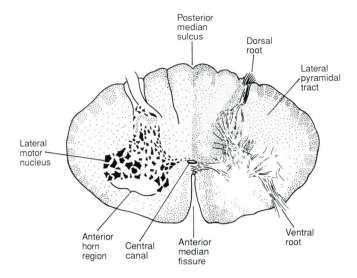

**Figure 8-3** Schematic cross-section of the spinal cord at the fifth cervical vertebrae showing motor neurons (black) and other anatomic landmarks. Modified from Nieuwenhuys *et al.* (1981) and reproduced with permission.

weight. It also should be noted that the process of age-dependent neuronal regression shows significant individual variability. Finally, neuronal regression does not necessarily imply functional regression (i.e., failure of the target organ or system) and thus factors synergistic to this regression process are likely involved in functional maintenance of the remaining neurons (Butcher and Woolf, 1989).

It seems reasonable, therefore, to assume that the concepts of optimal and critical levels of neuronal density apply to the aging nervous system. What is unknown is the degree to which neuronal plasticity occurs in the nervous system, the conditions under which it occurs and the degree of neuronal adaptation that results in various populations of this post-mitotic cell type. Moreover, it should be emphasized that we have focused mainly on the morphometric correlates of aging and have not specifically addressed neurochemical alterations or the extent of alterations in neurotrophism in the aging nervous system.

## AGE-RELATED NEURODEGENERATIVE DISEASES

In view of the preceding discussion, the neuronal degeneration and loss that accompanies adult-onset neurodegenerative disorders might be viewed morphometrically as extremes of naturally occurring neuronal attrition. However, these disorders are also characterized by both ultrastructural and biochemical changes and are manifested by a progression of clinical symptoms.

The major adult-onset neurodegenerative disorders including amyotrophic lateral sclerosis (ALS), parkinsonism and Alzheimer's disease have in common fundamental abnormalities in neuronal cytoskeletal protein biosynthesis or catabolism, a prominent hallmark of which is an abnormal accumulation of intra- and extraneuronal cytoskeletal proteins, often accompanied by extreme degrees of neuronal loss and atrophy. This process is exemplified by ALS, a relentlessly progressive, uniformly fatal disorder affecting 1.6–2.4/100,000 individuals worldwide (Bobowick and Brody, 1973; Juergens et al., 1980; Hudson et al., 1986). In this disorder, death occurs within 2.5 years in 50% of cases and within the first decade in 90–95% (Boman and Meurman, 1967; Rosen, 1978). The majority of cases occur sporadically, but a familial variant of ALS, inherited predominantly as an autosomal dominant, has been well characterized (Strong et al., 1991). An early ultrastructural lesion characteristic of the disease is the accumulation of neurofilament subunit proteins within spinal motor neurons in quantities several fold greater than that present in age-matched controls (Carpenter, 1968; Hirano, 1976; Chou, 1979; Averback, 1981; Schmidt et al., 1987). A later appearing pathology is a reduction in the numbers of motor neurons in the cervical spinal cord (level C6 and C8) to less than half that of age-matched controls (Tsukagoshi et al., 1980). In an electrophysiological analysis of motor unit numbers of the biceps brachii and brachialis in sporadic ALS, Strong et al. (1988) reported motor unit estimates that were often several standard deviations below normal values.

ALS also occurs in hyperendemic foci in islands of the Western Pacific (Guam and West New Guinea) as well as in the Kii Peninsula of Southern Japan. In these regions, the clinical manifestations differ little from the classic (sporadic) form of ALS present in North America and Europe. However, the hallmark pathological change of this western Pacific variant of ALS is the extensive development of neurofibrillary tangles (discussed below) in the brain as well as the spinal cord. Prior to the Westernization of these cultures, the incidence rates of ALS and a second neurological disorder, parkinsonism-dementia (PD), ranged from 50/100,000 to as high as 1,300/100,000 population compared to rates of 1.6–2.4/100,000 in cosmopolitan Western communities (Kurland and Mulder, 1954; Gajdusek and Salazar, 1982; Garruto et al., 1985). While ALS and PD in these foci were initially considered to be genetic disorders, subsequent studies have clearly demonstrated them to be "place-specific" disease foci, induced by environmental factors (Garruto, 1991). The study of these foci, of the relationship of environmental factors to the incidence rates, and of the factors leading to the subsequent decline in incidence rates, has provided significant insights into the impact of exogenous factors on the naturally occurring loss of motor and pyramidal neuron populations.

It has been postulated that the degenerative process of ALS is an augmentation of the normal abiotrophy or attrition of motor neurons irrespective of the ALS variant (Eisen and Calne, 1990). While an attractive hypothesis, the rates of loss of motor neurons in ALS are precipitous and exceed by several fold naturally occurring rates. Moreover, ALS is an age-related phenomenon with progressively increasing incidence rates beginning in the sixth decade of life, and as discussed previously, motor neuron estimates remain essentially stable until this time, thereafter declining in neurologically intact individuals. The threshold of motor neuron loss required to develop clinically overt muscle weakness is very large and in the extensor digitorum brevis, has been estimated to be a reduction to 10% of the original motor unit pool (McComas *et al.*, 1971). It would seem improbable, therefore, that such a precipitous drop in motor neuron numbers could occur as a manifestation of normal abiotrophy; yet, this does not imply that the process of normal abiotrophy does not in some way "prime" the neurons to render them more susceptible to some external insult which is causally related to the disease.

This superimposition of an extrinsic insult on the normal attrition of motor neurons can be illustrated by late onset muscular atrophy following recovery from poliomyelitis. This syndrome manifests as progressive muscular atrophy, weakness and fasciculations (muscle twitches) following an interval of one to two decades of normal or near-normal neuromuscular function (Dalakas *et al.*, 1986). It seems likely that this represents the cumulative effects of an acute insult to the motor neuron population, with an attendant loss of neurons, followed thereafter by normal rates of neuronal attrition that ultimately reduce the neuronal population to levels insufficient to maintain neuromuscular function (Swash and Schwartz, 1988).

The above hypothesis that an infection may affect neuronal function and/or number is not without precedence. With a latency of approximately 30 years following the 1918 influenza pandemic, Parkinson's disease, indistinguishable from idiopathic parkinsonism, was observed in epidemic proportions. Recently, it has been postulated that a similar viral phenomenon might underlie the Western Pacific variant of ALS (Hudson and Rice, 1990), although to date no evidence exists for the involvement of conventional or unconventional viruses in its etiology (Garruto, 1991).

The occurrence of accelerated neuronal aging is even less well defined in Alzheimer's disease. Like ALS, Alzheimer's disease, the most common of the adult onset neurodegenerative disorders, has age-specific prevalence rates with estimates of 10–20% of the population clinically affected by age 80 and up to 47% by age 85 (Jorm *et al.*, 1987; Evans *et al.*, 1989). Similar to ALS and Parkinson's disease, the underlying pathophysiology of Alzheimer's disease is morphologically highlighted by the accumulation of several cytoskeletal proteins in addition to an extensive cortical atrophy and neuronal loss disproportionate to that due to aging. The neuropathological features of Alzheimer's disease include neuronal degeneration, gliosis, and a complex array of intra- and extraneuronal cytoskeletal protein accumulations (e.g., neurofibrillary tangles, granulovacuolar degeneration, Hirano bodies, cerebrovascular and parenchymal $\beta$/A4 amyloid protein deposits) Terry, 1985; Wisniewski, 1991). To a large degree, these proteinaceous accumulations are present as phenomena of the "normal" aging process, but occur to a much greater extent and often at an earlier age in Alzheimer's disease (Tomlinson *et al.*, 1968; Mann *et al.*, 1985, 1990). More striking, however, is the absolute reduction of select neuronal populations. Whereas normal aging is accompanied by a 45–50% reduction in pyramidal cells of the temporal and hippocampal cortex by age 90 in controls (a 6–12% decline per decade after age 60), by age 75, a 60–80% reduction has occurred in individuals with Alzheimer's disease (Mann *et al.*, 1985).

The concept of a neurodegenerative disease continuum is also relevant. For example, the neuropathological hallmark of Guamanian ALS and PD, Alzheimer's disease and late Down's syndrome is the extensive development of neurofibrillary tangles (intra- and extraneuronal accumulations of highly insoluble fibrillar material). Their presence establishes an important link among these disorders. Ultrastructurally and immunocytochemically, the neurofibrillary tangles in these disorders are, in most instances, identical (Hirano *et al.*, 1961; Guiroy *et al.*, 1987, 1990; Shankar *et al.*, 1989). Biochemical and molecular characterization of these lesions show that they contain a low molecular weight (42 amino acid) hydrophobic polypeptide that forms paracrystalline arrays of $\beta$-pleated sheets designated amyloid $\beta$-protein or $\beta$/A4 protein (Guiroy *et al.*, 1987, 1990).

It has been widely held that a key to understanding the disease process in Guamanian ALS and PD and Alzheimer's disease will be through understanding the biosynthesis or catabolism of the proteins that accumulate to form neurofibrillary tangles. The lesions likely result from aberrant post-translational processing, phosphorylation, and co-polymerization of microtubule-associated protein-tau, ubiquitin, heavy and medium neurofilament subunit proteins, and $\beta$-amyloid (Garruto, 1991). Therefore, it is possible that these disorders (or some of their subtypes) form a biological continuum linked in their pathogenic process by a common pathway and/or initiating insult(s).

## CONCEPT OF AGE-RELATED DISEASE CONTINUUMS

It is becoming increasingly clear that many disorders with long latency and late onset may represent disease syndromes rather than single disease entities. This should not be unexpected given the limited phenotypic repertoire of the adult nervous system. Part of the difficulty in understanding the pathogenesis of these syndromes lies in the utilization of categorical clinical criteria to define continuous processes, that while superficially similar, may reflect varied pathophysiological processes. Returning to the examples above, ALS is defined by a clinical profile that includes the presence of progressive bulbar palsy and multi-segmental spinal muscular atrophy, accompanied by corticospinal tract dysfunction. While phenomenologically similar, the classical sporadic, familial and Western Pacific variants of ALS are typified by differing neuropathological features (Hudson, 1990). In this example, phenotypic homogeneity does not predict pathophysiological homogeneity.

Additionally, within the familial variant of ALS, two distinct groups appear to exist that can be defined on the basis of disease duration (<10 years and >10 years) (Strong *et al.*, 1991). While this finding can be statistically argued to represent the existence of a continuum of disease duration, dependent on the age of onset, with a younger age of onset predicting a longer survival, it can also be argued that it represents distinct clinical subpopulations within a given ALS variant (Horton *et al.*, 1976). It would be of interest to determine if the rate of neuronal loss in each disease duration sub-population is linear (as measured by electrophysiological techniques), and to what extent the rate of loss follows that of normal neuronal attrition. Theoretically, there should be no parallel to age-related neuronal attrition in the short duration sub-variant, whereas this might be expected in those with long-term survival. As discussed above for the post-polio muscular atrophy syndrome, superimposing an acute neurotoxic insult upon a neuronal population, followed thereafter by "normal" age-related neuronal attrition may be sufficient to produce an age-related neurodegenerative process. The nature of the neurotoxic insult can be expected to be highly variable given the limited phenotypic responses of the human nervous system. The interval at which the insult occurs and its magnitude (the "set point" from which neuronal regression will occur) would be of paramount importance.

The issue is no less complex for senile dementia of the Alzheimer type. To simply combine all adult-onset dementias under this heading obscures the multiple pathological processes which can induce this syndrome. Thus, as clinical/pathological correlates improve, even within disorders such as typical sporadic Alzheimer's disease, it is increasingly important to "tease out" previously unknown conditions such as diffuse Lewy body disease (Byrne *et al.*, 1989; Gibb *et al.*, 1989; Dickson *et al.*, 1991), focal neuronal achromasia (Lippa *et al.*, 1991) and regionally accentuated Alzheimer's disease with progressive aphasia (Mesulam, 1982). Few would suggest that these latter entities, like other age-related neurodegenerative diseases (e.g., Pick's disease, Creutzfeld–Jakob disease or Gerstmann–Sträussler–Sheinker disease), represent accelerations of normal neuronal attrition. However, when these clinical variants are excluded, the clinician is left with an aging population, in whom a number display a global cognitive and functional decline, and in whom, at autopsy, some of the pathological features of Alzheimer's disease are found. The challenge will be to determine if decrements in mentation in this population occur at a rate similar to that expected for normal neuronal attrition although starting with a smaller or damaged neuronal pool distinct from that of an age and sex-matched cognitively intact population.

However these diseases are ultimately classified, it is likely that the process of "pathological" neuronal degeneration is one with a long temporal sequence starting either *in utero*, during infancy, childhood, or adolescence or even at a later time, but long before onset of clinical disease (Garruto, 1991). Thus when these disorders are characterized, it is the end-stage of a long temporal sequence that manifests itself by the onset of clinical symptoms that will be described. If the disease process is to be truly understood, an appropriate methodology must be used which allows evaluation of the total life course of the individual and the identification of time-related risk factors and accumulating insults (see Brandt and Pearson, this volume). The multi-hit model discussed by Wood and colleagues (this volume) and the "thrifty-pleiotropic" model discussed by Crews and Gerber (this volume) are also highly relevant to this endeavour.

## THEORETICAL IMPLICATIONS AND FUTURE RESEARCH PERSPECTIVES

Several concepts relative to neuronal proliferation and regression during aging and the onset of age-related neurodegeneration have been discussed. It is obvious that the aging of the nervous system is quite different from that of systems involving mitotic cell types. Emphasis was placed on neuronal cell populations rather than on non-neuronal cell types, and included the processes of proliferation and regression in neurogenesis, the development of age-related neuronal regression post-natally, age-related disorders and the concepts of disease syndromes and continuums.

Future implications and perspectives relevant to an emerging synthesis between biological anthropology, gerontology and neurology include:

- An understanding of the mechanisms modulating selective developmental regression that may provide therapeutic insights into neuronal aging and neurodegenerative disease states.
- A need for the physician dealing with human neurodegenerative disease states to recognize the limited phenotypic plasticity of the nervous system, the concept of accelerated neuronal abiotrophy and the concept of altered disease "set-points".
- A need for the biological anthropologist and human population biologist to look for "triggers", either endogenous or exogenous, that may contribute to the altered "set-point" discussed above. Here also should be an understanding of synergism and the application of mathematical modelling to evaluate the possibility of a major gene defect in combination with an environmental trigger (Garruto, 1989; Bailey–Wilson *et al.*, 1992) as well as the search for biomarkers of individual exposure.
- A search for high-incidence foci of age-related neurodegenerative disorders worldwide in non-Western anthropological populations where confounding factors are less likely to occur compared with large, genetically diverse cosmopolitan communities.

What is not needed is emphasis on concepts, approaches, and methods which have yielded little beyond their own initial value. We must be willing to break with the past when necessary and to return to at least a modicum of "high-risk" research problems and approaches in furthering our understanding of the human nervous system, its plasticity and response to stress, and its ultimate degeneration and failure in later life. We cannot and should not be content to necessarily follow the same path as we did before, for what once worked may not work again, and what was once innovative and creative may no longer be so in the future.

## REFERENCES

Anderson, J. M., Hubbard, B. M. and Coghill, G. R. (1983) The effect of advanced old age on the neurone content of the cerebral cortex. *Journal of the Neurological Sciences* **58** 233–244.

Averback, P. (1981) Unusual particles in motor neuron disease. *Archives of Pathology and Laboratory Medicine* **105**, 490–493.

Bailey-Wilson, J. E., Plato, C. C., Elston, R. C. and Garruto, R. M. (1993) Potential role of an additive genetic component in the cause of amyotrophic lateral sclerosis and parkinsonism-dementia in the western Pacific. *American Journal of Medical Genetics* **45**, 68–76.

Baker, P. T. and Garruto, R. M. (1992) Health transition: examples from the western Pacific. *Human Biology* **64**, 785–789.

Ball, M. J. (1977) Neuronal loss, neurofibrillary tangles and granulovacuolar degeneration in the hippocampus with aging and dementia. *Acta Neuropathologica (Berlin)* **37**, 111–118.

Barr, M. L. and Kiernan, J. A. (1983) *The Human Nervous System—An Anatomical Viewpoint*, 4th edn. New York: Harper and Row.

Bobowick, A. J. and Brody, J. A. (1973) Epidemiology of motor-neuron diseases. *New England Journal of Medicine* **288**, 1047–1055.

Boman, K. and Meurman, T. (1967) Prognosis of amytrophic lateral sclerosis. *Acta Neurologica Scandinavia* **43**, 489–498.

Brody, H. (1955) Organization of the cerebral cortex. III. A study of the aging in the human cerebral cortex. *Journal of Comparative Neurology* **102**, 511–556.

Brody, H. (1970) Structural changes in the aging nervous system. *Interdisciplinary Topics in Gerontology* **7**, 9–21.

Brown, W. F., Strong, M. J. and Snow, R. (1988) Methods for estimating numbers of motor units in biceps-brachialis muscles and losses of motor units with aging. *Muscle & Nerve* **11**, 423–432.

Butcher, L. L. and Woolf, N. J. (1989) Authors response to commentaries. *Neurobiology of Aging* **10**, 588–590.

Byrne, J. E., Lennox, G., Lowe, J. and Godwin-Austen, R. B. (1989) Diffuse Lewy body disease: clinical features in 15 cases. *Journal of Neurology, Neurosurgery, and Psychiatry* **52**, 709–717.

Carpenter, S. (1968) Proximal axonal enlargement in motor neuron disease. *Neurology* **18**, 841–851.

Carpenter, M. B. and Sutin, J. (1983) *Human Anatomy*, 8th edn. Baltimore: Williams and Wilkins.

Chou, S. M. (1979) Pathognomy of intraneuronal inclusions in ALS. In: *Amyotrophic Lateral Sclerosis* (ed. Tsabaki, Y. and Toyokura, T.). Tokyo: University of Tokyo Press, pp. 135–176.

Chu-Wang, I.-W. and Oppenheim, R. W. (1978a) Cell death of motoneurons in the chick embryo spinal cord. I. A light and electron microscopic study of naturally occurring and induced cell loss during development. *Journal of Comparative Neurology* **177**, 33–58.

Chu-Wang, I.-W. and Oppenheim, R. W. (1978b) Cell death of motoneurons in the chick embryo spinal cord. II. A quantitative and qualitative analysis of degeneration in the ventral root, including evidence for axon outgrowth and limb innervation prior to cell death. *Journal of Comparative Neurology* **177**, 59–86.

Coleman, P. D. and Flood, D. G. (1987) Neuron numbers and dendritic extent in normal aging and Alzheimer's disease. *Neurobiology of Aging* **8**, 521–545.

Cowan, W. M., Fawcett, J. W., O'Leary, D. D. M. and Stanfield, B. B. (1984) Regressive events in neurogenesis. *Science* **225**, 1258–1265.

Cunningham, T. J. (1982) Naturally occurring neuron death and its regulation by developing neural pathways. *International Review of Cytology* **74**, 163–186.

Dalakas, M. C., Elder, G., Hallet, M., Ravits, J., Baker, M., Papadopoulos, N.,

Albrecht, P. and Sever, J. (1986) A long-term follow-up study with post-poliomyelitis neuromuscular symptoms. *New England Journal of Medicine* **315**, 959–963.

Dam, A. M. (1979) The density of neurons in the human hippocampus. *Neuropathology and Applied Neurobiology* **5**, 249–264.

Dickson, D. W., Ruan, D., Crystal, H., Mark, M. H., Davies, P., Kress, Y. and Yen, S.-H. (1991) Hippocampal degeneration differentiates diffuse Lewy body disease (DLBD) from Alzheimer's disease: light and electron microscopic immuno-cytochemistry of CA2-3 neurites specific to DLBD. *Neurology* **41**, 1402–1409.

Durrleman, S. and Alperovitch, A. (1989) Increasing trend of ALS in France and elsewhere: are the changes real? *Neurology* **39**, 768–773.

Eisen, A. A. and Calne, D. B. (1990) Latent neuro-abiotrophies: a clue to amyotrophic lateral sclerosis. In: *Amyotrophic Lateral Sclerosis. Concepts in Pathogenesis and Etiology* (ed. Hudson, A. J.). Toronto: University of Toronto Press, pp. 296–316.

Ellis, R. S. (1919) A preliminary quantitative study of the Purkinje cells in normal, subnormal and senescent human cerebella, with some notes on functional localization. *Journal of Comparative Neurology* **30**, 229–252.

Ellis, R. S. (1920) Norms for some structural changes in the human cerebellum from birth to old age. *Journal of Comparative Neurology* **32**, 1–33.

Evans, D. A., Funkenstein, H. H., Albert, M. S., Sherr, P. A., Cook, N. R., Chown, M. J., Hebert, L. E., Hennekens, C. H. and Taylor, J. O. (1989) Prevalence of Alzheimer's disease in a community population of older persons; higher than previously reported. *JAMA* **262**, 2551–2556.

Gadjusek, D. C. and Salazar, A. M. (1982) Amyotrophic lateral sclerosis and parkinsonian syndromes in high incidence among the Auyu and Jakai people in West New Guinea. *Neurology* **32**, 107–126.

Garruto, R. M. (1989) Amyotrophic lateral sclerosis and parkinsonism-dementia of Guam: clinical, epidemiological, and genetic patterns. *American Journal of Human Biology* **1**, 367–382.

Garruto, R. M. (1991) Pacific paradigms of environmentally-induced neurological disorders: clinical, epidemiological and molecular perspectives. *Neurotoxicology* **12**, 347–378.

Garruto, R. M., Yanagihara, R. and Gajdusek, D. C. (1985) Disappearance of high-incidence amyotrophic lateral sclerosis and parkinsonism-dementia on Guam. *Neurology* **35**, 193–198.

Gibb, W. R. G., Mountjoy, C. Q., Mann, D. M. A. and Lees, A. J. (1989) A pathological study of the association between Lewy body disease and Alzheimer's disease. *Journal of Neurology, Neurosurgery, and Psychiatry* **52**, 701–708.

Glücksmann, A. (1951) Cell deaths in normal vertebrate ontogeny. *Biological Reviews* **26**, 59–86.

Gowers, W. R. (1902) Abiotrophy. *Lancet*, 12th April, 1003–1007.

Gross, C. M. (1959) *Gray's Anatomy*, 27th edn. Philadelphia: Lea and Febiger.

Guiroy, D. C., Miyazaki, M., Multhaup, G., Fisher, P., Garruto, R. M., Beyreuther, K., Masters, C., Simms, G., Gibbs, C. J. and Gajdusek, D. C. (1987) Amyloid of neurofibrillary tangles of Guamanian Parkinsonism-dementia and Alzheimer disease share an identical amino acid sequence. *Proceedings of the National Academy of Sciences, USA* **84**, 2073–2077.

Guiroy, D. C., Miyazaki, M., Garruto, R. M., Yanagihara, R. and Gajdusek, D. C. (1990) Amyloid of neurofibrillary tangles of Guamanian amyotrophic lateral sclerosis contains low molecular weight proteins. *Annals of Neurology* **28**, 228.

Gunnarsson, L.-G., Lindberg, G., Söderfelt, B. and Axelson, O. (1990) The mortality of motor neuron disease in Sweden. *Archives of Neurology* **47**, 42–46.

Hall, T. C., Miller, A. K. H. and Corsellis, J. A. N. (1975) Variations in the human Purkinje cell population according to age and sex. *Neuropathology and Applied Neurobiology* **1**, 267–292.

Hamburger, V. (1939) Motor and sensory hyperplasia following limb-bud transplantation in chick embryos. *Physiological Zoology* **12**, 268–284.

Hamburger, V. (1975) Cell death in the development of the lateral motor column of the chick embryo. *Journal of Comparative Neurology* **160**, 535–546.

Hamburger, V. and Levi-Montalcini, R. (1949) Proliferation, differentiation and degeneration in the spinal ganglia of the chick embryo under normal and experimental conditions. *Journal of Experimental Zoology* **111**, 457–501.

Harris-Flanagan, A. E. (1969) Differentiation and degeneration in the motor horn of the foetal mouse. *Journal of Morphology* **129**, 281–306.

Hefti, F., Hartikka, J. and Knusel, B. (1989) Function of neurotrophic factors in the adult and aging brain and their possible use in the treatment of neurodegenerative diseases. *Neurobiology of Aging* **10**, 515–533.

Henderson, G., Tomlinson, B. E. and Gibson, P. H. (1980) Cell counts in human cerebral cortex in normal adults throughout life using an image analyzing computer. *Journal of Neurological Sciences* **46**, 113–136.

Herzog, A. G. and Kemper, T. L. (1980) Amygdaloid changes in aging and dementia. *Archives of Neurology* **37**, 625–629.

Hirano, A. (1976) Some current concepts in amyotrophic lateral sclerosis. *Neurological Medico (Tokyo)* **4**, 43–51.

Hirano, A., Malamud, N. and Kurland, L. T. (1961) Parkinsonism-dementia complex, an endemic disease on the island of Guam. I. clinical features. *Brain* **84**, 662–679.

Horton, W. A., Eldridge, R. and Brody, J. A. (1976) Familial motor neuron disease. Evidence for at least three different types. *Neurology* **26**, 460–465.

Hubbard, B. M. and Anderson, J. M. (1981) A quantitative study of cerebral atrophy in old age and senile dementia. *Journal of Neurological Sciences* **50**, 135–145.

Hudson, A. J. (1990) Amyotrophic lateral sclerosis: clinical evidence for differences in pathogenesis and etiology. In: *Amyotrophic Lateral Sclerosis* (ed. Hudson, A. J.). Toronto: University of Toronto Press, pp. 108–143.

Hudson, A. J., Davenport, A. and Hader, W. J. (1986) The incidence of amyotrophic lateral sclerosis in southwestern Ontario, Canada. *Neurology* **36**, 1524–1528.

Hudson, A. J. and Rice, G. P. A. (1990) Similarities of Guamanian ALS/PD to post-encephalitic parkinsonism/ALS: possible viral cause. *Canadian Journal of Neurological Sciences* **17**, 427–433.

Hughes, A. F. W. (1968) *Aspects of Neurontology*. New York: Academic Press.

Jeurgens, S. M., Kurland, L. T., Okazaki, H. and Mulder, D. W. (1980) ALS in Rochester, Minnesota, 1925–1977. *Neurology* **30**, 463–470.

Jorm, A. F., Korten, A. E. and Henderson, A. S. (1987) The prevalence of dementia: a quantitative integration of the literature. *Acta Psychiatrica Scandinavica* **76**, 465–479.

Kawamura, R., O'Brien, P., Okazaki, H. and Dyck, P. J. (1977) Lumbar motoneurons of man II: the number and diameter distribution of large- and intermediate-diameter cytons in "motoneuron columns" of spinal cord of man. *Journal of Neuropathology and Experimental Neurology* **36**, 861–870.

Konigsmark, B. W. and Murphy, E. A. (1972) Volume of ventral cochlear nucleus in man, its relation to neuronal population and age. *Journal of Neuropathology and Experimental Neurology* **31**, 305–316.

Kurland, L. T. and Mulder, D. W. (1954) Epidemiologic investigations of amyotrophic lateral sclerosis. 1. Preliminary report on geographic distributions, with special reference to the Marianas Islands, including clinical and pathological observations. *Neurology* **4**, 355–378, 438–448.

Lamb, A. H. (1974) The timing of the earliest motor innervation in the hind-limb bud in the *Xenopus* tadpole. *Brain Research* **67**, 527–530.

Lamb, A. H. (1977) Neuronal death in the development of the somatotopic projections of the ventral horn in *Xenopus*. *Brain Research* **134**, 145–150.

Lilienfeld, D. E., Ehland, J., Landrigan, P. J., Chan, E., Golbold, J., Marsh, G. and Perl, D. P. (1989) Rising mortality from motorneuron disease in the USA, 1962–84. *Lancet* **1**, 710–712.

Lippa, C. F., Cohen, R., Smith, T. W. and Drachman, D. A. (1991) Primary progressive aphasia with focal neuronal achromasia. *Neurology* **41**, 882–886.

Lumsden, A. (1990) The cellular basis of segmentation in the developing hindbrain. *Trends in Neuroscience* **3**, 329–335.

Mann, D. M. A. (1983) The locus coeruleus and its possible role in ageing and degenerative disease of the human central nervous system. *Mechanisms of Ageing and Development* **23**, 73–94.

Mann, D. M. A., Yates, P. O. and Marcyniuk, B. (1985) Some morphometric observations on the cerebral cortex and hippocampus in presenile Alzheimer's disease, senile dementia of Alzheimer type and Down's syndrome in middle age. *Journal of Neurological Science* **69**, 139–159.

Mann, D. M. A., Brown, A. M. T., Prinja, D., Jones, D. and Davies, C. A. (1990) A morphological analysis of senile plaques in the brains of nondemented persons of different ages using silver, immunocytochemical and lectin histochemical staining techniques. *Neuropathology and Applied Neurobiology* **16**, 17–25.

McComas, A. J., Sica, R. E. P., Campbell, M. J. and Upton, A. R. M. (1971) Functional compensation in partially denervated muscles. *Journal of Neurology, Neurosurgery and Psychiatry* **34**, 453–460.

Mesulam, M. M. (1982) Slowly progressieve aphasia without generalized dementia. *Annals of Neurology* **11**, 592–598.

Miller, A. K. H., Alston, R. L. and Corsellis, J. A. N. (1980) Variation with age in the volumes of grey and white matter in the cerebral hemispheres of man: measurements with an image analyser. *Neuropathology and Applied Neurobiology* **6**, 119–132.

Miller, A. K. H., Alston, R. L., Mountjoy, C. W. and Corsellis, J. A. N. (1984) Automated differential cell counting on a sector of the normal human hippocampus: the influence of age. *Neuropathology and Applied Neurobiology* **10**, 123–141.

Monagle, R. D. and Brody, H. (1974) The effects of age upon the main nucleus of the inferior olive in the human. *Journal of Comparative Neurology* **155**, 61–66.

Nieuwenhuys, R., Voogd, J. and van Huijzen, C. (1981) *The Human Central Nervous System—A Synopsis and Atlas*. New York: Springer-Verlag.

Okado, N. and Oppenheim, R. W. (1984) Cell death of motoneurons in the chick embryo spinal cord. The loss of motoneurons following removal of afferent inputs. *Journal of Neuroscience* **4**, 1639–1652.

Oppenheim, R. W. (1975) Progress and challenges in neuroembryology. *BioScience* **25**, 28–36.

Oppenheim, R. W. (1989) the neurotrophic theory and naturally occurring motoneuron death. *TINS* **12**, 252–255.

Oppenheim, R. W., Haverkamp, L. J., Preverte, D., McManaman, J. L. and Appel, S.

H. (1988) Reduction of naturally occurring motoneuron death in vivo by a target-derived neurotrophic factor. *Science* **240**, 919–922.

Oppenheim, R. W., Cobe, T. and Prevette, D. (1989) Early regional variations in motoneuron numbers arise by differential proliferation in the chick embryo spinal cord. *Developmental Biology* **133**, 468–474.

Pfeffer, R. I., Afifi, A. A. and Chance, J. M. (1987) Prevalence of Alzheimer's disease in a retirement community. *American Journal of Epidemiology* **125**, 420–436.

Prestige, M. C. (1967) The control of cell number in the lumbar ventral horns during the development of *Xenopus laevis* tadpoles. *Journal of Embryology and Experimental Morphology* **18**, 359–387.

Prestige, M. C. and Wilson, M. A. (1972) Loss of axons from ventral routes during development. *Brain Research* **41**, 467–470.

Rohrer, H. (1990) The role of growth factors in the control of neurogenesis. *European Journal of Neuroscience* **2**, 1005–1015.

Rootman, D. S., Tatton, W. G. and Hay, M. (1981) Postnatal histogenetic death of rat forelimb motoneurons. *Journal of Comparative Neurology* **199**, 17–27.

Rosen, A. D. (1978) Amyotrophic lateral sclerosis. Clinical features and prognosis. *Archives of Neurology* **35**, 638–642.

Schmidt, M. L., Carden, M. J., Lee, V.-Y. and Trojanowski, J. Q. (1987) Phosphate dependent and independent neurofilament epitopes in the axonal swellings of patients with motor neuron disease and controls. *Laboratory Investigation* **56**, 282–294.

Schoenberg, B. S., Kokmen, E. and Okazaki, H. (1987) Alzheimer's disease and other dementing illnesses in a defined United States population: incidence rates and clinical features. *Annals of Neurology* **22**, 724–729.

Shankar, S., Yanagihara, R., Garruto, R. M., Grundke-Iqbal, I., Kosik, K. S. and Gajdusek, D. C. (1989) Immunocytochemical characterization of neurofibrillary tangles in amyotrophic lateral sclerosis and parkinsonism-dementia on Guam. *Annals of Neurology* **25**, 146–151.

Shefer, V. F. (1972) Absolute number of neurons and thickness of the cerebral cortex during aging. Senile and vascular dementia and Pick's and Alzheimer's diseases. *Zhurnal Nevropatologii i Psikhiatrii Imeni S.S. Korsakova* **72**, 1024–1029.

Strong, M. J., Brown, W. F., Hudson, A. J. and Snow, R. (1988) Motor unit estimates in the biceps-brachialis in amyotrophic lateral sclerosis. *Muscle & Nerve* **11**, 415–422.

Strong, M. J., Hudson, A. J. and Alvord, W. G. (1991) Familial amyotrophic lateral sclerosis, 1850–1989: a statistical analysis of the world literature. *Canadian Journal of of Neurological Sciences* **18**, 45–58.

Swash, M. and Schwartz, M. S. (1988) Diseases of anterior horn cells. In: *Neuromuscular Diseases* (ed. Swash, M. and Schwartz, M. S.). London: Springer-Verlag, pp. 85–112.

Tada, K., Ohshita, S., Yonenobu, K., Ono, K., Satoh, K. and Shimizu, N. (1979) Development of spinal motoneuron innervation of the upper limb muscle in the rat. *Experimental Brain Research* **35**, 287–293.

Terry, R. D. (1985) Alzheimer's disease. In: *Textbook of Neuropathology* (ed. Davis, R. L. and Robertson, D. M.). Baltimore: Williams and Wilkins, pp. 824–841.

Tomlinson, B. E. and Irving, D. (1977) The number of limb motor neurons in the human lumbosacral cord throughout life. *Journal of Neurological Sciences* **34**, 213–219.

Tomlinson, B. E., Blessed, G. and Roth, M. (1968) Observations on the brains of non-demented old people. *Journal of Neurological Sciences* **7**, 331–356.

Torvik, A., Torp, S. and Lindboe, C. F. (1986) Atrophy of the cerebellar vermis in ageing. A morphometric and histologic study. *Journal of Neurological Sciences* **76**, 283–294.

Tsukagoshi, H., Yanagisawa, N., Ogushi, K., Nagashima, K. and Murakami, T. (1979) Morphometric quantification of the cervical limb motor cells in controls and in amyotrophic lateral sclerosis. *Journal of Neurological Sciences* **41**, 287–297.

Tsukagoshi, H., Yanagisawa, N. and Ogushi, K. (1980) Morphometric quantification of the cervical limb motor cells in various neuromuscular diseases. *Journal of Neurological Sciences* **47**, 463–472.

Van Stratten, H. W. M., Hekking, J. W. M., Beursgens, J. P. W. M., Terwindt-Rouwenhorst, E. and Drukker, J. (1990) Effect of the notochord on proliferation and differentiation in the neural tube of the chick embryo. *Development* **107**, 793–803.

Vijayashankar, N. and Brody, H. (1979) A quantitative study of the pigmented neurons in the nuclei locus coeruleus and subcoeruleus in man as related to aging. *Journal of Neuropathology and Experimental Neurology* **38**, 490–497.

Vogt, C. and Vogt, O. (1946) Ageing of nerve cells. *Nature* **158**, 304.

Williams, R. W. and Herrup, K. (1988) The control of neuron number. *Annual Review of Neuroscience* **11**, 423–453.

Wisniewski, H. M. (1991) Neuropathology and biochemistry of Alzheimer's disease and aluminium encephalopathy. In: *Proceedings of the Royal Society of Medicine, Round Table Series: Alzheimer's Disease and the Environment*. London: Royal Society of Medicine Services Ltd, pp. 35–41.

# 9

# Nutrition and Aging: Intraindividual Variation

WILLIAM A. STINI

## INTRODUCTION

Although it would not be accurate to characterize human dietary versatility as unique, it is nonetheless true that the human digestive system is remarkably tolerant with respect to the range of foods that can be processed to extract the nutrients needed to sustain homeostasis. A survey of dietary practices among human populations, past and present, would reveal some that are almost totally vegetarian while others are, or have been in the recent past, nearly totally carnivorous.

Along with dietary versatility, human nutritional requirements are notable for the presence of certain stringent constraints that define the limits of tolerance. It is still uncertain whether populations differ in any fundamental way in their ability to compensate for reduced intakes in any of the essential nutrients. For instance, it is not known what, if any, physiological adjustments permit some populations to subsist on diets yielding 300–400 mg of calcium per day on the average (Food and Agriculture Organization of the United Nations, 1977; Hegsted, 1986) while others, including that of the United States, are thought to require 1,000 mg per day. The essential amino acids which make up half of the total list of amino acids present in animal proteins must be consumed in amounts and at times that satisfy the requirements of complementarity in order to sustain protein synthesis. The demand for essential amino acids places serious constraints on the range of choices available in selecting a nutritionally adequate vegetarian diet, since most vegetable sources do not provide complete proteins. Most populations "living on the nutritional edge" of vegetarianism have evolved methods of satisfying the complementary requirement by combining foods that, in their totality, yield all of the essential amino acids. For instance, corn has a low lysine content but adequate amounts of methionine. Beans have adequate lysine but little methionine. Together, corn and beans can satisfy essential amino-acid requirements. Thus, most human populations have solved the problem of nutritional balance by exploiting the resources available to them in the assemblage of combinations constituting a cuisine.

Human ingenuity and physiological adaptability have made it possible to survive and reproduce in the face of periodic food shortages, although sometimes at considerable cost in mortality and morbidity (Stini, 1988). It is likely that the occurrence of famines and nutritional imbalances have had an evolutionary impact on human nutritional requirements. Indeed the ability to grow, mature, and reproduce depends upon success in extracting nutrients from the environment. Success is, of course, expressed as fitness, or the ability to produce viable offspring who, in turn, reproduce successfully. However, traits that favor reproductive success do not necessarily guarantee a long life, at least not a long postreproductive life when the intensity of natural selection diminishes markedly. Some population geneticists argue convincingly that aging is to some extent the result of pleiotropies that, while conferring a selective advantage early in life, lead to diminished capacities later (Rose, 1991; see also Crews and Gerber, and Wood et al., this volume). With this perspective on aging in mind it is instructive to examine the changing nature of human nutritional requirements over the life span, in particular the changes experienced in middle and old age.

## THE ROLE OF BIOLOGICAL ANTHROPOLOGY AND HUMAN POPULATION BIOLOGY IN AGING RESEARCH

Biological anthropologists and human population biologists have traditionally been concerned with human variation, its origins, and its significance. As new methodologies have become available, new dimensions of variability have come under scrutiny. Variation in biochemical traits and nuclear and mitochondrial DNA have become areas of research in which biological anthropology has made major contributions. The measurement of the processes of growth and development with associated changes in body composition is also an area in which biological anthropologists and human population biologists have long been active. The process of aging, with the physiological and anatomical changes it produces, calls attention to the fact that human variation has an important intraindividual dimension in addition to the interindividual and inter-populational ones. Idiosyncratic characteristics become accentuated with age so that variation is maximized among the aged. In this chapter, changes in human nutritional needs that occur during aging will be examined. Since some of the disease states associated with pathological aging have nutritional origins, failure to accommodate changing nutritional requirements can contribute materially to senescence, morbidity, and mortality. Changes in body composition can be seen as both cause and effect of changes in nutritional requirements. Whether the pathological changes that will be touched on in this chapter should be considered environmental or intrinsic in origin remains to be determined. Opportunities to address major theoretical and practical questions concerning intrinsic limits on human longevity can be found in the examination of changing nutritional requirements over the span of a lifetime. Biological anthropology and human population biology have much to contribute to this vital area of scientific inquiry.

## CHANGES IN BODY COMPOSITION DURING THE LIFE CYCLE

Loss of muscle and body fat is an aspect of the aging process common to all mammals. In most species living in the wild, the final stages of shrinkage or wasting are not usually seen since the associated vulnerability to predation and disease leads to mortality before the process has run its course. In domesticated animals, which live long enough to become senescent, age-related loss of muscle and fat is a frequent occurrence. Changes in body composition in most respects similar to those seen in humans are not uncommon in dogs and cats, for instance. Such changes in body composition, involving decreases in muscle mass, are reflected in altered nutritional requirements.

## NUTRITIONAL REQUIREMENTS

Human nutritional requirements change over time, creating changes in the demands made on the alimentary tract (see Table 9-1). Growth of human infants, much of it being protein synthesis, also relies heavily on fatty acid metabolism. There is still much to be learned about the mechanisms underlying the changes in metabolism from early infancy to adulthood, but there is no doubt that infant nutritional requirements are strikingly different than those of the adult and that a diet appropriate at one stage of life would be profoundly inappropriate at another.

During later infancy and childhood, it is recommended that a protein intake of 2.0–2.2 g per kg body weight be maintained. This is approximately 8% of total energy intake, a level similar to that recommended for adults, although their caloric requirements are proportionately higher than in adulthood. From the ages of one–three years, an energy intake of 100 kcal per kg body weight is recommended. The energy requirement declines to 85 kcal from four to ten years of age and further declines to 60 kcal per kg body weight from ages 11 to 14, and 42 kcal per kilogram by age 18. Male/female differences in energy requirements per kg body weight are relatively slight in adulthood, with male requirements being on the average slightly higher due to differences in body composition. The sex hormone-mediated adolescent growth spurt, which produces a greater increase in muscle mass in males and a greater increase in adiposity in females, underlies these sex differences in adult energy requirements.

Adult energy requirements continue to decline (Table 9-1), while protein requirements remain stable, with an intake of 0.75 g per kg body weight being recommended for both sexes throughout early and middle adulthood. An important point, which will be discussed in a later section, is that the need for ample protein, even while energy requirements are declining, mandates a change in dietary patterns. For a variety of reasons, the appropriate adjustments are often not made. The result is a surprisingly high frequency of protein-energy malnutrition among older adults, even in affluent industrial societies. Protein, carbohydrate, and fats are, of course, not the only nutrients that can become deficient in the diet of the elderly. Some of the vitamins and minerals

**Table 9-1**  Mean adult weights, heights, energy and protein requirements.

| Age (years) | Weight (kg) | Height (cm) | Daily energy allowance (kcal) | Daily protein allowance (g/kg) |
|---|---|---|---|---|
| *Male* | | | | |
| 18–24.9 | 70 | 177 | 2,800 | 0.75 |
| 25–49.9 | 69 | 176 | 2,600 | 0.75 |
| 50–69.9 | 68 | 173 | 2,300 | 0.75 |
| >70 | 66 | 171 | 2,000 | 0.75[a] |
| *Female* | | | | |
| 18–24.9 | 58 | 163 | 2,300 | 0.75 |
| 25–49.9 | 59 | 163 | 2,200 | 0.75 |
| 50–69.9 | 59 | 160 | 2,000 | 0.75 |
| >70 | 59 | 158 | 1,700 | 0.75[a] |

[a]May require upward adjustment.
Source: Adapted from Pellett (1990a,b).

known to be involved in nutritional deficiencies in the aged will be briefly reviewed next.

## Vitamins

### Thiamin

Although it is generally thought that vitamin requirements of the elderly are essentially the same as those of the young adult, there are circumstances which lead to a need for altered intakes in older individuals. In a recent study conducted in Ireland, Smidt *et al.* (1991) found that thiamin supplementation improved the appetite and energy intake of elderly women. As a result, body weight increased and the women expressed an improvement in general well-being. Associated with the feeling of well-being, these women also reported improved sleep patterns and less fatigue and daytime sleeping. The overall result was an increase in activity level. The beneficial effects of thiamin supplementation may arise from a correction of thiamin deficiency which has been shown to be associated with lowered alpha-wave activities in the electroencephalograph tracings of elderly subjects (Tucker *et al.*, 1990).

### Vitamin A and the Carotenoids

Elderly individuals often exhibit elevated serum levels of vitamin A, thought to reflect greater absorption from dietary sources. The presence of higher levels of retinyl esters in the plasma of older people may be the result of poorer clearance of chylomicron-bound esters by the aging liver. Persistently poor clearance can lead to high serum concentrations of free retinol which is toxic to tissues. Consequently, a high vitamin A intake can be potentially toxic to the elderly. In view of the tendency to take large quantities of vitamins exhibited by many older people, vitamin A toxicity is a risk that merits concern (Hollander and Dadufalza, 1990).

It also seems likely that the rate of absorption of $\beta$-carotene is enhanced with increasing age (Maiani et al., 1989). $\beta$-carotene has been shown to have anti-cancer properties where it is effective in reversing pre-cancerous conditions such as leukoplakia (Garewal, 1991; Krinsky, 1991; Stich et al., 1991). It is possible that the cancer-preventing attributes of the carotenoids involve immunomodulation, there being evidence of a dose-dependent increase in the percentage of circulating white cells with natural killer (NK) markers and expressing interleukin-2 receptors following $\beta$-carotene administration (Watson et al., 1991). On the basis of a steadily mounting body of information, the carotenoids, available from a number of dietary sources, have substantial anti-cancer potential. The lipid-soluble carotenoids also have the property of quenching singlet molecular oxygen, an antioxidant effect that is believed to have anti-cancer properties quite apart from their immunomodulatory ones (DiMascio et al., 1991). These antioxidant properties are shared by several other biologically active compounds, all of which may stop the chain reaction of free radical formation (Niki et al., 1991).

## Other Antioxidants

Beside the carotenoids, the tocopherols, which are also lipid soluble, are an important category of antioxidant compounds. They are probably the most efficient scavengers of hydroperoxyl radicals in membranes. Vitamin E ($\alpha$-tocopherol), being a lipophilic antioxidant that is present within the membrane itself, has the ability to suppress oxidative damage to membranes with maximum effectiveness (Niki et al., 1991; Packer, 1991). Like $\beta$-carotene, vitamin E is also believed to have a role in the improvement of the immune response. This role is thought to be effected through suppression of prostaglandin E-2 ($PGE_2$) and possibly other lipid peroxidation products in older subjects (Meydani et al., 1990).

In addition to the fat-soluble antioxidants there are a number of water-soluble compounds as well as the mineral selenium that all have antioxidant properties (Diplock, 1991). Among the water-soluble compounds are included ascorbic acid (vitamin C) and certain cellular thiols. One of the latter, glutathione, is an important substrate for antioxidant enzymes and is also capable of nonenzymatic scavenging of radicals. Thiols that are associated with membrane proteins are also believed to have antioxidant properties (DiMascio et al., 1991). Interactions of lipid-soluble and water-soluble antioxidants with other compounds at the membrane can enhance the effectiveness of cellular antioxidant defense. Cancers of the esophagus, stomach, liver, colon, breast, and prostate may all eventually be shown to be responsive to antioxidants used singly or in combination (Weisburger, 1991).

Both the lipid-soluble carotenoids and water-soluble ascorbic acid are believed to be capable of slowing or stopping the sequence of events culminating in multi-focal gastric carcinoma. Fahn (1991) reports that the progression of Parkinson's disease may also be slowed by administration of high doses of lipid-soluble tocopherol and ascorbate and there is evidence that inflamed human knee joints, in which some of the damage may be caused by radical-mediated lipid peroxidation, also respond to antioxidant treatment (Merry *et al.*, 1991).

One of the properties of vitamin C which is thought to underlie some of its beneficial effects is its ability to suppress the formation of *N*-nitroso compounds which are often the product of bacterial metabolism (Tannenbaum *et al.*, 1991). In the etiology of gastric carcinoma, ascorbic acid is secreted directly into the gastric lumen when gastric acidity is normal and is present in concentrations much higher than in plasma. However, under conditions of hypochlorhydria, the concentration of ascorbic acid in gastric juice declines sharply and the vulnerability of the gastric mucosa to metaplasia and ultimately dysplasia is the result (Schorah *et al.*, 1991). Schorah *et al.* have also shown that chronic gastritis reduces the vitamin C concentration of gastric juice and induced hypochlorhydria can drive its concentration down to virtually zero.

Vitamin C is also thought to be protective against the occurrence of cataracts, a condition that becomes virtually universal in people over 85 years of age. Jacques and Chylack (1991) cite epidemiologic evidence of a high risk of cataract when vitamin C and other antioxidant intakes are low. The etiology of cataract formation involves oxidation in the early stages of loss of transparency. Risk factors include diabetes, radiation (UV-B and X-ray), some drugs, nutritional status and, possibly, episodes of acute dehydration (Bunce *et al.*, 1990). Diabetes alone increases the risk by a factor of three to four. The onset of cataract shows a close association with the duration and intensity of ultraviolet radiation exposure, but part of the damage is also derived from the pressure of oxyradicals. Antioxidant scavenging of oxyradicals can be accomplished by a combination of compounds which includes ascorbate, riboflavin, vitamin E, and pyruvate (Varma, 1991). In a recent comparison of supplementation patterns of 175 cataract patients and 175 cataract-free individuals, Robertson *et al.* (1991) found that the cataract-free individuals used significantly more vitamin C and vitamin E. These investigators conclude that a reduction of cataract occurrence approximating 50% can be accomplished by supplementation with these antioxidant vitamins. It appears that the intake of vitamin C is the determinant of its pharmacokinetics and that age itself does not reduce its effectiveness, encouraging news indeed for potential cataract patients (Blanchard *et al.*, 1990).

## Vitamin D

Vitamin D is produced in the skin when sufficient ultraviolet radiation is present to irradiate ergosterol. People who spend relatively brief periods of time outdoors usually produce enough vitamin D to satisfy their requirements. However, in higher latitudes during the winter months, short days and unpleasant weather can combine to reduce vitamin D synthesis below critical levels. This is especially true of elderly people who are apprehensive of falls under icy and snowy conditions. Thus, there is a growing population at risk for vitamin D deficiency and vitamin D supplementation may frequently be necessary. The importance of vitamin D in the absorption of calcium in the intestine is well known. However, cells of a number of other tissues, including bone and kidney, have vitamin D receptors (Norman, 1979, 1984, 1985; Walters, 1985; Haussler, 1986). Receptors have recently been identified in the skin, brain, pancreas, pituitary and gonads, and in several cancer cell lines (Norman, 1990). The functions of many of these receptors are still unknown, but with increasing information, it has become evident that the vitamin D endocrine system is extensive. It is likely that some elements of immune regulation are within its purview (Rigby, 1988), as is regulation of insulin secretion and, possibly, oncogene expression (Nemere and Norman, 1982; Reichel *et al.*, 1989).

The regulation of serum calcium levels is perhaps the best understood function of vitamin D. By direct interaction with the DNA of intestinal mucosal cells, vitamin D facilitates synthesis of a binding protein which transports calcium from the intestinal lumen to the bloodstream. Under extreme circumstances, vitamin D also acts to stimulate rapid movement across the intestinal-cell membrane through a mechanism called transcaltachia, which is thought to involve interaction of vitamin D with the cholesterol component of the target cell membrane (Nemere *et al.*, 1987).

Vitamin D levels are themselves regulated by a negative-feedback system modulated by serum calcium levels. The most active form of vitamin D is $1,25(OH)_2D_3$. It is produced by twice hydroxylating cholecalciferol that had been produced in the skin by ultraviolet radiation of ergosterol. The first hydroxylation takes place in the liver, producing $25(OH)D_3$. The second hydroxylation occurs in the proximal tubules of the kidney. Although the predominant form of vitamin D leaving the kidney is $1,25(OH)_2D_3$, there is a second form, $24,25(OH)_2D_3$, also produced. Therefore, four different forms of vitamin D, all having different potential functions, may be simultaneously present in the blood of a normal individual.

It has been noted that vitamin D supplementation of elderly nursing-home patients may increase the serum concentration of $25(OH)D_3$ without an increase in the concentration of $1,25(OH)D_3$ (Himmelstein *et al.*, 1990). The significance of this effect for bone mineral status is presently unknown, but it has been shown that the receptors of intestinal mucosal cells bind 1,000 times more tightly to $1,25(OH)_2D_3$ than to $25(OH)D_3$ and that no binding at all takes place with the unhydroxylated precursor cholecalciferol (Norman, 1990). It is therefore possible that supplementation may only be effective at high dosages. Since vitamin D is fat soluble and therefore stored in the body, overdosing can produce toxic effects. When dietary sources of vitamin D are the only source and when minimal outdoor activity is experienced, supplementation has been shown to be essential (Webb *et al.*, 1990). A dose of 10 mg (400 IV) per day has been suggested as adequate.

## Calcium

The many roles that calcium performs in human physiology assures its status as a major macronutrient. Serum calcium levels are regulated to stay within limits of 7–13 mg. Any sustained deviations outside these limits can lead to dire consequences. Bone is the ultimate reservoir of calcium, and under most circumstances, the physiological functions of calcium are assigned a higher priority than its structural role as a component of calcium hydroxyapatite, or bone mineral. Consequently, any derangement of calcium homeostasis or of the regulatory systems monitoring it has the potential to produce bone loss. The clinical conditions arising from such derangements include rickets, osteomalacia, and osteoporosis. Osteoporosis is quite common among the elderly, especially among women, and is present to some degree in all humans living beyond the age of 90 years (see Plato *et al.*, this volume). For this reason, the increase in the number of people living beyond the age of 70 years has led to much concern about calcium homeostasis. One result of this concern has been an increase in the recommended daily allowance for all elderly people from 800 mg to 1,000 mg per day. Many physicians now recommend 1,500 mg per day for postmenopausal women and 2,000 mg per day is not an uncommon recommendation for the high-risk age–sex group.

As mentioned in the preceding section, absorption of dietary calcium is, in large part, vitamin D-dependent. Although some absorption occurs in the absence of vitamin D, it would not be sufficient to maintain homeostasis. Even when abundant calcium is present in the diet and when vitamin D is present in normal concentrations, calcium absorption may occur at a very low rate if serum calcium levels are high. As seen in Figure 9-1, net calcium absorption rises very little with increasing calcium intake but the absorption curve does vary to reflect different physiological states such as puberty, pregnancy, and lactation when women become highly "calcium efficient." The efficiency of absorption declines in the elderly, so that what may have been considered an adequate intake becomes inadequate and supplementation may not achieve its goal of restoring homeostatic balance.

There is a highly significant inverse correlation between calcium intake and the fraction absorbed (Heaney *et al.*, 1989). The mean absorption fraction declines from 0.45 at approximately 200 mg calcium per day to 0.15 at 2 g per day. The fall in absorptive efficiency with age has been calculated to be 0.0021 per year with an additional one-time decrease of 0.022 at the time of menopausal estrogen loss in women.

Even in younger individuals, dietary factors can reduce the efficiency of calcium absorption quite sharply. Phytates and oxalates can bind calcium and prevent its absorption. A high-protein diet can lead to urinary excretion of calcium, presumably through the mechanism of increased phosphate excretion, although insulin may play a role in the process as well (Howe, 1990).

Despite the lack of efficiency associated with calcium supplementation, it does produce measurable changes that are desirable. Calcium carbonate supplementation has been shown to lower the serum concentrations of parathyroid hormones in subjects at risk for Type II (senile) osteoporosis (Kochersberger *et al.*, 1990). This effect would tend to reduce bone reabsorption and thereby lower the risk of non-traumatic fractures.

Low calcium intakes are associated with increased risk of hypertension. Therefore supplementation to achieve intakes at or above the recommended

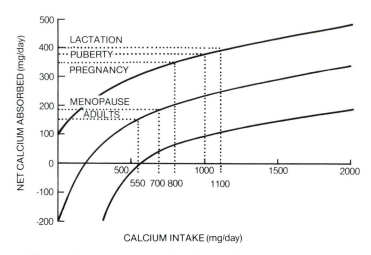

**Figure 9-1** Calcium absorption as related to calcium intake and physiological states. From Norman (1990).

daily allowance (RDA) may be essential in high-risk populations (McCarron *et al.*, 1991). One mechanism by which calcium prevents sodium chloride-sensitive hypertension is through increasing noradrenergic input to the hypothalamus, enhancing its ability to adjust fluid volume rapidly through diuresis and urinary salt excretion (Oparil *et al.*, 1991).

Although the benefits of sufficient calcium intake seem quite clear, it has also been shown that, on occasion, calcium supplements can interfere with absorption of other nutrients. One such nutrient is iron. All calcium supplements, including calcium carbonate, calcium phosphate, calcium citrate, and calcium chloride inhibit absorption of iron supplements when taken with a meal (Cook *et al.*, 1991). Even the calcium in milk and cheese can interfere with iron absorption, the effect possibly arising from impaired mucosal transfer of iron (Hallberg *et al.*, 1991). There has been considerable discussion of the possible effects of caffeine and alcohol use on calcium absorption. Barger-Lux *et al.* (1990) found little effect from caffeine consumption by postmenopausal women, while Hernandez-Avila *et al.* (1991) found that both caffeine and alcohol increased the risk of osteoporotic fractures in middle-aged women. They report an increase in urinary calcium excretion associated with caffeine use and cite an inverse relationship between amount of alcohol consumed and bone density in women.

## Alcohol

The effects of alcohol consumption may be of considerable nutritional significance among the elderly. Use of alcohol by the elderly is quite common both in the United States and in European populations. Sulsky *et al.* (1990) report that among a non-institutionalized, non-alcoholic population of men and women aged 60–95 years, 53% of the men and 42% of the women drank at least 2 g of alcohol per week, the equivalent of two 4 oz glasses of wine. The men drank more than the women and, in both sexes, intake tended to decrease with age. While alcohol averaged 6.2% of total caloric intake in the 60–69-year age group it made up only 3.8% of total calories among those over 80 years of age. It should be recalled, however, that decreasing lean body mass and age-related loss of fluid could result in even the lowered consumption in the 80-year-olds having equal or greater pharmacological impact.

Holbrook *et al.* (1990) have found that men, but not women, who developed non-insulin-dependent diabetes (NIDDM), used significantly more alcohol than those who did not. The highest rate of NIDDM incidence was, in this study, found among heavy-drinking men. It has been found that in women, energy consumed in the form of alcohol tends to displace the amount consumed in the form of sucrose (Colditz *et al.*, 1991). Men, on the other hand, tend to add their alcohol-derived energy intake to their total. There is a possibility, perhaps most likely in women, that there is a relationship between the appetite for sugar and the appetite for alcohol and that satisfaction of this appetite from one source will reduce intake of the other. The long-term effects of heavy alcohol consumption on pancreatic and liver function may derive from physiological events related to the satisfaction of these appetites.

In terms of the sex difference in energy intakes associated with alcohol consumption, the observations of Garn and colleagues (1989) on the relationship between socioeconomic status and degree of fatness are of interest. These investigators found that in Western industrialized nations socioeconomic status is inversely related to fatness in women, but in men the relationship is positive. In addition, the relationship of fatness to educational level is parabolic in men with the lowest fatness levels occurring in men with 9–12 years of education. Sulsky *et al.* (1990) found a positive correlation between alcohol consumption and educational level and there is a strong positive correlation between educational attainment and socioeconomic status. Men tend to add their alcohol-derived calories to their intake from other dietary sources and thus gain weight, while alcohol-consuming women tend to maintain the level of energy intake and thereby hold their weight constant. The observation by Garn and his colleagues that better educated men may be fatter than their spouses quite possibly reflects the nature of drinking patterns characterizing contemporary American society.

It has long been known that alcohol consumption has the effect of elevating serum uric acid levels. Although uric acid can act as an antioxidant and thereby have some beneficial effects, excessively high levels can become a major concern in the elderly and recent studies have shown that alcohol restriction, weight control, and diuretics may all be necessary to keep uric acid levels under control (Loenen *et al.*, 1990).

Along with its acknowledged deleterious effects on human health, alcohol consumption has some effects that appear to be beneficial. The amount of high-density lipoprotein cholesterol (HDL-C) present in the blood an hour after a meal at which alcohol is consumed has been found to exceed the amount following a meal without alcohol by more than 11% (Veenstra *et al.*, 1990). This increase appeared mainly in the HDL2-C subfraction and the increase is most pronounced in middle-aged males. The HDL2-C fraction does appear to be the most environmentally sensitive fraction of the HDL-C component as Christian *et al.* (1990) found in a comparison of aging male dizygotic and monozygotic twins. In view of the fact that healthy octogenarians, at least those in the Framingham Heart Study (Schaefer *et al.*, 1989), are exceedingly unlikely to have reduced HDL-C levels, factors that increase those levels appear to have a positive association with survivorship.

## Malnutrition Among the Elderly

In nursing homes and among the elderly living independently, protein-energy malnutrition (PEM) is not uncommon in the United States and in generally well-fed western European populations. One study (Thorslund *et al.*, 1990) estimates the prevalence of PEM in a European population of elderly people living at home at around 5%, unrelated to age or sex. There are many reasons for the occurrence of malnutrition in the elderly. Socioeconomic factors such as poverty and inabilities to shop for or to prepare well-balanced meals, lack of social stimulus for eating, depression, and anxiety may all function singly or in combination to suppress food intake. Other factors, such as tooth loss and poorly fitted dentures, can severely limit the variety of foods consumed. Fifty per cent of all Americans over age 65 have lost all of their teeth (Fischer and Johnson, 1990), an important factor in their selection of foods. Nearly one in five older adults suffers from xerostomia (dry mouth), a condition arising from salivary gland dysfunctions associated with aging and leading to problems in lubricating, masticating, tasting, and swallowing food (Rhodus and Brown, 1990). Food tolerance is affected adversely by these factors and loss of appetite and reduced food intake often is the result. Dry mouth sufferers have been found to exhibit significant deficiencies in intakes of fiber, potassium, vitamin $B_6$, iron, calcium, and zinc (Rhodus and Brown, 1990), deficiencies that clearly threaten overall nutritional status and health.

Chemosensory dysfunction is also common among the elderly. This condition can be the result of decline in the sensitivity of the sense of smell and the loss of taste buds associated with aging. Interestingly, loss of taste sensitivity has on occasion been shown to be associated with an increase in food consumption, perhaps as a compensatory response, while distorted taste perception most often leads to reduced food intake and weight loss (Mattes *et al.*, 1990).

Whatever the cause, anorexia in the elderly has serious implications for health status. Protein-energy malnutrition, in particular, has been shown to be highly correlated with risk of mortality when disease or trauma is experienced (Sullivan *et al.* 1990). In a study of mortality risk among patients at a geriatric rehabilitation center, Sullivan *et al.*, (1990, 1991) found that the best predictor of mortality was the percentage of weight lost in the year preceding admission. Even where factors such as diagnostic category, age, co-existing morbid conditions, indicators of disease severity, and functional status were controlled for, involuntary weight loss during the year preceding admission remained the strongest predictor of mortality and the amount of weight lost was positively correlated with the level of risk. Even when factors such as the risk of developing infections following trauma such as a bone fracture are assessed, it is found that indicators of nutritional status are effective predictors of patient outcome (Puskarich *et al.*, 1990).

While much emphasis has been placed on risk factors for cardiovascular diseases and cancer, the spectrum of nutritional factors implicated in morbidity and mortality among the elderly is much broader than frequently recognized. In a recent study of Dutch vegetarians aged 65–97 years, comparison with omnivores showed that while the vegetarians had aged successfully with respect to cardiovascular risk factors, they exhibited a higher risk for marginal iron, zinc, and vitamin $B_{12}$ status (Lowik *et al.*, 1990).

In a middle-aged Netherlands population studied by Kramhout *et al.* (1990) it was found that nutritional patterns have undergone some distinct changes since 1960, with decreases in consumption of bread, potatoes, and edible fats, and increases in fruits, pastries, and animal protein. In Warsaw, Poland, it was found that fat intakes in middle age remain high at about 137% of RDA in men and about 108% in women. However, in this population, intakes of carbohydrates, calcium, vitamin A, vitamin $B_1$, and vitamin C were all well below recommended values for both sexes (Pardo *et al.*, 1991). The marked contrast in mortality rates for cardiovascular diseases and cancer in eastern and central Europe compared to those in central America and the United States clearly reflects these differences in dietary patterns in middle age (see Table 9-2), although these associations are much less clear and predictable in the older age groups.

The voluminous literature (Metropolitan Life Insurance Company, 1959, 1984; Van Itallie, 1979; Hirsch *et al.*, 1985; Van Itallie and Abraham, 1985; Battenelli *et al.*, 1986) on the association of high-fat diets and obesity with coronary heart disease, some types of cancer, and diabetes documents obesity's relationship with reduced life expectancy. Recent increases in the recommended weights for height for older people (US Department of Agriculture,

**Table 9-2** Major causes of mortality in selected populations of Central Europe, Central and North America (deaths per 100,000 population).

| Country | Total deaths | Cardiovascular disease | Cancer | Diabetes | Influenza and pneumonia | Infectious diseases of the GI tract |
|---|---|---|---|---|---|---|
| Austria | 1,232.0 | 658.4 | 279.2 | 16.1 | 26.6 | 0.1 |
| Czechoslovakia | 1,178.7 | 611.5 | 254.9 | 17.5 | 43.4 | 0.3 |
| Hungary | 1,348.1 | 714.1 | 299.0 | 17.9 | 14.9 | 0.2 |
| El Salvador | 625.3 | 59.2 | 17.1 | 5.4 | 13.6 | 46.5 |
| Guatemala | 1,031.7 | 52.3 | 30.7 | 5.2 | 144.0 | 203.9 |
| Mexico | 595.5 | 98.0 | 33.7 | 21.7 | 47.8 | 50.7 |
| United States | 817.9 | 361.4 | 203.0 | 15.8 | 29.4 | 0.2 |

GI = gastrointestinal.
Sources: United Nations (1986) and National Center for Health Statistics (1991).

**Table 9-3** Major causes of death in the United States, 1900–1991 (deaths per 100,000 population).

| Cause of death | 1900 | 1960 | 1970 | 1980 | 1990 | 1991 (Feb) |
|---|---|---|---|---|---|---|
| Cardiovascular disease | 345.2 | 515.1 | 496.0 | 436.4 | 377.1 | 361.4 |
| Cancer | 64.0 | 149.2 | 162.8 | 183.9 | 199.9 | 203.0 |
| Pneumonia and influenza | 202.0 | 37.3 | 37.0 | 24.1 | 31.9 | 29.4 |
| Tuberculosis | 194.0 | 6.1 | 2.6 | 0.9 | 0.7 | 0.7 |

Sources: US Bureau of the Census (1986) and National Center for Health Statistics (1991).

1990) have sparked vigorous and sometimes acrimonious debate in the nutritional literature (see Stampfer *et al.*, 1991; Willett *et al.*, 1991). Although well-intentioned, several arguments apparently fail to account for changing human nutritional characteristics over the life span or that among the oldest-old (persons over 85 years of age), the risk of mortality from causes other than cardiovascular disease is important (Table 9-3). In the United States deaths due to cardiovascular diseases declined steadily after the mid-1950s, while cancer deaths, which are also age-associated, have increased. Importantly, while cardiovascular diseases and cancer remained the leading causes of death, jointly accounting for about 66% of all mortality, cardiovascular diseases alone accounted for 42% of the total. In other words, currently 58% of deaths in the United States arise from causes other than cardiovascular. Therefore any discussion of nutritional recommendations for the elderly must consider factors beyond those emphasized by the "cardiocentric majority."

In a recent analysis of trends in vital statistics in the United States, Olshansky and colleagues (1990) point out that if all circulatory disease, cancer, and diabetes deaths were eliminated, the expectation of life at age 50 would increase by only about 15 years. As the number of people aged 85 and over increases, enhancing immune system function becomes a major concern. Since immune function plays an important role in cancer etiology, any factors that enhance its effectiveness may potentially increase life expectancy. It is imperative that research in geriatric nutrition addresses itself toward realization of this potential.

## BODY COMPOSITION AND DISEASE RESISTANCE

The foregoing discussion addressed the nutritional requirements experienced at various stages in the human life span and the major causes of mortality which are generally acknowledged to have important nutritional correlates. It has already been pointed out that involuntary weight loss in older patients is frequently associated with poor survival during and following treatment. A possible explanation for these observations lies in the changes that occur in human body composition with aging. Age and activity levels interact to elicit

**Table 9-4**  Ratio of adipose tissue to total body weight in humans.

| Age | Total body fat/total body weight | |
| --- | --- | --- |
| | Male | Female |
| 25 | 0.14 | 0.25 |
| 40 | 0.22 | 0.32 |
| 55 | 0.25 | 0.38 |

Source: Masoro (1972).

changes in body composition even when nutritional factors are held constant. Does human adiposity increase because of decreased exercise or do humans exercise less because of increased adiposity? There is no totally correct answer to this question because the two alternatives are not mutually exclusive. Closely related physiological processes such as the supply of oxygen to tissues during maximal exercise ($VO_2$ max), undergo a steady decline with age even in individuals who continue to exercise vigorously. The difference between exercisers and non-exercisers is in the slope of the curve. Even with continued vigorous exercise, the proportion of skeletal muscle decreases and the proportion of fat increases with age (see Table 9-4). Again, this trend can be modified but apparently not avoided and, as always, human variation in all such traits is considerable.

In a recent study of healthy persons aged 60–83 years, total body fat averaged 31% of total body weight in men and 44% in women (Deurenberg *et al.*, 1989, 1990), indicating that the trend seen in Table 9-4 continues into old age (see Garn, this volume).

Differences in published values for total body fat (TBF), total body water (TBW), and lean body mass (LBM) arise from the use of different methods to estimate them. For a number of years, estimates based on calculations of body density through hydrostatic weighing were thought to be the most accurate. Using overall density and known values for density of muscle as opposed to adipose tissue, the ratio of fat to lean was calculated using equations developed by Siri (1956a, 1956b). This method formed the basis of the two-compartment model for estimation of body composition in living individuals. In recent years it has become increasingly recognized that the two-compartment model, long the "gold standard" of body composition analysis, has serious shortcomings, and methods less dependent on the two-compartment model have gained increasing favor (Slaughter *et al.*, 1988). One source of error in the two-compartment model lies in variations in the aqueous fraction of the LBM or fat-free mass (Baumgartner *et al.*, 1991). Combinations of hydrodensitometry, dual-photon absorptiometry and dilution methods have shown that the two-compartment model can produce very misleading results. However, a number of investigators have found that a relatively simple method for determining total body water (bioelectrical impedance) has proven useful, especially when used in conjunction with other techniques (Heitman, 1990). In fact, one group of investigators reports success in predicting 24-hour energy expenditure, basal energy expenditure, and sleeping energy expenditure using estimates of LBM attained through bioelectrical impedance (Astrup *et al.*, 1990).

Estimation of body composition is often limited to the calculation of the body mass index (BMI). This is simply done by dividing weight (kg) by height (m) squared. While such a calculation clearly ignores the important differences in the density of muscle, fat, and bone, estimation of BMI has the attractive advantages of being noninvasive and based on easily accessible information. Consequently, there has been considerable interest in the use of the BMI as a basis for body composition estimates. Much controversy has developed as a result. Some investigators defend the BMI as an estimate of obesity because of its high correlation with weight and relatively low correlation with height (Billewicz *et al.*, 1962; Khosla and Lowe, 1967; Rao and Singh, 1970; Cerovska *et al.*, 1977; Babu and Chuttani, 1979; Roche *et al.*, 1981). Others cite the high correlation of BMI values with skinfold thickness, another indicator of obesity (Florey, 1970; Frisancho and Flegel, 1982). Yet others have found acceptable correlations of BMI with a combination of skinfold thickness and hydrostatically determined weight (Benn, 1971; Goldbourt and Medalie, 1974; Revicki and Israel, 1986). However, a large and growing contingent finds the BMI seriously deficient as an indicator of obesity. Durnin *et al.* (1985) warn against its use for this purpose and Garn (1986) and Micozzi *et al.* (1986) make the point that BMI is as much a measure of muscle as it is of fat. McLaren (1987) and Micozzi and Albanes (1987) especially discourage the use of the BMI for individual assessment (the use to which it is most commonly put). As Garn and Pesick (1982) have pointed out, BMI can be misleading because composition of the body varies considerably, even in individuals of identical weight and height. Moreover, lean tissue is heavier than fat and, even within the lean tissue mass itself, there are components that may vary in weight and thereby alter the BMI in misleading ways (Smalley *et al.*, 1990). Acknowledging these shortcomings in the use of the BMI for individual estimates of adiposity, it is still a useful device for assessing population phenomena such as the ongoing trend of increasing BMI with increasing age in the US population (Rossman, 1977; Kahn and Williamson, 1990).

The most severe critic of the use of BMI for diagnosing obesity in the individual is W. L. Ross who, with his colleagues (Ross *et al.*, 1986, 1987, 1988), has demonstrated that the prediction of skinfold values using BMI is only 21.5% better than chance in males and 15.9% better in females. Muscularity and bone density can influence the BMI value far more than fat. As a result, a high BMI value can at times be a function of high muscularity (Hirsch *et al.*, 1985). Basing a diagnosis of obesity on such BMI values would obviously be a serious error and a recommendation to lose weight under such circumstances would, in effect, be a recommendation to lose muscle. The consequences of acting on such a recommendation would be undesirable at any age, but for reasons that will be explored presently, the loss of muscle mass in the elderly is an especially serious matter.

## MUSCLE MASS AND AGING

Loss of muscle mass appears to be an inevitable component of the aging process. This loss is related to whole-body protein turnover and the rate of protein synthesis (Uauy *et al.*, 1978). As a result, aging humans experience a change in amino-acid requirements (Young *et al.*, 1982). With increasing age, the concentration of serum albumin also declines as the rate of albumin syntheses falls (Gersovitz *et al.*, 1980; Pellett, 1990a). It has been shown that even high-quality egg protein, consumed at a rate of 0.8 g per kg body weight per day, is insufficient to maintain nitrogen balance in most elderly men and women over a 30-day period (Gersovitz *et al.*, 1981). There is some evidence that maintenance of a favorable energy balance may have a mitigating effect, increasing the amount of dietary protein retained (Zanni *et al.*, 1979). Usually, however, while muscle-protein turnover accounts for 30% of total protein turnover in the young adult, it represents only 20% of the total in the healthy elderly adult (Munro, 1983; Pellett, 1990a).

As muscle mass declines, so does the basal metabolic rate (BMR). It has been estimated that BMR declines from 3 to 5% per decade from age 55 to age 75 and as much as 7% per decade beyond age 75 (National Research Council, 1980). The amount by which physical activity increases energy expenditure also declines with age. Light to moderate activity raises the metabolic rate to a level 1.6 times BMR in individuals 50–70 years old, but only 1.5 times BMR beyond age 70 (Pellett, 1990b). Still, despite lower BMR, sedentary energy expenditure in older people appears to decline only in proportion to diminished body size, indicating that their lower energy intakes may relate mainly to lower activity levels (Vaughan *et al.*, 1991). There is evidence that age-related decline in muscle mass is related to a decline in growth hormone levels. Marcus *et al.* (1990) report that administration of a recombinant human growth hormone to elderly people resulted in a dose-dependent increase in somatomedin-C, and increased nitrogen retention. When malnourished (20% below average body weight) older persons were similarly treated, arm muscle circumference increased, and weight gain averaged 2.2 kg (Kaiser *et al.*, 1991). There was also a significant association between weight gain and interstitial growth factor-1 concentration.

In a study of the loss of muscle mass in women, Aloia *et al.* (1991) found that the loss of total body potassium (a reliable measure of cell loss) was negligible before menopause, but accelerated at menopause. Although loss of potassium was significantly related to declines in bone density and total body calcium, it was totally unrelated to total body fat. Lack of association with total body fat is an indication that there is little or no protective value to adiposity with respect to postmenopausal bone loss.

Diversion of exchange amino acids freed from muscle to other uses when protein intake is inadequate or when trauma or infection increases the demand for amino acids has been well documented (Young and Marchini, 1990). Newsholme *et al.* (1988) outline a system in which enhanced muscle protein degradation serves to provide amino acids for tissue repair and to sustain the immune response. Some amino acids are also directed to the liver where they are converted to an energy source through gluconeogenesis. Branched-chain amino acids serve as donors of nitrogen for the syntheses of glutamine in muscle. Glutamine, when released from muscle, may be used to support the function of cells of the immune system as well as for tissue repair. This response assumes added importance when a superimposed infectious disease, even a mild one, adversely affects nutritional condition and magnifies the effect of a protein deficient diet (Frenk, 1986).

Animal research on the role of protein turnover after trauma (Cammisa and Tischler, 1982; Tischler, 1983, 1984; Tischler et al., 1986a, 1986b) has shown that increased urinary nitrogen excretion after severe injury results from muscle proteolysis. In humans, such proteolysis arises from muscle insensitivity to insulin following trauma (Brandi et al., 1990). Following the trauma of surgery, patients often become hyperglycemic to the extent that eight times the normal insulin dose is required to return blood glucose levels to normal. When such insulin doses are used, protein loss and lipolysis can be normalized. It has also been shown that administration of $\alpha$-ketoglutarate will maintain nitrogen balance following surgery. $\alpha$-Ketoglutarate has a carbon skeleton corresponding to glutamine. The fact that a normal polyribosome count can be maintained in the muscles of $\alpha$-ketoglutarate-supplemented surgery patients is evidence of continued protein synthesis instead of the shift to proteolysis that would occur in the unsupplemented patient (Hammarquist et al., 1991).

While the benefits of proteolysis following trauma derive from the use of amino acids for energy and tissue repair, loss of amino acids in the urine appears to be clearly maladaptive. Paauw and Davis (1990) postulate a secondary impairment of renal tubule absorption to explain its occurrence. These investigators also report an early decline in serum taurine levels in trauma patients indicating that taurine may play a special role in the post-injury state. Increased excretion of orotic and uric acids, evidence of enhanced pyrimidine and purine liberation associated with protein mobilization, is also seen in trauma victims (Jeevanandam et al., 1991). Age-associated decreases in lean body mass appear to affect the response to trauma, producing a sluggish rise in plasma free amino acids in the early "flow" (catabolic) phase following injury (Jeevanandam et al., 1990).

The evidence for an adaptive response to injury through the release of amino acids from muscle comes from both animal experiments and clinical experience. The use of muscle protein as a reserve to be drawn upon when tissue repair and/or immune response is imperative could mean the difference between life and death in the absence of sophisticated and timely medical intervention. Such exploitation of exchange amino acids is probably an adaptive response of considerable antiquity. Moreover, it is likely that support of the immune response alone is of sufficient importance to warrant diversion of amino acids for its use even in the absence of trauma. Here, however, the evidence is only indirect, in that reduced vigor of the immune response is associated with reduced lean body mass and a shrinking pool of amino acids (Young et al., 1989). Young (1990) argues that older people have generally increased protein needs compared to younger ones. Protein, according to Young, should make up 10% to 12% of total energy intake in the elderly, and essential amino-acid intake should be equal to that of schoolchildren.

While it may not be possible to sustain muscle mass with increasing age, steady supply of essential amino acids through dietary intake could at least furnish the resources needed to repair damage and mount an effective immune response when infections occur. The most desirable situation, of course, would be preservation of muscle mass and effective support of the wound healing process and the immune response. All the evidence supports the argument that it is important for the elderly to preserve muscle mass through an appropriate diet and exercise. Avoidance of obesity to reduce the risks of cardiovascular diseases and certain cancers remains important, but weight loss programs that result in loss of muscle mass may do more harm than good in the long run (Stini, 1991). Elderly people should be encouraged to control their weight, but advice to lose weight should be accompanied by a workable plan to assure preservation of muscle mass. Such a plan requires considerable individual monitoring. It has been argued that exercise can facilitate weight loss without compromising muscle mass (King and Katch, 1986). However, it is doubtful that the right combination of diet and exercise can be achieved when a substantial weight loss is attempted. In a recent study of the effect of high- and low-intensity exercise on the ratio of fat to lean tissue loss experienced by obese women on a 1,200 kcal per day diet, Ballor and colleagues (1990) found that whatever the exercise level, these women reduced lean body mass by 10% while reducing fat mass by 16%. A 16% loss of fat mass was clearly a desirable outcome. It is, however, questionable whether the overall outcome was beneficial, especially in view of the high likelihood that at least some weight gain will occur in the future, a gain that is more likely to be fat than muscle.

The location of fat deposits appears to have a bearing on certain clinical conditions. Fat deposits on the trunk, a pattern most commonly seen in males, relate to risk factors for cardiovascular disease and diabetes to a much greater extent than limb fat deposits or subcutaneous fat (Feldman et al., 1969; Vague et al., 1979: Baumgartner et al., 1986). In truly obese individuals there is a relatively low correlation between the amount of subcutaneous fat and the amount of internal fat (see Garn, this volume). Not only is a predominance of trunk fat a risk factor for coronary heart disease (Blair et al., 1988), but its association with poor glucose tolerance and diabetes adds a whole list of morbidity risk factors (Newell-Morris et al., 1989). Repeated weight-gain and weight-loss cycles have the potential of redistributing body fat in the direction of the trunk, enhancing these risk factors beyond the level of genetic predisposition.

Even in the absence of cycles of weight gain and weight loss, loss of muscle and fat deposition, largely in the trunk, are an aspect of human aging that has proven exceedingly difficult to control. As a result, there is a general tendency for the body mass index to increase with age (Keys et al., 1972; Rossman, 1977).

Using categories derived from the Metropolitan tables for recommended weights (Metropolitan Insurance Company, 1959, 1984), Bray (1978) de-

**Table 9-5**   Body mass index values at several heights and weights.[a]

| Height (cm) | Body mass index (BMI)[b] | | | |
|---|---|---|---|---|
| | 19 Weight (kg) | 20–24 Weight (kg) | 25–27 Weight (kg) | 28 Weight (kg) |
| 160 | 48.6 | 51.2–61.4 | 64.0–69.0 | 71.6 |
| 170 | 54.9 | 57.8–69.4 | 72.3–78.0 | 80.9 |
| 180 | 61.6 | 64.8–77.8 | 81.0–87.5 | 90.7 |
| 190 | 68.6 | 72.2–86.6 | 90.3–97.5 | 101.1 |

[a]Designations according to the Metropolitan Life Insurance Tables of Recommended Weights for Height.
[b]BMI: 19 = excessively lean; 20–24 = acceptable; 25–27 = mildly obese; 28 = obese.

veloped a scale of recommended BMI values. The range of acceptable BMI values using this approach lies between 20 and 24. Values under 20 can be considered excessively lean, values from 25 to 27 are categorized as mildly obese, and those over 27 are designated obese. Table 9-5 shows the BMI values for individuals whose heights are 160, 170, 180, and 190 cm at various weights. It can be seen from these values that a man 180 cm tall (5′ 10″) would be considered mildly obese when his weight exceeds 81 kg (178.5 pounds), and obese at 90.7 kg (200 pounds). While in many instances these designations would be quite acceptable, a number of very fit athletes would also fall well within the obese category, since muscle mass has greater density than fat. On 28 June 1991, a heavyweight championship fight between Mike Tyson and James Rudduck was won by Tyson. The winner, whose height was 180.3 cm and weight was 98 kg, had a BMI of 30.15, while the loser, whose height was 190.5 cm and whose weight was 108 kg, had a BMI of 29.75. In this matchup of two "obese" individuals, the more obese one emerged victorious.

The body mass index at which minimal mortality occurs tends to increase consistently with age between the ages of 29 and 69 years (Society for Actuaries, 1979). Other investigators (Keys, 1980a, 1980b) also found that survival rates were highest among individuals in the mildly obese category. Andres (1980, 1981, 1985) has shown that the relationship between BMI and mortality can be graphed as a "U"- or "J"-shaped curve, with the greatest risk of mortality occurring among the very thin and the very obese. The lowest risk in Andres' U-shaped curve, is again experienced by individuals falling in the "mildly obese" category.

In a study of 8,428 patients admitted to the University of Nebraska Medical Center Hospital at Omaha, Potter et al. (1988) reported survival outcomes that strongly support Andres' conclusions. Moreover, these investigators found the U-shaped distribution of mortality risk was accentuated as age increased. When they split their population into two groups, one whose BMI values were less than 34 and the other with values greater than 34, they found that while thin patients were at significant risk at all ages, the risk for the obese was greater only in the 20–29 year and 50–59 age categories. The relationship of

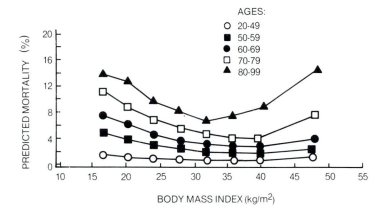

**Figure 9-2**  Predicted probability of death as a function of body mass index (BMI) calculated from the logistic model for each of five age groups. The plotted points are mean values for subjects in a given weight group. Highest mortality almost always occurs at lowest BMI and mortality also increases at greatest BMI.

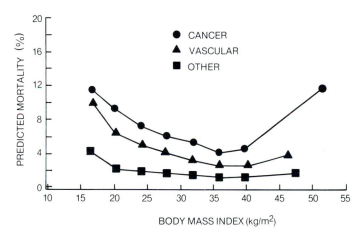

**Figure 9-3**  Predicted probability of death as a function of body mass index (BMI) calculated from the logistic model for each of three disease categories. The plotted points are mean values for subjects in a given weight group. Highest mortality occurs at the extremes of BMI.

obesity to mortality decreased with increasing age, being the weakest of all in the 80–99 year age group (see Figures 9-2 and 9-3).

Most of the hospital patients in the Potter *et al.* study were subjected to trauma of one form or another. Muscle proteolysis in response to trauma was undoubtedly a factor in their survival. That the survival of individuals in the oldest age groups was most closely related to BMI values is added evidence that retention of amino-acid reserves gains importance with age. In view of these findings, the aforementioned relationship between wasting and increased mortality risk can be linked to an adaptive mechanism (muscle proteolysis) that has been compromised to an extent where it is no longer capable of meeting a serious challenge.


## THE AGING DIGESTIVE SYSTEM

A number of anatomical changes occur in the human digestive system with age, some of which have the potential to alter nutritional requirements or intakes. The loss of taste buds and altered perception of taste and smell can have the effect of reducing appetite and food enjoyment (Balogh and Lelkes, 1961; Hermel et al., 1970; Grzegorczyk et al., 1979; Hay and Coons, 1979). Similar effects can arise from dental and periodontal problems and xerostomia. In addition, changes in the tissue layers of the esophagus can make swallowing difficult and reduce food intake. Hiatus hernia, the weakening of the sphincter through which food passes from the esophagus into the stomach, can lead to acid reflux, heartburn, and difficulties in consumption of certain foods. Hiatus hernia is a condition that becomes increasingly common with age and overweight, causing a restriction of dietary choices because of the tendency for certain dense, fibrous foods to block the emptying of the esophagus. Thus, foods that might be considered desirable from the standpoint of their nutritional value for the aging individual are often avoided. Barrett's osephagus, a pre-cancerous change in the cellularity of the esophagus, also becomes more frequent with age. It, too, can lead to avoidance of foods that would otherwise be valuable components of the diet.

In addition to changes in the esophagus, there are a number of predictable changes in gastric secretion and emptying, intestinal and pancreatic morphology, colorectal motility and hepatic mass and blood flow with aging. However, although predictable, the functional significance of any or all of these changes varies greatly from person to person (Altman, 1990). One consequence of this constellation of changes is an alteration of the pharmacokinetics of many medications (Feely and Coakley, 1990).

Both physiological factors and changes in eating habits in response to previously mentioned conditions may lead to an increasing prevalence of glucose intolerance in the aging individual (Fiskens et al., 1991). It is possible that a high-carbohydrate, high-fiber diet in the elderly can improve carbohydrate economy through enhancement of peripheral sensitivity to insulin (Fucagawa et al., 1990). There has been considerable interest in the substitution of fructose for other sugars in the diet, particularly in the elderly, to avoid some of the effects of glucose intolerance. The consumption of fructose has increased dramatically in the United States since 1970 (Hallfrisch, 1990). Fructose is sweeter and less glycogenic than either glucose or sucrose, hence it has been frequently recommended for diabetics and the obese. Fructose is absorbed mainly in the jejunum and metabolized in the liver. Unfortunately, when fructose is consumed in excess of dietary glucose, malabsorption may occur. Also, fructose is more lipogenic than glucose or starches, usually causing greater elevation of serum triglycerides and, sometimes, cholesterol than other carbohydrates. Dietary fructose has resulted in increases in blood pressure and serum uric and lactic acids. Most susceptible to these effects are individuals who already show hypertension, hyperinsulinemia, non-insulin-dependent diabetes, and/or are postmenopausal. On the basis of these factors, deliberate addition of fructose to the diet beyond that contained in fruits and vegetables does not seem advisable for older people (Hallfrisch, 1990).

Another concern for all age groups, but one that is especially felt by the elderly, is the control of cholesterol levels. It would be beyond the scope of this survey to explore the many facets of cholesterol metabolism and nutritional factors that could interact with them. Nevertheless, it should be noted that alterations in intestinal absorption, liver and pancreatic function, and gut flora that occur with age add additional elements of unpredictability to the control of serum cholesterol levels. Lichtenstein (1990) points out that the handling of cholesterol in the intestine involves maintenance of a balance between absorption, excretion, and metabolism by gut microflora. Of ingested cholesterol, between 34% and 57% is actually absorbed. The amount absorbed is affected by the amount consumed, the simultaneous presence of certain plant sterols in the gut, dietary fiber, intestinal motility/transit time and, quite possibly, the relative proportions of fatty acids present in ingested food.

About 150 mg of cholesterol is excreted daily in the feces. This excreted component is derived from bile secreted into the gut as well as from sloughed intestinal epithelial cells and the unabsorbed fraction of ingested cholesterol. The major products of cholesterol metabolism in the gut are coprostanol, cholestanol, cholestanone, and epicoprostanol. The degree to which bacteria in the gut metabolize cholesterol is influenced by dietary intake, with dairy products having a major effect. Some alterations of bacterial cholesterol metabolism in the intestine can increase the risk of a number of colon disorders. Age-associated changes in the number, species, and locations of bacteria in the alimentary tract have considerable potential for affecting cholesterol metabolism in unpredictable ways.

## Diverticulosis

Another characteristic of the aging gut that may alter dietary habits is a tendency toward diverticulosis. The impact of Western diets, which have been characterized by low-fiber intakes, increased transit times, and reduced fecal volume, has been the subject of considerable discussion (Burkitt, 1977), particularly with respect to its potential to increase intra-abdominal pressure and its sequelae of hiatus hernia, diverticulosis, hemorrhoids, and assorted other conditions. However, other age-related changes are now being identified as having a role in the occurrence of diverticulosis. The mechanical properties of the wall of the intestine itself appears to be subject to alterations that are part of the aging process. The tensile strength and elasticity of the intestinal wall decline with age. This decline is most marked in the left colon, which is the narrowest and thickest part (Watters and Smith, 1990). It appears that addition of fiber to the diet can mitigate the effects of this change, lending support to Burkett's earlier recommendations but for quite different reasons.

Diverticulosis is generally not of clinical significance and may exist for some considerable time without symptoms. However, some diverticula may become large and may be entered by seeds or other small elements of food. With sufficient build up of such material in the intestinal outpocketings, infection can ultimately occur, producing diverticulitis, which can be extremely uncomfortable and, if a diverticulum ruptures into the abdominal cavity, life threatening.

## Hypochlorhydria and Achlorhydria

A widespread condition associated with aging is a reduction in the amount of hydrochloric acid produced by the parietal cells of the stomach. This condition, designated hypochlorhydria, can have far-reaching effects on the digestive process. About 30% of elderly Americans are known to have a clinically significant loss of hydrochloric acid production (Champagne, 1989). In addition to affecting intestinal absorption of a number of nutrients, hypochlorhydria potentiates pathological changes that range from merely unpleasant to life threatening. For instance, prolonged hypochlorhydria can result in bacterial colonization of the stomach. Some of these bacteria may generate carcinogens during their metabolism of stomach contents. If for no other reason, this possibility warrants caution when long-term suppression of gastric acid production is elected as a therapeutic measure to treat heartburn or gastritis of certain forms (Karnes and Walsh, 1990; Selway, 1990).

An age-related increase in the frequency of *Helicobacterium pylori* infection in the elderly parallels an increase in the prevalence of gastritis. Gastritis is, in turn, closely associated with hypochlorhydria and gastric carcinoma (Green and Graham, 1990). When hypochlorhydria progresses to achlorhydria, a number of events ensue. Prolonged achlorhydria stimulates hypergastrinemia, which produces a steady oversupply of gastrin accompanied by chronically elevated mRNA levels in secretory cells (Dockray *et al.*, 1991). Hypergastrinemia is thought to be the result of hyperplasia of antral G-cells in the atrophic and occasionally metaplastic cells of the gastric body mucosa (Kern *et al.*, 1990). One symptom of this series of events is pernicious anemia. A failure of atrophic gastric mucosa to produce sufficient intrinsic factor leads to deficient absorption of vitamin $B_{12}$. Vitamin $B_{12}$ deficiency usually develops through a slowly progressive continuum in the older patient (Goodman and Salt, 1990). The early signs are a generalized fatigue, weakness, diarrhea, and indigestion. Although pernicious anemia is the classic cause of this cluster of symptoms, achlorhydria alone may produce a similar symptomology, as can fish tapeworm infestation and a strictly vegetarian diet. Iron deficiency often co-exists in all of these conditions. In patients with low serum vitamin $B_{12}$, gastrointestinal abnormalities are always a prime suspect and atrophy of the gastric mucosa is a major etiologic factor (Nilsson-Ehle *et al.*, 1989) (see Table 9-6).

Achlorhydria is also associated with greater loss of dietary nitrate, presumably resulting from metabolic activity of nitrate-reducing bacteria in the stomach (Packer *et al.*, 1990). Calcium absorption is often adversely affected by a reduction in stomach acid production. When achlorhydria is diagnosed, it

**Table 9-6**  Prevalence of gastric atrophy (USA).

| Age (years) | % affected |
|-------------|------------|
| 60–69       | 24         |
| 70–79       | 32         |
| >80         | 37         |

is generally recommended that calcium carbonate supplements be taken with food or that some more readily absorbed calcium compound, such as calcium citrate malates (Dawson-Hughes *et al.*, 1990), be used instead. It is also recommended that supplementation be divided into two or three doses spread out over the day (Trachtenbarg, 1990).

There has also been some concern about the simultaneous effects of hypochlorhydria or achlorhydria and high-fiber diets on calcium absorption. However, Knox *et al.* (1991) report that the reduction in calcium absorption associated with high-fiber diets is unaffected by the level of stomach acidity. Since calcium is absorbed both in the small intestine and in the colon, a compensatory increase in colonic absorption can offset reduced absorption in the small intestine when pH in the stomach rises. In fact, colonic calcium absorption might be especially important when the diet is high in fiber since bacterial metabolism breaks down fiber–calcium complexes there, increasing ionized calcium available for absorption. This can be a very important aspect of calcium absorption when hypochlorhydria occurs, since fiber–calcium binding is pH dependent, increasing as pH rises. *In vitro* experiments to measure the effect of pH on calcium–phytase binding have shown that complexes begin to precipitate when pH rises to 4.5. At a pH of 6, 70% of the calcium present is bound and at pH 7, less than 10% is soluble. Clearly, absorption in the small intestine would be inadequate to support metabolic requirements under such conditions if other factors, such as bacterial action, did not come into play. Therefore the inhibitory effect of a high phytate diet is sufficiently marked to be of nutritional significance to the elderly (Rossander-Hulthen *et al.*, 1990).

## Stomach Cancer

In addition to their effects on the absorption of vitamin $B_{12}$ and calcium, hypochlorhydria and achlorhydria have a known association with atrophic gastritis and gastric carcinoma. Simultaneous occurrence of achlorhydria and low serum ferritin levels are associated with a risk of cancer ten times normal (Akiba *et al.*, 1991). Lipkin (1991), in tracing the etiology of stomach cancer, identifies an early event involving modification of gastrointestinal epithelial cells in which proliferation in the basal epthelium is a major factor. Subsequently, increasing numbers of cells experience continued synthesis of DNA and delayed terminal differentiation. This may constitute a pre-cancerous state. These events can occur in the esophagus (Barrett's esophagus), in the stomach, or in the colon. Singh and Gaby (1991) link gastritis and stomach cancer through mucosal changes that make tissues more susceptible to damage by genotoxic agents such as $N$-nitroso compounds.

Intestinal metaplasia, in which cells of the gastric mucosa take on characteristics of intestinal cells, is induced by genotoxins eventually leading to further damage producing dysplasia and, ultimately, cancer. Correa (1985) also points out the close relationship between intestinal-type gastric carcinoma and intestinal metaplasia associated with chronic atrophic gastritis. They point out that intestinal metaplasias increase in frequency with increasing age and that they are predominantly found in the antral location, a site which defines Type B gastritis. As a rule, the first metaplasia occurs around the incisura and the lesser curvature of the stomach. In intestinal metaplasia, the muscular walls of the stomach are invaded by glandular tissue and the invading cells adhere to each other forming junctions. When the change has progressed to the multi-focal stage, glands of the stomach are lost and replaced by intestinalized cells. At this stage gastric pH rises from about 1 to near 6 (Correa, 1982, 1983, 1985; Correa et al., 1985). The internal surface of the stomach takes on an intestinal appearance and, in complete metaplasia, all enzymes produced by the small intestine can be present. One explanatory hypothesis concerning this series of events is that gastric carcinoma involves a regression of cells to the stem-cell phase in which there is a progressive loss of differentiation.

In certain populations where gastric carcinoma occurs in high frequency, it is believed that early childhood infections by *Helicobacterium pylori* may act as a promoter. The association of high *H. pylori* IgG serum antibody titers in populations at high risk for gastric carcinoma provides presumptive evidence for this connection. The transition from normal to a stage of superficial gastritis would occur only when the stomach lining was exposed to certain irritants such as aspirin and high sodium chloride concentrations. With continued irritation, superficial gastritis progresses to atrophic gastritis and gastric pH rises, permitting increased bacterial colonization of the stomach and, through bacterial metabolism, increased presence of nitrites. In some populations with high stomach cancer frequency, the diet includes items such as fava beans, whose nitrosated metabolites are known to be highly mutagenic. Figure 9-4 presents a proposed etiology.

Table 9-7 compares the incidence of gastric and colorectal cancers in a number of populations. The high rate of stomach cancer seen in Japan is particularly notable, especially when Japan's position as the world's longest-lived population is considered. The lifelong consumption of a very salty diet is thought to be an important factor in the etiology of stomach cancer in Japan. The death rate appears to be declining gradually in Japan as well as other countries where stomach cancer has been most frequent. It is possible that changing dietary patterns are responsible for the decline.

A number of dietary constituents appear to have potential for reducing the incidence of stomach cancer. Among these are ascorbic acid (in its reduced form) consumed in fresh fruits and vegetables, and $\beta$-carotene. Ascorbic acid appears to play a protective or preventive role, while $\beta$-carotene is thought to suppress carcinoma in its early stages. Lipkin (1991) reports that compounds from more than 20 classes of chemicals have potential chemopreventive

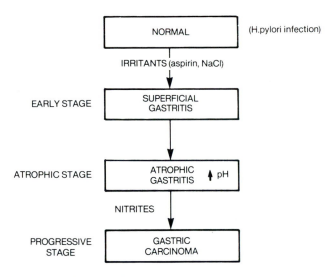

**Figure 9-4** Proposed etiology of gastric carcinoma.

properties. Some of these preventive compounds, like ascorbic acid and β-carotene, occur naturally in foods. One group of compounds acts to inhibit formation or activation of tumor-initiating agents (genotoxins). The second group inhibits tumor promoters.

In addition to ascorbic acid the first group includes tocopherol and certain plant phenols, caffeic, and ferulic acids, all of which prevent formation of carcinogens from their precursors. Also included in the first group are compounds that prevent carcinogens from reaching or reacting with their targets. Compounds that afford this kind of protection include phenols and some plant flavinoids, flavins, coumarins, and isothiocyanates. Compounds that act after exposure to a carcinogen to suppress expression of neoplasia include, beside the carotenes, retinoids, selenium salts, protease inhibitors, inhibitors of arachidonic acid metabolism, sterols, and steroid hormones.

Inhibition of tumor promotion is a property of a second group of

**Table 9-7** Mortality rates (per 100,000 population) for stomach and colon cancer.

| Population | Stomach cancer | Colon cancer |
|---|---|---|
| Japan (1988) | 39.1 | 18.2 |
| Italy (1977) | 25.1 | 23.4 |
| United Kingdom (1988) | 18.7 | 34.2 |
| France (1988) | 13.1 | 27.5 |
| Canada (1988) | 8.2 | 22.3 |
| United States (1991) | 5.8 | 22.5 |
| Mexico (1986) | 4.8 | 1.8 |

Source: United Nations (1990) and National Center for Health Statistics (1991).

compounds, a number of which are also included in the first group, such as the retinoids, protease inhibitors, inhibitors of arachidonic acid metabolism, and phenols as well as agents that increase intracellular c-AMP activity and modulators of calcium metabolism.

## Colon Cancer

While the incidence of stomach cancer appears to be on the decline in the United States, Japan, and several other countries, the incidence of colon cancer, which is also age- and diet-related, is on the rise virtually everywhere. This trend is at least in part attributable to the increase in the number of older people in the world's population. As a cause of death, cancer of the colon ranks second only to lung cancer among all neoplastic diseases in the United States. This is also true in Canada, the United Kingdom, and most of western Europe. The etiology of colon cancer, as in the case of stomach cancer, appears to involve metaplasia, reversion to a stem-cell phase and absence of terminal differentiation producing dysplasia. Fat and phosphates are etiological factors in colon cancer (Newmark et al., 1991). The mechanism includes a highly surfactant effect of fatty acids and bile acids on the colonic mucosa leading to cell loss and compensatory hyperproliferation (Wargovich et al., 1991). It is thought that a high-fiber diet, through its effect of increasing stool bulk and decreasing transit time, reduces the opportunity for damage to mucosal cells (Burkitt, 1971; Kritchevsky, 1984). Dietary fiber may also act directly by absorbing bile acids (Story, 1986) or by altering them chemically to a form that is no longer carcinogenic (Cheah and Bernstein, 1990). Fermented dairy products also seem to have a beneficial effect; in part through their capacity to reduce the concentrations of potentially carcinogenic enzymes in the colon (Marteau et al., 1990).

The role of calcium and vitamin D in the lowering of colon cancer risk is an area of increasing interest, with several investigators reporting substantial reductions in incidence as a result of calcium and vitamin supplementation (Garland et al., 1991). In this case, the mechanism is thought to be the formation of soaps by the complexing of calcium and lipids. The reduced presence of free lipids in the colon reduces surfactant cell damage and compensatory hyperproliferation. While fats are widely viewed as the villain in the etiology of colon cancer, there is reason to believe that their irritant interaction promotes carcinogenesis only when a genetic predisposition is also present (Hill, 1986; Cheah, 1990).

## SUMMARY AND CONCLUSIONS

The recommended dietary allowances that have been developed for the United States increasingly acknowledge that certain nutritional needs change substantially with increasing age. While the body probably needs no more vitamins and minerals in old age than it did in youth, the amount that can be extracted from food may vary considerably. The absorption of nutrients requires effective function of highly specialized tissues that come into play sequentially. Changes that take place in the mouth, including reduced salivary gland output, altered sensory input and loss of teeth can affect nutritional intake both quantitively and qualitatively. Difficulties in swallowing and discomfort can further alter enthusiasm for eating, and functional changes in the stomach, intestines, pancreas, and liver can alter the bioavailability of a number of nutrients. Changes in microflora present in the gastrointestinal tract create a drastically altered environment with bacterial metabolism at times competing with and at other times reinforcing the absorptive process. In some areas, such as in the stomach, bacterial colonization arises because of altered environments. In the small intestine it may be the result of impaired local immunity (Smith et al., 1990). Whatever the cause, the effect is an altered absorption pattern that, in the older individual, may be highly idiosyncratic. There is a geriatric truism that the older a person becomes the more marked is his or her individuality. Nowhere is this more true than in the area of nutritional needs. Consequently, blanket recommendations for people over 50, 60, 70, or 80 years of age become progressively more error prone.

One factor, however, appears to be quite universal. That is the need to maintain a reserve to deal with trauma and infection. Since the ultimate reserve to be drawn on is muscle tissue, preservation of muscle mass is an important element of survival. Wasting, in humans just as in other mammals, is a sign of future trouble. Voluntary loss of muscle mass through ill-advised weight reduction programs is increasingly a threat to health and survival with increasing age. Some changes, like those occurring in the liver, where reduced fluidity of hepatocyte plasma membranes alters membrane transfer (Gentile et al., 1990), are poorly understood and may be irreversible. Other changes may be preventible. Emotional problems, such as depression, may play a major role in pathological aging (Van Vort et al., 1990), and may be treatable.

Much remains to be learned about the factors underlying sex differences in the aging process. Women live longer than men, but experience more morbidity in their later years (Verbrugge, 1989). Male eating and drinking patterns differ from female throughout life as does body composition. Can better understanding of the causes and effects of these differences provide leads for more effective nutritional recommendations for the elderly? As mortality patterns change with one category of nutritionally related mortalities, from cardiovascular diseases to cancer, attention should shift to dietary factors that have until recently been ignored. For instance, is there a nutritional component in the decreasing effectiveness of human thermoregulation in old age? The thermogenic response to food intake declines with age (Golay et al., 1983). Some investigators attribute the blunted thermic effect of food intake to alterations in the sympathetic nervous response with age (Schwartz et al., 1990). However, it has also been shown that the thermogenic response remains more vigorous in more active elderly males than in sedentary ones (Lundholm et al., 1986). Just as in the case of retention of muscle mass, exercise is an important modulator of the physiological response.

The basic relationships between energy intake and energy expenditure remain the same throughout life. Keeping the equation balanced requires knowledge of the many facets of individual uniqueness. It is unlikely that the average human life span will ever exceed 100 years (Olshansky *et al.*, 1990). As the major diseases causing death come increasingly under control, intrinsic life-limiting factors will emerge, revealing the essential nature of our species' evolutionary heritage of mortality. The phenomenon of wasting, wherein humans effectively starve in the midst of abundance, may be an important aspect of that heritage.

## REFERENCES

Akiba, S., Nerüshi, W., Blot, W. J., Kabuto, M., Stevens, R. G., Kato, H. and Land, C. E. (1991) Serum ferretin and stomach cancer risk among a Japanese population. *Cancer* **67**, 1707–1712.

Aloia, J. F., McGowan, D. M., Voswane, A. N., Ross, P. and Cohn, S. H. (1991) Relationship of menopause to skeletal and muscle mass. *American Journal of Clinical Nutrition* **53**. 1378–1383.

Altman, D. F. (1990) Changes in gastrointestinal, pancreatic, biliary and hepatic function with aging. *Gastroentology Clinics of North America* **19**, 227–234.

Andres, R. (1980) Effect of obesity on total mortality. *International Journal of Obesity* **4**, 381–386.

Andres, R. (1981) Influence of obesity on longevity in the aged. In: *Ageing: A Challenge to Science and Society. Vol. 1: Biology* (ed. Marvis, M.). Oxford: Oxford University Press, pp. 196–203.

Andres, R. (1985) Mortality and obesity: the rationale for age-specific height-weight tables. In: *Principles of Geriatric Medicine* (ed. Andres, R., Bierman, E. L. and Hazzard, W. R.). New York: McGraw-Hill, pp. 311–318.

Astrup, A., Thorbek, G., Lind, J. and Isaksson, B. (1990) Prediction of 24-h energy expenditure and its components from physical characteristics and body composition in normal-weight humans. *American Journal of Clinical Nutrition* **52**, 777–783.

Babu, D. S. and Chuttani, C. S. (1979) Antropometric indices independent of age for nutritional assessment in school children. *Journal of Epidemiology and Community Health* **33**, 177–179.

Ballor, D. L., McCarthy, J. P. and Wilterdink, E. J. (1990) Exercise intensity does not affect the composition of diet- and exercise-induced body mass loss. *American Journal of Clinical Nutrition* **51**, 142–146.

Balogh, K. and Lelkens, K. (1961) The tongue in old age. *Gerontologia Clinica* **3**, 38–54.

Barger-Lux, M. J., Heaney, R. P. and Stegman, M. R. (1990) Effects of moderate caffeine intake on the calcium economy of premenopausal women. *American Journal of Clinical Nutrition* **52**, 722–725.

Battinelli, T., Gleason, R. E., Ganda, O. P. and Cunningham, L. N. (1986) Height–weight indices and blood lipid levels in normal controls and offspring of conjugal diabetics. *Human Biology* **58**, 601–614.

Baumgartner, R. N., Roche, A. E., Guo, S., Lohman, T., Boeleau, R. A. and Slaughter, M. H. (1986) Adipose tissue distribution: the stability of principal components by sex, ethnicity, and maturation age. *Human Biology* **58**, 719–735.

Baumgartner, R. N., Heymefield, S. B., Lichman, S., Wang, J. and Pierson, R. N., Jr

(1991) Body composition in elderly people: affect of criterion estimates on predictive equations. *American Journal of Clinical Nutrition* **53**, 1345–1353.

Benn, R. T. (1971) Some mathematical properties of weight-for-height indices used as measures of adiposity. *British Journal of Preventive Social Medicine* **25**, 42–50.

Billewicz, W. Z., Kemsley, W. F. F. and Thompson, A. M. (1962) Indices of obesity. *British Journal of Preventive Social Medicine* **16**, 183–188.

Blair, N., Ludwig, D. A. and Goodyear, N. N. (1988) A canonical analysis of central and peripheral subcutaneous fat distribution and coronary heart disease risk factors in men and women aged 18–65 years. *Human Biology* **60**, 111–122.

Blanchard, J., Conrad, K. A., Mead, R. A. and Garry, P. J. (1990). Vitamin C disposition in young and elderly men. *American Journal of Clinical Nutrition* **51**, 837–845.

Brandi, L. S., Frediani, M., Oleggini, M., Mosca, F., Cerri, M., Boni, C., Pecori, N., Buzzigoli, G. and Ferrannini, E. (1990) Insulin resistance after surgery: normalization by insulin treatment. *Clinical Science* **79**, 443–450.

Bray, G. A. (1978) Definitions, measurements, and classifications of the syndromes of obesity. *International Journal of Obesity* **2**, 99–121.

Bunce, G. E., Kinoshita, J. and Horwitz, J. (1990) Nutritional factors in cataracts. *Annual Reviews of Nutrition* **10**, 233–254.

Burkitt, D. P. (1971) Epidemiology of cancer of the colon and rectum. *Cancer* **28**, 3–13.

Burkitt, D. P. (1977) Relationships between diseases and their etiological significance. *American Journal of Clinical Nutrition* **30**, 262–267.

Cammisa, H. and Tischler, M. E. (1982) Protein turnover in skeletal muscles and myocytes of traumatized and normal rats. *Federation Proceedings* **41**, 866.

Cerovska, J., Petrasek, R., Hajino, K. and Kauka, J. (1977) Indices of obesity and body composition in four groups of Czech population. *Zeitschrift of Morphological Anthropology* **68**, 213–219.

Champagne, E. T. (1989) Low gastric hydrochloric acid secretion and mineral bioavailability. *Advances in Experimental Medicine and Biology* **249**, 173–184.

Cheah, P. Y. (1990) Hypothesis for the etiology of colorectal cancer: an overview. *Nutrition and Cancer* **14**, 5–13.

Cheah, P. Y. and Berstein, H. (1990) Colon cancer and dietary fiber: cellulose inhibits the DNA-damaging ability of bile acids. *Nutrition and Cancer* **13**, 51–57.

Christian, J. C., Carmelli, D., Castelli, W. P., Fabsitz, R., Grim, C. E., Meaney, F. J., Norton, J. A., Jr, Reed, T., Williams, C. P. and Wood, P. D. (1990) High density lipoprotein cholesterol. A 16-year longitudinal study in aging male twins. *Arteriosclerosis* **10**, 1020–1025.

Colditz, G. A., Giovannucci, E., Rimm, E. B., Stampfer, M. J., Rosner, B., Speiser, F. E., Gordes, E. and Willett, W. C. (1991) Alcohol intake in relation to diet and obesity in women and men. *American Journal of Clinical Nutrition* **54**, 49–55.

Cook, J. D., Dassenko, S. A. and Whittaker, P. (1991) Calcium supplementation: effect on iron absorption. *American Journal of Clinical Nutrition* **53**, 106–111.

Correa, P. (1982) Precursors of gastric and esophageal cancer. *Cancer* **50**, 2554–2565.

Correa, P. (1983) The gastric precancerous process. *Cancer Surveys* **2**, 437–450.

Correa, P. (1985) Mechanisms of gastric carcinogenesis. In: *Diet and Human Carcinogenesis* (eds Joossens, J. V., Hill, M. J. and Gebbers, J.). New York: Elsevier Science Publishers BV, pp. 109–115.

Correa, P., Fontham, E., Pickle, L. W., Chen, V., Lin, Y. and Haenszel, W. (1985) Dietary determinants of gastric cancer in south Louisiana inhabitants. *American Journal of Clinical Nutrition* **75**, 645–654.

Dawson-Hughes, B., Dalla, G. E., Sadowski, L., Sahyoun, N. and Tannenbaum, S. (1990) A controlled trial of the effect of calcium supplementation on bone density in postmenopausal women. *New England Journal of Medicine* **323**, 878–883.

Deurenberg, P., vander Kooij, K., Hulshof, J. and Evers, P. (1989) Body mass index as a measure of fatness in the elderly. *European Journal of Clinical Nutrition* **43**, 231–236.

Deurenberg, P., vander Kooij, K., Evers, P. and Hulshof, T. (1990) Assessment of body composition by bioelectrical impedance in a population aged >60 y. *American Journal of Clinical Nutrition* **51**, 3–6.

DiMascio, P., Murphy, M. E. and Sies, H. (1991) Antioxidant defense systems: the role of carotenoids, tocopherols and thiols. *American Journal of Clinical Nutrition* **53**, 194s–200s.

Diplock, A. T. (1991) Antioxidant nutrients and disease prevention: an overview. *American Journal of Clinical Nutrition* **53**, 189s–193s.

Dockray, G. J., Hamer, C., Evans, D., Varro, A. and Dimaline, R. (1991) The secretory kinetics of the G-cell in omeprazole-treated rats. *Gastroenterology* **100** (pt 1), 1187–1194.

Durnin, J. V. G. A., McCay, F. C. and Webster, C. I. (1985) *A New Method of Assessing Fatness and Desirable Weight for Use in the Armed Services*. Technical Report, University of Glasgow.

Fahn, S. (1991) An open trial of high-dosage antioxidants in early Parkinson's disease. *American Journal of Clinical Nutrition* **53**, 380s–382s.

Feely, J. and Coakley, D. (1990) Altered pharmacodynamics in the elderly. *Clinical Geriatric Medicine* **6**, 269–283.

Feldman, M., Sender, A. J. and Siegelaub, A. B. (1969) Difference in diabetic and non-diabetic fat distribution patterns by skinfold measurements. *Diabetes* **18**, 478–486.

Fischer, J. and Johnson, M. A. (1990) Low body weight and weight loss in the aged. *Journal of the American Dietetic Association* **90**, 1697–1706.

Fiskens, E. J. M., Bowles, C. H. and Kromhout, D. (1991) Carbohydrate intake and body mass index in relation to the risk of glucose intolerance in an elderly population. *American Journal of Clinical Nutrition* **54**, 136–140.

Florey, C. D. V. (1970) The use and misuse of ponderal index and other weight-height ratios in epidemiological studies. *Journal of Chronic Diseases* **23**, 93–103.

Food and Agriculture Organization of the United Nations (1977) *The Fourth FAO World Food Survey*. Rome: Food and Agriculture Organization of the United Nations.

Frenk, S. (1986) Metabolic adaptation in protein-energy malnutrition. *Journal of the American College of Nutrition* **5**, 371–381.

Frisancho, A. R. and Flegel, P. N. (1982) Relative merits of old and new indices of body mass with reference to skinfold thickness. *American Journal of Clinical Nutrition* **36**, 697–699.

Fucagawa, N. K., Anderson, J. W., Hageman, G., Young, V. R. and Minaker, K. L. (1990) High-carbohydrate, high-fiber diets increase peripheral insulin sensitivity in healthy young and old adults. *American Journal of Clinical Nutrition* **52**, 524–528.

Garewal, H. S. (1991) Potential role of B-carotene in prevention of oral cancer. *American Journal of Clinical Nutrition* **53**, 294s–297s.

Garland, C. F., Garland, F. C. and Gorham, E. D. (1991) Can colon cancer incidence and death rates be reduced with calcium and vitamin D? *American Journal of Clinical Nutrition* **54**, 193s–201s.

Garn, S. M. (1986) Who is obese? *Current Controversies* **2**, 26–27.

Garn, S. M. and Pesick, S. D. (1982) Comparison of the Benn and other body mass indices in nutritional assessment. *American Journal of Clinical Nutrition* **36**, 573–575.

Garn, S. M., Sullivan, T. V. and Hawthorne, V. M. (1989) Educational level, fatness, and fatness differences between husbands and wives. *American Journal of Clinical Nutrition* **50**, 740–745.

Gentile, S., Persico, M., Orlando, C., LeGrazie, C., Di Padova, C. and Coltorte, M. (1990) Age-associated decline of hepatic handling of cholephilic anions in humans is reverted by S-adenosyl methionine (SAMe). *Scandinavian Journal of Clinical Laboratory Investigations* **50**, 565–571.

Gersovitz, M., Munro, H. N., Udall, J. and Young, V. R. (1980) Albumin synthesis in young and elderly subjects using a new stable isotope methodology: response to level of protein intake. *Metabolism* **29**, 1075–1086.

Gersovitz, M., Motil, K., Munro, H. N., Scrimshaw, N. S. and Young, V. R. (1981) Human protein requirements: assessment of the adequacy of the current recommended dietary allowance for dietary protein in elderly men and women. *American Journal of Clinical Nutrition* **35**, 6–14.

Golay, A., Schutz, Y., Broquet, C., Moeri, R., Felber, J. P. and Jequier, E. (1983) Decreased thermogenic response to an oral glucose load in older subjects. *Journal of the American Geriatric Society* **31**, 144–148.

Goldbourt, U. and Medalie, J. (1974) Weight–height indices. *British Journal of Preventive Social Medicine* **16**, 116–126.

Goodman, K. I. and Salt, W. B., II (1990) Vitamin B-12 deficiency: important new concepts in recognition. *Postgraduate Medicine* **88**, 147–150, 153–158.

Green, L. K. and Graham, D. Y. (1990) Gastritis in the elderly. *Gastroenterology Clinics of North America* **19**, 273–292.

Grzegorczyk, P. B., Jones, S. W. and Mistnetta, C. M. (1979) Age-related differences in salt taste acuity. *Journal of Gerontology* **34**, 834–840.

Hallberg, L., Brune, M., Erlandsson, A.-S., Sandberg, L. and Rossander-Hultén, L. (1991) Calcium: effect of different amounts on nonheme- and heme-iron absorption in humans. *American Journal of Clinical Nutrition* **53**, 112–119.

Hallfrisch, J. (1990) Metabolic effects of dietary fructose. *FASEB Journal* **4**, 2652–2660.

Hammarquist, F., Wernerman, J., von der Deckan, A. and Vinnars, E. (1991) Alpha-ketoglutarate preserves protein synthesis and free glutamine in skeletal muscle after surgery. *Surgery* **109**, 28–36.

Haussler, M. R. (1986) Vitamin D receptors: nature and function. *Annual Reviews of Nutrition* **6**, 527–562.

Hay, S. S. and Coons, D. H. (eds) (1979) *Special Senses in Aging: A Current Biological Assessment*. Ann Arbor: University of Michigan Press.

Heaney, R. P., Recker, R. R., Stegman, M. R. and Moy, A. J. (1989) Calcium absorption in women: relationships of calcium intake, estrogen status, and age. *Journal of Bone Mineral Research* **4**, 469–475.

Hegsted, D. M. (1986) Calcium and osteoporosis. *Journal of Nutrition* **116**, 2316–2319.

Heitmann, B. L. (1990) Prediction of body water and fat in adult Danes from measurement of electrical impedance: a validation study. *International Journal of Obesity* **14**, 789–802.

Hermel, J., Schonwetter, S. and Samueloff, S. (1970) Taste sensation and age in man. *Journal of Oral Medicine* **25**, 39–42.

Hernandez-Avila, M., Colditz, G. A., Stampfer, M. J., Rosner, B., Speizer, F. E. and Willett, W. C. (1991) Caffeine, moderate alcohol intake, and risk of fractures of the hip and forearm in middle-aged women. *American Journal of Clinical Nutrition* **54**, 157–163.

Hill, M. J. (1986) Bile acids and colorectal cancer in humans. In: *Dietary Fiber—Basic and Clinical Aspects* (eds Vahouny, G. V. and Kritchevsky, D.). New York: Plenum, pp. 497–513.

Himmelstein, S., Clemens, T. L., Rubin, A. and Lindsay, R. (1990) Vitamin D supplementation in elderly nursing home residents increases 25(OH)D but not 1,25(OH)$_2$D. *American Journal of Clinical Nutrition* **52**, 701–706.

Hirsch, J., Bell, C. H. and Dwyer, J. T. (1985) Health implications of obesity. National Institutes of Health consensus development conference statement. *Annals of Internal Medicine* **103**, 147–151.

Holbrook, T. L., Barrett-Connor, E. and Wingard, D. L. (1990) A prospective population-based study of alcohol use and non-insulin-dependent diabetes mellitus. *American Journal of Epidemiology* **132**, 902–909.

Hollander, D. and Dadufalza, V. (1990) Influence of aging on vitamin A transport into the lymphatic circulation. *Experimental Gerontology* **25**, 61–65.

Howe, J. C. (1990) Postprandial response of calcium metabolism in postmenopausal women to meals varying in protein level/source. *Metabolism* **39**, 1246–1252.

Jacques, P. F. and Chylack, L. T., Jr (1991) Epidemiologic evidence of a role for the antioxidant vitamins and carotenoids in cataract prevention. *American Journal of Clinical Nutrition* **53**, 352s–355s.

Jeevanandam, M., Young, D. H., Ramias, L. and Schiller, W. R. (1990) Effect of major trauma on plasma free amino acid concentrations in geriatric patients. *American Journal of Clinical Nutrition* **51**, 1040–1045.

Jeevanandam, M., Hsu, Y.-C., Ramias, L. and Schiller, W. R. (1991) Mild orotic aciduria and uricosuria in severe trauma victims. *American Journal of Clinical Nutrition* **53**, 1242–1248.

Kahn, H. S. and Williamson, D. F. (1990) The contributions of income, education, and changing marital status to weight change among US men. *International Journal of Obesity* **14**, 1057–1068.

Kaiser, F. E., Silver, A. J. and Morley, J. E. (1991)) The effect of recombinant human growth hormone on malnourished older individuals. *Journal of the American Geriatrics Society* **39**, 235–240.

Karnes, W. E., Jr and Walsh, J. H. (1990) The gastrin hypothesis implications for anti-secretory drug selection. *Journal of Clinical Gastroenterology* **12** (Suppl. 2), S7–S12.

Kern, S. E., Yardley, J. H., Lazenby, A. J., Boitnott, J. K., Yang, V. W., Bayless, T. M. and Sitzmann, J. V. (1990) Reversal by antrectomy of endocrine cell hyperplasia in the gastric body in pernicious anemia: a morphometric study. *Modern Pathology* **3**, 561–566.

Keys, A. (1980a) Overweight and obesity. In: *Seven Countries: A Multivariate Analysis of Death and Coronary Heart Disease* (ed. Keys, A.). Cambridge, MA: Harvard University Press, pp. 161–195.

Keys, A. (1980b) Overweight, obesity, coronary heart disease, and mortality. *Nutrition Reviews* **38**, 297–307.

Keys, A., Fidanza, F., Karvonen, M. J., Kimura, N. and Taylor, H. L. (1972) Indices of relative weight and obesity. *Journal of Chronic Diseases* **25**, 239–243.

Khosla, T. and Lowe, C. R. (1967) Indices of obesity derived from body weight and height. *British Journal of Preventive Social Medicine* **21**, 122–128.

King, M. A. and Katch, F. I. (1986) Changes in body density, fatfolds, and girths at 2.3 kg increments of weight loss. *Human Biology* **58**, 709–718.

Knox, T. A., Kassarjian, Z., Dawson-Hughes, B., Golner, B. B., Dallal, G. E., Arora, S. and Russell, R. M. (1991) Calcium absorption in elderly subjects on high- and low-fiber diets: effect of gastric acidity. *American Journal of Clinical Nutrition* **53**, 1480–1486.

Kochersberger, G., Bates, C., Lobaugh, B. and Lyles, K. W. (1990) Calcium supplementation lowers serum parathyroid hormone levels in elderly subjects. *Journal of Gerontology* **45**, M159–M162.

Kramhout, D., Coulander, C. L., Obermann-deBoer, G. L., van Kampen-Donker, M., Goddijn, E. and Bloemberg, B. P. M. (1990) Changes in food and nutrient intake in middle-aged men from 1960 to 1985 (The Zeitphen Study). *American Journal of Clinical Nutrition* **51**, 123–129.

Krinsky, N. I. (1991) Effects of carotenoids in cellular and animal systems. *American Journal of Clinical Nutrition* **53**, 238s–246s.

Kritchevsky, D. (1984) Dietary fiber and cancer. *Nutrition and Cancer* **6**, 213–219.

Lichtenstein, A. H. (1990) Intestinal cholesterol metabolism. *Annals of Medicine* **22**, 49–52.

Lipkin, M. (1991) Application of intermediate biomarkers to studies of cancer prevention in the gastrointestinal tract: introduction and perspective. *American Journal of Clinical Nutrition* **54**, 188s–192s.

Loenen, H. M., Eshuis, H., Lowik, M. R., Schouten, E. G., Hulshof, K. F., Odink, J. and Kok, F. J. (1990) Serum uric acid correlates in elderly men and women with special reference to body composition and dietary intake (Dutch Nutrition Surveillance System). *Journal of Clinical Epidemiology* **43**, 1297–1303.

Lowik, M. R., Schryver, J., Odink, J., vanden Berg, H. and Wedel, M. (1990) Long-term effects of a vegetarian diet on the nutritional status of elderly people (Dutch Nutrition Surveillance System). *Journal of the American College of Nutrition* **9**, 600–609.

Lundholm, K., Holm, G., Lindmark, L., Larsson, B., Sjöström, L. and Björntorp, P. (1986) Thermogenic effect of food in physically well-trained elderly men. *European Journal of Applied Physiology* **55**, 486–492.

Maiani, G., Mobarhan, S., Ceccanti, M., Ranaldi, L., Gettner, S., Bowen, P., Friedman, H., DeLorenzo, A. and Ferro-Luzzi, A. (1989) Beta-carotene response in young and elderly females. *European Journal of Clinical Nutrition* **43**, 749–761.

Marcus, R., Butterfield, G., Holloway, L., Gilliland, L., Baylink, D. J., Hintz, R. L. and Sherman, B. M. (1990) Effects of short-term administration of recombinant human growth hormone to elderly people. *Journal of Clinical Endocrinology and Metabolism* **70**, 519–527.

Marteau, P., Pockart, P., Flourie, B., Pellier, P., Santos, L., Desjeux, O.-F. and Rambaud, J.-C. (1990) Effect of chronic ingestion of a fermented dairy product containing *Lactobacillis acidophilus* and *Bifidobacterium bifidium* on metabolic activities of the colonic flora in humans. *American Journal of Clinical Nutrition* **52**, 685–688.

Masoro, E. (1972) Other physiologic changes with age. In: *Epidemiology of Aging* (eds Ostfeld, A. M., Gibson, D. C. and Donnelly, C. P.). Bethesda, MD: US Department of Health, Education and Welfare, DHEW publication no. (NIH) 77-711, pp. 137–155.

Mattes, R. D., Cowart, B. J., Schiavo, M. A., Arnold, C., Garrison, B., Kare, M. R. and Lowry, L. D. (1990) Dietary evaluation of patients with smell and/or taste disorders. *American Journal of Clinical Nutrition* **51**, 233–240.

McCarron, D. A., Morris, C. D., Young, E., Roullet, C. and Drüeke, T. (1991) Dietary calcium and blood pressure: modifying factors in specific populations. *American Journal of Clinical Nutrition* **54**, 215s–219s.

McLaren, D. S. (1987) Body mass index and the obesities. *American Journal of Clinical Nutrition* **46**, 121.

Merry, P., Grootveld, M., Lunec, J. and Blake, D. R. (1991) Oxidative damage to lipids within the inflamed human joint provides evidence of radical-mediated hypoxic–reperfusion injury. *American Journal of Clinical Nutrition* **53**, 362s–369s.

Metropolitan Life Insurance Company (1959) New weight standards for men and women. *Statistical Bulletin of the Metropolitan Insurance Company* **40**, 11–14.

Metropolitan Life Insurance Company (1984) Metropolitan height and weight tables, 1983. *Statistical Bulletin of the Metropolitan Insurance Company* **64**, 2–9.

Meydani, S. N., Borklund, M. P., Liu, S., Meydani, M., Miller, R. A., Cannon, J. G., Morrow, F. D., Rocklin, R. and Blumberg, J. B. (1990) Vitamin E supplementation enhances cell-mediated immunity in healthy older subjects. *American Journal of Clinical Nutrition* **52**, 557–563.

Micozzi, M. S. and Albanes, D. (1987) Three limitations of the body mass index (letter). *American Journal of Clinical Nutrition* **46**, 376.

Micozzi, M. S., Albanes, D., Jones, D. Y. and Chumlea, W. C. (1986) Correlations of body mass indices with weight, stature, and body composition in men and women. In NHANES I and II. *American Journal of Clinical Nutrition* **44**, 725–731.

Munro, H. N. (1983) Protein nurtriture and requirement in elderly people. *Bibliography of Nutrition and Dietetics* **33**, 61–74.

National Center for Health Statistics (1991) Births, marriages, divorces, and deaths for 1990. *Monthly Vital Statistics Report* Vol. 40, 7 July 1991. Hyattsville, MD: Public Health Service.

National Research Council (1980) *Recommended Dietary Allowances* 9th revised edn. Washington, DC: National Academy of Sciences.

Nemere, I. and Norman, A. W. (1982) Vitamin D and intestinal cell membranes. *Biochemica et Biophysica Acta* **694**, 307–327.

Nemere, I., Theofan, G. and Norman, A. W. (1987) 1,25-Dihydroxyvitamin $D_3$ regulate tubuline expression in chick intestine. *Biochemistry and Biophysics Research Communications* **148**, 1270–1276.

Newell-Morris, L. L., Treder, R. P., Shuman, W. P. and Fujimoto, W. Y. (1989) Fatness, fat distribution, and glucose tolerance in second-generation Japanese-American (Nisei) men. *American Journal of Clinical Nutrition* **50**, 9–18.

Newmark, H. L., Lipkin, M. and Makeshwari, N. (1991) Colonic hyperproliferation induced in rats by nutritional-stress diets containing four components of a human Western-style diet. *American Journal of Clinical Nutrition* **54**, 209s–214s.

Newsholme, E. A., Newsholme, P., Curie, R., Challoner, E. and Ardawi, M. S. M. (1988) A role for muscle in the immune system and its importance in surgery, trauma, sepsis, and burns. *Nutrition* **4**, 261–268.

Niki, E., Yamamoto, Y., Komuro, E. and Sato, K. (1991) Membrane damage due to lipid oxidation. *American Journal of Clinical Nutrition* **53**, 201s–205s.

Nilsson-Ehle, H., Landahl, S., Lindstedt, G., Netterblad, L., Stockbruegger, R., Westin, J. and Ahren, C. (1989) Low serum cobalamin levels in a population study of 70- and 75-year-old subjects. Gastrointestinal causes and hematological effects. *Digestive Disease Science* **34**, 716–723.

Norman, A. W. (1979) *Vitamin D: The Calcium Homeostatic Steroid Hormone.* New York: Academic Press.

Norman, A. W. (1984) The role of receptors in mediating the biologial responses to 1,25-dihydroxyvitamin D: the hormonally active form of vitamin D. In: *Steroid Hormone Receptors: Structure and Function* (ed. Gustafson, J. A. and Erikson, H.). Amsterdam: Elseveir Biomedical Press, pp. 479–493.

Norman, A. W. (1985) The vitamin D endocrine system. *Physiologist* **28**, 219–232.

Norman, A. W. (1990) Intestinal calcium absorption: a vitamin D-hormone mediated adaptive response. *American Journal of Clinical Nutrition* **51**, 290–300.

Olshansky, S. J., Carnes, B. A. and Cassel, C. (1990) In search of Methuselah: estimating the upper limits to human longevity. *Science* **250**, 634–640.

Oparil, S., Chen, Y.-F., Jin, H., Yang, R.-H. and Wyse, J. M. (1991) Dietary $Ca^{2+}$ prevents NaCl-sensitive hypertension in spontaneously hypertensive rats via sympatholytic and renal effects. *American Journal of Clinical Nutrition* **54**, 227s–236s.

Paauw, J. D. and Davis, A. T. (1990) Taurine concentrations in serum of critically injured patients and age- and sex-matched healthy control subjects. *American Journal of Clinical Nutrition* **52**, 657–660.

Packer, L. (1991) Protective role of vitamin E in biological systems. *American Journal of Clinical Nutrition* **53** (Suppl.), 1050s–1055s.

Packer, P. J., Van Acker, B., Reed, P. I., Haines, K., Thompson, M. H., Hill, M. J. and Leach, S. A. (1990) The effect of gastric achlorhydria on the urinary recovery of nitrate in man: relevance to urinary nitrate as a measure of dietary nitrate exposure. *Carcinogenesis* **11**, 1373–1376.

Pardo, B., Sygnowska, E., Rywik, S., Kulesza, W. and Waskiewicz, A. (1991) Dietary habits of the middle-aged Warsaw population in 1984 relative to nutritional guidelines. *Appetite* **16**, 1–15.

Pellett, P. L. (1990a) Protein requirements in humans. *American Journal of Clinical Nutrition* **51**, 723–737.

Pellett, P. L. (1990b) Food energy requirements in humans. *American Journal of Clinical Nutrition* **51**, 711–722.

Potter, J. F., Schafer, D. F. and Bohi, R. L., (1988) In-hospital mortality as a function of Body Mass Index: an age-dependent variable. *Journal of Gerontology: Medical Sciences* **43**, M59–M63.

Puskarich, C. L., Nelson, C. L., Nusbickel, F. R. and Stroope, H. F. (1990) The use of two nutritional indicators in identifying long bone fracture patients who do and do not develop infections. *Journal of Orthopedic Research* **8**, 799–803.

Rao, R. K. and Singh, D. (1970) An evaluation of the relationship between nutritional status and anthropometric measurements. *American Journal of Clinical Nutrition* **23**, 83–93.

Reichel, H., Koeffler, H. P. and Norman, A. W. (1989) The role of the vitamin D endocrine system in health and disease. *New England Journal of Medicine* **320**, 980–991.

Revicki, D. A. and Israel, G. R. (1986) Relationships between body mass indices and measures of body adiposity. *American Journal of Public Health* **76**, 992–994.

Rhodus, N. L. and Brown, J. (1990) The association of xerostomia and inadequate intake in older adults. *Journal of the American Dietetic Association* **90**, 1688–1692.

Rigby, W. F. C. (1988) The immunology of vitamin D. *Immunology Today* **9**, 54–58.

Robertson, J. McD., Donner, A. P. and Trevthick, J. R. (1991) A possible role for vitamins C and E in cataract prevention. *American Journal of Clinical Nutrition* **53**, 346s–351s.

Roche, A. F., Siervogel, R. M., Chumlea, W. C. and Webb, P. (1981) Grading body fatness from limited anthropometric data. *American Journal of Clinical Nutrition* **34**, 2831–2838.

Rose, M. R. (1991) *Evolutionary Biology of Aging.* New York: Oxford University Press.

Ross, W. D., Eiben, O. G., Ward, R., Martin, A. D., Drinkwater, D. T. and Clarys, J. P. (1986) Alternatives for the conventional methods of human body composition and physique assessment. In: *New Perspectives in Kinanthropometry* (ed. Day, J. A. P.). Champaign: Human Kinetics Press, pp. 203–220.

Ross, W. D., Martin, A. D. and Ward, R. (1987) Body composition and aging: theoretical and methodological implications. *Collegium Antropologicum* **11**, 15–44.

Ross, W. D., Crawford, S. M., Kerr, D. A., Ward, R., Bailey, D. A. and Mirwald, R. M. (1988) Relationship of the Body Mass Index with skinfolds, girths, and bone breadths in Canadian men and women aged 20–70 years. *American Journal of Physical Anthropology* **77**, 169–173.

Rossander-Hulthan, L., Gleerup, A. and Hallberg, L. (1990) Inhibitory effect of oat products on non-haem iron absorption in man. *European Journal of Clinical Nutrition* **44**, 783–791.

Rossman, I. (1977) Anatomic and body composition changes with aging. *Handbook of the Biology of Aging* (eds Finch, C. E. and Hayflick, L.). New York: Van Nostrand Reinhold, pp. 189–221.

Schaefer, E. J., Moussa, P. B., Wilson, P. W., McGee, D., Dallal, G. and Castelli, W. P. (1989) Plasma lipoproteins in healthy octogenarians: lack of reduced high density lipoprotein cholesterol levels: results from the Framingham Heart Study. *Metabolism* **38**, 293–296.

Schorah, C. J., Sobala, G. M., Sanderson, M., Collis, N. and Primrose, J. N. (1991) Gastric juice ascorbic acid: effects of disease and implications for gastric carcinogenesis. *American Journal of Clinical Nutrition* **53**, 287s–293s.

Schwartz, R. S., Jaeger, L. F. and Veith, R. C. (1990) The thermic effect of feeding in older men: the importance of the sympathetic nervous system. *Metabolism* **39**, 733–737.

Selway, S. A. (1990) Potential hazards of long-term acid suppression. *Scandinavian Journal of Gastroenterology* **178** (Suppl.) 85–92.

Singh, V. N. and Gaby, S. N. (1991) Premalignant lesions: role of antioxidant vitamins and B-carotene in risk reduction and prevention of malignant transformation and prevention of malignant transformation. *American Journal of Clinical Nutrition* **53** (Suppl.), 386s–390s.

Siri, W. E. (1956a) The gross composition of the body. *Advances in Biology and Medical Physics* **4**, 239–280.

Siri, W. E. (1956b) Apparatus for measuring human body volume. *Reviews of Scientific Instrumentation* **27**, 729–738.

Slaughter, M. H., Lohman, T. G., Boeleau, R. A., Horswill, C. A., Stillman, R. J., Van Loan, M. D. and Bemben, D. A. (1988) Skinfold equations for estimation of body fatness in children and youth. *Human Biology* **60**, 709–723.

Smalley, K. J., Knerr, A. N., Kendrick, Z. V., Colliver, J. A. and Owen, O. E. (1990) Reassessment of body mass index. *American Journal of Clinical Nutrition* **52**, 405–408.

Smidt, L. J., Cremin, F. M., Grinetti, L. E. and Clifford, A. J. (1991) Influence of thiamin supplementation on the health and general well-being of an elderly Irish population with marginal thiamin deficiency. *Journal of Gerontology* **46**, M16–M22.

Smith, G. M., Chesner, K. M., Asquith, P. and Leyland, M. J. (1990) Small intestinal bacterial overgrowth in patients with chronic lymphocytic leukemia. *Journal of Clinical Pathology* **43**, 57–59.

Society of Actuaries and Association of Life Insurance Medical Directors of America Build Study, 1979. Chicago, 1980.

Stampfer, M., Manson, J. and Van Itallie, T. (1991) Reply to C. W. Calloway. *American Journal of Clinical Nutrition* **54**, 173–174.

Stich, H. F., Mathew, B., Sankaranarayanan, R. Nair, M. K. (1991) Remission of precancerous lesions in the oral cavity of tobacco chewers and maintenance of the protective effect of B-carotene or vitamin A. *American Journal of Clinical Nutrition* **53**, 298s–304s.

Stini, W. A. (1988) Food, seasonality, and human evolution. In: *Coping with Uncertainty in Food Supply* (eds de Garine, I. and Harrison, G. A.). Oxford: Oxford University Press, pp. 32–51.

Stini, W. A. (1991) Body composition and longevity: is there a longevous morphotype? *Medical Anthropology* **13**, 215–229.

Story, J. A. (1986) Modification of steroid excretion in response to dietary fiber. In: *Dietary Fiber—Basic and Clinical Aspects* (eds Vahouny, G. V. and Kritchevsky, D.). New York: Plenum, pp. 253–274.

Sullivan, D. H., Patch, G. A., Walls, R. C. and Lipschitz, D. A. (1990) Impact of nutrition status on morbidity and mortality in a select population of geriatric rehabilitation patients. *American Journal of Clinical Nutrition* **51**, 749–758.

Sullivan, D. H., Walls, R. C. and Lipschitz, D. A. (1991) Protein–energy malnutrition and the risk of mortality within 1 y of hospital discharge in a select population of geriatric rehabilitation patients. *American Journal of Clinical Nutrition* **53**, 599–605.

Sulsky, S. I., Jacques, P. F., Otradovic, C. L., Hartz, S. C. and Russell, R. M. (1990) Descriptors of alcohol consumption among non-institutionalized non-alcoholic elderly. *Journal of the American College of Nutrition* **9**, 326–331.

Tannenbaum, S. R., Wishnok, J. S. and Leaf, C. D. (1991) Inhibition of nitrosomine formation by ascorbic acid. *American Journal of Clinical Nutrition* **53**, 247s–250s.

Thorslund, S., Toss, G., Nilsson, I., von Schenok, H., Symreng, T. and Zetterquist, H. (1990) Prevalence of protein–energy malnutrition in a large population of elderly people at home. *Scandinavian Journal of Primary Health Care* **8**, 243–248.

Tischler, M. E. (1983) Responses of carbohydrate and amino acid metabolism in rat skeletal muscle to injury and trauma. *Federation Proceedings* **42**, 2816.

Tischler, M. E. (1984) Metabolic response of muscle to trauma. In: *Branched-Chain Amino and Keto Acids in Health and Disease* (eds Adibi, S. A., Fekl, W., Langenbeck, U. and Schander, P.). Basel: Karger, pp. 361–383.

Tischler, M. E., Eisenfeld, S., Rosenberg, S. and Henriksen, E. J. (1986a) Role of lysosomal proteolysis in soleus muscle atrophy by unloading. *American Society of Gravitational and Space Biology Meeting*, Charlottesville, VA.

Tischler, M. E., Leng, E., Al-Kanhal, M., Mnichoevicz, J., Reiser, J. and Norton. L. W. (1986b) Metabolic response of muscle to trauma: altered control of protein turnover. In: *Clinical Nutrition and Metabolic Research* (eds Dietze, G., Grunert, A., Kleinberger, G. and Wolfram, G.). Basel: Karger, pp. 40–53.

Tischler, M. E., Rosenburg, S., Satarug, S., Henriksen, E. J., Kirby, C. R., Tome, M. and Chase, P. (1990) Different mechanisms of increased proteolysis in atrophy induced by denervation or unweighting of rat soleus muscle. *Metabolism* **39**, 756–763.

Trachtenbarg, D. E. (1990) Treatment of osteoporosis: what is the role of calcium? *Postgraduate Medicine* **87**, 263–266, 269–270.

Tucker, D. M., Penland, J. G., Sandstead, H. H., Milne, D. B., Heck, D. G. and Klevay, L. M. (1990) Nutrition status and brain function in aging. *American Journal of Clinical Nutrition* **52**, 93–102.

Uauy, R., Winterer, J. C., Belmazeo, C., Haverberg, L. N., Scrimshaw, N. S., Munro, H. N. and Young, V. R. (1978) The changing pattern of whole body protein and metabolism in aging humans. *Journal of Gerontology* **33**, 663–671.

United Nations (1986) *Demographic Yearbook 1984*.

United Nations (1990) *Demographic Yearbook 1988*.

US Bureau of the Census (1986) *Statistical Abstract of the United States*, 106 edn. Washington, DC, 1985.

US Department of Agriculture, US Department of Health and Human Services (1990) *Nutrition and Your Health: Dietary Guidelines for Americans*, 3rd edn. Washington, DC: US Government Printing Office.

Vague, J. R., Combes, R., Tramoni, M., Angeletti, S., Rubin, Ph., Hachem, A., Perey, D., Lansade, M. F., Zeras, Ch., Ramahandridona, G., Jouve, R., Sambuc, R. and Jubelin, J. (1979) Clinical features of diabetogenic obesity. In: *Diabetes and Obesity Exerpta Media* (eds Vague, J., Vague, Ph. and Eblin, F. J. G.). Amsterdam: Excerpta Medica, pp. 127–147.

Van Itallie, T. B. (1979) Obesity: adverse effects on health and longevity. *American Journal of Clinical Nutrition* **32**, 2723–2733.

Van Itallie, T. B. and Abraham, S. (1985) Some hazards of obesity and its treatment. In: *Recent Advances in Obesity Research IV* (eds Hirsch, J. and Van Itallie, T. B.). London: John Libbey, pp. 1–19.

Van Vort, W. B., Rubenstein, M. and Rose, R. P. (1990) Osteoporosis with pathologic hip fractures in major depression. *Journal of Geriatric Psychiatry and Neurology* **3**, 10–12.

Varma, S. D. (1991) Scientific basis for medical therapy of cataracts by antioxidants. *American Journal of Clinical Nutrition* **53**, 335s–345s.

Vaughan, L., Zurlo, F. and Ravussin, E. (1991) Aging and energy expenditure. *American Journal of Clinical Nutrition* **53**, 821–825.

Veenstra, J., Ockhuizen, T., van de Pol, H., Wedel, M. and Schaafsma, G. (1990) Effects of a moderate dose of alcohol on blood lipids and lipoprotein postprandially and in the fasting state. *Alcohol-Alcoholism* **25**, 371–377.

Verbrugge, L. M. (1989) Gender, Aging, and Health. In: *Aging and Health: Perspectives on Gender, Race, Ethnicity, and Class* (ed. Markides, K. S.). Newbury Park, CA: Sage Publications, Inc., pp. 23–78.

Walters, M. R. (1985) Steroid hormone receptors and the nucleus. *Endocrinological Reviews—1985*, 512–543.

Wargovich, M. J., Lynch, P. M. and Levin, B. (1991) Modulating effects of calcium in animal studies of colon carcinogenesis and short-term studies in subjects at increased risk for colon cancer. *American Journal of Clinical Nutrition* **54**, 202s–205s.

Watson, R. R., Prabhala, R. H., Plezia, P. M. and Alberts, D. S. (1991) Effect of B-carotene on lymphocyte subpopulations in elderly humans: evidence for a dose–response relationship. *American Journal of Clinical Nutrition* **53**, 90–94.

Watters, D. A. and Smith, A. N. (1990) Strength of the colon wall in diverticular disease. *British Journal of Surgery* **77**, 257–259.

Webb, A. R., Pilbeam, C., Hanafen, N. and Holick, M. (1990) An evaluation of the relative contributions of exposure to sunlight and of diet to the circulating concentrations of 25-hydroxy vitamin D in an elderly nursing home population in Boston. *American Journal of Clinical Nutrition* **51**, 1075–1081.

Weisburger, J. H. (1991) Nutritional approach to cancer prevention with emphasis on vitamins, antioxidants, and carotenoids. *American Journal of Clinical Nutrition* **53**, 226s–237s.

Willett, W. C., Stampfer, M., Marison, J. and Van Itallie, T. (1991) New weight guidelines for Americans: justified or injudicious? *American Journal of Clinical Nutrition* **53**, 1102–1103.

Young, V. R. (1990) Amino acids and proteins in relation to the nutrition of elderly people. *Age and Aging* **19**, 510–524.

Young, V. R. and Marchini, J. S. (1990) Mechanisms and nutritional significance of metabolic responses to altered intakes of protein and amino acids with reference to nutritional adaptation in humans. *American Journal of Clinical Nutrition* **51**, 270–289.

Young, V. R., Gersovitz, M. and Munro, H. N. (1982) Human aging, protein, and amino acid metabolism and implications for protein and amino acid requirements. In: *Nutritional Approaches to Aging Research* (ed. Moment, G. B.). Boca Raton, FL: CRC Press, pp. 47–81.

Young, V. R., Bier, D. M. and Pellett, P. L (1989) A theoretical basis for increasing current estimates of the amino acid requirements in adult man with experimental support. *American Journal of Clinical Nutrition* **50**, 80–92.

Zanni, E., Calloway, D. H., Zezulka, A. Y. (1979) Protein requirements of elderly men. *J. Nutr.* **109**, 513–524.

# 10
# Skeletal Changes in Human Aging

CHRIS C. PLATO, KATHLEEN M. FOX AND JORDAN D. TOBIN

## INTRODUCTION

Changes in bone and cartilage take place during all stages of the human life span. During childhood and through adolescence, these changes are cumulatively characterized as growth and development. They are relatively fast and are usually beneficial to the individual. The maturing human skeleton undergoes a large increase in bone size and volume during pubertal development (Garn, 1981). Individuals will attain their full adult skeletal size by the age of 35 (Exton-Smith et al., 1969; Garn, 1970; Albanese, 1977). Skeletal changes, brought about by aging, progress at a slower rate, are less uniform, and are associated with decreasing levels of adaptability and performance.

After the third decade of life, the human skeleton begins to undergo two diverse changes: (1) it gains bone matter by forming osteophytes at the joints; and (2) it loses endosteal cortical and trabecular bone from both the axial and peripheral areas of the skeleton. While age-related bone loss and joint cartilage degeneration usually do not interfere with the normal function of the individual, occasionally, these changes progress to a stage where they become deleterious and significantly affect the individual's normal functioning. These pathological changes are then considered to be diseases, and referred to as osteoporosis and osteoarthritis.

## BONE LOSS AND OSTEOPOROSIS

Loss of bone mass begins as early as the third decade of life as bone resorption exceeds the acquisition of new bone (Garn et al., 1967a; Garn, 1972; Riggs et al., 1973; Heaney, 1981; Parfitt, 1981; Mazess, 1982). Bones lose both mineral and organic matrix but retain their basic organization. Bone loss is universal and an inevitable consequence of aging (Garn et al., 1972a; Cummings et al., 1985). It occurs in both sexes and in all human populations studied thus far (Trotter et al., 1960; Nordin, 1966; Spencer et al., 1966; Garn et al., 1969; Garn, 1970; Newton-John and Morgan, 1970; Frisancho et al., 1971; Cohn et al., 1977; Riggs et al., 1981; Mazess, 1982; Plato et al., 1982; Kusec et al., 1988,

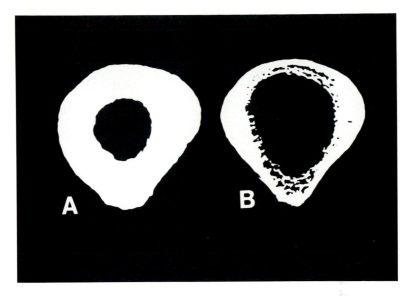

**Figure 10-1** Cross-sections of tabular bone showing vertebrae with (A) normal young bone and (B) osteoporotic bone. From Plato and Tobin (1990).

1989, 1990). Furthermore, bone loss with age was also demonstrated on archaeological specimens from three Nubian groups who lived in Sudan as early as 350BC (Dewey *et al.*, 1969; Armelagos *et al.*, 1972; Carlson *et al.*, 1974; Martin *et al.*, 1981).

**Pathological Signs**

Bone is a dynamic tissue that constantly undergoes remodeling throughout life (Garn, 1970). This remodeling entails resorption of old bone by osteoclasts and formation of new bone by osteoblasts. It is the coupling/uncoupling of bone formation and resorption that plays a key role in the pathogenesis of bone loss and osteoporosis. As bone resorption exceeds bone formation, the inner surface of cortical bone becomes progressively thinner (Figure 10-1) even though outer surface apposition continues throughout life (Sedlin *et al.*, 1963; Smith and Walker, 1964; Epker *et al.*, 1965; Arnold *et al.*, 1966; Garn *et al.*, 1967b, 1968, 1972; Garn, 1970, 1972; Parfitt, 1981; Milhaud *et al.*, 1983). Trabecular bone, the spongy series of thin plates forming the interior meshwork of bones (Figure 10-2), also decreases with increasing age.

The process of bone remodeling is complex. Calcium, phosphorus, and endocrine hormones operating at the system level, as well as local regulating factors, influence bone cells during the formation and breakdown of bone (Canalis, 1983). While the effects of systemic hormones such as parathyroid hormone, vitamin D, calcitonin, growth hormone, and sex steroids have been investigated extensively, much of the current research in bone remodeling is directed toward the effects of local factors such as insulin-like growth factors,

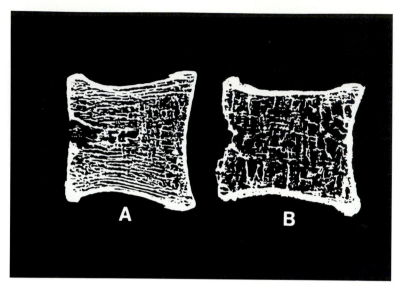

**Figure 10-2** Section of normal human vertebral body (A). Osteoporotic vertebra (B) with almost complete absence of horizontal trabeculae and increased prominence of vertical trabeculae. From Plato and Tobin (1990).

transforming growth factors, and fibroblast growth factors whose operation and effect on bone metabolism are not yet clearly understood (Canalis, 1990).

## Bone Mass Measurements

To determine the amount of bone loss, bone mineral determinations are made by calculating the cortical thickness and percentage cortical area from hand–wrist X-ray measurements of the second metacarpal or from direct bone mineral density evaluations of the radius, lumbar spine, and proximal evaluations of the radius, lumbar spine, and proximal femur through absorptiometry. Second metacarpal bone measurements include total bone diameter ($T$), medullary width ($M$) and cortical thickness, measured directly from radiographs (Figure 10-3A). Percentage cortical area (PCA), derived from total and medullary area measurements (Figure 10-3B), is utilized as the indicator of bone mass. However, at least 30% of the bone mineral in the metacarpal must be lost before a change can be detected by radiography (Mazess, 1978; Cohn, 1981). Single- and dual-photon absorptiometry and more recently dual-energy X-ray absorptiometry are used to provide accurate measurements of bone loss over time in the radius, spine, and femur. Absorptiometry uses a narrow collimated beam of low-energy photons or X-rays to estimate the mineral content of bone as well as bone width. Bone mineral density (g/cm$^2$) is estimated by dividing bone mineral content by bone width.

The rate of bone loss is not equal for cortical and trabecular bone. Bone mineral density (BMD) in the radius, spine, and proximal femur, and the PCA

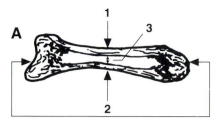

Total Width (**T**) = Distance 1 to Distance 2

Medullary Width (**M**) = Distance 3

Cortical Thickness (**CT**) = **T - M**

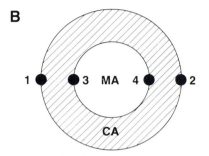

Total Width (**T**) = Distance 1 to 2
Medullary Width (**M**) = Distance 3 to 4
Cortical Thickness (**CT**) = Distance (1 to 3) + (2 to 4)
Total Area (**TA**) = Area with Diameter 1 to 2
Medullary Area (**MA**) = Open Area with Diameter 3 to 4
Cortical Area (**CA**) = Cross Hatched Area = **TA - MA**
Percent Cortical Area (**PCA**) = (**CA/TA**) x 100

**Figure 10-3**   Cross-sections of the second metacarpal bone indicating the measurements used in bone mass estimates. (A) Longitudinal section; (B) transverse section at the midshaft.

of the second metacarpal are shown for each decade of age in male and female participants of the Baltimore Longitudinal Study of Aging (BLSA) (Figure 10-4). The ages of the participants ranged from 20 to 90 years of age. Observations were available from the second metacarpal of 1,192 males and 415 females, from the radius of 528 males and 344 females, from the spine of 529 males and 309 females, and from the femur (femoral neck, Ward's triangle and greater trochanter) of 188 males and 215 females. Neither the mean levels of bone mineral at each age group, nor the decrease in bone mineral with age are the same in different parts of the skeleton (Figure 10-4). Cortical bone loss, at a rate of 0.5–1% per year, appears to be linear for both men and women, starting around age 40 (Riggs *et al.*, 1982; Fox *et al.*, 1986; Riggs and Melton, 1986). Trabecular bone loss starts earlier than cortical loss, around age 35 and sometimes as early as the mid-twenties (Plato *et al.*, 1990). It is linear for men at a rate of about 1–1.2% per year (Riggs *et al.*, 1973, 1981, 1982). In women, the loss is also linear, at a rate of about 1–4% per year but the pattern is

# Hand, Forearm and Spine

# Hip

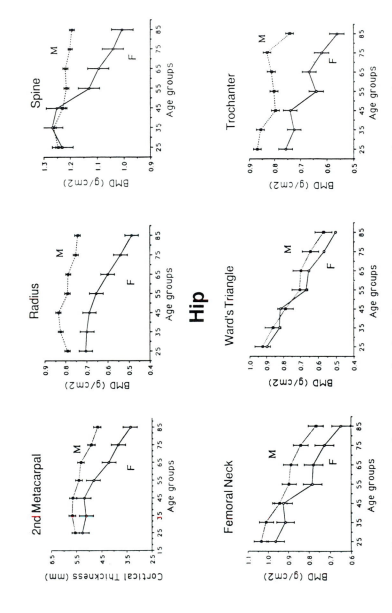

**Figure 10-4** Mean bone mineral values for each age group at (A) the second metacarpal, the radius, the spine, and (B) the hip of male and female participants of the Baltimore Longitudinal Study of Aging.

characterized by a rapid postmenopausal acceleration in loss (Riggs *et al.* 1982; Parfitt, 1984). Bone mass is lost at a rate of up to 10% per year 3–7 years after menopause (Riggs *et al.*, 1982; Parfitt, 1984; Riggs and Melton, 1986). Men (with the exception of ages 35–45 in the spine and Ward's triangle) have more bone mineral in all age groups than females (Figure 10-4).

In a recent cross-sectional study, Plato *et al.* (1990) tested the linearity of bone loss at different skeletal sites; the second metacarpal and the radius, lumbar spine and the proximal femur of young (ages 20–48) and older (ages 60+) men and women. Women in their perimenopausal years (49–59) and men of the same age group were excluded. The results indicated that contrary to common belief, younger women showed no significant change (gain or loss) in bone mineral density in any of the skeletal sites studied, while younger men showed significant linear loss in the two femoral sites (femoral neck and Ward's triangle) and curvilinear change (increase then decrease in bone mineral) in the lumbar spine, the radius, and the second metacarpal. Only in the radius did young women have less bone than young men. Furthermore, older men and women showed significant linear bone loss at all skeletal sites studied. Neither men nor women, young or old, showed significant change in bone density in the greater femoral trochanter area. Overall, bone diminution in women throughout life was found to be 22–47% for the vertebrae, 30% for the midradius, 39% for the distal radius, 30–58% for the femoral neck, 25–53% for the intertrochanteric region of the femur, 41% for Ward's triangle and 25% for the second metacarpal (Riggs *et al.*, 1981, 1982; Mazess, 1982; Plato *et al.*, 1993). For men, the overall decline in bone mass is 14% for the vertebrae, 22–39% in the femoral neck, 33% for Ward's triangle, 9% for the greater trochanter, 11% for the second metacarpal, and 12% for the midradius (Horsman *et al.*, 1981; Riggs *et al.*, 1982; Plato *et al.*, 1993).

It is not clear what brings about the differences in the rate of bone loss at the different skeletal sites. While differential ratios of cortical to trabecular bone may explain a portion of the differences between the second metacarpal and radius on one hand and the spine and femur on the other, this cannot be the only factor involved. The largest difference in both the total amount as well as the rate of bone loss is seen between the greater trochanter and the other two femoral sites. What brings about an almost 40% reduction in bone density from age 30 to 90 in the Ward's triangle and only 9% in the adjacent greater trochanter is not understood. Developmental, structural, and biomechanical differences may contribute to inter-site variation in bone mineral density. Despite their physical proximity, the femoral neck and the greater trochanter have different developmental origins. The arrangement of the cancelli in the neck of the femur differs from that of the greater trochanter to accommodate the different types of tension encountered in each region. In the femoral neck and Ward's triangle, the stress is more of the shearing and weight-bearing (pressure) type while in the greater trochanter, where muscles holding the erect body posture are attached, the stress is principally of the tension type. In addition, bone responds to the stresses placed on it from activity level and exercise (Nilsson and Westlin, 1971; Plato and Norris, 1980; Brewer *et al.*, 1983; Block *et al.*, 1986). Notwithstanding the above inter-site differences, there is a significantly high, albeit variable, correlation in the amount of bone mineral density at different skeletal sites of the same individual (Aitken *et al.*, 1974; Plato, 1987).

Bone mass also demonstrates bilateral asymmetry. It has been shown that the right second metacarpal has higher cortical thickness than the left (Garn, 1970; Plato *et al.*, 1980). This is in part a reflection of the right-hand dominance and hence higher activity of the right hand among the majority of humans. However, since most left-handed people also have higher cortical thickness in the right hand, one must suspect an inherent predisposition of humankind to have more bone on the right side which may be enhanced or decreased by hand dominance (Plato *et al.*, 1980). This predisposition is supported by limited experiments in rats that showed higher bone mineral in the left side (opposite to what we find in humans) or most bilateral bones of this animal (S. Kimura, personal communication).

## Clinical and Epidemiological Characteristics

Some individuals will lose extreme amounts of bone and become osteoporotic to the extent that their bones lose mechanical integrity and fracture more readily. Osteoporotic bone is susceptible to fracture, especially that of the hip, vertebrae, and radius. More than 220,000 hip fractures occur in individuals over age 65 each year in the United States alone (Cummings *et al.*, 1985; National Center for Health Statistics (NCHS), 1985). Over 90% of these femoral fractures and 75% of all Colles' fractures (fractures of the distal radius) in adults are due to osteoporosis (Melton *et al.*, 1988). Fractures of the femur are associated with more deaths, disability and medical costs than all other osteoporotic fractures combined. At least half of the hip-fracture patients ambulating before sustaining a hip fracture cannot walk independently afterward (Miller, 1978; Jette *et al.*, 1987; Mossey *et al.*, 1989; Magaziner *et al.*, 1990). In the first year after fracture, mortality is 12–20% higher in hip-fracture patients than in persons of similar age and gender (Gallagher *et al.*, 1980; Lewinnek *et al.*, 1980; Magaziner *et al.*, 1989).

After age 50, the incidence rate of hip fracture rises dramatically with age (Figure 10-5). Almost 50% of hip fractures occur among individuals 80 years of age and older (Alffram, 1964; Gallagher *et al.*, 1980). Age-specific incidence rates for hip fracture are 2–3 times higher in women than in men (Alffram, 1964; Gallagher *et al.*, 1980). The lifetime risk of a hip fracture has been estimated to be 15% in white women and 5% in white men (Cummings *et al.*, 1985). This risk is equivalent to the combined lifetime risk of developing breast, uterine, or ovarian cancer in women (Seidman *et al.*, 1978). The lifetime risk of Colles' fracture from age 50 is also 15% in white women and about 2% in white men (Cummings *et al.*, 1985). Until age 75, fractures of the distal forearm (Colles' fractures) are the most common fracture among white women in the United States (Alffram and Bauer, 1962; Owen *et al.*, 1982).

The severity and the high cost of managing hip fractures notwithstanding, the spine is the skeletal site principally affected by osteoporosis. Almost one

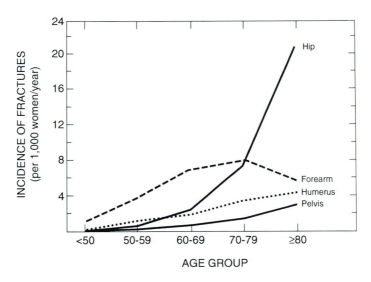

**Figure 10-5**   Age-specific incidence rates of hip fracture per 1,000 women per year. From Cummings *et al.* (1985).

third of women age 65 years and older will have one or more vertebral fractures (Melton *et al.*, 1989). Among women 50 years of age and older, new vertebral fractures are nearly three times as frequent as hip fractures. As many as 500,000 white women are newly affected by vertebral fractures each year (Melton, 1987). As trabeculae diminish in numbers and size, vertebrae become deformed. Vertebrae collapse upon one another and take on a wedge-shaped form. These vertebral deformities accumulate in some women and eventually cause a kyphotic "Dowager's hump" posture. Each complete vertebral compression fracture causes the loss of about 1 cm in height (Parfitt and Duncan, 1982).

## Cross-cultural Variability

Little data are available on cross-cultural differences in bone density levels. Data from several countries, however, are available from radiographic studies of the second metacarpal. Garn and his associates published detailed data on bone gain and loss from a number of Central American populations (Garn *et al.*, 1969, 1976; Garn, 1970). In general, among Western populations, blacks have higher bone density than whites (Trotter *et al.*, 1960; Nordin, 1966; Johnston *et al.*, 1968; Garn *et al.*, 1972b; Cohn *et al.*, 1977). In men from Jamaica and from Gambia, Africa, metacarpal measurements are clustered above the mean measurements for white United States men (Nordin, 1966). Cross-cultural data from Central and North America indicate that males and females from Mexico, Guatemala, and El Salvador have metacarpal measurements similar to US males and females (Table 10-1) (Garn *et al.*, 1967a, 1967b). Additionally, Yugoslavians have metacarpal measurements that are

**Table 10-1** Percentage cortical area of the second metacarpal by region, age group, and sex.

| Region (Reference) | Percentage cortical area | | | | | |
|---|---|---|---|---|---|---|
| | Males | | | Females | | |
| | Age | | | Age | | |
| | 60 | 70 | 80 | 60 | 70 | 80 |
| Scotland | 52.0 | 52.0 | 52.0 | 50.0 | 46.0 | — |
| Japan (Nordin, 1966) | 51.0 | 52.0 | — | 52.0 | — | — |
| USA (Garn, 1970) | 79.4 | 78.0 | 78.6 | 81.3 | 71.8 | 63.7 |
| Guatemala (Garn, 1970) | 83.5 | 79.0 | 80.3 | 76.8 | 72.9 | 66.9 |
| El Salvador (Garn, 1970) | 83.4 | 77.7 | 76.4 | 78.4 | 73.4 | 62.9 |
| Mexican American (Garn et al., 1972a) | 82.3 | 85.5 | 81.9 | 85.0 | 77.0 | 69.6 |
| Yugoslavia (Kusec et al., 1988) | 79.0 | 76.0 | 75.0 | 77.0 | 71.0 | 67.0 |

similar but slightly lower than US populations (Table 10-1). Additional studies on Yugoslavia were published by Kusec and associates (Kusec et al., 1988, 1989, 1990; Simic et al., 1992) and in Albania by Behluli and his colleagues (1991). A comparative study of bone mass between male and female inhabitants of the island of Guam and Caucasians of the Baltimore Longitudinal Study of Aging (Plato et al., 1984), matched for sex, age and menopausal status (among females) indicated that Caucasians had longer and larger (in total width) second metacarpals than their Guamanian counterparts. However, despite the differences in length and total width, Guamanians and Caucasians showed no significant differences in percentage cortical area. This suggests that larger bones do not always indicate greater cortical mass. Bone measurements of the second metacarpal of Guamanian children, ages 5–17 years, who lived during the nutritional deprivation of the Japanese occupation of the island of Guam during World War II, were also studied (Plato et al., 1984). The results indicated that the second metacarpals of Guamanian boys and girls had narrower width and shorter length and less percentage cortical area than their black, white, or Mexican American counterparts reported by Garn and colleagues (1976). It was unclear whether the lower bone values of the Guamanian children were due to the nutritional deprivation or to genetic variability. Cross-sectional and longitudinal studies of Guamanian patients with amyotrophic lateral sclerosis (Lou Gehrig's disease) showed that these patients, who eventually developed paralysis and complete immobility, had significantly lower percentage cortical area than nonaffected, age-matched Guamanian controls (Yanagihara et al., 1984; Garruto et al., 1989).

Cross-cultural studies also included archaeological data. Dewey et al. (1969) excavated femoral sections from three Nubian cultural groups who lived in Sudan during three prehistoric periods (350BC–AD350, AD350–AD550, and AD550–AD1300). The results revealed no statistical differences in femoral cortical thickness between corresponding age groups from the three prehistoric sites. However, they found significant differences in bone loss between males

**Table 10-2**   Incidence rates of hip fracture per 100,000 age-adjusted to the 1970 US population by region and sex (adapted from Cummings *et al.*, 1985).

| Region | Women | Men | Female/male ratio |
|---|---|---|---|
| United States | 101.6 | 50.5 | 2.01 |
| New Zealand | 96.8 | 35.2 | 1.79 |
| Sweden | 87.2 | 38.2 | 2.75 |
| Jerusalem | 69.9 | 42.8 | 1.63 |
| United Kingdom | 63.1 | 29.3 | 2.15 |
| Holland | 51.1 | 28.5 | 1.80 |
| Finland | 49.9 | 27.4 | 1.78 |
| Yugoslavia[a] | 39.2 | 37.9 | 1.03 |
| Hong Kong | 31.3 | 27.2 | 1.15 |
| Yugoslavia[b] | 17.3 | 18.2 | 0.95 |
| Singapore | 15.3 | 26.5 | 0.58 |
| South African Bantu | 5.3 | 5.6 | 0.94 |

[a]Low-calcium diet.
[b]High-calcium diet.

and females. Females showed significant bone loss with age ($P<0.001$), while males showed no significant age-related bone loss. Bone loss in females of ages 20–41 was twice as much as that of males of the same age. Furthermore, the total percentage of bone loss among Nubians was similar to that of modern populations. However, the Nubian females started losing bone much earlier than women of modern populations. Our data (Plato *et al.*, 1990) showed no significant bone loss in females prior to 45 years of age. Dewey and his colleagues (1969) suggested that the observed early onset of bone loss in Nubian women is due to nutritional factors, long lactation periods (2–4 years) and more pregnancies rather than due to estrogen hormonal changes and menopause. In a follow-up study (Mielke *et al.*, 1972) of one of these groups (AD350–AD550), investigators found that both males and females lost trabecular bone at the head of the femur (16% in males and 13% in females) as age increased from 17 to 50 years.

Incidence rates of hip fracture also vary considerably from one geographic area to another. Age- and sex-adjusted hip fracture incidence rates in the United States are higher than those in any other region from which data have been published (Table 10-2) (Nordin, 1966; Lewinnek *et al.*, 1980). New Zealand and Western Europe also have high rates while the lowest reported rates are found among the South African Bantu (Bloom and Pogrund, 1982). Age-specific incidence rates of hip fracture are about twice as high in white women as in black women. Most studies also indicate a higher risk for hip fractures among white men as compared with black men (Bollet *et al.*, 1965; Engh *et al.*, 1968; Farmer *et al.*, 1984). Mexican American populations have lower fracture rates than whites but slightly higher rates than blacks (Bauer *et al.*, 1986; Bauer, 1988). These large geographic variations may be attributable to genetic variability or differences in diet, degree of physical activity, and exposure to sunlight or to differences in reporting fracture cases.

Additional factors that may influence the geographic variability as well as sex differences in bone mass levels and fracture rates are reproductive characteristics. The rate of cortical and trabecular bone loss accelerates around the time of menopause (Cann *et al.*, 1980; Christiansen *et al.*, 1980; Mazess, 1982). Reduced estrogen production at menopause is the suspected cause of this accelerated bone loss. Current data indicate that additional reproductive factors, such as parity, menarche, and menstrual history, influence bone density. High parity (three or more births) has been shown to be associated with increased bone density (Smith, 1967; Nilsson, 1969; Frisancho *et al.*, 1971; Fox, 1990). A history of breast feeding was found to have no effect on bone density, neither detrimental nor beneficial (Sowers *et al.*, 1985; Byrne *et al.*, 1987; Fox, 1990; Bauer *et al.*, 1992). Menstrual cycle characteristics tend to have profound effects on bone density. An early age at menarche, more years menstruating, and longer periods of bleeding during each menstrual cycle have been associated with higher levels of bone density of the distal radius (Smith, 1967; Fox, 1990). Amenorrhea, on the other hand, places a woman at risk of osteoporosis due to estrogen deficiency (Drinkwater *et al.*, 1984, 1990). Women athletes who exercise excessively and become amenorrheic actually negate the benefits of mechanical loading on the bone. If exercise is reduced and normal menses resume, bone loss slows (Drinkwater *et al.*, 1986; Lindberg *et al.*, 1987). These reproductive factors may serve as markers of estrogen levels with estrogen deficiency leading to bone loss and osteoporosis.

## JOINT DEGENERATION AND OSTEOARTHRITIS

Like bone loss, every human skeleton is subjected to some degree of joint degeneration and osteophyte formation after the middle years of life are reached. In certain individuals, these changes become excessive and the disease, osteoarthritis, develops.

Osteoarthritis has been well known since the ancient times. Hippocrates made reference to its occurrence among the aged. Evidence of the disease has also been found in Egyptian mummies (Osgood, 1940) and in remains of prehistoric American Indians (Hooton, 1930). Chapman (1972) also reported the presence of vertebral osteoarthritis in five prehistoric populations of central and southern Mexico. It is the most common rheumatic disease worldwide and one of the most common chronic diseases, affecting over 40 million Americans in the United States alone (NCHS, 1966a; Dawson and Adams, 1987).

### Pathological Signs

While discussion of the pathological signs of osteoarthritis is beyond the scope of this paper, the general pathological appearance of the joints is outlined here because they are related to the clinical and radiological signs which follow them. Osteoarthritis is a chronic, noninflamatory, usually benign form of arthritis. It is characterized by abrasion and degeneration of cartilage and bone hypertrophy at or near the movable joints of the skeleton. Initially, there occurs a softening, roughening, and fibrilization of the articular cartilage with the appearance of clefts and fissures (Brandt and Fife, 1986). As the disease progresses, the articular cartilage erodes irregularly until it is eventually worn down. Sometimes this erosion may be complete thus exposing the underlying bone. The latter in such cases becomes dense and hard. Paralleling the articular cartilage degeneration, there is a proliferation of the cellular components of the cartilage, forming a dense layer. The intracellular substance swells while individual cells enlarge and form clusters. These eventually spread to the areas of the clefts and fissures. This is believed to be a vain attempt by the system to regenerate lost matter through enhanced cell division. Marginal proliferations eventually develop in the form of osteophytes, spurs, lipping, or exostoses. Heberden's nodes are the specific enlargements seen at the terminal joints of the fingers due to bone proliferation. Pathological changes in the joints as seen from autopsies appear as early as the second decade of life (Lowman, 1955). By the ninth decade of life, the pathological signs of osteoarthritis become practically universal.

## Clinical Signs

Clinically, the cardinal symptom of osteoarthritis is pain as well as soreness and stiffness which increases with use and subsides with rest. Osteoarthritis not only involves the weight-bearing joints but also the interphalangeal joints of the fingers. The joints most commonly involved are the interphalangeal joints of the hands, the knees, the spine, hips, the sacro-iliac and the shoulders. Osteoarthritis very rarely involves the wrists or elbows. It should be noted here that even though almost all people beyond the age of 50 show pathological signs of osteoarthritis in one or more joints, clinical manifestations occur only in about 5–10% of the cases and are very rare prior to the age of 40.

## Roentgenographic Signs

In the very early stages of the disease and in mild cases, the X-ray appearance of the joints may be normal. As the disease progresses, the radiological signs become more pronounced. The cardinal X-ray sign of degenerative joint disease, especially in the early stages, is the narrowing of the joint space which is a result of the degeneration and gradual elimination of the articular cartilage. However, since this criterion is not specific to osteoarthritis and is very difficult to evaluate, most investigators consider the beginning of the disease with the appearance of marginal osteophytes (Kellgren et al., 1963). These are formed on or near the joint and result from the pathological bone or cartilage proliferations. Gradual sclerosis of the subchondral bone follows as new bone material is deposited in the sub-articular areas. Small cysts may also appear in some cases. All these changes will eventually alter the overall shape and appearance of the bone ends and the joint in general. In Heberden's nodes, one also encounters spur formation (Stecher and Hauser, 1948). These spurs usually develop at the attachments of the flexor and extensor tendons of the distal phalanx.

## Epidemiological Characteristics

Several multi-disciplinary studies have reported on the epidemiological aspects of osteoarthritis. They include the Tecumseh, Michigan study (Mikkelsen *et al.*, 1967, 1970; Butler *et al.*, 1988), the NCHS (1966a, 1966b, 1966c, 1979), Framingham study (Felson, 1990), the Baltimore Longitudinal Study of Aging (Plato and Norris, 1979a, 1979b; Busby *et al.*, 1991; Hochberg *et al.*, 1991), Ten State Nutritional survey (Hollingsworth, 1974), and several additional general reports (Kraus *et al.*, 1978; Lawrence *et al.*, 1989; Van Sasse *et al.*, 1989; Hochberg, 1993). Most epidemiological studies on osteoarthritis have been based on roentgenographic data, mainly from hand–wrist X-rays evaluated through the use of the Kellgren scale (Table 10-3 and Figure 10-6) which considers the oesteophyte formation as the cardinal criterion for the process (Kellgrenand Lawrence, 1957; Kellgren, 1963). Grades 0 and 1 of the Kellgren scale are considered negative (normal) while grades 2, 3 and 4 are accepted as positive (affected). While it is relatively easy to discriminate between widely separated grades, discrimination between consecutive grades is not always clear and is subject to considerable inter-investigator error. The classification of both grades 0 and 1 as negative does not mean that they are the same. Busby *et al.* (1991) in a longitudinal study involving 386 normal male participants of the Baltimore Longitudinal Study of Aging concluded that grade 1 is an intermediate step in the progression of osteoarthritis of the interphalangeal joint and is not synonymous with grade 0.

There is preferential involvement of the distal interphalangeal joints of the fingers in osteoarthritis (Radin *et al.*, 1971; Plato and Norris, 1979a). Prevalence of osteoarthritis of the hands and feet in the adult US population is

**Table 10-3** Main criteria for osteoarthritis classification of the joints of the hand (adapted from Kellgren, 1963).

| Classification | | Criteria for classification |
|---|---|---|
| Kellgren grade | Clinical classification | Radiographic appearance of the joints |
| 0 | Negative | Normal |
| 1 | Negative | Presence of a minimal osteophyte at one point. Otherwise a normal joint. |
| 2 | Positive | Definite osteophyte at two points. Minimal subchondral sclerosis. Fairly good joint space. No deformity at bone ends. |
| 3 | Positive | Moderate osteophytes at two or more places. Considerable narrowing of the joint space. Some deformity of the bone ends. |
| 4 | Positive | Presence of large osteophytes. Loss of joint space. Sclerosis. Gross deformity of the bone ends and the joint in general. Cysts may be present. |

grade 0          grade 1

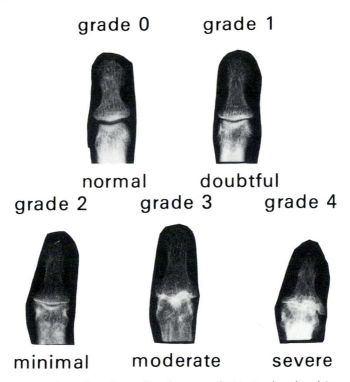

normal          doubtful
grade 2      grade 3      grade 4

minimal     moderate     severe

**Figure 10-6**  Examples of each grade of osteoarthritis in the distal interphalangeal joints of the hand (see Table 10-2 and the text).

37%. About 23% of these cases had moderate or severe osteoarthritis (Scott and Hochberg, 1984). Prevalence rates as well as severity of osteoarthritis increase with age. In a longitudinal study of osteoarthritis of the hand, it was shown that only 3.8% of subjects under 40 years of age had any sign of osteoarthritis while 33.3% of the middle-aged and 70.6% of the elderly subjects had osteoarthritis of the distal interphalangeal joints of the hand (Busby *et al.*, 1991). The incidence of new cases of osteoarthritis is higher and disease progression more rapid in the hand with increasing age (Kallman *et al.*, 1990; Busby *et al.*, 1991; Verbrugge *et al.*, 1991). The median time for development of an additional affected joint in the hand was about 15 years for young subjects versus 9.4 years for elderly subjects (Plato and Norris, 1979b; Busby *et al.*, 1991). These longitudinal results suggest that even individuals who reached old age with minimal or no radiographic signs of osteoarthritis are still at an accelerated risk for developing the disease. However, osteoarthritis progresses very slowly. It takes approximately 10–20 years for any feature of osteoarthritis to progress to the next grade (Plato and Norris, 1979b; Kallman *et al.*, 1990). It takes even longer for subjects to progress from the intermediate to late stages of osteoarthritis (Kallman *et al.*, 1990). The prevalence of osteoarthritis varies from one digit to another. In the general population, the fifth digit is the most frequently affected, regardless of age or joint (Plato and Norris, 1979a). The first digit is the least frequently affected.

Although osteoarthritis of the hip and knee is less prevalent than that of the hand, a substantial number of individuals are incapacitated from knee and hip osteoarthritis. Substantial disability (chronic back pain) also results from osteoarthritis of the spine. In the United States, prevalence of severe or moderate osteoarthritis of the knee is 0.9% while an additional 2.9% have minimal knee osteoarthritis (NCHS, 1979). Rates of osteoarthritis of the hip are 1.3% (NCHS, 1979). Osteoarthritis progresses more rapidly in the knees than in the elbow and in the hips more rapidly than in the shoulder (Mikkelsen *et al.*, 1970).

## Etiological Considerations
### General

There are two types of osteoarthritis: (1) primary or idiopathic; and (2) secondary or traumatic. The latter type is usually a consequence of direct or indirect injuries or insults to the joint areas and generally remain localized to the joints originally involved. The idiopathic forms are produced spontaneously without history of injury and gradually extend to other joints. The etiology of the idiopathic forms remains elusive but probably is multi-factorial. A number of factors, including physical and biomechanical stress, endocrine disturbances, and heredity have been found to contribute to the development of osteoarthritis.

### Physical and Biomechanical Stress

It is generally accepted by most investigators and supported by laboratory and epidemiological studies that chronic irritation to a joint can and often does produce osteoarthritis. The irritation may either be a result of injury or due to excessive stress because of occupational habits, sports activities, obesity, poor posture or simply the wear and tear of the joints in everyday life. Several studies (Copeman, 1940; Kellgren and Lawrence, 1952; Lawrence *et al.*, 1963; NCHS, 1966a, 1966b; Gordon and Engel, 1968; Partridge and Duthie, 1968; Hadler *et al.*, 1978; Lindberg and Montgomery, 1987; Hochberg, 1992) indicated that osteoarthritis is more prevalent among craftsmen, farmers, heavy machinery operators, and laborers than among salesmen, clerical and house workers. Studies on the effects of regimented exercise and sports activities on the development of osteoarthritis gave variable results (Puranen *et al.*, 1975; Klunder *et al.*, 1980; Lane *et al.*, 1986, 1990; Panush *et al.*, 1986). Hochberg (1993) summarizes the results of some of these studies. Mechanical stresses increase the prevalence of osteoarthritis in the involved joints (Radin *et al.*, 1971). Radin and his associates (1971) suggested that the differential involvement of the distal interphalangeal joints may be due to biomechanical or functional mechanical factors, such as higher pressure per unit area exerted on these small joints by the muscles that govern them. It seems that the critical factor is not the force, rather it is longitudinal pressure on the joint brought about by normal functions of the joints. Plato and Norris (1979a) suggested that osteoarthritis of the proximal interphalangeal joints of the hand may be caused by trauma and other exogenous factors. Conversely, osteoarthritis of the distal interphalangeal joints, a more prevalent condition, may be due to factors related to the process of aging.

### Endocrine and Physiological Factors

There is evidence that the endocrine system is involved in the development of osteoarthritis. The close association of osteoarthritis with menopause has been noted by a number of investigators dating back to the 1920s (Cecil and Archer, 1925; Hall, 1939; Stecher et al., 1949). This association holds true whether the menopause is normal or induced by disease or surgery.

Some investigators reported association between osteoarthritis and several body measurements (NCHS, 1966c; Felson et al., 1988; Felson, 1990). Obesity was reported to be associated with osteoarthritis of the knee (Engel, 1966; Acheson and Collart, 1975; Hartz et al., 1986; Anderson and Felson, 1988; Van Saase et al., 1988; Davis et al., 1989). However, the association between obesity and osteoarthritis of the hand and hip remains debatable (Hochberg, 1993). Davis and colleagues (1989) found obesity to be a stronger predictor of bilateral rather than unilateral osteoarthritis of the knee. Muscle strength was also reported to be associated with osteoarthritis (Acheson et al., 1970). Hochberg and colleagues (1991) studied the association between osteoarthritis of the hand and body mass index, waist to hip ratio, percentage body fat, grip strength, and forearm circumference in a group of 888 male Caucasian volunteers between 17 and 102 years of age. They found that a higher grade of (more severe) osteoarthritis was associated with increasing mean levels of waist-to-hip ratio and percentage body fat, as well as decreasing mean values in grip strength, forearm circumference, and bone mass of the second metacarpal. However, after adjusting for age, none of the above physiological and metabolic parameters remained significantly associated with hand osteoarthritis. It appears that the observed associations are due to the mutual relationship of these variables to age (Hochberg et al., 1991).

### Heredity

It is the impression of most investigators of osteoarthritis that heredity plays a role in the etiology of the idiopathic forms. The genetic contribution may be either direct or indirect, through the inheritance of poor grades of cartilage (Bauer and Bennett, 1936). Stecher and his associates (Stecher, 1940; Stecher and Hauser, 1941; Stecher et al., 1953) and Radin and his colleagues (1971) showed that the idiopathic form of degenerative joint disease of the fingers (Heberden's nodes) is due to genetic factors. Kellgren et al. (1963) found familial tendencies in generalized arthritis but could not establish a mode of inheritance. It has also been suggested that there is an inheritance of increased susceptibility to the wear and tear of daily life and an inheritance of factors known to contribute to the development of osteoarthritis such as congenital hip dislocation (Radin et al., 1971; Moscowitz, 1972; Jurmain, 1977; Hollander, 1980).

More recently, genetic studies of osteoarthritis have focused on the molecular, biological level, especially the linkage between cartilage specific genes and the disease (Palotie *et al.*, 1989; Ala-Kokko *et al.*, 1990; Knowlton *et al.*, 1990; Jimenez, 1991). Palotie and his colleagues (1989), through restriction fragment length polymorphism analysis on chromosome 12, were able to demonstrate genetic linkage between the cartilage specific gene (type II collagen gene) and primary osteoarthritis. These studies open new avenues toward the elucidation of the genetic contributions in the etiology of osteoarthritis.

## Cross-cultural Variability

While all human populations demonstrate joint degeneration, the limited cross-cultural data available suggest that the age–sex-specific prevalence varies among the major racial groups (Table 10-4). Eskimos have the lowest prevalence of the disease while the American Indians have the highest (Blumberg *et al.*, 1961; Bennett and Burch, 1968). American whites and blacks have intermediate rates of disease. Osteoarthritis of the knee was more frequent in US blacks while osteoarthritis of the distal interphalangeal joints of the hands and the first metatarsophalangeal joint was more frequent in US whites (NCHS, 1966a; Mikkelsen *et al.*, 1970; Hollingsworth, 1974). Solomon and colleagues (1975) reported that osteoarthritis of the hands, feet, and hips was less common among South African black females than among white females, while South African black males had greater hand involvement than white males. The prevalence of osteoarthritis of the hip has been reported to be low in Asian peoples (Hoaglund *et al.*, 1973) and natives of India (Mukhopadhaya and Barooah, 1967). Some studies suggest that osteoarthritis may be less prevalent in cold climates, such as in Alaska or Finland (Blumberg *et al.*, 1961; Lawrence *et al.*, 1963). However, comparisons by latitude show no gradient in prevalence of osteoarthritis (Lawrence, 1977). Other cross-sectional studies on osteoarthritis were reported for Jamaicans (Bremmer *et al.*, 1968), for Africans (Beighton *et al.*, 1985), and for Bulgarians (Tzonchev *et al.*, 1968).

Lethbridge-Cejku and colleagues (1992) completed a comparative study of the prevalence of osteoarthritis of the hand in two phenotypically healthy male Caucasian samples; one from the Baltimore Longitudinal Study of Aging (BLSA) and the other from the island of Brac in Croatia. The BLSA sample was composed mainly of highly educated urban professionals while the Brac sample consisted of individuals from a mostly rural environment with diverse socioeconomical and occupational levels. While both groups demonstrated an increase in osteoarthritis with increasing age, the Brac sample had a significantly larger number of joints affected and more severely affected joints at all ages than the BLSA sample. The authors suggested differential life styles and occupations as a reason for the differences in the occurrence and severity of osteoarthritis. It is therefore important that life style, occupation, and leisure activities, as well as ethnic and genetic variation, be taken into consideration when assessing cross-cultural differences.

**Table 10-4** Age- and sex-specific prevalence of osteoarthritis (grades 2–4) of the hands and the hands and/or feet in United States samples.

| Sex/Age | Hands affected (with or without involvement of the feet) | | | | | | | | | Hands and/or feet affected | | | |
|---|---|---|---|---|---|---|---|---|---|---|---|---|---|
| | Whites | | | | | | Mostly Whites | Blacks | Eskimos | Whites | Blacks | American Indians | |
| | Tecumseh[a] | Ten State[b] | BLSA[c] | USPHS Indiana/Idaho[d] | West Virginia Non-Miners[c] | West Virginia Miners[c] | NHES[f] | Ten State[g] | Alaska[d] | NHES[f] | NHES[f] | Black-feet[g] | Pima[g] |
| *Male* | | | | | | | | | | | | | |
| <25 | 0.0 | | | | | | 2.8 | | | 6.6 | 11.4 | | |
| 25–34 | 1.0 | 1.0 | 0.0 | 4.9 | 1.5 | 0.0 | 4.8 | 3.0 | 0.0 | 13.5 | 20.0 | 34.0 | 28.0 |
| 35–44 | 5.5 | 3.0 | 3.9 | 12.8 | 2.0 | 7.7 | 17.5 | 9.0 | 0.0 | 29.1 | 41.2 | 58.0 | 49.0 |
| 45–54 | 25.1 | 34.0 | 29.4 | 23.9 | 15.2 | 24.5 | 38.2 | 18.0 | 7.0 | 47.8 | 44.7 | 82.0 | 92.0 |
| 55–64 | 57.4 | 58.0 | 59.7 | 57.1 | 50.0 | 51.9 | 54.4 | 46.0 | 19.6 | 63.4 | 66.3 | 91.0 | 99.0 |
| 65–74 | 78.2 | 76.0 | 77.9 | 69.2 | 75.0 | 75.6 | 68.5 | 66.0 | 50.0 | 77.5 | 55.6 | 100.0 | 96.0 |
| 75+ | 88.0 | 88.0 | 93.3 | | | | 78.7 | 76.0 | | 81.1 | 78.6 | | |
| *Female* | | | | | | | | | | | | | |
| <25 | 0.0 | | | | | | 0.4 | | | 1.4 | 3.4 | | |
| 25–34 | 0.0 | 0.0 | | | | | 2.2 | 0.0 | 0.0 | 5.4 | 12.0 | 21.0 | 12.0 |
| 35–44 | 3.8 | 0.0 | | 2.1 | | | 11.2 | 5.0 | 4.3 | 19.8 | 19.3 | 37.0 | 25.0 |
| 45–54 | 31.5 | 20.0 | | 5.2 | | | 32.9 | 10.0 | 10.5 | 45.1 | 55.0 | 72.0 | 68.0 |
| 55–64 | 70.6 | 48.0 | | 26.2 | | | 65.4 | 52.0 | 28.0 | 75.9 | 66.4 | 93.0 | 93.0 |
| 65–74 | 90.5 | 92.0 | | 56.8 | | | 76.4 | 58.0 | 57.1 | 85.7 | 75.9 | 99.0 | 95.0 |
| 75+ | 78.0 | | | 84.6 | | | 85.0 | 83.0 | | 90.6 | 78.0 | | |

[a] From Mikkelsen et al. (1970).

[b] From Hollingsworth (1974).

[c] From Plato et al. (unpublished); ages: 20–29, 30–39, 40–49, 50–59, 60–69, 70+ years.

[d] From Blumberg et al. (1961); ages: 20–29, 30–39, 40–49, 50–59, 60+ years.

[e] From Lockshin et al. (1969); ages 20–29, 30–39, 40–49, 50–59, 60+ years.

[f] From US Dept Health Education and Welfare (1966); National Center for Health Statistics (1966a).

[g] From Bennett and Burch (1968); ages: 30–34, 35–39, 40–44, 45–49, 50–54, 55–59, 60–64, 65+ years.

## OVERVIEW

Skeletal changes in bone and cartilage, bone loss and osteoarthritis, in the non-traumatic forms, are very closely associated with age and the aging process. They are gradual and erosive. They are universal to the extent they occur in individuals of either sex and in all populations studied thus far, although there is variability among individuals, between sexes, and among populations. This is largely due to the multi-factorial nature of these pathogenic processes. The association between aging and skeletal changes is also seen in epidemiological studies, not only because the prevalence of these processes increases with age, but also because of the abrupt increase in prevalence after the onset of female menopause. This association is further reinforced by the fact that skeletal changes are an almost inevitable occurrence in old age. If a person lives long enough (past the age of 80), he or she will develop some degree of osteoarthritis and bone loss.

Numerous factors influence the development and progression of bone loss and osteoarthritis. The level of activity, stress, injuries, nutrition, occupational conditions, obesity, personal life style and habits are suspected to contribute to the etiology of both pathogenic processes. Lateral dominance has been shown to be related to bilateral asymmetry in both osteoarthritis and bone loss. Right hands of right-handed persons demonstrate more bone and higher frequency of osteoarthritis than the left hands. Among left-handed persons, the bilateral differences were reduced in both processes, although the right hands still had more bone (Plato and Norris, 1980; Plato *et al.*, 1980) and more osteoarthritis than the left hands (Acheson *et al.*, 1970).

In both pathogenic processes, family data have been utilized only to a limited extent. Because of the universality of degenerative joint disease and bone loss, the issue becomes not so much the actual presence of the disease in sib or parent–offspring pairs but the study of quantitative aspects of concordance in regard to the rate of progression and degree or pattern of involvement at a given age. This brings to the foreground the need for more longitudinal studies. Longitudinal data until recently were lacking. However, longitudinal studies which were initiated 20 or 30 years ago are now maturing and data should be available soon for extensive longitudinal evaluations of skeletal changes.

## ACKNOWLEDGMENTS

The authors are indebted to Drs Stanley M. Garn and Marc C. Hochberg for reviewing an early draft of the manuscript and for their invaluable comments and suggestions. We also thank Mrs Margaret Lethbridge-Cejku and Ms Jennifer Meyers for their assistance in the preparation of the manuscript.

# REFERENCES

Acheson, R. and Collart, A. B. (1975) New Haven survey of joint diseases. XVII. Relationship between some systemic characteristics and osteoarthrosis in a general population. *Annals of Rheumatic Disease* **34**, 379–387.

Acheson, R. M., Chan, Y.-K. and Clemett, A. (1970) New Haven survey of joint diseases. XIII. Distribution and symptoms of osteoarthritis in the hands with reference to handedness. *Annals of Rheumatic Disease* **29**, 275–286.

Aitken, J. W., Smith, C. B., Horton, P. W., Clark, D. L., Boyd, J. F. and Smith, D. A. (1974). The interrelationships between bone mineral at different skeletal sites in male and female cadavera. *Journal of Bone and Joint Surgery* **56B**, 370.

Ala-Kokko, L., Baaldwin, C. T., Moskowitz, R. W. and Prockop, D. J. (1990) Single base mutation in the type II procollagen gene (COL2A1) as a cause of primary osteoarthritis associated with a mild chondrodysplasia. *Proceedings of the National Academy of Sciences, USA* **87**, 6565–6568.

Albanese, A. A. (1977) *Bone Loss: Causes, Detection, and Therapy*. New York: Alan R. Liss.

Alffram, P. (1964) An epidemiologic study of cervical and trochanteric fractures of the femur in an urban population. *Acta Orthopaedica Scandinavica. (Suppl.)* **65**, 1–109.

Alffram, P. A. and Bauer, C. H. (1962) Epidemiology of fractures of the forearm: a biomechanical investigation of bone strength. *Journal of Bone and Joint Surgery (Am.)* **44A**, 105–114.

Anderson, J. J. and Felson, D. T. (1988) Factors associated with osteoarthritis of the knee in the First National Health and Nutrition Examination Survey (HANES I): evidence for an association with overweight, race and physical demands of work. *American Journal of Epidemiology* **128**, 179–189.

Armelagos, G. J., Mielke, J. H., Owen, K. H., Van-Gerven, D. P., Dewey, J. R. and Mahler, R. E. (1972) Bone growth and development in prehistoric populations from Sudanese Nubia. *Journal of Human Evolution* **1**, 89–119.

Arnold, J. S., Bartley, M. H., Tont, S. A. and Jenkins, D. P. (1966) Skeletal changes in aging and disease. *Clinical Orthopedics* **49**, 17–38.

Bauer, R. L. (1988) Ethnic differences in hip fracture: a reduced incidence in Mexican Americans. *American Journal of Epidemiol.* **127**, 145.

Bauer, W. and Bennett, G. A. (1936) Experimental and pathological studies in the degenerative type of arthritis. *Journal of Bone and Joint Surgery* **18**, 1–18.

Bauer, R. L., Diehl, A. K., Barton, S. A., Brender, J. and Dayo, R. A. (1986) Risk of postmenopausal hip fracture in Mexican American women. *American Journal of Public Health* **76**, 1020.

Bauer, D. C., Browner, W. S., Cauley, J. A., Orwoll, E. S., Scott, J. C., Black, D. M., Tao, J. L. and Cummings, S. R. (1993) Factors associated with appendicular bone mass in older women. *Annals of Internal Medicine* **118**, 657–665.

Behluli, I., Lethbridge-Cejku, M., Plato, C. C., Rudan, P., Rudan, I., Stini, W. A. and Tobin, J. D. (1991) Percent cortical area (PCA) of metacarpal bones in adult Albanian population — preliminary report. *Medica Jadertina* **21**, 55–60.

Beighton, S. W., DeLa Harpe, A. L. and VanStaden, D. A. (1985) The prevalence of osteoarthritis in a rural African community. *British Journal of Rheumatology* **24**, 321–325.

Bennett, P. H. and Burch, T. A. (1968) Osteoarthrosis in the Blackfeet and Pima

Indians. In: *Population Studies of the Rheumatic Diseases* (ed. Bennett, P. H. and Wood, P. H.). Amsterdam: Excerpta Medica, pp. 407–412.

Block, J. E., Genant, H. K. and Black, D. (1986) Greater vertebral bone mineral mass in exercising young men. *Western Journal of Medicine* **145**, 39.

Bloom, R. A. and Pogrund, H. (1982) Humeral cortical thickness in female Bantu: its relationship to the incidence of femoral neck fracture. *Skeletal Radiology* **8**, 56–62.

Blumberg, B. S., Block, K. J., Black, R. L. and Dotter, C. (1961) A study of the prevalence of arthritis in Alaskan Eskimos. *Arthritis and Rheumatism* **4**, 325-340.

Bollett, A. J., Engh, G. and Parson, W. (1965) Epidemiology of osteoporosis. *Archives of Internal Medicine* **16**, 191–194.

Brandt, K. D. and Fife, R. S. (1986) Ageing in relationship to the pathogenesis of osteoarthritis. *Clinical Rheumatic Disease* **12**, 117–130.

Bremner, J. M., Lawrence, J. S. and Miall, W. E. (1968) Degenerative joint disease in a Jamaican rural population. *Annals of Rheumatic Disease* **27**, 326–332.

Brewer, V., Meyer, B. M., Keele, M. S., Upton, S. J. and Hagan, R. D. (1983) Role of exercise in prevention of involutional bone loss. *Medicine and Science in Sports and Exercise* **15**, 445.

Busby, J., Tobin, J. D., Ettinger, W., Roadarmel, K. and Plato, C. C. (1991) A longitudinal study of osteoarthritis of the hand: the effect of age. *Annals of Human Biology* **18**, 417–424.

Butler, W. J., Hawthorne, V. M., Mikkelsen, W. M., Carman, W. J., Bouthillier, D. L., Lamphiear, D. E. and Kazi, I. U. (1988) Prevalence of radiologically defined osteoarthritis in the finger and wrist joints of adult residents of Tecumseh, Michigan, 1962–65. *Journal of Clinical Epidemiology* **41**, 467–473.

Byrne, J., Thomas, M. R. and Chan, G. M. (1987) Calcium intake and bone density of lactating women in their late childbearing years. *Journal of the American Dietetic Association* **87**, 883–887.

Canalis, E. (1983) The hormonal and local regulation of bone formation. *Endocrinology Review* **4**, 62–77.

Canalis, E. (1990) Regulation of bone remodelling. In: *Primer on the Metabolic Bone Diseases and Disorders of Mineral Metabolism* (ed. Favus, M. J.). Richmond, VA: William Byrd Press, pp. 23–26.

Cann, C. E., Genant, H. K., Ettinger, B. and Gordan, G. S. (1980) Spinal mineral loss in oophorectomized women. *JAMA* **244**, 2056.

Carlson, D. S., Armelagos, G. J. and Van Gerven, D. P. (1974) Factors influencing the etiology of Cribra Orbitalia in Prehistoric Nubia. *Journal of Human Evolution* **3**, 405–410.

Cecil, R. L. and Archer, A. H. (1925) Arthritis of the menopause: a study of fifty cases. *JAMA* **84**, 75–79.

Chapman, F. H. (1972) Vertebral osteophytosis in prehistoric populations of central and southern Mexico. *American Journal of Physical Anthropology* **36**, 31–37.

Christiansen, C., Christiansen, M. S., McNair, P., Hagen, C., Stocklund, K. E. and Transbol, I. (1980) Prevention of early postmenopausal bone loss: controlled 2-year study in 315 females. *European Journal of Clinical Investigation* **10**, 273–279.

Cohn, S. H. (1981) *Non-invasive Measurements of Bone Mass and their Clinical Application*. Boca Raton, Florida: CRC Press.

Cohn, S. H., Abesami, C., Yasumur, S. *et al.* (1977) Comparative skeletal mass and radial bone mineral content in black and white women. *Metabolism* **26**, 171–178.

Copeman, W. (1940) The arthritis sequelae of pneumatic drilling. *Annals of Rheumatic Disease* **2**, 141–146.

Cummings, S. R., Kelsey, J. L., Nevitt, M. C. and O'Dowd, K. J. (1985) Epidemiology of osteoporosis and osteoporotic fractures. *Epidemiology Reviews* **7**, 178–208.

Davis, M. A., Ettinger, W. H., Neuhaus, J. M., Cho, S. A. and Hauck, W. W. (1989) The association of knee injury and obesity with unilateral and bilateral osteoarthritis of the knee. *American Journal of Epidemiology* **132**, 701–707.

Dawson, D. A. and Adams, P. F. (1987) Current estimates from the National Health Interview Survey, United States, 1986. *Vital and Health Statistics*, Series 10, No. 164, National Center for Health Statistics, US Department of Health and Human Services, Hyattsville, Maryland.

Dewey, J. B., Armelogos, G. H. and Bartley, M. H. (1969) Femoral cortical involution in three Nubian archaeological populations. *Human Biology* **41**, 13–28.

Drinkwater, B. L., Nilson, K., Chesnut, C. H., Bremner, W. J., Shainholtz, S. and Southworth, M. B. (1984) Bone mineral content of amenorrheic and eumenorrheic athletes. *New England Journal of Medicine* **311**, 277.

Drinkwater, B. L., Nilson, K., Ott, S. and Chesnut, C. H. (1986) Bone mineral density after resumption of menses in amenorrheic women. *JAMA* **256**, 380.

Drinkwater, B. L., Bruemmer, B. and Chesnut, C. H. (1990) Menstrual history as a determinant of current bone density in young athletes. *JAMA* **263**, 545.

Engel, A. (1966) Osteoarthritis and body measurements. *Vital Health Statistics*, Series 11, No. 29. Washington, DC: Department of Health, Education and Welfare.

Engh, G., Bollett, A. J., Hardin, G. and Parson, W. (1968) Epidemiology of osteoporosis. II. Incidence of hip fractures in mental institutions. *Journal of Bone and Joint Surgery (Am.)* **50A**, 557–562.

Epker, B. N., Kelin, M. and Frost, H. (1965) Magnitude and location of cortical bone loss of bone with aging. *Clinical Orthopedics* **41**, 198–203.

Exton-Smith, A. N., Millard, P. H., Payne, P. R. and Wheeler, E. F. (1969) Pattern of development and loss of bone with age. *Lancet* **2**, 1154–1157.

Farmer, M. E., White, L. R., Brody, J. A. and Bailey, K. R. (1984) Race and sex difference in hip fracture incidence. *American Journal of Public Health* **74**, 1374–1380.

Felson, D. T. (1990) The epidemiology of knee osteoarthritis: results from the Framingham Osteoarthritis Study. *Seminars on Arthritis and Rheumatism* **20** (Suppl. 1), 42–50.

Felson, D. T., Anderson, J. J., Naimark, A. A., Walker, A. M. and Meenan, R. F. (1988) Obesity and knee osteoarthritis. *Annals of Internal Medicine* **109**, 18–24.

Fox, K. M. (1990) *Reproductive Factors in Osteoporosis*. Ph.D. dissertation, University of Maryland.

Fox, K. M., Tobin, J. D. and Plato, C. C. (1986) Longitudinal study of bone loss in the second metacarpal. *Calcified Tissue International* **39**, 218–225.

Frisancho, R. A., Garn, S. M. and Ascoli, W. (1971) Unaltered cortical area of pregnant and lactating women. Studies of the second metacarpal bone in North and Central American populations. *Investigative Radiology* **6**, 119–121.

Gallagher, J. C., Melton, L. J., Riggs, B. L. and Bergstrath, E. (1980) Epidemiology of fractures of the proximal femur in Rochester, Minnesota. *Clinical Orthopedics* **150**, 163–171.

Garn, S. M. (1970) *The Earlier Gain and Later Loss of Cortical Bone*. Springfield, IL: Charles C. Thomas.

Garn, S. M. (1972) The course of bone gain and the phases of bone loss. *Orthopedic Clinics of North America* **3**, 503–519.

Garn, S. M. (1981) The phenomenon of bone formation and bone loss. In: *Osteoporosis: Recent Advances in Pathogenesis and Treatment* (ed. DeLuca, H. F., Frost, H. M., Jee, W. S., Johnston, C. and Parfitt, A. M.). Baltimore: University Park Press, pp. 3–16.

Garn, S. M., Rohmann, C. G. and Wagner, B. (1967a) Bone loss as a general phenomenon in man. *Federation Proceedings* **26**, 1729–1736.

Garn, S. M., Rohmann, C. G., Wagner, B. and Ascoli, W. (1967b) Continuing bone growth throughout life: a general phenomenon. *American Journal of Physical Anthropology* **26**, 313–317.

Garn, S. M., Wagner, B., Rohmann, C. G. and Ascoli, W. (1968) Further evidence for continuing bone expansion. *American Journal of Physical Anthropology* **28**, 219–221.

Garn, S. M., Rohmann, C. G., Wagner, B., Davila, G. H. and Ascoli, W. (1969) Populations similarities in the onset and rate of adult endosteal bone loss. *Clinical Orthopedics* **65**, 51–60.

Garn, S. M., Frisancho, A. R., Sandusky, S. T. and McCann, S. T. (1972a) Confirmation of the sex difference in continuing subperiosteal apposition. *American Journal of Physical Anthropology* **36**, 377–380.

Garn, S. M., Sandusky, S. T., Magy, J. M. and McCann, S. T. (1972b) Advanced skeletal development in low income Negro children. *J. Pediatr.* **80**, 965–969.

Garn, S. M., Poznaski, A. K. and Larson, K. (1976) Metacarpal lengths, cortical diameters and areas from the 10-state nutritional survey, including: estimated skeletal weights, weight and stature for whites, blacks and Mexican-Americans. In: *Proceedings of Workshop in Bone Morphometry* (ed. Jaworski, Z. F.). Ottawa: University of Ottawa Press, pp. 367–391.

Garruto, R. M., Plato, C. C., Yanagihara, R., Fox, K. M., Dutt, J., Gajdusek, D. C. and Tobin, J. D. (1989) Bone mass in Guamanian patients with amyotrophic lateral sclerosis and Parkinsonism-dementia. *American Journal of Physical Anthropology* **80**, 107–113.

Gordon, T. and Engel, A. (1968) Osteoarthritis in U.S. adults. In: *Population Studies of the Rheumatic Diseases* (ed. Bennett, P. and Woods, P.). Amsterdam: Excerpta Medica, pp. 391–397.

Hadler, N. M., Gillings, D. B., Imbus, H. R., Levitin, P. M., Macuc, D., Utsinger, P. D., Yount, W. J., Slusser, D. and Moskovitz, N. (1978) Hand structure and function in an industrial setting. *Arthritis and Rheumatism* **21**, 210–220.

Hall, F. C. (1939) Menopause arthritis. *Proceedings of the American Rheumatism Association* **113**, 1061.

Hartz, A. J., Fischer, M. E., Brill, G., Kelber, S., Rupley, D., Jr, Oken, B. and Rimm, A. A. (1986) The association of obesity with joint pain and osteoarthritis of the knee in the HANES data. *Journal of Chronic Diseases* **39**, 311–319.

Heaney, R. P. (1981) Unified concept of the pathogenesis of osteoporosis: updated. In: *Osteoporosis: Recent Advances in Pathogenesis and Treatment* (ed. DeLuca, H. F., Frost, H. M., Jee, W. S., Johnston, C. and Parfitt, A. M.). Baltimore: University Park Press, pp. 3–16.

Hoaglund, F. T., Yau, A. C. and Wong, W. L. (1973) Osteoarthritis of the hip and other joints in southern Chinese in Hong Kong. *Journal of Bone and Joint Surgery* **55A**, 545–557.

Hochberg, M. C. (1993) Osteoarthritis. In: *Epidemiology of the Rheumatic Diseases* (eds Silman, A. and Hochberg, M. C.). Oxford: Oxford University Press (in press).

Hochberg, M. C., Lethbridge-Cejku, M., Plato, C. C., Wigley, F. M. and Tobin, J. D.

(1991) Factors associated with osteoarthritis of the hand in males: data from the Baltimore Longitudinal Study of Aging. *American Journal of Epidemiology* **134**, 1121–1127.

Hollander, J. L. (1980) Osteoarthritis: perspectives on treatment. *Postgraduate Medicine* **68**, 161–168.

Hollingsworth, C. G. (1974) *Osteoarthrosis in the Ten State Nutrition Survey Populations, 1968–1970*. Doctoral thesis, University of Michigan.

Hooton, E. A. (1930) *The Indians of Pecos Pueblo: A Study of their skeletal remains*. New Haven: Yale University Press.

Horsman, A., Nordin, B. E. C., Aaron, J. *et al.* (1981) Cortical and trabecular osteoporosis and their relation to fractures in the elderly. In: *Osteoporosis: Recent Advances in Pathogenesis and Treatment* (eds DeLuca, H. F., Frost, H. M., Jee, W. S., Johnston, C. and Parfitt, A. A.). Baltimore: University Park Press, pp. 175–184.

Jette, A. M., Harris, B. A., Cleary, P. D. and Campiol, E. W. (1987) Functional recovery after hip fracture. *Archives of Physical and Medical Rehabilitation* **68**, 735–740.

Jimenez, S. A. (1991) Molecular biological approaches to the study of heritable osteoarthritis. *Journal of Rheumatology* **18** (Suppl. 27), 7–9.

Johnston, C. C., Smith, D. M., Yu, P. L. and Deiss, W. P., Jr (1968) *In vivo* measurement of bone mass in the radius. *Metabolism* **17**, 1140.

Jurmain, R. D. (1977) Stress and the etiology of osteoarthritis. *American Journal of Physical Anthropology* **46**, 353–365.

Kallman, D. A., Wigley, F. M., Scott, W. W., Hochberg, M. C. and Tobin, J. D. (1990) The longitudinal course of hand osteoarthritis in a male population. *Arthritis and Rheumatism* **33**, 1323–1332.

Kellgren, J. H. (1963) Atlas of standard radiographs for arthritis. In: *The Epidemiology of Chronic Rheumatism*, Vol. II (ed. Kellgren, I. H.). Philadelphia: F. A. Davis Company, pp. 1–44.

Kellgren, J. H. and Lawrence, J. S. (1952) Rheumatism in coal miners II: X-ray study. *British Journal of Industrial Medicine* **9**, 197–207.

Kellgren, J. H. and Lawrence, J. S. (1957) Radiological assessment of osteoarthrosis. *Annals of Rheumatic Disease* **16**, 494–501.

Kellgren, J. H., Lawrence, J. S. and Bier, F. (1963) Genetic factors in generalized osteoarthrosis. *Annals of Rheumatic Disease* **22**, 237–255.

Klunder, K., Rud, B. and Jorgen, H. (1980) Osteoarthritis of the hip and knee joint in retired football players. *Acta Orthopaedica Scandinavica* **51**, 925–927.

Knowlton, R. G., Katzenstein, P. L., Moskowitz, R. W., Weaver, E. J., Malemud, C. J., Pathria, M. N., Jimenez, S. A. and Prockop, D. J. (1990) Demonstration of genetic linkage of the type II procollagen gene (COL2A1) to primary osteoarthritis associated with a mild chondrodysplasia. *New England Journal of Medicine* **322**, 526–530.

Kraus, J. F., D'Ambrosia, R. D., Smith, E. G., Van Meter, J., Borhani, D. O., Franti, C. E. and Lipscomb, P. R. (1978) An epidemiological study of severe osteoarthritis. *Orthopedics* **51**, 925–927.

Kusec, V., Simic, D., Chaventre, A., Tobin, J. D., Plato, C. C. and Rudan, P. (1988) Age, sex and bone measurements of the second, third and fourth metacarpal. *Collegium Antropologicum* **2**, 309–322.

Kusec, V., Simic, D., Chaventre, A., Tobin, J. D., Plato, C. C. and Rudan, P. (1989) Age, sex and bone measurements of the second, third and fourth metacarpal. *Collegium Antropologicum* **1**, 163–169.

Kusec, V., Simic, D., Chaventre, A., Tobin, J. D., Plato, C. C., Turek, S. and Rudan, P. (1990) Asymmetry of metacarpal skeleton — analyses of second, third and fourth metacarpal bone dimensions. *Collegium Antropologicum* **14**, 273–281.

Lane, N. E., Bloch, D. A., Jones, H. H., Marshall, W. H., Wood, P. D. and Fries, J. F. (1986) Long distance running, bone density and osteoarthritis. *JAMA* **255**, 1147–1151.

Lane, N. E., Bloch, D. A., Hubert, H. B., Jones, H., Simpson, U. and Fries, J. F. (1990) Running, osteoarthritis, and bone density: initial 2-year longitudinal study. *American Journal of Medicine* **88**, 452–459.

Lawrence, J. S. (1977) *Rheumatism in Populations*. London: Heimmann.

Lawrence, J. S., Degraaf, R. and Laine, V. A. (1963) Degenerative joint disease in random samples and occupational groups. In: *The Epidemiology of Chronic Rheumatism* (eds Kellgren, J. H., Jeffrey, M. R. and Ball, J.). Oxford: Blackwell Press, pp. 98–120.

Lawrence, R. C., Hochberg, M. C., Kelsey, J. L., McDuffie, F. C., Medsger, T. A., Jr, Felts, W. R. and Shulman, L. E. (1989) Estimates of the prevalence of selected arthritis and musculoskeletal disease in the United States. *Journal of Rheumatology* **16**, 427–441.

Lethbridge-Cejku, M., Plato, C. C., Rudan, P., Tobin, J. D. and Hochberg, M. C. (1992) Cross-cultural comparison of radiographic hand osteoarthritis in males. Presented at the *Annual Meeting of the International Genetic Epidemiology Society*, Minneapolis, 12–13 June, 1992.

Lewinnek, G., Kelsey, J., White, A. and Kreiger, N. J. (1980) The significance and comparative analysis of the epidemiology of hip fractures. *Clinical Orthopedics* **152**, 35–43.

Lindberg, H. and Montgomery, F. (1987) Heavy labor and the occurrence of gonarthritis. *Clinical Orthopedics* **214**, 235–236.

Lindberg, J. S., Powell, M. R., Hunt, H. M., Ducey, D. E. and Wade, C. E. (1987) Increased vertebral bone mineral in response to reduced exercise in amenorrheic runners. *West Journal of Medicine* **146**, 39.

Lockshin, M., Higgins, I., Higgins, M., Dodge, H. and Canale, N. (1969) Rheumatism in mining communities in Marion County, West Virginia. *American Journal of Epidemiology* **90**, 17–29.

Lowman, E. W. (1955) Osteoarthritis. *JAMA* **157**, 487–488.

Magaziner, J., Simonsick, E. M., Kashner, T. M., Hebel, J. R. and Kenzora, J. E. (1989) Survival experience of aged hip fracture patients. *American Journal of Public Health* **79**, 274–278.

Magaziner, J., Simonsick, E., Kashner, M., Hebel, J. R. and Kenzora, J. E. (1990) Predictors of functional recovery one year following hospital discharge for hip fracture: a prospective study. *Journal of Gerontology* **45**, 101–107.

Marti, B., Knobloch, M., Tschoph, A., Jucker, A. and Howald, H. (1989) Is excessive running predictive of degenerative hip diseases *British Medical Journal* **299**, 91–93.

Martin, D. L., Armelagos, G. J., Mielke, J. H. and Meindl, R. (1981) Bone loss and dietary stress in an adult skeletal population from Sudanese Nubia. *Bulletin et Memoire de la Société d'Anthropologie de Paris* **8** (Series XIII), 307–319.

Mazess, R. B. (1978) Non-invasive measurement of bone. In: *Osteoporosis II* (ed. Barzel, U.S.). New York: Grune and Stratton, pp. 5–26.

Mazess, R. B. (1982) On aging bone loss. *Clinical Orthopedics* **165**, 239–252.

Melton, L. J. (1987) Epidemiology of vertebral fractures. In: *Osteoporosis 1987* (eds

Christiansen, C., Johansen, J. S. and Riis, B. J.). Copenhagen: Osteopress A/S, pp. 33–37.

Melton, L. J., Kan, S. H., Wahner, H. W. and Riggs, B. L. (1988) Lifetime fractures risk: an approach to hip fracture risk assessment based on bone mineral density and age. *Journal of Clinical Epidemiology* **41**, 985–994.

Melton, L. J., Wahner, H. W., O'Fallon, W. M. and Riggs, B. L. (1989) Epidemiology of vertebral fractures in women. *American Journal of Epidemiology* **129**, 1000–1011.

Mielke, J. H., Armelagos, G. J. and Van Gerven, D. P. (1972) Trabecular involution in femoral heads of a prehistoric (X-group) population from Sudanese Nubia. *American Journal of Physical Anthropology* **36**, 39–44.

Mikkelsen, W. M., Dodge, H. J., Duff, I. F. and Kato, H. (1967) Estimates of the prevalence of rheumatic diseases in the population of Tecumseh, Michigan, 1959–1960. *Journal of Chronic Diseases* **20**, 351–369.

Mikkelsen, W. M., Duff, I. F. and Dodge, H. J. (1970) Age-sex specific prevalence of the radiographic abnormalities of the joints of the hands, wrists and cervical spine of adult residents of the Tecumseh, Michigan Community Health Study Area, 1962–1965. *Journal of Chronic Diseases* **23**, 151–159.

Milhaud, G., Christiansen, C., Gallagher, J. C., Reeve, J., Seaman, E., Chesnut, C. and Parfitt, A. (1983) Pathogenesis and treatment of postmenopausal osteoporosis. *Calcified Tissue International* **35**, 708–711.

Miller, C. W. (1978) Survival and ambulation following hip fracture. *Journal of Bone and Joint Surgery (Am)* **60A**, 930–934.

Moskowitz, R. W. (1972) Clinical and laboratory findings in osteoarthritis. In: *Arthritis and Allied Conditions, Part VIII* (eds Hollander, J. L. and McCarty, D. J.). Philadelphia: Lea & Febiger, pp. 1032–1053.

Mossey, J. M., Mutran, E., Knott, K. and Craik, R. (1989) Determinants of recovery 12 months after hip fracture: the importance of psychosocial factors. *American Journal of Public Health* **79**, 279–286.

Mukhopadhaya, B. and Barooah, B. (1967) Osteoarthritis of the hip in Indians. An anatomical and clinical study. *Indian Journal of Orthopaedics* **1**, 55–62.

National Center for Health Statistics (1966a) *Prevalence of Osteoarthritis in Adults by Age, Sex, Race, and Geographic Area, United States, 1960–1962*. Public Health Service Series 11, no. 15, US Government Printing Office.

National Center for Health Statistics (1966b) *Osteoarthritis in Adults by Selected Demographic Characteristics: United States 1960–1962*. Public Health Service Series 11, no. 29, US Government Printing Office.

National Center for Health Statistics (1966c) *Osteoarthritis and Body Measurements. United States 1960–1962*. Public Health Service Series 11, no. 29, US Government Printing Office.

National Center for Health Statistics (1979) *Basic Data on Arthritis: Knee, Hip and Sacroiliac Joints in Adults Ages 25–74 Years, United States, 1971–1975*. Public Health Service Series 11, no. 213, US Government Printing Office.

National Center for Health Statistics (1985) *Utilization of Short-stay Hospitals*. US Department of Health and Human Services, Public Health Service Series 13, no. 19, US Government Printing Office.

Newton-John, H. F. and Morgan, D. B. (1970) The loss of bone with age, osteoporosis, and fractures. *Clinical Orthopedics* **71**, 229–252.

Nilsson, B. E. (1969) Parity and osteoporosis. *Surgical Gynecological Obstetrics* **129**, 27–28.

Nilsson, B. E. and Westlin, N. E. (1971) Bone density in athletes. *Clinical Orthopedics* **77**, 179.

Nordin, B. E. C. (1966) International patterns of osteoporosis. *Clinical Orthopedics* **45**, 17–30.

Osgood, R. B. (1940) The medical and social approaches to the problem of chronic rheumatism. *American Journal of Medical Science* **200**, 429–445.

Owen, R. A., Melton, L. J., Johnson, K. A., Ilstrup, D. M. and Riggs, B. L. (1982) Incidence of Colles' fracture in a North American community. *American Journal of Public Health* **72**, 604–607.

Palotie, A., Vaisaner, P., Ott, J., Ruhanen, L., Elima, K., Vikkula, M., Cheah, K., Vuorico, E. and Peltonen, L. (1989) Predisposition to familial osteoarthrosis is linked to type II collagen gene. *Lancet* **1**, 924–927.

Panush, R. S., Schmidt, C., Caldwell, J. R., Edwards, N. L., Longley, S., Yonker, R., Webster, E., Nauman, J., Stork, J. and Pettersson, H. (1986) Is running associated with degenerative joint disease? *JAMA* **255**, 1152–1155.

Parfitt, A. M. (1981) Bone remodeling in the pathogenesis of osteoporosis. *Resident and Staff Physician* **1**, 60–72.

Parfitt, A. M. (1984) Age related structural changes in trabecular and cortical bone: cellular mechanisms and biomechanical consequences. *Calcified Tissue International* **36** (Suppl.), 123.

Parfitt, A. M. and Duncan, H. (1982) Metabolic bone disease affecting the spine. In: *The Spine* (eds Rothmanand, R. H. and Simeone, F. A.). Philadelphia: W. B. Saunders Company, pp. 775–905.

Partridge, R. E. H. and Duthie, J. J. R. (1968) Rheumatism in dockers and civil servants: a comparison of heavy manual and sedentary workers. *Annals of the Rheumatic Diseases* **27**, 559–568.

Plato, C. C. (1987) The effects of aging on bioanthropological variables: changes in bone mineral density with increasing age. *Collegium Anthropologicum* **11**, 59–72.

Plato, C. C. and Norris, A. H. (1979a) Osteoarthritis of the hand: age-specific joint-digit prevalence rates. *American Journal of Epidemiology* **109**, 169–180.

Plato, C. C. and Norris, A. H. (1979b) Osteoarthritis of the hand: longitudinal studies. *American Journal of Epidemiology* **110**, 740–746.

Plato, C. C. and Norris, A. H. (1980) Bone measurements of the second metacarpal and grip strength. *Human Biology* **52**, 131–149.

Plato, C. C. and Tobin, J. D. (1990) Bone loss and cartilage degeneration of the joints: Diseases or normative aging processes. *Collegium Antropologicum* **14**, 57–65.

Plato, C. C., Wood, J. L. and Norris, A. H. (1980) Bilateral asymmetry in bone measurements of the hand and lateral hand dominance. *American Journal of Physical Anthropology* **52**, 27–31.

Plato, C. C., Garruto, R. M., Yanagihara, R. T., Chen, K. M., Wood, J. L., Gajdusek, D. C. and Norris, A. H. (1982) Cortical bone loss and measurements of the second metacarpal bone. I. Comparisons between adult Guamanian Chamorros and American Caucasians. *American Journal of Physical Anthropology* **59**, 461–465.

Plato, C. C., Greulich, W. W., Garruto, R. M. and Yanagihara, R. (1984) Cortical bone loss and measurements of the second metacarpal bone. II. Hypodense bone in postwar Guamanian children. *American Journal of Physical Anthropology* **63**, 57–63.

Plato, C. C., Roy, T. Sherman, S. and Tobin, J. D. (1990). Bone mineral density in normal men and women: the effect of age at different bone sites. *Journal of Bone Mineral Research* **5** (Suppl. 2), 248.

Plato, C. C., Tobin, J. D., Roy, T. A. (1993) Age specific bone mineral evaluations in the femur, spine, radius and the second metacarpal bone of normal white American men: an interskeletal site assessment. (Manuscript in preparation.)

Puranen, J., Ala-Ketola, L., Peltokallio, P. and Saarela, J. (1975) Running and primary osteoarthritis of the hip. *British Medical Journal* **1**, 424–435.

Radin, E. L., Parker, H. G. and Paul, I. L. (1971) Pattern of degenerative arthritis: preferential involvement of distal finger-joints. *Lancet* **1**, 377–379.

Riggs, B. L. and Melton, L. J. (1986) Involutional osteoporosis. *New England Journal of Medicine* **314**, 1676.

Riggs, B. L., Jowsey, J., Kelly, P. J., Hoffman, D. L. and Arnaud, C. D. (1973) Studies on pathogenesis and treatment in postmenopausal and senile osteoporosis. *Clinical Endocrinology and Metabolism* **2**, 317–332.

Riggs, B. L., Wahner, H. W., Dunn, W. L., Mazess, R. B., Offord, K. P. and Melton, L. J. (1981) Differential changes in bone mineral density of the appendicular and axial skeleton with aging. *Journal of Clinical Investigation* **67**, 328–335.

Riggs, B. L., Wahner, H. W., Seeman, E., Offord, K. P., Dunn, W. L., Mazess, R. B., Johnson, K. A. and Melton, L. J. (1982) Changes in bone mineral density of the proximal femur and spine with aging: differences between the postmenopausal and senile osteoporosis syndromes. *Journal of Clinical Investigation* **70**, 716–723.

Scott, J. C. and Hochberg, M. C. (1984) Osteoarthritis I: epidemiology. *Maryland State Medical Journal* **33**, 712–716.

Sedlin, E., Frost, H. M. and Villanueva, A. R. (1963) Variation in cross-section area of rib cortex with age. *Journal of Gerontology* **18**, 9–13.

Seidman, H., Silverberg, E. and Bodden, A. (1978) Probabilities of eventually developing and dying of cancer. *CA-A Cancer Journal for Clinicians* **28**, 33–44.

Simic, D., Kusek, V., Chaventre, A., Plato, C. C., Tobin, J. D. and Rudan, P. (1992) Factor structure and morphometric variables measured on six metacarpal bones. *Annals of Physiological Anthropology* **10**, 3–12.

Smith, R. W. (1967) Dietary and hormonal factors in bone loss. *Federation Proceedings* **26**, 1737–1746.

Smith, R. W., Jr and Walker, R. R. (1964) Femoral expansion in aging women: implications for osteoporosis and fractures. *Science* **145**, 156–157.

Solomon, L., Beighton, P. and Lawrence, J. S. (1975) Rheumatic disorders in the South African Negro. Part II. Osteo-arthrosis. *South African Medical Journal* **49**, 1373–1340.

Sowers, M. F., Wallace, R. B. and Lemke, J. H. (1985) Correlates of forearm bone mass among women during maximal bone mineralization. *Preventative Medicine* **14**, 585–596.

Spencer, R. P., Garn, S. M. and Coulombe, M. J. (1966) Age-dependent changes in metacarpal cortical thickness in two populations. *Investigative Radiology* **1**, 394–397.

Stecher, R. M. (1940) Herberden's nodes. Their incidence of hypertrophic arthritis of the fingers. *New England Journal of Medicine* **22**, 300–308.

Stecher, R. M. and Hauser, H. (1941) Heberden's nodes. Heredity in hypertrophic arthritis of the finger joints. *American Journal of Medicial Science* **201**, 801–809.

Stecher, R. M. and Hauser, H. (1948) Herberden's nodes. VII. The roentgenological and clinical appearance of degenerative joint disease of the fingers. *American Journal of Roentgenology* **59**, 326–337.

Stecher, R. M., Beard, E. E. and Hersh, A. H. (1949) Heberden's nodes: the relationship of menopause to degenerative joint disease of the fingers. *Journal of Laboratory and Clinical Medicine* **34**, 1193–1202.

Stecher, R. M., Hersh, A. H. and Hauser, H. (1953) Heberden's nodes. The family history and radiographic appearance in a large family. *American Journal of Human Genetics* **5**, 46–60.

Trotter, M., Bromen, G. E. and Peterson, R. R. (1960) Densities of bones of white and negro skeletons. *Journal of Bone and Joint Surgery (Am.)* **42A**, 50–58.

Tzonchev, V. T., Pilossoff, T. and Kanev, K. (1968) Prevalence of osteoarthritis in Bulgaria. In: *Population Studies of the Rheumatic Diseases*. (eds Bennett, P. H. and Wood, P. H. N.). Amsterdam: Exerpta Medica Foundation, pp. 413–416.

Van Saase, J. L. C. M., Vandenbroucke, J. P., van Romunde, L. K. J. and Valkenburg, H. A. (1988) Osteoarthritis and obesity in the general population: a relationship calling for an explanation. *Journal of Rheumatology* **15**, 1152–1158.

Van Saase, J. L. C. M., Van Romunde, L. K. J., Cats, A., Vandenbroucke, J. P. and Valkenburg, H. A. (1989) Epidemiology of osteoarthritis: Zoertermeer survey. Comparison of radiologic osteoarthritis in a Dutch population with that in 10 other populations. *Annals of Rheumatic Disease* **48**, 271–280.

Verbrugge, L. M., Lepkowski, J. M. and Konkol, L. L. (1991) Levels of disability among U.S. adults with arthritis. *Journal of Gerontology* **46**, S71–83.

Yanagihara, R., Garruto, R. M., Gajdusek, C. D., Tomita, A., Konagaya, Y., Uckikawa, T., Chen, G. M., Plato, C. C. and Gibbs, C. J. (1984) Calcium and vitamin D metabolism in Guamanian Chamorros with amyotrophic lateral sclerosis and Parkinsonism-dementia. *Annals of Neurology* **15**, 42–48.

# 11

# Fat, Lipid, and Blood Pressure Changes in Adult Years

## STANLEY M. GARN

## INTRODUCTION

In Westernized countries such as the United States, Canada, and Great Britain, the thickness of outer fat and the weight of fat increase in both sexes during adulthood, until the sixth decade at least. These increases are so well replicated in the mass-data statistics from the Ten-State Nutrition Survey (TSNS), National Health and Nutrition Examinations (NHANES I) and NHANES II, and the Tecumseh Community Health Survey, and with the same points of inflection, that the age-specific trend lines appear as slightly out-of-register copies of each other (cf., Garn, 1991, and Figure 11-1). Despite sampling and measurement differences, data from the Bogalusa Heart Study, from Muscadine and from the Charleston (S.C.) Heart Study reiterate the adiposity trends shown in the figure. So do Polish data, as shown graphically by Wolanski and identically labeled with respect to points of inflection (Wolanski, 1979). One might therefore assume that the gain in fatness from 20 to 50 and beyond represents the human condition, were it not for the highly divergent trends shown by third-world and marginal peoples, and different rates of increase in poor and rich North Americans (Garn *et al.*, 1992).

Our adult gains in outer and inner fatness are not replicated by many third-world populations. Among some such groups (as among the Au in New Guinea) the level of fatness actually decreases from 20 to 50, in striking contrast to the systematic gains shown in massed data from the United States. Limited weight data from preindustrial Europe also suggest that the adult gains in fatness that we experience and consider to be natural and physiological were not the rule little more than a century ago.

In the United States (and in other Westernized countries) the poor and the rich do not follow identical adult courses, either in the amount of fat or the changes during the adult years. More affluent, better-educated women are leaner than their less educated and less affluent peers from mid-adolescence onward. Moreover, women of high socioeconomic status (SES) gain less fat during the fat-gaining years and attain their peak fatness earlier (see Figure

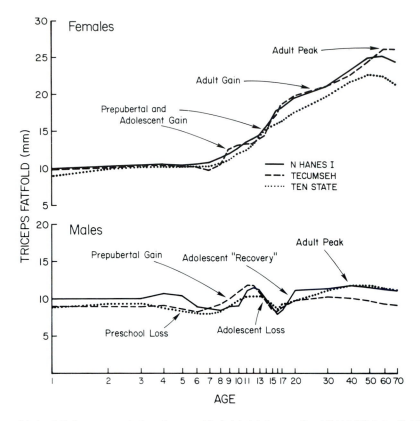

**Figure 11-1**  Lifelong trends in triceps skinfold thickness for NHANES-I (solid line), Tecumseh (dashed line) and the Ten State Nutrition Survey (dotted line). The age trends are very much the same in all three surveys, with similar inflections and similarities in the age at peak adult fatness. However, the adult gain in fatness is not necessarily the "human condition" (see text and Garn, 1991).

11-2). There are also SES-related differences in fatness, fatness gain, and the attainment of peak adult fatness in men as well. Though men tend to gain less fat (on the average), they appear to attain peak fatness earlier (Garn *et al.*, 1988a, 1988b) and the SES-related differences are in a diametrically opposite direction from those in women (cf., Figure 11-2, and Garn *et al.*, 1989a, 1992).

Given population differences in adult fatness trends, sex differences and in the amount of gain among us, and the SES-related differences in the rates of gain and in peak attainment, it is obviously premature to describe the "human condition" with respect to fat accumulation and aging. Though most of us do gain fat from 20 to 60, as suggested by the massed-data trends, some of us do not gain and some actually lose fat during these adult years. The fat data from the many surveys, neatly graphed and tabulated, tell us rather little about aging, or the intent of our genes.

Lipid levels (both serum cholesterol and the serum triglycerides) also increase with age, in Westernized populations. Despite differences in analytic

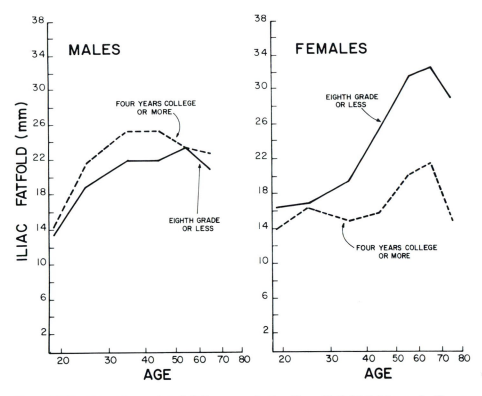

**Figure 11-2** Education-related differences in the iliac skinfold thickness in Tecumseh, Michigan. Throughout adulthood and into advanced age, college-educated women are 10–30% leaner than their less educated peers. In contrast, college-educated men are systematically fatter than their less educated peers (Garn *et al.*, 1977, 1988b, 1989a; Garn and Clark, 1974; Garn, 1981; Garn and Ryan, 1981).

techniques that complicate laboratory comparisons, even of the same cohorts over time, the adult trend for cholesterol, cholesterol esters, and the triglycerides is upward from adolescence through the sixth decade of life, in Westernized peoples (cf., Figure 11-3). However, the age trends also differ between the sexes, between first-world and third-world peoples, and between the obese and the lean. Becoming older and becoming hyperlipidemic are not necessarily the same.

In many third-world peoples serum cholesterols are far lower than among those in the first-world. In San Antonio La Paz, Guatemala, adult cholesterols rarely exceed 100–120 mg/dl (about half the comparable United States values). In San Antonio La Paz and in many other places, the adult increase in cholesterol is small, whereas in the United States it averages over 1 mg/dl per year in both sexes. Of course such Central American peoples are habituated to chronic malnutrition. They experience recurrent acute malnutrition, and their parasitic load is often very high. They may be as atypical as people of the first world are, with respect to lipid trends, but in the opposite direction.

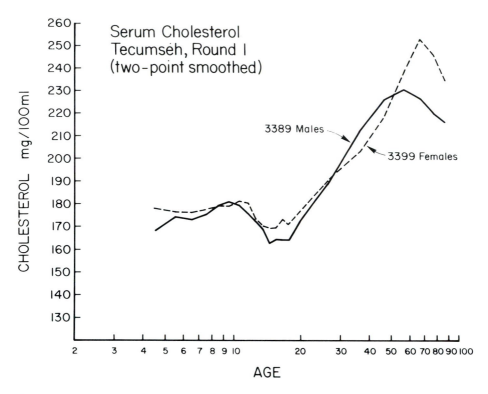

**Figure 11-3** Age trends and sex differences in serum cholesterol in Tecumseh, Michigan showing (1) a 60–70 mg/dl increase in cholesterol from early adulthood onwards and (2) the continuing increase in women after age 50 so that cholesterol peaks later in them and at a higher level. Cholesterol data shown are based on the Abel-Kendall technique in the laboratory of Dr Walter Block (cf., Garn *et al.*, 1975, 1979, 1980; Bailey *et al.*, 1977).

In the United States, serum cholesterol levels tend to be slightly lower in women than in men, though on the average they increase, through age 50 or so. Thereafter, cholesterol levels in women continue to increase, but not so in men. Some workers attribute the continuing elevation of cholesterol levels in women to the event of menopause or its endocrine determinants, though the female increase in cholesterol levels begins long before the average age at menopause and continues far longer. Some investigators attribute the earlier peak and decline in cholesterol levels in men to selective mortality and loss of the hypercholesterolemics, but the cumulative cardiovascular mortality in men is still too low to explain the lipid decline after age 50.

When we turn to the triglycerides, which include a variety of glycerides as measured, we again discover an age-associated increase, and a near-doubling in values from age 20 through age 50 in both sexes, as shown in Figure 11-4. We also discover a marked sex difference, as much as 70 mg/dl, with far higher values in males until very late in life. Though triglyceride levels are clearly associated with age, the differences in trend seen in Figure 11-3 (for

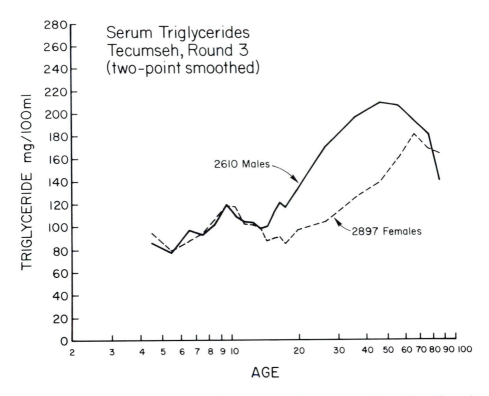

**Figure 11-4**  Age increases and sex differences in the serum triglycerides. Though triglycerides increase some 100–120 mg/dl after age 20 in both sexes, triglyceride values are as much as 60 mg/dl higher in males 40 years old. As with cholesterol, the serum triglycerides peak by age 50 in the male and then decline, whereas the triglyceride peak is much later in the female (cf., Garn *et al.*, 1988a).

cholesterol) and Figure 11-4 (for the triglycerides) are so large as to suggest quite different controlling mechanisms even in the same demographic population and between husbands and wives, who share the same diets and are reasonably similar in serum and urinary vitamins, as we have shown (Garn *et al.*, 1975).

As a further complication, as if there were not enough complications already, correlations between lipid levels and fatness levels are systematically positive, though the apparent correlations are low (0.2–0.3 as shown in Figure 11-5). However, the true lipid–fatness correlations are probably much higher, given the imperfect replicability of skinfold measurements (say 0.9) and the still poorer replicability of cholesterol levels where the standard error of estimate is ±11 mg/dl in our Tecumseh data (provided by Dr Walter Block), ±15 mg/dl in the better hospital laboratories but often closer to ±30 mg/dl in some commercial laboratories. Also, individuals tend to be inconstant in both lipid and fatness levels, cycling in both, so any given measurement may be at either extreme of the individual cycle. In all likelihood, the *true* triglyceride–

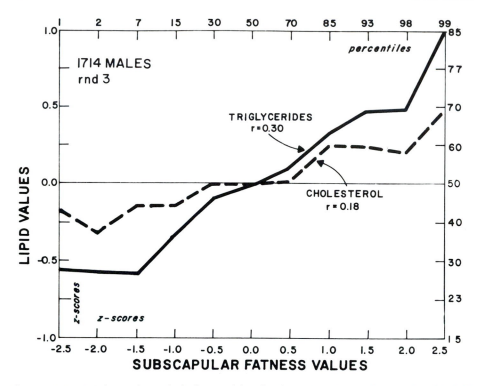

**Figure 11-5**   Triglyceride and cholesterol levels plotted against subscapular skinfold values. Though the correlations are relatively low (0.18 for cholesterol and 0.30 for the triglycerides), the lipid differences at the extremes of fatness exceed 1Z or 30 centile points (cf., Garn *et al.*, 1979).

fatness correlation is well in excess of 0.5, and the age-associated trends in lipid levels are therefore confounded by the equally non-linear age-associated trends in fatness levels.

Though we can provide very impressive age-trends for cholesterol and the triglycerides, derived from numerically large adult samples (*N*>2,000), and with impressive technical accuracy, the complications introduced by fatness changes and the low and nearly flat age curves from third-world populations together force us to ponder the relationship between age and lipid levels, and its implications to aging *per se*.

## BLOOD PRESSURE AND AGE

As we all know, blood pressure values (both systolic and diastolic) increase during adulthood in the USA and in similarly Westernized countries. With the progress of years, a larger and larger proportion of the population becomes hypertensive, by definition. (Hypertension is currently defined as a diastolic blood pressure in excess of 90 mm of mercury as used by Garn *et al.*, 1988a,

1988b). Even at 90 mm, however, the probability of stroke is greater than at lower blood pressure values.

The clear-cut and systematically positive correlations between the level of fatness (as variously measured) and blood pressure do not exclude the confounding effects of other risk variables such as electrolyte intakes, exercise or "stress." In comparison, however, the weightings exhibited by subcutaneous fat thickness (FW) etc., greatly exceed the apparent weightings of Na and K intakes derived from self-reported dietary histories and so-called self-perceived stress is admittedly difficult to validate. Moreover, the contribution of age-associated increases in FW to the elevated blood pressures seen in older individuals in the USA can not be separated from structural changes in the arterial system and the venous incompetencies that are concomitants of age in Westernized countries.

How the level of fatness and systolic and diastolic blood pressure effectively interact in preindustrial populations is also difficult to evaluate as pointed out by James and Pecker in this volume and by Little and Haas (1989). Though leaner agriculturalists and hunter–gatherers may have lower blood pressures that do not increase with age simply because they do not gain in fat weight or percentage fat, such peoples also differ from us in so many respects (cf., Page in Hunt, 1979). Studies on Pacific populations including the Western and Eastern Samoans remain equivocal because there are still so many unmeasured differences in diet, climate, and life style (cf., Friedlaender, 1987). The role of "modernization" on blood pressure and the age-associated increase in blood pressure can only be elucidated by attention to its components which may include clock-watching, deadlines, workplace competition, the daily news, and fear of failure. Similarly the genetic component remains a potential complication, both on a population basis (as we know for Blacks in the USA) and, alternatively, for those familial hypotensives and hypertensives among the categorized "Whites." For these various reasons, the age-associated increase in blood pressure so typical of the United States and Western Europe, need not be viewed as the human condition, but its absence in specific populations may not be the hominid norm either.

Though increased blood pressure levels appear to be positively associated with sodium intakes and negatively associated with potassium intakes, the beta weightings are low and may be attributable to a minority of susceptible individuals. Both systolic and diastolic blood pressures are statistically associated with self-perceived "stress," which again may be attributable to a minority of the population, especially the poor and impoverished. However, blood pressure levels are systematically related to the level of fatness, in both sexes, and at every adult age. Roughly speaking, systolic blood pressure increases 1 mm of mercury for each mm of triceps or subscapular skinfold in Tecumseh (Garn et al., 1988a, 1988b).

If we compare the lean (i.e., the lowest 16%) and the obese (the highest 16%), blood pressure values are systematically different from 20 through 60, in both sexes. Obese men and obese women both average close to or above 90 mm of mercury by the time they are age 55 or so (see Figure 11-6). Fatter individuals are much more likely to be hypertensive, which is why fatness-

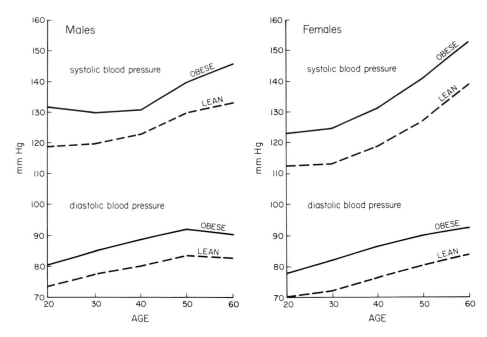

**Figure 11-6**  Systolic blood pressure (upper pairs of lines) and diastolic blood pressure (lower lines) in obese individuals (solid lines) and lean individuals (dashed lines). In both sexes, but especially in women, the obese exceed the lean in systolic and diastolic blood pressure by as much as 30 mm of mercury (see Garn *et al.*, 1988b).

reduction is the first order of therapy for the hypertensive adult, and—in many cases—it is successful, by itself (cf., Garn *et al.*, 1988b).

In our studies, we find that the obese are—at every adult age—more likely to be on prescription anti-hypertensives. In fact, more than half of the obese women in Tecumseh aged 50 and up have been given such prescriptions. Ignoring compliance, which is far from perfect, this complicates all attempts to study aging and blood pressure now. Should those on anti-hypertensives be excluded from consideration, thereby excluding many hypertensives?

We have also explored the possibility that the age-associated increases in systolic and diastolic blood pressure are simply a function of fatness, by plotting the blood pressures of individuals at the same low level of fatness throughout the adult years. So partitioned, the age increase in systolic and diastolic blood pressures from 20 to 40 disappears, although from age 40 onward, systolic and diastolic blood pressures do increase with age even at the same low and constant level of fatness. Nevertheless very lean individuals, and especially very lean women, often approximate the desirable blood pressure levels of 130/70 through the eighth and ninth decades while their obese sisters survive on diuretics, calcium blockers, and venous relaxants, but still with far higher blood pressure levels.

As with lipid levels, it is unclear just how adiposity is involved in blood pressure, including the purely mechanical diffusing effect of a thick paniculus on the pressure exerted by the inflated cuff. It is not quite possible to blame all of the age-associated increase in blood pressure on the fat increase alone, though much of the age increase in blood pressure has just such an origin. The greater risk of hypertension faced by women may be at least a partial function of their outer adiposity; at constant skinfold thickness the sex differences in blood pressure nearly disappear.

Our (Western) habit of adding fat during adulthood does explain part of our (Western) habit of becoming hypertensive and, hence, part of the association between hypertension and age. However, the association may be less with fatness *per se* than the factors that make for a more positive energy balance, among them decreased activity. The possibility of a separate, purely dietary, explanation also exists if there is an increased proportion of calories supplied by fats and oils, and if a higher proportion of fat calories is itself a factor in blood pressure elevation.

## AGING AND FAT PLACEMENT

As subcutaneous fat is added, it adds all over, literally from head to foot. The cephalic fat pad becomes larger, especially in the male, one of the two reasons why one needs a larger hat in later life (cf., Garn, 1989a). Subcutaneous fat around the feet also gains in thickness, one of two reasons why most of us need larger shoes after the mid-century mark. In between, increases in subcutaneous fat thickness can be documented for the neck, chest, arms, and back, and for the abdominal, iliac, thigh, and calf sites. Shirt sizes, coat sizes, and trouser sizes become larger with the progress of years for most of us, reflecting the addition of subcutaneous fat from scalp to toe (and intrathoracic and omental fat as well).

However, subcutaneous fat is not added at a uniform rate (mm/kg) at all bodily sites. The addition (mm/kg) is relatively small on the scalp and on the feet, somewhat larger (mm/kg) on the upper arm and larger still for the abdominal site, technically midway between the iliac crest and the umbilicus (Garn et al., 1988c). That is why the waist circumference (and trouser size and belt size) are such useful non-technical and therefore popular measures of adiposity and of changes in adiposity (Garn, 1989b). That is why Morris used trouser size so successfully in his cardiovascular comparisons of London tram drivers and conductors (cf., Garn, 1989b).

With more subcutaneous fat on it and more omental fat under it, the abdominal area becomes more convex and more protuberant in older, fatter individuals. The "waist" constriction may entirely disappear. This is equally true in both sexes, so both men and women tend to look more "android" as they get older and fatter. In the super-obese, those above the 95th centile for fatness, the subcutaneous fat thickness often exceeds the jaw capacity of the Lange–Cambridge and similar skinfold calipers, which is why the simple waist circumference is so useful as an index of fatness for them. The fact that abdominal fat adds at a greater rate (mm/kg) than does fat at the trochanteric level, also provides a sartorial challenge for older, fatter men, whose trousers are therefore at continual risk of slipping downward, and their underpants (or drawers) become geotrophic, too. The abdominal fat deposit primarily accounts for the utility of the waist/hip circumference as a measure of adiposity.

The waist/hip ratio is effective as an obesity measure, simply because it compares two sites with differing rates of fat gain (delta fat/delta kg). Similar circumferential ratios document the greater rate of fat addition about the abdomen as compared with the chest, i.e., the waist/chest ratio, once widely used as a measure of "fitness." Ignoring differences in the bony frame size, the waist/chest ratio can be said to indicate the relative amounts of upper-body and lower-body fat, though this ratio, like the waist/hip ratio, is highly fatness dependent.

Ratios involving subcutaneous fat thicknesses are also used to document the changing relative thicknesses of subcuteanous fat on different parts of the body, and therefore differences in the placement of fat. While one can argue whether subscapular fat is truly "central" and whether upper arm fat is properly "peripheral," such ratios have been much used to describe the changing placement of fat during the fat-gaining phase which characterizes most of us in the Western world. Yet all of these ratios are fatness dependent (Figure 11-7).

All of the ratios (waist/hip, or triceps/subscapular or abdominal/thigh) are demonstrably fatness dependent, in a direction determined by their construction (Garn et al., 1982, 1988c, 1988d). One can also show, quite simply, that the triceps skinfold is usually the thickest, in leaner individuals (young or old). With advancing age, and increasing fatness, the abdominal and iliac skinfolds tend to be the thickest. In obese children the abdominal skinfold exceeds the triceps skinfold, but in the lean elderly the triceps skinfold is still thicker than the abdominal skinfold (cf., Tables 11-1 and 11-2). Fatness dependence of these ratios therefore complicates their use both as descriptive devices and in relation to other risk factors and to lipid levels, blood pressure values or diabetes.

Individuals with a high waist/hip circumferential ratio (for their age) will have higher cholesterol and triglyceride levels, simply because they are fatter as mentioned above. Women with a larger waist/hip ratio are more likely to be diabetic, not because they are "android" but because they are fatter. Differences in the relative thickness of the triceps and subscapular skinfolds are associated with differences in systolic and diastolic blood pressure measurements not so much because fat placement is a risk factor by itself, but because such ratios do reflect differences in the level of fatness. A 50-inch trouser size is a very potent risk factor because individuals so larded are fat all over.

There are, of course, individuals whose outer fat thicknesses at particular sites are exceptional for their level of fatness (cf., Garn, 1977). Expressed at centiles or as normalized Z-scores, some women do have excessive thigh and lower leg fat deposits (>2 Z-scores above the average for all sites). There are also individuals who are excessively fat below the navel, yet truly lean above,

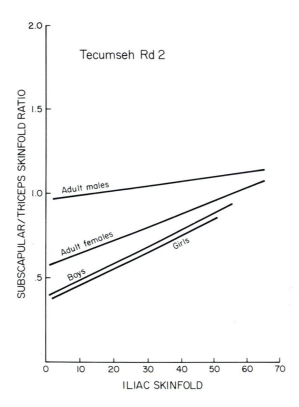

**Figure 11-7** Fatness dependence of the subscapular–triceps skinfold ratio in both sexes and in children and adults alike shown in reference to the iliac skinfold. All skinfold ratios are fatness dependent, in a direction determined by their construction, and therefore related to lipid levels, blood pressure values, and glucose tolerance values as well (cf., Garn *et al.*, 1982, 1988b).

**Table 11-1** Location of the thickest skinfold in children aged 5–9 and in adults aged 50–75.

| | Percentage thickest by site | | | |
| | Children 5–9 | | Adults 50–75 | |
| Thickest skinfold | Boys (N = 633) | Girls (N = 631) | Men (N = 578) | Women (N = 631) |
|---|---|---|---|---|
| Triceps | 86.8[a] | 82.7 | 4.8[a] | 12.8 |
| Subscapular | 0.5 | 0.2 | 9.4 | 1.7 |
| Iliac | 7.7 | 8.0 | 14.6 | 8.4 |
| Abdominal | 4.9 | 9.2 | 71.4 | 77.2 |

[a]e.g., in 86.8% of boys the triceps skinfold was the thickest of the four, whereas the triceps was thickest in only 4.8% of men aged 50–75.

**Table 11-2**  Summed skinfold thicknesses by thickest skinfold in 50–75-year-old men and women.

| | Summed skinfolds (mm) | | | |
| --- | --- | --- | --- | --- |
| | Men | | Women | |
| Thickest skinfold | N | Mean | N | Mean |
| Triceps | 28 | 60.2[a] | 81 | 76.0[a] |
| Subscapular | 53 | 75.2 | 10 | 155.7 |
| Iliac | 84 | 88.8 | 53 | 149.1 |
| Abdominal | 413 | 97.0 | 487 | 126.4 |

[a]Individuals in whom the triceps skinfold was thickest tended to be lean individuals for their age and sex.

but such individuals are so rare that they are not regularly included in most study or survey populations. There are individuals with excessive fat on the upper arm for their average level of fatness, but they constitute too small a fraction for study. True differences in relative fat patterning corrected for the amount of fat do exist, but their numbers are small and the implications of such relative fat patterns to aging and mortality therefore remain obscure.

## MENOPAUSE AND FAT ACCUMULATION

As a group, and in conventional mass-data statistics, American women do gain in fatness level after age 50, i.e., the median age at menopause. As a group, they develop double chins, fatter arms and (with marked increases in abdominal fat deposits) they come to look much the same fore and aft, i.e., coming and going. The increases in the thickness of fat and total body weight are well documented in the data from all national surveys but the fat and weight increases after 50 are especially marked for women of low income and less than high-school education.

Since outer fat is added after 50 in most American women and since the median age at which menopause is approximately that, it has been common thinking to attribute those fatness changes after 50 to the changes in ovarian function. Analogy is drawn to fatness changes in "polled" or caponized domestic animals including fowl and to the fatness changes supposedly common in castrate males, as in the Chinese court eunuchs, the Ottoman harem eunuchs, and the *castrati* who lent their arrested voices to the glory of the Church and Italian opera.

There are, however, numerous objections to the popular notion of menopausal-onset obesity. First, mass-data statistics do not reveal an inflection in the weight-for-age data corresponding to age 50, nor any such inflection in the triceps, subscapular, iliac, or abdominal thickness-for-age plots. Second, high SES women tend to achieve a weight and fatness plateau by the time of menopause, so the postmenopausal increase (if it actually exists) is not

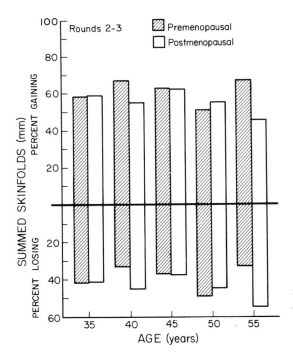

**Figure 11-8** Five-year skinfold losers and gainers among premenopausal women (shaded bars) and postmenopausal women (open bars) arranged by entry-age intervals from age 35 onwards. Though the proportion of skinfold gainers tends to exceed the proportion of skinfold losers consistent with the general gain in fatness during this age period, premenopausal and postmenopausal women are not systematically different in incremental trend. In short, there is no "menopausal" effect.

applicable to them. Third, male castrates do not necessarily gain in fatness following orchidectomy, whatever may have been the case for the prepubertally castrated *castrati* of opera fame. Of the 81 castrate males we studied in Winfield, Kansas in 1949, some were obese for their age and others were very lean.

If we compare actual 5-year fatness changes for premenopausal and postmenopausal women at different ages from 35 on, we find no clear evidence of a "menopausal" effect. Age for age, the proportion of fat gainers and fat losers is much the same for the premenopausal and postmenopausal women alike (see Figure 11-8). Evidently, menopause does not automatically produce fatness gain.

The question of a "menopausal effect" has also been raised with respect to the lipids—cholesterol and triglycerides—and the elevated levels of both that go with advancing age in the female. However, as shown in the earlier figures (Figures 11-3 and 11-4) the age-associated increase in serum cholesterol long antedates the mid-century mark and continues for two decades thereafter. Cross-sectional data, therefore, show no evidence of an inflection or "spurt" in serum cholesterol levels among women that could truly be called a "menopaus-al effect." With respect to cholesterol, where the levels are consistently lower in women until the senior ages, it is again difficult to document a menopausal effect, either in cross-sectional comparisons (as in the earlier figures) or by comparison of lipid gainers and losers over successive half-decade periods as in Tecumseh, Michigan, Examination Rounds 2 and 3.

There are, of course, obvious complications to the testing of a menopausal effect on weight or fat or cholesterol or the triglycerides. First, lower and upper economic groups differ in the magnitude of these values (kilograms of fat or millimoles of cholesterol) and they differ in the peak ages of attainment as well. Second, even within a socioeconomic group, there are the losers and there are the gainers at the very time when fatness-gaining or lipid-gaining is modal behavior. Further to complicate such mass-data statistics, even within socioeconomic groupings, the fact that the gainers usually gain more than the losers lose results in an upward trend with respect to median or (especially) mean values, even though the number of losers actually exceeds the number of gainers. Accordingly, analyses of semi-longitudinal data with respect to the proportion gaining and the proportion losing at each successive half-decade grouping—and for a defined period of time—are necessary to show whether there is any menopausal effect at all. Our data, to date, argue against such an effect. However, and by analogy with menarche, it is possible that women with early and precipitous menopauses may still show such a "menopausal effect."

## EXPLANATIONS FOR THE FATNESS CHANGES THROUGH THE OLDER YEARS

Granted that the weight of fat (FW) and the thicknesses of the *tela subcutanea* at most sites all increase (on the average) during the first four adult decades in US Whites, explanations are surely in order. While such gains in stored fat necessarily result from a more positive energy balance (energy in minus energy out), the possible reasons for the more positive energy balance are numerous, and it is difficult to weight them or arrange them in a hierarchical order (cf., Table 11-3). Voluntary activity does decrease, during the adult years, but the caloric intake does not diminish in proportion. The basal energy production decreases, as the metabolic fires die (to use Raymond Pearl's descriptive phrase) but most of us do not compensate at the table. This problem of adjusting food intake to decreased energy expenditure is especially apparent in some individuals who become immensely obese when they are forced to assume a wheelchair or bedridden existence or are otherwise activity-restricted—as in severe arthritis or following hip-joint replacement or multiple amputations.

Still, it is true that some of us weigh no more at 70 than at 20, somehow having learned to adjust appetites to meet lowered energy needs. More affluent women somehow adjust their energy balance so as to have less fat and also to gain less fat, as the years go on. Moreover, the lean, in general, add less fat with the progress of time than do the obese. By peer-pressure, by the influence

**Table 11-3**   Possible explanations for the earlier increase and later decrease in fat during adulthood.

| Explanation | Comment |
|---|---|
| *The earlier increase in FW* | |
| 1. Decreased lean body mass | Proportional decrease in energy requirements |
| 2. Decreased thyroid activity | Decrease in thyroid hormone (TH) and therefore in basal energy production |
| 3. Decreased levels of estrogens and anrogens | Decreased energy requirements for tissue maintenance and repair |
| 4. Decreased activity levels | Decreased energy expenditure, lesser decrease in intake[a] |
| *The later decrease in FW and % fat* | |
| 1. Reduced energy intake | Poorer appetite due to inactivity, decreased sensory activities (taste and smell) |
| 2. Diminished absorption | Changes in absorptive efficiency, morphology of the gut, and gastrointestinal functioning in general |
| 3. Reduced levels of HGH and other pituitary hormones | Older individuals approach the panhypopituitary state |

[a]Though energy intakes clearly decrease after age 25, energy expenditures presumably decrease to a greater extent, so that the energy balance becomes increasingly positive with increasing age.

of the media, and perhaps because they have other things to do, some individuals do not gain much fat for decades while most gain in adiposity. The sex differences in the age at peak fatness and the timing of the decline also merit explanation (cf., Table 11-3) but the explanations are both few and dubious. Why women continue to add fat longer than men do, by a decade at least, might seem to be a simple matter of "sex differences," except for the fact that high SES women attain the fatness peak and then begin to decline long before their low-SES sisters.

Fat weight does enter a period of decrease late in life, after which time previously plump men and women all become scrawny and emaciated. Lipid levels also decrease, rather precipitously as shown in the figures, and so do the common hematologic values (Hct and Hgb) as well. The lean body mass (LBM) obviously decreases, and some older individuals become totally bed-bound for lack of supporting muscle mass. It is not clear how much the age-associated diminution of intestinal mass and reduction of intestinal villi is involved, resembling the situation in protein-energy malnutrition. It is not clear whether a program of heroic hypernutrition associated with forced activity can remedy or reverse this last declining phase of aging.

When we study the octogenarians and the nonagenarians, we study a mixed lot. Some are simply survivors, men and women that have lasted that long because they have enjoyed lower lipid levels and are not cancer-prone. Others are aged marvels, more like far-younger individuals with a surprisingly high lean body mass for their age and with appetites to match. Some older men still have respectable sperm counts and can become progenitors so late that we still honor the children of Civil War veterans conceived after 1940! True, those aged progenitors were mere drummer-boys at Appomattox and Gettysburg, but they remained potent for more than 75 years. They had the energy (and interest) for fatherhood long after the usual time, which gives us interest in following survivors of World War I who are still similarly active, now and through the remainder of this century.

## GENETIC AND NON-GENETIC FACTORS IN AGING

Having noted the considerable extent to which fat weights and fat thicknesses of older adults may differ when socioeconomic or educational subgroups are compared, one might assume that rather little of the total interpersonal variance in fatness can be under genetic control. Given the fact that poor and affluent sexagenarian women differ by some 6 kg in weight and even more in the weight of fat, the genetic hypothesis would seem unlikely for them. Moreover, the inverse relationship between SES and fatness in older women, and the positive relationship in older men, would preclude any easy genetic explanation.

However, grandparents do show systematically positive weight and fat correlations with their adult grand-children, even though these correlations are usually far lower than for parents and children still living together (cf., Garn, 1985, 1986). Even more interesting is the fact that grandparent–grandchild fatness correlations are all positive, though low, and for all skinfold sites considered. In our data, from the Tecumseh Community Health Survey, grandparent–grandchild fatness correlations start at 0.05 (for one grandparent) and increase to 0.25 when all four grandparents are taken into account (Figure 11-9). Taking the median age for the grandchildren as close to 10 years and the median age for the grandparents as close to 60, these inter-generational correlations are impressive and they quite delight our colleagues in human genetics. For one, two, three and four grandparents the values of the Z-scored grandparent–grandchild fatness correlations come close to genetic expectancy (cf., Garn *et al.*, 1984a).

To the good, most of the grandparents in Tecumseh are separately domiciled from their grandchildren, thereby minimizing the living-together explanation. However, we do not have data on the number of meals actually shared in common, or the extent to which grandmothers (on both sides) also serve as mother-surrogates and built-in babysitters. We do not know the extent to which eating habits and activity levels are passed down from grandparent to parent to grandchild. From these grandparent–grandchild fatness correlations we rediscover the same problem that goes with stature, i.e., that stature is influenced both by socioeconomic status and family line. Some part of the fatness variance of older adults is certainly a function of education, occupation, and income. Some part is obviously familial, but conventional heritability ($H^2$) calculations as presently calculated are ineffective in telling us how much.

In similar vein, some part of the fat distribution (e.g., fat patterning) of elderly individuals must be uniquely familial, after correcting for the amount of

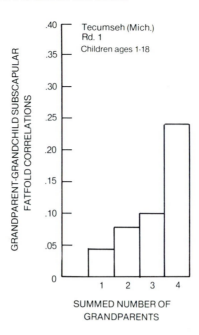

**Figure 11-9** The "grandparent effect" on fatness level in Tecumseh. Although grandparent–grandchild correlations for the subscapular skinfold are only 0.05 for a single grandparent–grandchild pair, the correlations increase in magnitude with the number of grandparents, achieving an *r* of 0.25 when all four grandparents are included.

fat. This is certainly true in the radiogrammetric data from the Baltimore Aging Study of the National Institute of Aging, and for the various arm, chest, hip, and calf sites. From their data, using soft-tissue radiographs following our Fels model of 1960, adult fathers do resemble their adult sons in relative (Z-scored) fat patterns (cf., Garn, 1977). The use of age-specific Z-scores corrects for the amount of fat, so the Z-scored pattern comparisons and the statistic $r_Z$ effectively compare older fathers and their younger adult sons. In other and fewer words, there are familial and presumably genetic determinants for the relative (Z-scored) fat patterns of older men.

It is also true that parents and their children show similarities in 5-year and 10-year fatness *changes* (delta fat) which defy any simple genetic explanation, for the parents and their children are at very different ages and at very different points in their life cycles. Grandparents and grandchildren also exhibit significant but low order similarities in long-term fatness change (delta fat) even though they are separately domiciled. Extended families as a whole tend to change fatness in concert, perhaps intentionally (by adopting a prudent diet and a healthier life style), or for economic reasons, and the grandparental generation is not exempt (cf., Garn and Pilkington, 1984; Garn *et al.*, 1984a, 1984b).

It is tempting to wonder whether the fatness peak of older adults and its later decline is also under genetic control, at least in part. True, there are the pervasive sex differences. Men peak in fatness earlier and then decline earlier, as they do in lipid levels as well. True, there are the socioeconomic differences: affluent women peak earlier and poor women peak later. However, the peak age of fatness or lipid levels does appear to be familial, recalling sister–sister similarities in the age at menarche even for female siblings living apart.

The pendulum of accepted thinking is ever-swinging with respect to the concomitants of aging and the timing of the ultimate decline. There are significant parent-child correlations with respect to longevity, and for siblings, too. However, there are statistically significant spousal correlations for longevity as well. When we consider the fatness and lipid and blood pressure changes in adults and older adults, we have evidence that points both ways. Fatter teenagers do have fatter grandparents, on the average. However, the poorer and richer elderly also differ in how fat they are and when they attain peak fatness and then begin to decline. The evidence points both ways and we can not yet calculate the proper weightings to apply, even with mathematically sophisticated estimates of $H^2$ that purport to take "environment" into account.

## THE ARGUMENTS FOR FATNESS REDUCTION IN THE SENIOR YEARS

Given the fact that lipid levels tend to be elevated in the elderly, at least through the 70th year in women, the potential value and the disadvantages of intervention have been warmly debated. On the one hand we might agree with Raymond Pearl that those who have lived so long, with such elevated risk factors, are the tougher and more resistant of the elderly. If so, why subject them to low-fat and low-cholesterol diets of diminished palatability, and to cholesterol-lowering agents with their various side effects? The same argument applies to the fatter older men and women, who will enter an irreversible fatness-reduction phase in just a few years.

To be sure, the evidence that greater fatness is morbidogenic becomes increasingly poor as the years go on. Our most-cited evidence stems from 40-year-old insured men, then followed for 30 years. Evidence for women is poorer both because of their longer span of life and because early obesity is seemingly less morbidogenic for them, at least for coronary artery disease.

The elderly now arc on a heavy diet of prescription medications, of which anti-hypertensives constitute a considerable part, especially in women. (More than half of the older women we have followed have been given prescription anti-hypertensives, though compliance is far less than perfect.) Anti-arthritic drugs further complicate the picture, for the salicylates may minimize the prevalence of strokes, and episodes of cardiac ischemia. Fatness reduction may be an un-needed step for obese septuagenarians and octogenarians, but it may also eliminate the need for many other medications. For a portly 75-year-old, a reduction in fat weight may diminish the discomfort of knee and hip arthritis and allow a return to greater activity (beneficial both to the joints and to maintenance of a lower level of fatness).

The well-to-do elderly in Sun City and other retirement communities constitute a surprisingly active group, able to travel and to keep up with younger peers on their excursions and cruises. They may show how continued leaness of body allows a greater enjoyment of life and reduced age-specific mortality, they may be the affluent elderly lean, or those survivors who are active beyond the expectancy for their years (and remarried to other survivors who then keep each other "young").

# REFERENCES

Bailey, S. M., Garn, S. M., Block, W. D. and Cole, P. E. (1977) Definitive estimate of fatness lipid relationships in the normal adult population. *Federation Proceedings* **37**, 593.

Friedlaender, J. S. (1987) *The Solomon Islands Project: A Long-Term Study of Health, Human Biology and Culture Change.* Oxford: Clarendon Press.

Garn, S. M. (1977) Patterning in ontogeny, taxonomy, phylogeny and dysmorphogenesis. In: *Colloquia in Anthropology*, Vol. 1 (ed. Wetherington, R. K.). The Fort Burgwin Research Center, pp. 83–106.

Garn, S. M. (1981) Socioeconomic aspects of obesity. *Contemporary Nutrition* **6**, 1–2.

Garn, S. M. (1985) Continuities and changes in fatness from infancy through adulthood. *Current Problems in Pediatrics* **15**, 1–47.

Garn, S. M. (1986) Family-line and socioeconomic factors in fatness and obesity. *Nutrition Reviews* 41, 381–386.

Garn, S. M. (1989a) Directions of aging. In: *Orthodontics in an Aging Society* (ed. Carlson, D. S.). Ann Arbor, MI: Center for Human Growth and Development, pp. 33–39.

Garn. S. M. (1989b) The return of circumferences in health appraisal. *American Journal of Public Health* **79**, 688.

Garn, S. M. (1991) Implications and applications of subcutaneous fat measurement to nutritional assessment and health risk evaluation. In: *Anthropometric Assessment of Nutritional Status* (ed. Himes, J. H.). New York: Wiley-Liss, pp. 123–140.

Garn, S. M. and Clark, D. C. (1974). Economics and fatness. *Ecology of Food and Nutrition* **3**, 19–20.

Garn, S. M. and Pilkington, J. J. (1984) Comparison of three-year weight and fat change distributions of lean and obese individuals. *Ecology, Food and Nutrition* **15**, 7–12.

Garn, S. M. and Ryan, A. S. (1981) Replicating the income related reversal of fatness. *Ecology, Food and Nutrition* **10**, 237–239.

Garn, S. M., Block, W. D. and Clark, D. C. (1975) Level of fatness and lipid levels. *Ecology, Food and Nutrition* **4**, 235–236.

Garn, S. M., Bailey, S. M., Cole, P. E. and Higgins, I. T. T. (1977) Level of education, level of income, and level of fatness in adults. *American Journal of Clinical Nutrition* **30**, 721–725.

Garn, S. M., Bailey, S. M. and Block, W. D. (1979) Relationships between fatness and lipid levels in adults. *American Journal of Clinical Nutrition* **32**, 733–735.

Garn, S. M., Hopkins, P. J. and Block, W. D. (1980) Parental lipid levels and lipid continuities in their children. *American Journal of Clinical Nutrition* **33**, 2214–2216

Garn, S. M., Ryan, A. S. and Robson, J. R. K. (1982) Fatness-dependence and utility of the subscapular/triceps ratio. *Ecology, Food and Nutrition* **12**, 173–177.

Garn, S. M., LaVelle, M. and Pilkington, J. J. (1984a) Obesity and living together. *Marriage and Family Reviews* **7**, 33–47.

Garn, S. M., Pilkington, J. J. and LaVelle, M. (1984b) Relationship between initial fatness level and long term fatness change. *Ecology, Food and Nutrition* **14**, 85–92.

Garn, S. M., Sullivan, T. V. and Hawthorne, V. M. (1988a) Age changes in hard and soft tissues and lipids. *New York Medical Quarterly* **8**, 40–46.

Garn, S. M., Sullivan, T. V. and Hawthorne, V. M. (1988b) Effect of skinfold levels on lipids and blood pressure in younger and older adults. *Journal of Gerontology* **43**, 170–174.

Garn, S. M., Sullivan, T. V. and Hawthorne, V. M. (1988c) Persistence of relative fatness at different body sites. *Human Biology* **60**, 43–53.

Garn, S. M., Sullivan, T. V. and Hawthorne, V. M. (1988d) Fatness dependence of skinfold ratios and its implications to fat patterning. *Ecology, Food and Nutrition* **21**, 151–158.

Garn, S. M., Sullivan, T. V. and Hawthorne, V. M. (1989) The education of one spouse and the fatness of the other spouse. *American Journal of Human Biology* **1**, 223–238.

Garn, S. M., Sullivan, T. V. and Hawthorne, V. M. (1992) The impermanence of obesity and its temporal variations as studied in family context. In: *Health Implications of Obesity* (ed. Enwonwu, E. O.). Nashville, Tenn: Center for Nutrition Research, Meharry Medical College, pp. 41–52.

Little, M. A. and Haas, J. D. (1989) *Human Biology: A Transdisciplinary Science*. New York: Oxford University Press.

Page, L. B. (1979) Hypertension and atherosclerosis in primitive and acculturating societies. In: *Dialogues in Hypertension: Hypertension Update*, Vol. 1 (ed. Hunt, J. C.). Bloomfield, NJ: Health Learning Systems, pp. 1–12.

Wolanski, N. (1979) Genetic control of bone, cartilaginous and adipose tissues growth. *Anthropos* **6**, 115–127.

# 12

# Aging and Blood Pressure

## GARY D. JAMES AND MARK S. PECKER

## INTRODUCTION

On average, the blood pressure of individuals in industrialized societies increases with age (Lew, 1990). In these people, mean systolic pressure increases until the seventh decade of life, while mean diastolic pressure increases until the sixth decade of life and thereafter levels off or even declines slightly (Lew, 1990; see Figure 12-1). These findings are consistent among industrialized societies and raise the question: is this increase in blood pressure part of the natural aging process? Since the level of blood pressure considered to constitute hypertension is fixed [140/90 mm of mercury (mmHg)] and independent of age, a further question arises: is the development of hypertension, in part, simply a facet of the normal aging process? Over the past several decades, surveys of casual blood-pressure measurements in a variety of non-Westernized people with traditional lifestyles suggest that the answer to these questions may be no. These populations, living in a diversity of environments and climates, with different diets and customs, have been reported to show no blood pressure increase with age in adults (Waldron *et al.*, 1982; Henry, 1988; James and Baker, 1990).

The level of a blood pressure measurement, physiologically, is determined by the integrated effects of endocrinological, renal, neurological, and cardiovascular systems and their interactions with environmental factors including diet, activity level, and climate. In modern Western populations, these systems undergo several age-associated changes which can influence the level and variability of blood pressure (Laragh and Brenner, 1990). From this perspective, any age-related increase in blood pressure is not a primary process but rather reflects these underlying changes. A consequence of this perspective is that if, as reported, pressure does not increase with age in some traditionally living people, then one must presume they do not undergo the same physiological changes seen in the people of modern Western societies.

How certain is it, that traditional non-Western populations do not have an age increase in pressure? Can anything be learned about the aging process and blood pressure by studying traditionally living, non-Western people? This chapter will explore these questions and discuss the phenomenon of increasing blood pressure with age in culturally and genetically diverse populations. The

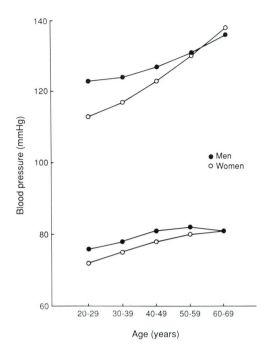

**Figure 12-1**   Average blood pressures by sex and age for the US White population [averaged data from the NHANES II survey (1976–1980) (US Department of Health and Human Services, 1986) and Society of Actuaries and the Association of Lifes Insurance Medical Directors of America, 1979].

discussion will center on the physiological and ecological aspects of blood pressure variation. The reason for this perspective is that these aspects are rarely, if ever, considered in population studies of blood pressure and aging.

## WHAT IS BLOOD PRESSURE?

In a rhythmic fashion, the left ventricle of the heart ejects blood into the aorta, resulting in a pulse wave which is propagated throughout the arterial system. The most common characterization of this pulse wave is the quantification of its maximum (systolic) and minimum (diastolic) pressure (Blank, 1987). Systolic pressure corresponds to that pressure exerted by the pulse wave against the arterial wall at the peak of ventricular contraction, and diastolic pressure corresponds to that pressure when the heart is at rest just prior to the next heart beat. Since every heart beat has a corresponding pulse wave and hence blood pressure, the average person experiences some 90,000 to more than 100,000 blood pressures over the course of a single day (James *et al.*, 1988a).

The most common means of measuring blood pressure in medical practice

Cuff
pressure        Systolic
                pressure

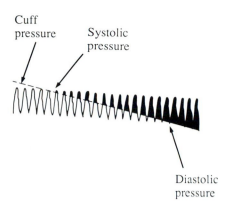

Diastolic
pressure

**Figure 12-2** An illustration of arterial pulse waves showing a decreasing cuff (bladder) pressure and the recorded systolic (appearance of sound) and diastolic (disappearance of sound) pressure using the auscultatory method of blood pressure measurement.

as well as anthropological studies is the auscultatory method. In this procedure, a bladder attached to either a mercury column or gauge is inflated to occlude the brachial artery. A listener places a stethoscope just distal to the occlusion and the pressure in the bladder is slowly released. At the first appearance of sound (Korotkoff phase I) systolic pressure is recorded and at the disappearance of sound (Korotkoff phase V) diastolic pressure is recorded. The deflation of the bladder usually takes about 20 seconds, during which time there are from 20 to 40 ventricular contractions. Therefore, the systolic and diastolic pressures that are recorded are not derived from the same pulse waves. Thus, the "traits" systolic and diastolic pressure, as they are measured in anthropological studies, defines semi-independent estimates of the maximum and minimum pressure exerted by a periodic, continuous series of pulse waves (see Figure 12-2).

It should also be noted that the pulse waves are not generated in a regular harmonic fashion (all with the same amplitude and frequency). Minima (diastolic) and maxima (systolic) can, and do change by 10% or more within seconds (a few heart contractions). Several behavioral and environmental factors have been associated with both systolic and diastolic variation. These include physical activity (van Egeren and Madarasmi, 1988; James and Pickering, 1991), postural change (James et al., 1988b), respiration (Dornhurst et al., 1952), emotional state (James et al., 1986a), temperature (Rose, 1961; Hata et al., 1982; James et al., 1990), the nature of the physical surroundings (Harshfield et al., 1982, 1990) and sodium intake (Pecker and Laragh, 1991). Because of the many factors that affect it, a single determination is unlikely to reflect accurately the average blood pressure of the individual.

Among the elderly, the ability to make accurate blood pressure measurements using the auscultatory method may also be impaired (Spence et al., 1980). Specifically, blood pressure has been shown to be overestimated in some elderly people (Hla *et al.*, 1985). It is postulated that this occurs because the cuff (bladder) pressure needed to occlude sclerotic or calcified arteries (which are more common in the elderly) is much greater than that required by the actual pressure within the artery (Taguchi and Suwangool, 1974; Hla *et al.*, 1985). Furthermore, as people age, the skin wrinkles and loses turgor (Harshfield *et al.*, 1989). In many people, there is a reduction of subcutaneous tissues (such as fat, see Garn, this volume) and skeletal muscle which maintain the structural integrity of the arm (Harshfield *et al.*, 1989). Vessels, including the brachial artery, become more mobile as a result of the hypotrophy of the adjacent sustaining soft tissues (Harshfield *et al.*, 1989). This change in morphology may further contribute to an increasing inaccuracy of blood pressure measurements with age because the altered shape and decreased elasticity of the tissues may compromise the ability of the bladder to properly occlude the brachial artery. The issue of accuracy in measurement among the elderly has only been systematically examined in modern Western societies, so that it is unknown if the decreased ability to measure blood pressure accurately in older people occurs in all populations.

## BLOOD PRESSURE REGULATION

Physically, the extent of pressure variability and the level of average pressure depend upon the lumenal diameter and elasticity of the arteries and the volume of fluid within them. Intrinsic (local, autoregulatory), extrinsic (neurohumoral), and humoral (hormonal) factors regulate these parameters (Rowell, 1986). In addition, control of extracellular fluid volume is exerted by the kidney. Myocardial (heart) function *per se* is a factor only in the presence of marked heart disease, although changes in myocardial contractility can affect blood pressure variability.

The intrinsic control of blood pressure includes a basal tone which is an inherent property of the arterial smooth muscle cells. It is caused by coordinated contractions that propagate from cell to cell producing a partial constriction of the artery (Rowell, 1986). This tonic constriction is important in that it allows the cells to further contract or expand (decreasing or increasing the arteriolar lumen).

The extrinsic control refers to the central innervation (sympathetic and parasympathetic) that, when excited, locally alters arteriolar tone (Rowell, 1986). Finally, the humoral factors refer to several circulating systemic hormones (such as epinephrine, angiotensin II, kinins, vasopressin, and atrial natriuretic factor) which regulate fluid volume, lumen diameter, or arterial rigidity through their effects on receptors located in the various tissues of the body (Rowell, 1986).

From an aging perspective, changes in basal tone, receptor sensitivity or blood-flow dynamics are what probably cause an age increase in blood pressure. Any elevation in blood pressure must reflect changes in the regulatory mechanisms. To understand why blood pressure may increase with age, the effects of aging on the regulatory mechanisms must be understood.

## AGING AND BLOOD-PRESSURE REGULATORY MECHANISMS

As blood pressure is dynamic, so too are the mechanisms that regulate it. Furthermore, these mechanisms are not independent of one another. They continuously interact to maintain the arterial pressure (Rowell, 1986; O'Rourke, 1990). A major difficulty in understanding the blood pressure of an aging cardiovascular system is that as one mechanism loses functional capacity, another compensates so that the net effect is no change in blood pressure (the system maintains homeostasis). The development of higher blood pressure with age, therefore, may be thought of as a loss of the ability to compensate. When regulatory mechanisms cannot compensate, pressure rises.

Because any one of several structural or hormonal systems can be the first to "break down," normal aging of the vessels and hormones is difficult to determine. Given the complexity of the mechanisms and their interaction, an exhaustive description of their age-related changes is impractical for this discussion. However, as examples, age-associated changes in the sympathetic adrenal medullary system and the renin–angiotensin–aldosterone system will briefly be discussed.

### Sympathetic Adrenal Medullary System

The sympathetic adrenal medullary system affects arterial pressure largely through the actions of the catecholamines epinephrine and norepinephrine which are secreted into the blood from chromaffin cells located primarily in the adrenal medullae (Guyton, 1981). In addition, substantial amounts of norepinephrine are released into the blood from sympathetic nerve endings as this hormone also functions as a primary neurotransmitter for the sympathetic nervous system. The specific action of epinephrine and norepinephrine on the vasculature (and blood pressure) depends upon the sensitivity and distribution of catecholamine-specific receptors (alpha and beta) (Guyton, 1981). Epinephrine excites both types of receptors approximately equally. Norepinephrine excites mainly alpha receptors, but also beta receptors to a lesser extent (Guyton, 1981). An important point about these receptors is that they can be excitatory or inhibitory depending upon the tissue in which they are located.

During periods of stress, epinephrine and norepinephrine are released, constricting peripheral arterioles and increasing heart rate, the net effect of which is to increase blood pressure (Kaplan, 1978; James et al., 1989). Continued elicitation of this "fight or flight" response over decades has been suggested to be one way the sympathetic system contributes to the age increase in pressure. It has been hypothesized that the repeated response leads to an attenuation of the baroreceptor reflex, which normally relaxes the heart and dilates the peripheral vessels when blood pressure rises (Kaplan, 1978). Over the years, the baroreceptors which would normally counteract the elevated pressure due to the vasoconstriction caused by the catecholamines, become less sensitive to pressure, thus the average pressure in the system is increased.

Several studies have shown that plasma levels of epinephrine remain constant with aging (Barnes *et al.*, 1982; Goldstein and Kopin, 1990), while norepinephrine levels increase (Ziegler *et al.*, 1976; Goldstein and Kopin, 1990). This increase may occur because of a decreased capacity for uptake by sympathetic nerve endings, or because of an impaired ability to catabolize the norepinephrine, or because of increased secretion consequent to desensitization of the alpha and/or beta receptors with age (Goldstein and Kopin, 1990). The increased circulating catecholamine levels may reflect impaired function of the sympathetic system. However, this elevation in catecholamines with age may not be relevant to age-related increases in blood pressure since the levels of the hormones are not directly related to the mean level of blood pressure (Goldstein and Kopin, 1990).


## Renin–Angiotensin–Aldosterone System

The control of arterial pressure by the renin–angiotensin–aldosterone system (RAAS) is exerted through the several actions of angiotensin II which influences the circulation directly and indirectly through its effects on the kidney and other hormonal systems (Hall and Guyton, 1990). The RAAS is a major regulator of body fluid volume both by its actions on fluid intake via the stimulation of thirst and by altering the renal excretion of electrolytes (sodium and potassium) and water (Hall and Guyton, 1990). Except under extreme conditions, the latter mechanisms are more important since food intake in many circumstances is habitual or preferential (Hall and Guyton, 1990).

The rate-limiting step in the production of circulating angiotensin II is the secretion of renin by the kidney (assayed by plasma renin activity) (see Figure 12-3). The secretion of renin is altered by several negative feedback mechanisms as well as by direct stimulation from the sympathetic nervous system (Laragh and Sealey, 1973).

There is no simple relationship between the RAAS and age-related increases in pressure, except that when it functions inappropriately, pressure may rise. There is no direct relationship between plasma renin activity and the absolute level of blood pressure (Sealey *et al.*, 1990). Blood pressure could increase with age when plasma renin activity increases (due to the enhanced amount and action of angiotensin II, which is a powerful vasoconstrictor) or when plasma renin activity decreases [relating to pathology in the kidney caused by a heterogeneity in the function of nephrons, see Sealey *et al.* (1990) for discussion.]

From the standpoint of "normal" aging, plasma renin activity tends to be lower in older than younger individuals (James *et al.*, 1986b). In addition, renin measurements over 9 years in adults whose blood pressure remained within "normal" limits are quite stable, regardless of the age of the individual at the beginning of the interval or the initial level of plasma renin activity (James *et al.*, 1986b). What this observation suggests is that while people differ in the amount of plasma renin activity, as long as the activity remains relatively stable, pressure may not rise with age.

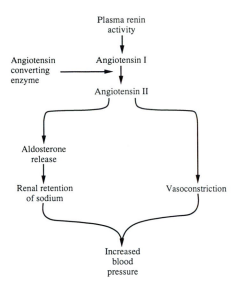

Plasma renin
activity

Angiotensin
converting          Angiotensin I
enzyme

Angiotensin II

Aldosterone
release

Renal retention                    Vasoconstriction
of sodium

Increased
blood
pressure

**Figure 12-3**   The regulation of blood pressure by the RAAS as initiated by plasma renin activity.

In summary, blood pressure is a physiological measurement that describes a pulsatile phenomenon. The extent, amplitude, and frequency of the pulses is determined by several regulatory mechanisms including circulating hormones such as epinephrine, norepinephrine, and angiotensin II. Blood pressure is a continuously varying function which changes with ambient conditions as part of the adaptive, homeostatic processes of the body. It is not a stable trait, although methodologically it has generally been treated as such in most population research. The following sections discuss the population perspective in the study of blood pressure and age concentrating on methodological issues and the interpretation of cross-cultural data.

## METHODOLOGICAL ISSUES IN BLOOD PRESSURE STUDIES

In nearly all studies of non-Western traditionally living populations where blood pressure has been reported not to increase with age, the sample of subjects studied is not random with regard to the population (James and Baker, 1990). People included in the surveys are often those who agreed to be measured or who were available when the researchers were there (Oliver *et al.*, 1975; James and Baker, 1990). Studies of blood pressure in non-Western societies also tend to concentrate in a single village or band, or at most a few such groups, which rarely represent the entire population (James and Baker, 1990).

"Low blood pressure" populations also tend to live in what might be termed "marginal" environments, where there are extremes of temperature, low-quality or poor availability of food, and pestilence. The blood pressure measurements taken in these conditions are clearly not directly comparable and cannot be interpreted in the same way as pressures taken under the "standard" conditions of studies in modern Western populations. It must also be noted, that even in the best large-scale epidemiological surveys of Western populations, there are several factors which influence the accuracy of blood pressure measurements. For example, pressure measurements by physicians at a clinic are higher than the readings taken at home (Ayman and Goldshine, 1940; Beckman et al., 1981). Measurements are also influenced by the relationship between listener and the subject (Shapiro et al., 1954) and even by whether these people are of the same or different sex (Comstock, 1957). There are often additional observer bias in the measurements in the form of digit preference (Rose, 1965; Armitage et al., 1966), and interobserver bias that results when more than one listener is taking measurements (McGarvey and Baker, 1979).

Finally, it is often the case in population studies of blood pressure that only a single measurement per subject is taken. As previously noted, such determinations do not accurately reflect the average pressure of the individuals.

## CROSS-CULTURAL STUDIES: INTERPRETATIONS AND CRITIQUE

Results from cross-cultural studies of blood pressure have been interpreted to show that there need not be an age increase in blood pressure. Is this true? In our opinion, with the available data, there is no way to ascertain with certainty that blood pressure remains stable with advancing age. There are several reasons for the uncertainty.

The first is that nearly all studies of aging and blood pressure in traditional population groups are cross-sectional. Generally speaking, in order to show the age relationship the average pressures of different individuals at different ages are plotted. If the slope of this line is zero, the population group is said to show no age-related increase in pressure. Obviously, a better approach would be to measure pressure continuously in the same persons for decades and examine their individual slopes. However, the main criticism against the interpretation of the cross-sectional studies is that the effect of differential mortality on the blood pressure pattern with age is not taken into consideration (James and Baker, 1990). For example, in many non-Western populations life expectancies are much less than they are in the industrialized Western societies (Teitlebaum, 1975). There is a substantial selective mortality in many traditionally living groups, much of which occurs in infancy (Baker and Dutt, 1972; Baker and Crews, 1986). The adults who are measured in blood pressure surveys (assuming that all of them have been included) are a select group of all those born. The individuals in the older age groups (the survivors) may have lower blood pressure because by definition they are a healthier and heartier group. The average individual in the population may actually have an increase in pressure with age. But, the fact that individuals over 70 years old have blood pressures similar to adults in their 20s and 30s suggests that blood pressure may not increase with age in all people.

A second reason why it is difficult to conclude, even in longitudinal studies (for example, Friedlander and Page, 1987, or Kannel, 1990) that blood pressure does not increase with age (or for that matter does increase), is the low frequency and inaccuracy of the blood pressure measurements. Specifically, systolic and diastolic pressure are estimates of the maximum and minimum of a continuous varying pulse wave. Over the course of 60 years, assuming 70 pulse waves per minute, an individual will experience approximately 2,207,500,000 blood pressures! Given the innate variability of the measurement, it is hard to accept that a periodic sample of one or two measurements every few years will provide a clear indication of the impact of normal aging on blood pressure or its regulatory mechanisms.

A final point about blood pressure among different population groups is that given the genetic diversity among them, it is possible that the mechanisms that either maintain or elevate pressure with age are different as a consequence of natural selection, drift, or other evolutionary forces. Cardiovascular systems that evolve, adapt, and develop in hypoxic, cold, or hot environments may age differently.

## GENETICS AND BLOOD PRESSURE

Blood pressure is not a quantitative trait in the same sense as height, where several genes contribute in an additive fashion to the measurement (Acheson and Fowler, 1967). As has been discussed, blood pressure is a dynamic result of the actions of multiple physiological functions. Intraindividually, blood pressure is maintained within an upper and lower limit. When compensatory mechanisms can no longer maintain the pressure within the appropriate limits, the variability and mean level of blood pressure rises. High blood pressure can thus be thought of as a symptom that reflects pathology in the regulatory mechanisms of the cardiovascular system (Laragh, 1987). To the extent that the pathological change of a given regulatory mechanism has a heritable component, the high blood pressure that results from it will aggregate in families. However, the pathology that is inherited in one family may not be the same as that inherited in another (James and Baker, 1990). The concept is also true of populations. That is, because geographically isolated populations of human beings have evolved under different circumstances and environments for different lengths of time, the genetic basis of their hypertension (or lack of it) may be different. Thus, the similarity of diverse populations with regard to their blood pressure distributions with age may occur because of different homeostatic mechanisms (James and Baker, 1990). In other words, evolutionary forces such as natural selection or random drift may affect the frequencies of alternative genes which determine the structural development of the cardiovascular system, the density or sensitivity of vasoactive hormonal receptors or the function of the hormones themselves which could cause differences in how blood pressure is maintained in individuals from populations living in different environments.


## BLOOD PRESSURE, ADAPTATION, AND THE ENVIRONMENT

Many of the traditionally living people who have been reported to show no age increase in pressure are found in environments far different than the temperate climates of North America, Western Europe, and Japan where most of the epidemiological evidence about age and blood pressure has been collected (James and Baker, 1990). Given their simple technologies, environmental stressors such as high-altitude hypoxia or hot climate have played a significant role in shaping their biology and culture. Adaptations to these stressors may affect blood pressure and impact on the age course of blood pressure as well. The following sections will briefly describe some of these adaptations and their possible effects on the age-related changes in blood pressure.


### High-altitude Hypoxia

The cardiovascular traits of traditionally living natives at altitudes of 4,000 meters above sea level and greater are markedly different than similar groups living at sea level. Much of the work on cardiovascular function in high-altitude natives has been conducted on South American Andean populations, such as the Quechua and Aymara (Baker and Little, 1976; Baker, 1978). Systemic blood pressure levels in adult high-altitude natives are lower than those of natives of similar background at sea level (Frisancho, 1979). Prolonged residence at altitude also results in a lowering of systolic and diastolic pressures in sojourners to high altitude (Marticorena et al., 1969; Frisancho, 1979). The decrease in pressure suggests that chronic hypoxia may have a relaxing effect on smooth muscle (a vasodilation of the arterial media) (Heath and Williams, 1977). Because exposure to high-altitude hypoxia may also increase peripheral vascularization (Valdivia et al., 1960; Tenney and Ou, 1970; Frisancho, 1979), it is possible that the lower blood pressure of high-altitude adult natives may be related to a reduction in peripheral vascular resistance, which might be considered a byproduct of tissue adaptation to the high-altitude hypoxia (Frisancho, 1979).

It has been suggested that native populations living in hypoxic environments at high altitude do not have an age increase in pressure, or more precisely, the blood pressure of old survivors is as low as that of young individuals in the population (Tenbrinck, 1964). Is the lower pressure at older ages due to a chronic vasodilation and decreased peripheral resistance? That is, as people age at altitude, do the adaptations to high-altitude hypoxia overwhelm other degenerations in the cardiovascular or other regulatory systems so that blood pressure does not rise? These questions are largely unanswered, and until they are, the phenomenon of no age increase in pressure in high-altitude native populations should probably not be considered an example of "normal" aging for low-altitude native populations.

## Hot Climate

Adaptation to heat stress requires increased blood flow from the body core and viscera to the skin and muscles of the extremities (Rowell, 1986). This alteration in flow is necessary to rid the body of excess heat, which is manifested as a rise in core temperature (Briggs, 1975). The chronic peripheral vasodilation associated with heat stress may have a lowering effect on blood pressure (Briggs, 1975). Sweating is increased during heat stress to better facilitate heat loss through evaporation of water from the skin. The increase in sweating also causes an increase in the loss of sodium, and a greater sweat output produces a greater sodium loss (Ladell, 1964).

Physiological studies among men from traditional non-Western populations who live in chronically hot environments [such as Bushmen, Aborigines, and Bantu Tribesmen (sub-Saharan Blacks)] show that the average sweat rates of each of the groups were lower during work in hot environments when compared to South African Whites, and that during and after the work load, the men from the traditional groups also maintained a tolerable core temperature (see Frisancho, 1979, for discussion). The implication of these findings is that populations indigenous to hot climates have adapted to heat stress by mechanisms which allow fluid and sodium retention while simultaneously maintaining a tolerable body core temperature. The sodium retention mechanism may have an added benefit in that the hot climate environments are also generally characterized by low availability of dietary salt (Gleibermann, 1973; Frisancho, 1979; Crews and Gerber, this volume).

Many populations that show no increase in blood pressure with age are found in tropical or desert environments (Huizinga, 1972; INTERSALT, 1988; James and Baker, 1990). It may be speculated that a hot climate maintains a continuous peripheral vasodilation over the life of the individual, and when combined with low salt availability in the environment, there is likely to be a relatively low fluid volume in the cardiovascular system as well. Thus, adaptations and conditions related to hot climate may override other degenerations in the cardiovascular system with a net effect of no increase in pressure with age.

However, if heat-adapted populations are moved to more temperate climates, with moderate to unlimited availability of salt, the aging profile of blood pressure may dramatically change. That is, the cardiovascular system of people whose physiology is adapted to the previously described conditions (hot climate with low salt availability) is now confronted with different circumstances (periodic cold with high salt availability), which may cause periodic vasoconstriction with an increase in body fluid volume (Hata *et al.*, 1982). The net effect of such a combination of environmental changes might be an earlier onset (by age) and more malignant form of hypertension in the individual. That is, it is possible that a heat-adapted cardiovascular system more rapidly loses the ability to compensate in a cold salt-rich environment when compared to a cardiovascular system that has evolved to survive in extremes of temperature and salt availability (that adapted to a temperate climate).

It may be speculated that the increased prevalence and earlier average onset of hypertension in Black populations in the United States may in part be related to the mismatch between a heat-adapted physiology and a colder salt-rich environment (see Crews and Gerber, this volume, for discussion). It is of interest that in recent reviews of skin color and blood pressure in US populations, relationships between darker skin color and higher blood pressure have been interpreted only in terms of social factors (Tyroler and James, 1978; Cooper, 1991; Dressler, 1991). The concept that individual Blacks in the United States with darker skin may retain a greater preponderance of an ancestral African genotype that may be more adaptive in a hot salt-poor environment and less so under the temperate salt-rich environmental conditions of the US is not discussed. Given the differences in cardiovascular disease course, clinical manifestations of hypertension, and morbid outcome of cardiovascular disease between Black and White hypertensive patients in the US (Thomson, 1981; McClellan et al., 1988; Aviv and Gardner, 1989; James, 1991), it is difficult to accept that the differences between the groups in the level of and age changes in blood pressure are wholly explainable by social processes.

Studies such as INTERSALT (INTERSALT, 1988; Stamler et al., 1989), which have focussed attention on the effects of salt on blood pressure in a worldwide context have not accounted for biological differences between populations that reflect adaptations to low-salt or hot-climate environments. Specifically, those populations with the lowest sodium excretion and blood pressure in the INTERSALT survey live in hot, tropical, salt-poor environments. Because these populations may have adapted to their environments, it is inappropriate to conclude from their data that removal of salt from diets of people in temperate climates will lower the average pressure of the population. This is not to say that salt plays no role in the development of hypertension in some people. Rather the point being made is that the cross-cultural data, as analyzed, neither supports or refutes the idea that excessive dietary salt causes hypertension. In fact, several studies have shown that many people from industrialized Western populations who dramatically increase or decrease dietary sodium (intraindividually) have no change in their casual blood pressure (Kawasaki et al., 1978; Moore et al., 1991).

## OVERVIEW

The lack of a blood pressure increase with age described in many traditionally living non-Western populations is equivocal. As mentioned earlier, it is difficult to conclude with any certainty that blood pressure does not increase with age because of several methodological problems in the research conducted to date. These include issues related to cross-sectional data, genetic differences among populations and the nature of blood pressure as a trait and its measurement. But, assuming that the data can be interpreted to show that blood pressure need not increase with age (because there are people in traditionally living populations who reach ages greater than 70 or even 80 years who have casual blood pressures similar to those of younger adults in their 20s and 30s), it is difficult to ascribe a single "natural" aging process that has led to the observed phenotypes. The reason, we suspect, is that it is possible that genes, the environment, or both act differently among populations to maintain low pressures in the surviving elderly. For example, it is possible that specific vascular adaptations to chronic hypoxic or hot environments in populations indigenous to the conditions may work to maintain lower blood pressures among the elderly, in spite of other degenerative changes. It is also possible that given the evolutionary timeframe (tens of thousands of years), and intense selective pressures in these environments, natural selection may have modified enzymes, hormones, or the rates of processes in the cardiovascular system which slow an age increase in blood pressure.

There is little evidence that natural selective processes have resulted in specific "low blood pressure" genotypes, not because there is none, but rather because there have been virtually no tests for any. For example, the hormones of the renin–angiotensin–aldosterone system which regulate fluid volume have not been examined, between populations, for genetic variants which may subtly alter their function. That is, the question of whether the potency of angiotensin II measured in Yanomamo indians (a low blood pressure, low sodium excreting population; Oliver *et al.*, 1975; INTERSALT, 1988) is different than that measured among white, Northern European populations (high blood pressure, high salt consumption populations; INTERSALT, 1988) has never been addressed. The concept that single mutations in the polypeptides that define the structure of vasoactive hormones which may render the compounds more or less effective has generally been overlooked. There has also been no assessment as to whether the receptors for vasoactive hormones vary among populations. It is unusual that this line of inquiry has generally been neglected since it is well known that there is a wide array of genotypic variants in plasma proteins, lipoproteins, the immune system, and blood cell antigens, many of which vary because of selective pressure, and which cause specific degenerative diseases (Siervogel, 1983; Crews and James, 1991; see also Crews and Gerber, this volume). It is incumbent upon biological anthropologists to pursue inquiry into possible genetic variants in vasoactive substances and the enzymes which manufacture them as differences may help explain variation in the aging of the cardiovascular system among populations.

The possibility that populations living in different environments may have different mechanisms that maintain lower blood pressure to more advanced age also presents an opportunity to study different mechanisms in the aging of the cardiovascular system. That is, specific populations could be studied as models for different mechanisms that cause hypertension (much like studies of different animal strains). For example, by designing natural experiments in hot climate traditional populations, the interaction among fluid volume, the RAAS and blood pressure with aging could be examined, since populations indigenous to hot climates may have either genetic or developmental adaptations to fluid and salt retention.

Finally, the most important point of this brief overview is that blood pressure *per se* should really not be a central focus of aging studies, since it is a dynamic physiological measurement that, when elevated, suggests change in other underlying mechanisms. In other words, it is a derived function. Research, instead, should concentrate on the structural, endocrinological, genetic, and environmental factors which regulate and modify this variable homeostatic function, and the possible changes in them that occur with age.

# REFERENCES

Acheson, R. M. and Fowler, G. B. (1967) On the inheritance of stature and blood pressure. *Journal of Chronic Diseases* **20**, 731–751.

Armitage, P., Fox, W., Rose, G. A. and Tinker, C. M. (1966) The variability of measurements of casual blood pressure II: survey experience. *Clinical Science* **30**, 337–344.

Aviv, A. and Gardner, J. (1989) Racial differences in ion regulation and their possible links to hypertension in blacks. *Hypertension* **14**, 584–589.

Ayman, D. and Goldshine, A. D. (1940) Blood pressure determinations by patients with essential hypertension I. The difference between clinic and home readings before treatment. *American Journal of Medical Science* **200**, 465–474.

Baker, P. T. (ed.) (1978) *The Biology of High Altitude Peoples.* New York: Cambridge University Press.

Baker, P. T. and Crews, D. E. (1986) Mortality patterns and some biological predictors. In: *The Changing Samoans: Behavior and Health in Transition* (eds Baker, P. T., Hanna, J. M. and Baker, T. S.). Oxford: Oxford University Press, pp. 93–122.

Baker, P. T. and Dutt, J. S. (1972) Demographic variables as measures of biological adaptation: a case study of high altitude human populations. In: *The Structure of Human Populations* (eds Harrison, G. A. and Boyce, A. J.). Oxford: Clarendon Press, pp. 352–378.

Baker, P. T. and Little, M. A. (ed.) (1976) *Man in the Andes: A Multidisciplinary Study of High Altitude Quechua.* Stroudsburg, PA: Dowden, Hutchinson and Ross.

Barnes, R. F., Raskind, M., Gumprecht, G. and Halter, J. B. (1982) The effects of age on the plasma catecholamine response to mental stress in man. *Journal of Clinical Endocrinology and Metabolism* **54**, 64–69.

Beckman, M., Panfilov, V., Sivertsson, R., Sannerstedt, R. and Anderson, O. (1981) Blood pressure and heart rate recordings at home and at the clinic. *Acta Medica Scandinavica* **210**, 97–102.

Blank, S. G. (1987) *The Korotkoff Signal and its Relationship to the Arterial Pressure Pulse.* Ph.D. thesis, Department of Physiology and Biophysics, Cornell University Medical College.

Briggs, L. C. (1975) Environment and human adaptation in the Sahara. In: *Physiological Anthropology* (ed. Damon, A.). New York: Oxford University Press, pp. 93–129.

Comstock, G. W. (1957) An epidemiologic study of blood pressure levels in a biracial community in the southern United States. *American Journal of Hygiene* **65**, 271–315.

Cooper, R. S. (1991) Celebrate diversity—or should we? *Ethnicity & Disease* **1**, 3–7.

Crews, D. E. and James, G. D. (1991) Human evolution and the genetic epidemiology of chronic degenerative diseases. In: *Applications of Biological Anthropology to Human Affairs* (eds Lasker, G. A. and Mascie-Taylor, N.). London: Cambridge University Press, pp. 185–206.

Dornhurst, A. C., Howard, P. and Leathart, G. L. (1952) Respiratory variations in blood pressure. *Circulation* 6, 553–558.

Dressler, W. W. (1991) Social class, skin color, and arterial blood pressure in two societies. *Ethnicity & Disease* 1, 60–77.

Friedlander, J. S. and Page, L. B. (1987) Blood Pressure changes in the survey populations. In: *The Solomon Islands Project: A Long-term Study of Health, Human Biology, and Culture Change* (ed. Friedlander, J. S.). Oxford: Clarendon Press, pp. 307–326.

Frisancho, A. R. (1979) *Human Adaptation: a Functional Interpretation*. St Louis: C. V. Mosby.

Gleibermann, L. (1973). Blood pressure and dietary salt in human populations. *Ecology, Food and Nutrition* 2, 83–90.

Goldstein, D. S. and Kopin, I. J. (1990) The autonomic nervous system and catecholamines in normal blood pressure control and in hypertension. In: *Hypertension: Pathophysiology, Diagnosis, and Management* (eds Laragh, J. H. and Brenner, B. M.). New York: Raven Press, pp 711–747.

Guyton, A. C. (1981) *Textbook of Medical Physiology*. Philadelphia: W. B. Saunders Company.

Hall, J. E. and Guyton, A. C. (1990) Control of sodium excretion and arterial pressure by intrarenal mechanisms and the renin-angiotensin system. In: *Hypertension: Pathophysiology, Diagnosis, and Management* (eds Laragh, J. H. and Brenner, B. M.). New York: Raven Press, pp. 1105–1129.

Harshfield, G. A., Pickering, T. G., Kleinert, H. D., Blank, S. and Laragh, J. H. (1982) Situational variation of blood pressure in ambulatory hypertensive patients. *Psychosomatic Medicine* 44, 237–245.

Harshfield, G. A., Hwang, C., Blank, S. G. and Pickering, T. G. (1989) Research techniques for ambulatory monitoring. In: *Handbook of Research Methods in Cardiovascular Behavioral Medicine* (eds. Schneidermann, N., Weiss, S. M. and Kaufmann, P. G.). New York: Plenum Press, pp. 293–309.

Harshfield, G. A., Pickering, T. G., James, G. D. and Blank, S. G. (1990) Blood pressure variability and reactivity in the natural environment. In: *Blood Pressure Measurements: New Techniques in Automatic and 24-hour Indirect Monitoring* (eds Meyer-Sabellek, W., Anlauf, M., Gotzen, R. and Steinfield, L.). New York: Springer-Verlag, pp. 241–251.

Hata, T., Ogihara, T., Maruyama, A., Mikami, H., Nakanaru, M., Naka, T., Kumahar, Y. and Nugent, C. A. (1982) The seasonal variation of blood pressure in patients with essential hypertension. *Clinical and Experimental Hypertension— Theory and Practice* A4(3), 341–354.

Heath, D. and Williams, D. R. (1977) *Man at High Altitude: the Pathophysiology of Acclimatization and Adaptation*. Edinburgh: Churchill Livingstone.

Henry, J. P., (1988) Salt, stress and hypertension. *Social Science and Medicine* 26, 293–302.

Hla, K. M., Vokaty, K. A. and Feussner, J. R. (1985) Overestimation of diastolic blood pressure in the elderly: magnitude of the problem and a potential solution. *Journal of the American Geriatric Society* 33, 659–663.

Huizinga, J. (1972) Casual blood pressures in populations. In: *Human Biology of Environmental Change* (ed. Vorester, D. J. M.). London: International Biological Programme, pp. 164–169.

INTERSALT Cooperative Research Group (1988) INTERSALT: an international study of eletrolyte excretion and blood pressure. Results for 24-hour urinary sodium and potassium excretion. *British Medical Journal* **297**, 319–330.

James, G. D. (1991) Race and perceived stress independently affect the diurnal variation of blood pressure in women. *American Journal of Hypertension* **4**, 382–384.

James, G. D. and Baker, P. T. (1990) Human population biology and hypertension: evolutionary and ecological aspects of blood pressure. In: *Hypertension: Pathophysiology, Diagnosis, and Management* (eds Laragh, J. H. and Brenner, B. M.). New York: Raven Press, pp. 137–145.

James, G. D. and Pickering, T. G. (1991) Ambulatory blood pressure monitoring: assessing the diurnal variation of blood pressure. *American Journal of Physical Anthropology* **84**, 343–349.

James, G. D., Yee, L. S., Harshfield, G. A., Blank, S. and Pickering, T. G. (1986a) The influence of happiness, anger and anxiety on the blood pressure of borderline hypertensives. *Psychosomatic Medicine* **48**, 502–508.

James, G. D., Sealey, J. E., Muller, F., Alderman, M., Madhaven, S. and Laragh, J. H. (1986b) Renin relationship to sex, race, and age in a normotensive population. *Journal of Hypertension* **4** (Suppl. 5), S328–S330.

James, G. D., Pickering, T. G., Yee, L. S., Harshfield, G. A., Riva, S. and Laragh, J. H. (1988a) The reproducibility of average ambulatory, home, and clinic pressures. *Hypertension* **11**, 545–549.

James, G. D., Yee, L. S., Harshfield, G. A. and Pickering, T. G. (1988b) Sex differences in factors affecting the daily variation of blood pressure. *Social Science and Medicine* **26**, 1019–1023.

James, G. D., Crews, D. E. and Pearson, J. (1989) Catecholamines and stress. In: *Human Population Biology: A Transdisciplinary Science* (eds Little, M. A. and Haas, J. D.). Oxford: Oxford University Press, pp. 280–295.

James, G. D., Yee, L. S. and Pickering, T. G. (1990) Winter–Summer differences in the effects of emotion, posture, and place of measurement on blood pressure. *Social Science and Medicine* **31**, 1213–1217.

Kannel, W. B. (1990) Hypertension and the risk of cardiovascular disease. In: *Hypertension: Pathophysiology, Diagnosis and Management* (eds Laragh, J. H. and Brenner, B. M.). New York: Raven Press, pp. 101–117.

Kaplan, N. M. (1978) Stress, the sympathetic nervous system and hypertension. *Journal of Human Stress* **4**, 29–34.

Kawasaki, T., Delea, C. S., Bartter, F. C. and Smith, H. (1978) The Effect of high sodium and low sodium intakes on blood pressure and other related variables in human subjects with idiopathic hypertension. *American Journal of Medicine* **64**, 193–198.

Ladell, W. S. S. (1964) Terrestrial animals in humid heat: man. In: *Handbook of Physiology*, Vol. 4: *Adaptation to the Environment* (eds Dill, D. B., Adolph, E. F. and Wilber, C. G.). Baltimore: Williams & Wilkins, pp. 625–659.

Laragh, J. H. (1987) Rounds with Laragh. *Cardiovascular Reviews and Reports* **8**, 38–39.

Laragh, J. H. and Brenner, B. M. (eds) (1990) *Hypertension: Pathophysiology, Diagnosis, and Management*. New York: Raven Press.

Laragh, J. H. and Sealey, J. E. (1973) The renin-angiotensin–aldosterone hormonal system and regulation of sodium, potassium, and blood pressure homeostatsis. In: *Handbook of Physiology: Renal Physiology* (eds Orloff, J. and Berliner, R. W.). Baltimore: Waverly Press, pp. 831–908.

Lew, E. A. (1990) Hypertension and longevity. In: *Hypertension: Pathophysiology, Diagnosis, and Management* (eds Laragh, J. H. and Brenner, B. M.). New York: Raven Press, pp. 175–190.

Marticorena, E., Ruiz, L., Severino, J., Galvez, J. and Penaloza, D. (1969) Systemic blood pressure in white men born at sea level: changes after long residence at high altitudes. *American Journal of Cardiology* **23**, 364–368.

McClellan, W., Tuttle, E. and Issa, A. (1988) Racial differences of hypertensive end-stage renal disease (ESRD) are not entirely explained by differences in the prevalence of hypertension. *American Journal of Kidney Disease* **xii**, 285–290.

McGarvey, S. T. and Baker, P. T. (1979) The effects of modernization and migration on Samoan blood pressure. *Human Biology* **51**, 461–479.

Moore, T. J., Malarick, C., Olmedo, A. and Klein, R. C. (1991) Salt restriction lowers resting blood pressure but not 24-H ambulatory blood pressure. *American Journal of Hypertension* **4**, 410–415.

Oliver, W. J., Cohen, E. L. and Neel, J. V. (1975) Blood pressure, sodium intake, and sodium related hormones in the Yanomamo Indians, a "no salt" culture. *Circulation* **52**, 146–151.

O'Rourke, M. F. (1990) What is blood pressure? *American Journal of Hypertension* **3**, 803–810.

Pecker, M. S. and Laragh, J. H. (1991) Dietary salt and blood pressure: a perspective. *Hypertension* **17**, I97–I99.

Rose, G. (1961) Seasonal variation in blood pressure in man. *Nature* **189**, 235.

Rose, G. (1965) Standardization of observers in blood pressure measurement. *Lancet* **1**, 673–674.

Rowell, L. B. (1986) *Human Circulation: Regulation During Physical Stress*. New York: Oxford University Press.

Sealey, J. E., Blumenfeld, J. D., Bell, G. M., Pecker, M. S., Sommers, S. C. and Laragh, J. H. (1990) On the renal basis for essential hypertension: nephron heterogeneity with discordant renin secretion and sodium excretion causing a hypertensive vasoconstriction–volume relationship. In: *Hypertension: Pathophysiology, Diagnosis, and Management* (eds Larah, J. H. and Brenner, B. M.). New York: Raven Press, pp. 1089–1103.

Shapiro, A., Meyers, T. and Reiser, M. F. (1954) Comparison of blood pressure response to veriloid and to the doctor. *Psychsomatic Medicine* **16**, 478–488.

Siervogel, R. M. (1983) Genetic and familial factors in essential hypertension and related traits. *Yearbook of Physical Anthropology* **26**, 37–63.

Society of Actuaries and the Association of Life Insurance Medical Directors of America (1980) *Blood Pressure Study, 1979*. Boston.

Spence, J. D., Sibbald, W. J. and Cape, R. D. (1980) Direct, indirect and mean blood pressure in hypertensive patients: the problem of cuff artifact due to wall stiffness, and a partial solution. *Clinical Investigation and Medicine* **2**, 165–173.

Stamler, J., Rose, G., Stamler, R., Elliot, P., Dyer, A. and Marmot, M. (1989) INTERSALT study findings: public health and medical care implications. *Hypertension* **14**, 570–577.

Taguchi, J. T. and Suwangool, P. (1974) Pipe-stem brachial arteries: a cause of pseudohypertension. *Journal of the American Medical Association* **228**, 733.

Teitlebaum, M. S. (1975) Relevance of demographic transition theory for developing countries. *Science* **188**, 420–425.

Tenbrinck, M. S. (1964) Blood pressure comparisons in tropical Africans and Peruvians. *New York State Journal of Medicine* October, 2584–2587.

Tenny, S. M. and Ou, L. C. (1970) Physiological evidence for increased tissue capillarity in rats acclimatized to high altitude. *Respiratory Physiology* **8**, 137–150.

Thomson, G. E. (1981) Hypertension in the black population. *Cardiovascular Reports & Reviews* **4**, 351–357.

Tyroler, H. A. and James, S. A. (1978) Blood pressure and skin color. *American Journal of Public Health* **68**, 1170–1172.

US Department of health and Human Services (1986) *Blood Pressure Levels in Persons 18–74 years of age in 1976–1980*. Data from National Health Survey, Series 11, no. 234. US Department of Health and Human Services, DHHS publication (PHS) 86–168, July.

Valdivia, E., Watson, M. and Dass, C. M. (1960) Histologic alterations in muscles of guinea pigs during chronic hypoxia. *Archives of Pathology* **69**, 199–208.

Van Egeren, L. F. and Madarasmi, S. (1988) A computer assisted diary (CAD) for ambulatory blood pressure monitoring, *American Journal of Hypertension* **1**, 179S–185S.

Waldron, I., Nowotarski, M., Freimer, M., Henry, J. P., Post, N. and Witten, C. (1982) Cross-cultural variation in blood pressure: a quantitative analysis of the relationships of blood pressure to cultural characteristics, salt consumption and body weight. *Social Science and Medicine* **16**, 419–430.

Ziegler, M., Lake, C. R. and Kopin, I. J. (1976) Plasma noradrenaline increases with age. *Nature (London)* **261**, 333–335.

# 13

# Aging and Adaptation to the Environment

CYNTHIA M. BEALL

## INTRODUCTION

Human adaptation to environmental stressors such as heat, cold, and high altitude has been studied for decades, but nearly all work has focussed on young adults and, to a lesser extent, on children (e.g., Dill, 1964; Baker and Weiner, 1966; Damon, 1975; Frisancho, 1985). This reflects the theoretical paradigm that evolutionary processes enhancing genetic fitness result in well-adapted individuals of reproductive age. In this context, a logical focus of enquiry to identify the results of evolutionary processes was to examine the group with the highest fertility and their offspring. However, the worldwide demographic aging transition in the past few decades has led to the realization that significant proportions of human populations can and do live past the usual reproductive years. This has raised theoretical and empirical questions regarding the evolution and biology of the late reproductive and postreproductive human life span.

Information on biological aging suggests that aged organisms may adapt (adjust beneficially) to environmental stressors differently from young ones because organ system function declines during adulthood. One view is that "Generally, the capacity of aged organisms to maintain homeostasis is impaired as compared to younger organisms." (Davis and Wood, 1985: vii) and homeostasis "is the sum total of all regulatory mechanisms that maintain a constant internal environment." (Davis and Wood, 1985: vii). Another view is that "In effect, any functional decrement is probably accompanied by compensatory processes which help to establish new equilibra and ensure maintenance of biological competence even in older age." (Collins, 1983a: 489). Whether adaptability is simply worse—less effective at restoring homeostasis—or simply different—establishes a different homeostasis or restores homeostasis using different means—is important for understanding and interpreting the human biology of the aging process.

If the adaptability of older adults is poorer, then there may be public health consequences. Another result of the worldwide demographic aging transition occurring today is tens of millions of older adults living in a variety of climates, including extreme climates, throughout the world. Social change producing

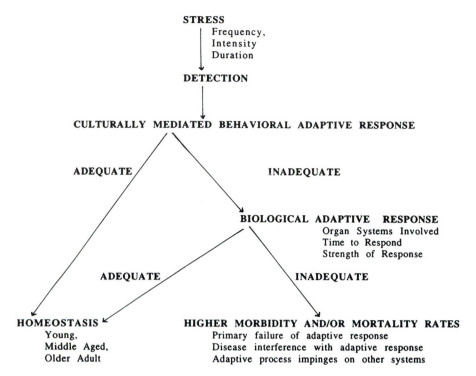

**Figure 13-1** Model of age differences in adaptation to environmental stress (based on Thomas, 1975).

more leisure time and money for travel and relocation throughout the life span acutely exposes an increasing number of older adults to environments unlike their own. If older adults are less able to adapt to their native environments or to environments to which they migrate or visit, then additional morbidity and premature mortality may result.

This chapter evaluates questions of adaptation to the environment in older individuals by reviewing published studies of adult age differences in adaptation to the environmental stresses of cold, heat, and hypoxia. Maintaining an adequate thermal environment and level of tissue oxygenation are vital homeostatic processes throughout the life span. Another chapter in this volume deals with the stress of disease.

This chapter uses the conceptual model of adaptation to environmental stress described in Figure 13-1 (based on Thomas, 1975). In this model, stresses move an organism away from homeostasis and are characterized by their frequency, intensity, and duration. For example, lifelong residence in the Arctic might elicit different responses than acute exposure to cold during a skiing vacation. Stress detection may be psychological and/or physiological. For example, cold stress may be detected by feeling cold while that sensation may be mediated by mental status as well as by the ability of receptors to respond. Detecting stress may prompt a behavioral adaptive response such as adding clothing or building a fire which may be adequate to maintain homeostasis. If inadequate, then a biological adaptive response is engaged which may be characterized by the organ systems involved as well as by the time required to respond, the time course and the strength of the response. An adequate adaptive response restores homeostasis. It is possible that the homeostatic state differs at different stages of the life cycle. An inadequate adaptive response leads to elevated morbidity or mortality. The degree of elevation may be influenced by aging changes in organ systems not directly involved in the adaptive response.

## THERMOREGULATION

Biological adaptations to thermal stress involve an integrated set of physiological responses that act to maintain deep body temperature within a narrow homeostatic range. Integrated systems may be particularly vulnerable to derangement because slow or incomplete response or failure of one component may alter the entire system. Age differences in the various components of thermoregulation have been studied, revealing important variation within the elderly population as well as age differences between "older" and "young" people.

### Detecting Thermal Stress

Two types of evidence demonstrate that detection of thermal stress is less precise among elderly men and women than younger adults. Nearly everyone below the age of 60 can detect temperature differences of less than 1°C. From 60 to 90 years, few can detect such small temperature differences. Most elderly detect temperature differences of 1–5°C (Collins and Exton-Smith, 1981). Other studies confirm these findings (Collins *et al.*, 1977, 1981, Collins and Hoinville, 1980). In one case, the age difference was accounted for by a subgroup of roughly one-third of the elderly who had particularly poor thermal discrimination of 3°C or more while the remainder did not differ from young adults (Collins and Hoinville, 1980).

Behavioral studies offer a second line of evidence for less precise detection of thermal stress by some elderly people. Given the opportunity to regulate room temperature in a temperature-controllable chamber, elderly and young adult men preferred the same room temperature. However, the elderly men allowed ambient temperatures to deviate further from their preferred levels before making adjustments (Collins *et al.*, 1981). Two groups of people in their 70s allowed a temperature oscillation of about 8°C, large compared with just 5°C allowed by a young adult control group. A subgroup of elderly with poor thermal distinction (>2°C) permitted an oscillation twice the size of the young adults, while those elderly with "normal-for-age" (≤2°C) were intermediate. This is evidence that varying ability to detect temperatures corresponds with different levels of behavioral response. Other studies confirm that older adults are likely to have less precise behavioral adaptations to thermal stress. Men in their 60s subjectively rated their physical condition the same as a group of young men even though the former had physiological signs of greater heat stress (Miescher and Fortney, 1989). Men in their 70s exposed to heat stress and provided with the opportunity to give themselves blasts of cool air responded later and at a higher deep-body temperature than young adult controls (Fennell and Moore, 1973).

Thus, some, although not all, older adults are poorer at detecting changes in environmental temperature, are less precise in evaluating their own conditions, and take longer to respond behaviorally. Consequently, behavioral adaptations are probably less effective at maintaining homeostasis with the result that these individuals probably have longer exposure to stress, greater deviation from homeostasis and more need for a biological adaptive response.

## Cold Stress

According to studies of young adult men, the normal adaptive responses to cold exposure act to conserve body heat by two mechanisms. First, vasoconstriction sharply decreases blood flow to the skin and heat loss to the environment. If this is inadequate, the second response is an increase in heat production by shivering and increasing metabolic rate (Weiner and Edholm, 1981).

The sole longitudinal study of aging changes in response to cold stress reports those occurring over 4 years as a cohort aged from a mean of 70–74 years (Collins et al., 1977) and from 74–78 years (Collins and Exton-Smith, 1986). The experimental protocol consisted of exposing 47 people to a cycle of brief total body exposure to thermoneutral, moderately cold, and hot conditions (14 minutes at 30°C, 16 minutes at 15°C, 46 minutes at 45°C, respectively). After 4 years, a retest showed that the group retained the ability to maintain deep-body temperatures during cold exposure although skin temperatures were higher, resulting in a smaller temperature gradient between the deep body and skin, a larger temperature gradient between the skin and the environment, and thus greater heat loss from the skin to the environment (Collins et al., 1977). The higher skin temperatures at the later testing appear to be explained by less vasoconstriction and therefore less reduction in blood flow to the extremities. Furthermore, while two-thirds of the group responded with a qualitatively normal pattern of vasoconstriction on cooling or heating, roughly one-third responded abnormally by failing to vasoconstrict. The number of "non-constrictors" increased from 6 to 14 of the 43 participants (14–33%) in the 4-year interval. [Just 3% of young adult controls were non-constrictors (Collins et al., 1977).] This suggests that aging changes rather than individual lifelong characteristics underlie the non-constricting response in the older group.

The logic of thermoregulation argues that simultaneously maintaining core temperature and relatively high skin temperature requires increasing heat production by shivering and elevating metabolic rate. This short exposure elicited shivering from only a few individuals, all non-constrictors (the number of shiverers increased from four to five during the 4-year interval), suggesting that the failure to vasoconstrict accelerated heat loss and hastened the onset of this second line of response. A few individuals neither vasoconstricted nor shivered. These findings indicate that the group became progressively more impaired in thermoregulation over 4 years and that the prevalence of failures of specific components increased with age.

These studies demonstrate that "older" adults are heterogeneous. The large range of variation and the distinctive subgroups of the older samples indicate the need for careful selection and description of "older" samples, and for relatively large samples to attain statistical power equal to that in studies of less variable young adults. Unfortunately, most samples used in studies of age differences in thermal adaptation are small and poorly described. About 275 men and women aged 46–91 have been studied cross-sectionally as "older adults" in experiments designed to detect age differences in adaptation to cold stress (Table 13-1). Sex was not specified for roughly 70% of those studied and about 10% were hospital patients. Nearly all studies have samples of fewer than 15 "older" individuals. Few very old individuals have been studied. About seven people in their 80s and 90s have been studied; two of these had diagnoses of "senile psychosis." This fairly small number of people spanning 5–6 decades in age participated in studies employing a variety of protocols ranging from 2 hours to 2 minutes exposure to temperatures from 20°C to 0°C and to air speeds from 0 to 40 miles per hour. Experimental protocols entailing 2 hour total body exposure provide opportunity for engaging the full adaptive response. Shorter exposures may be more lifelike.

With respect to maintaining deep body temperature, the objective of thermoregulation, studies are consistent in reporting a fall in deep body temperature of men and women in their 60s and older during 2 hours exposure to cold. For example, one study reports a significant fall of 0.4°C in deep body temperature at 6°C and 12°C among men with an average age of 67 years compared with an insignificant 0.1°C fall in young men with an average age of 21 (Collins *et al.*, 1985). Another study found that while older men consistently had slightly lower deep-body temperatures during cold exposure, older women had higher deep-body temperatures than their younger counterparts (Wagner and Horvath, 1985a). Methodologically, this finding signals that grouping samples on the basis of age alone may confound the effects of age and sex.

That older individuals' deep-body temperature tends to move further away from baseline values implies that vasoconstriction is less effective. Reduction in peripheral blood flow measured in the forearm, hand, or finger is a measure of vasoconstriction. Older men and women consistently exhibit a smaller reduction in peripheral blood flow (Collins *et al.*, 1985, 1986; Wagner and Horvath, 1985b; Collins and Exton-Smith, 1986.) For example, after 2 hours at 20°C the peripheral blood flow of men in their 60s fell to about 40% of the thermoneutral value while that of young men fell to 21% (Collins *et al.*, 1985). The same is observed during shorter exposures (Yoshimura and Iida, 1951-1952; Wagner *et al.*, 1974). The age changes may accelerate at higher ages. Peripheral flow after cooling, which averaged 34% of the thermoneutral value at a mean age of 72 years, increased to an average of 53% of the thermoneutral value at a mean age of 80 years (Collins and Exton-Smith, 1986). Vasoconstriction is even poorer among older adults with arterioscler-

**Table 13-1** Summary of participants and exposures used in published experiments designed to test for adult age differences in adaptation to cold stress.

| Source | Older | | | | Young | | | | Exposure | |
|---|---|---|---|---|---|---|---|---|---|---|
| | # M | # F | Age range | Mean age | # M | # F | Age range | Mean age | Time[b] | Temperature (°C) |
| *Longitudinal* | | | | | | | | | | |
| Collins et al. (1977) | 19 | 28 | 69–90 | 70/74 | 40 | [a] | <45 | | 14 min, 16 min, 46 min | 30, 15, 45 |
| Collins and Exton-Smith (1986) | (21) | [a] | — | 80 | 13 | [a] | — | 23 | | [c] |
| *Cross-sectional* | | | | | | | | | | |
| Collins et al. (1985) | 5 | 0 | 63–70 | 67 | 4 | 0 | 18–24 | 21 | 2 h | 6, 12, 15, 23 |
| Krag and Kountz (1950) | 6 | 7 | 57–91 | 73 | 3 | 3 | 23–36 | 28 | 2 h | 5–15 |
| Macmillan et al. (1967) | 2 | 9 | 66–94 | — | — | — | — | — | 20–70 min | 20 |
| Wagner and Horvath (1985a, 1985b) | 10 | 7 | 51–72 | 64 (M); 61 (F) | 10 | 10 | 20–29 | 22 (M); 24 (F) | 2 h | 10, 15, 20, 28 |
| Collins et al. (1981) | 7 | 0 | — | 80 | 6 | 0 | — | 26 | 1 h | 20 |
| Mathew et al. (1986) | 45 | 0 | 51–70 | — | 90 | 0 | 20–49 | — | 2 h, 30 min, 2 min | 10, 4 |
| Wagner et al. (1974) | 7 | 0 | 46–67 | — | 10 | 0 | 20–29 | — | 23 min | 10 |
| Hovarth et al. (1955) | 3 | 5 | 52–76 | 64 | 7 | 0 | 22–27 | 26 | [c] | 16–17 |
| Collins et al. (1980) | [46] | [a] | 63–91 | — | (10) | [a] | — | 24 | 30 min | 10 |
| Yoshimura and Iida (1951) | 12 | [a] | 50–79 | — | 46 | [a] | 25–49 | — | [c] | 0 |
| Collins and Exton-Smith (1981) | 144 | [a] | 60+ | — | 144 | [a] | — | — | | |
| Collins et al. (1986) | 10 | [a] | 68–88 | — | 10 | [a] | 19–31 | — | 15 min, 15 min, 15 min | 30, 15, 45 |
| Collins et al. (1989) | (5) | 0 | 63–70 | 67 | 4 | 0 | 18–24 | 21 | 6 min | 3.5 |
| LeBlanc et al. (1978) | 8 | [a] | 53–60 | 56 | 9 | [a] | 20–47 | 35 | 2 min | 5, 0[d] |

[a]Sex not stated, sample size listed under M (males). [b]min = minutes, h = hours. [c]Inferred to be the same as Collins *et al.* (1977). [d]40 miles per hour wind.
[ ] Second time this sample is listed in this table. F = females.

osis, perhaps due to structural changes in blood vessels (Collins, 1987). The high prevalence of non-constrictors, generally poorer vasoconstriction, plus evidence of differences in nerve-impulse patterns to the vasomotor system all contribute to the general evaluation that older adults have "impaired vasomotor control" (Collins *et al.*, 1982).

When warmer blood is flowing to the extremities, more heat can be lost to the cold environment and maintenance of deep-body temperatures requires greater heat production. Older men and women increase metabolic rate sooner and higher over a thermoneutral baseline (Krag and Kountz, 1950; Wagner and Horvath, 1985a). Because resting metabolic rates of older individuals are generally lower than those of young adults (e.g., Wagner and Horvath, 1985a; Poehlman and Horton, 1990), a greater increase over baseline may not necessarily result in a higher absolute metabolic rate.

Two early studies of short-term total body cooling report contradictory findings of negligible increase in the metabolic rate of older groups, the majority of whom were in their 50s and 60s (Horvath *et al.*, 1955; Wagner *et al.*, 1974). The reason for this inconsistency is not clear.

Shivering enhances metabolic heat production. In one study, only the non-vasoconstrictors shivered (Collins *et al.*, 1977). Older men and women shivered an average of 10–12 minutes later during exposure to 10°C (Wagner and Horvath, 1985a), perhaps because their metabolic rates increased more and thus the shivering back-up mechanism engaged later. Older adults do not achieve equally forceful muscle contraction while shivering (Collins *et al.* 1981).

Generally, it appears that the older groups are regulating body temperature slightly differently from their younger counterparts, losing more heat because of poor vasoconstriction and increasing heat production more in order to maintain the same or slightly lower deep-body temperature as young adults.

These biological adaptive responses can strain other systems not directly involved in thermoregulation. One consequence of vasoconstriction among older individuals with less distensible blood vessels is a rise in blood pressure. The pattern and magnitude of change in blood pressure upon exposure to cold differs consistently with age. Older men and women gradually increase systolic blood pressure throughout 2 hour cold exposures for a greater total rise than young controls who respond with an immediate, small increase in systolic blood pressure (Collins *et al.*, 1985; Wagner and Horvath, 1985b). In apparent contrast, a study of hand cooling for 2 minutes at 5°C reports no age differences in the blood pressure increase (LeBlanc *et al.*, 1978). This is probably explained by age differences in the onset of blood pressure rises. If the young group has a small rapid response and the older group has a larger slow response, then they may not differ after a very short exposure. Because older individuals tend to have higher resting blood pressures, elevating blood pressure during thermoregulation may precipitate or aggravate disease, thus linking these processes to the health of other physiological systems.

Studies of brief facial cooling, a common real-life exposure, report conflicting results. One reports that the response of older men to 6 minutes of 3.5°C air on the face is less vasoconstriction, a greater blood pressure increase and a smaller fall in heart rate than young men (Collins *et al.*, 1989). Another study reports that a 2 minute exposure to 0°C air blowing at 40 miles per hour produces a greater fall in heart rate of an older group (LeBlanc *et al.*, 1978). The different exposures and age range may account partly for the different results of these two studies.

The studies discussed above involve acute exposure to cold. In one case, an acclimatization procedure was undertaken to ascertain whether 7–10 days of repeated exposure to cold produced adaptive changes (Collins *et al.*, 1985). This study found little effect on either young or old. Evidence of seasonal natural acclimatization comes from the finding that blood pressures are generally higher in the winter in the United Kingdom. This effect is more pronounced in people over 65 and could be due to mild sustained vasoconstriction (Brennan *et al.*, 1982).

The biological adaptive response to cold stress of older people is different but not necessarily less efficient at restoring homeostasis. Indeed, one study concluded that its results brought into question the proper measure of homeostasis and noted "Young Caucasian males have generally been the typical subject not only for cold exposure studies but studies of any environmental stress. In view of the results of the present study, this concept needs to be reassessed, since the younger men in this study were clearly not typical of any of the other groups [young women, older men and women]" (Wagner and Horvath, 1985a, 185). The model presented in Figure 13-1 indicates that the effectiveness of the thermoregulatory response of older adults will be reflected in age differences in the association between cold exposure and morbidity and mortality.

Hypothermia is a clinical condition defined as deep-body temperature less than 35°C (Collins, 1983b, 1). If the different behavioral and biological adaptive responses to cold manifested by older adults are less effective, then the incidence of primary hypothermia (due to dysfunction of the thermoregulatory system) should increase with age. Unfortunately, few reports distinguish primary from secondary hypothermia (due to clinical conditions that lead to intolerance) from that due to behaviors such as alcohol and tranquilizer consumption and to socioeconomic conditions such as poverty which hamper effective behavioral adaptation.

Mortality rates due to hypothermia increase throughout adulthood in the United States (Figure 13-2 from Rango, 1985, 424–426). They increase by about 50% between age 25 and 74 and then sharply thereafter. The mortality rate in the 85+ age category is ten-fold higher than that of the 35–44 age category. This rise is larger than anticipated based on the data reviewed above. It may indicate that small physiological adaptive differences lead to large mortality rate differences or that confounding factors are operating in addition to age differences in thermoregulation. The finding that males have 3–5 times higher rates than females and "other" males and females have 4–6 times higher mortality than "Whites" suggests that factors other than age influence hypothermia mortality.

Social factors play an important role in morbidity due to hypothermia. A national survey of body temperature of the elderly in the United Kingdom

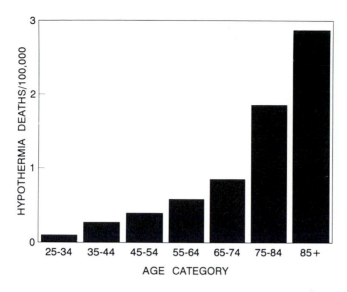

**Figure 13-2**   Hypothermia death rate/100,000 population in the United States, 1979. Data from Rango (1985: 424–426).

found that those with low morning body temperature (<35.5°C) tended to be poor (Fox *et al.*, 1973). A case control study of patients 65+ years admitted to a hospital with hypothermia revealed more social insolation and mental confusion among the patients than among controls (Dawson, 1987).

While social factors may influence the prevalence of hypothermia, age differences in thermoregulatory dysfunction can also be linked to its higher prevalence at older ages. For example, studies of elderly survivors of hypothermia reveal a very high prevalence of the non-constricting response (Macmillan *et al.*, 1967; Collins *et al.*, 1977). Similarly, 75% of a group 60+ years old with low deep-body temperature were non-constrictors, compared with about half in the general population (Collins and Exton-Smith, 1981). Because this response has been identified in healthy elderly, it is likely that it precedes rather than follows hypothermia or low body temperature. Consequently, it is important for future research to learn why some individuals respond this way and others do not, particularly since these risk factors occur in a substantial portion of the elderly population.

Hypothermia is not the only cause of morbidity and mortality associated with cold exposure. Indeed all causes of death (except cancers), and particularly deaths due to respiratory and arteriosclerotic disease, increase linearly with decreasing environmental temperatures from 20°C to −10°C in the United Kingdom and the United States (Bull and Morton, 1978). Figure 13-3 (from Bull and Morton, 1978, 214) illustrates this for myocardial infarction in New York State and illustrates also that the increase is greater among people 60+ years of age. The increase in arteriosclerotic deaths could be partly due to secondary effects of thermoregulation such as blood pressure and heart rate changes. Blood pressures are generally higher in the winter and this effect is

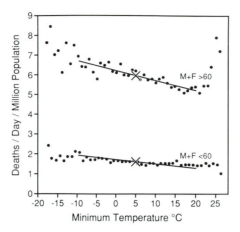

**Figure 13-3** Age differences in the relationship between myocardial infarction death rates and environmental temperature, New York State (1965–1968). From Bull and Morton (1978: 214); reproduced with permission of Oxford University Press.

more pronounced in people over 65 (Brennan *et al.*, 1982). If the higher blood viscosity following total cooling reported for young adults (Keating *et al.*, 1984) holds true for older adults, this would add to the strain on the cardiovascular system. These responses might precipitate disease in individuals with sub-clinical or clinical conditions. It therefore seems probable that cardiovascular health will influence the association between temperature and mortality rate. The chronically ill may be particularly vulnerable. Unfavorable temperatures in one nursing home played a part in 12% of the deaths in the 90–99 year age range (MacPherson *et al.*, 1967).

To summarize this discussion of age differences in adaptation to cold stress, there is an increase in the prevalence of cold-related morbidity and mortality with age and this is attributable to a variety of factors including an increase in the prevalence of abnormal thermoregulatory response, cascade effects on other systems, as well as the socioeconomic and health status of the older adult population. Because of all these confounding factors, it is not clear how much of the increase in mortality and morbidity is an inevitable consequence of the passage of time. All studies so far use samples from temperate latitude industrial populations with high rates of cardiovascular disease and seasonal exposure to cold. The sole exception is passing mention of progressively less "cutaneous reactivity" during 30 minutes of finger immersion in ice water among older Chinese coolies residing in Manchuria (Yoshimura and Iida, 1951–1952). Information from populations with low levels of cardiovascular disease or who are chronically exposed to unusual cold stress would be very useful.

## Heat Stress

The "usual" pattern of adaptation to heat stress, identified by studies of young adult men, acts to rid the body of heat by vasodilation of the blood vessels to the periphery which increases the flow of warm blood from the deep body to the skin where heat is lost to the environment. If this is inadequate to reduce body temperature, the second line of response is sweating to cool the body by the loss of latent heat energy from sweat evaporation (Weiner and Edholm, 1981). With repeated exposure and acclimatization to heat stress, a greater sweating response begins after a shorter time and the net rise in body temperature is smaller.

Longitudinal studies of age changes in response to heat stress reveal changes in the sweating response. One reported a higher deep body temperature at the onset of sweating after a 4-year interval when the average age was 74 years (Collins et al., 1977). Another reported that the overall sweat rate and the sweat loss per degree rise in deep body temperature were lower in a sample of four men 44–60 years old remeasured after 21 years (Robinson et al., 1965). These findings suggest that older adults move further away from homeostasis before sweating begins. Acclimatization to repeated exposure to work in dry heat, as measured by fall in deep body temperature and rise in sweat rate over the course of a week's time, was found to be little changed when repeated after 21 years (Robinson et al., 1965).

Because age differences in heat adaptation have been more widely studied than cold, more study protocols and conflicting results are available for review. Over 300 people aged 41–95 years of age have participated as "older adults" in cross-sectional studies assessing age differences in response to heat exposure (Table 13-2). As with studies of cold adaptation, few studies provide details of the age and sex composition of the sample and few include individuals over 80.

A general measure of the effectiveness of adaptation to heat is deep body temperature at the end of exposure. Older adults exhibit a 40–50% larger increase in body temperature during work and rest in hot-humid and hot-dry environments (Bernstein et al., 1956; Hellon et al., 1956; Hellon and Lind, 1958, Figure 4; Wagner et al., 1974, Figure 1; Yousef et al., 1984, Figure 7; Anderson and Kenney, 1987; Kenney and Anderson, 1988. Figure 1; Sagawa et al., 1988; Miescher and Fortney, 1989, Figure 1). For example, women in their 50s and 60s have a 0.2–0.4°C higher core temperature when exercising at submaximal levels in humid heat (Drinkwater and Horvath, 1979; Kenney and Anderson, 1988). Because these two experiments matched older women with younger controls on the basis of aerobic capacity (physical fitness) or had them perform exercise at the same relative intensities in order to control for the possible confounding effects of age differences in physical fitness, they concluded that the temperature differences were age-, not fitness-, related.

In apparent contrast, two studies report slightly less change in body temperature in older samples. These, however, may be explained by the very short 10 minute exposure time of one (Schoenfeld et al., 1978) and the small age difference (58 versus 38) of the other (Drinkwater et al., 1982). A study that reported no age differences in body temperature after an hour's walk in "desert" conditions is difficult to evaluate without information on actual heat exposure (Yousef et al., 1984). Generally, core temperatures of older adults rise farther above baseline than those of young adults exposed to the same heat stress.

**Table 13-2** Summary of participants and exposures used in published experiments designed to test for adult age differences in adaptation to heat stress.

| Source | Older # M | Older # F | Older Age range | Older Mean age | Younger # M | Younger # F | Younger Age range | Younger Mean age | Time | Exposure Type | Exposure Temperature (°C) | Exposure RH (%) |
|---|---|---|---|---|---|---|---|---|---|---|---|---|
| *Longitudinal* | | | | | | | | | | | | |
| Collins et al. (1977) | 19 | 28 | 69–90 | 70 | 40 | [a] | <45 | — | 14 min, 16 min, 46 min | Rest | 30, 15, 45 | — |
| Robinson et al. (1965) | 4 | 0 | 44–60 | — | [4] | — | 23–39 | — | 65 min, 85 min | Ex | 40 | 24 |
| Dill and Consolazio (1962) | [2] | 0 | 50, 70 | — | [2] | — | 21, 41 | — | <20 min | Ex | 0, 10, 20, . . 50 | 50 |
| Dill et al. (1966b) | 3 | 0 | 54–73 | — | [3] | — | 22–41 | — | 60–90 min | Ex | Desert[b] | |
| *Cross-sectional* | | | | | | | | | | | | |
| *Hot, Humid* | | | | | | | | | | | | |
| Kenney and Anderson (1988) | 0 | 8 | 52–62 | — | 0 | 8 | 20–30 | — | 2 h | Ex | 37 | 60 |
| Drinkwater and Horvath (1979) | 0 | ? | 12–68 | — | 0 | ? | 12–68 | — | 2 h | Ex | 35 | 65 |
| Hellon and Lind (1958) | 6 | 0 | 41–57 | 48 | 6 | 0 | 17–26 | — | 170 min | Ex | 38 | 59 |
| Kenney (1988) | 2 | 4 | 55–68 | — | 2 | 4 | 19–30 | — | 75 min | Ex | 37 | 60 |
| Hellon & Lind (1956) | 12 | 0 | 45–57 | — | 12 | 0 | 18–23 | — | 170 min | Ex | 38 | — |
| Gonzalez et al. (1980) | 7 | [c] | 54–67 | — | 11 | 8 | 16–50 | — | 55 min | Rest | 50 | Wet |
| Hellon et al. (1956) | 18 | 0 | 39–45 | 43 | 18 | 0 | 19–31 | 26 | 230 min | Ex | 38 | 54 |
| Tankersley et al. (1987) | 5 | 0 | 63–72 | — | 5 | 0 | 29–36 | — | 20 min | Ex | 30 | 50–60 |
| Drinkwater et al. (1982) | 0 | 10 | — | 58 | 0 | 10 | — | 38 | 2 h | Rest | 40 | 40 |
| Hellon and Lind (1958) | [6] | 0 | 41–57 | 48 | [6] | 0 | 17–26 | 20 | 150 min | Rest | 38 | 59 |
| Krag and Kountz (1950) | 6 | 8 | 57–95 | 74 | 6 | 6 | 21–36 | 27 | 60–90 min | Rest | 38–45 | 100 |

| | | | | | | | | | | | | Wet |
|---|---|---|---|---|---|---|---|---|---|---|---|---|
| Richardson (1989) | 40 | 0 | 40-79 | — | 20 | 0 | 20-39 | — | 15+ min | Rest | 35, 40 | 40 |
| Sagawa et al. (1988) | 6 | 0 | 61-73 | 66 | 10 | 0 | 21-39 | 27 | 130 min | Rest | 40 | d |
| Collins et al. (1980) | [46] | a | — | 71-87 | [10] | — | — | 24 | d | d | d | d |
| Shiraki et al. (1987) | 6 | 0 | 61-73 | — | 10 | 0 | 21-39 | — | 105 min | Rest | 40 | 40 |
| Bernstein et al. (1956) | 0 | 10 | 60-70 | — | 0 | 10 | 21-28 | — | 60 min | Rest | 38 | 66 |
| *Hot, Dry* | | | | | | | | | | | | |
| Anderson and Kenney (1987) | 0 | [8] | 52-62 | — | 0 | [8] | 20-30 | — | 2 h | Ex | 48 | 15 |
| Kenney and Anderson (1988) | 0 | [8] | 52-62 | — | 0 | [8] | 20-30 | — | 2 h | Ex | 48 | 15 |
| Drinkwater and Horvath (1979) | 0 | c | 12-68 | — | 0 | a | 12-68 | — | 2 h | Ex | 48 | 10 |
| Gonzalez and Pandolf (1989) | c | 0 | 19-55 | 35 | a | — | — | — | 110 min | Ex | 50 | 1 |
| Pandolf et al. (1988) | 9 | 0 | — | 46 | 9 | 0 | — | 21 | 110 min | Ex | 49 | 20 |
| Wagner et al. (1974) | 7 | 0 | 46-67 | — | 10 | 0 | 20-29 | — | 60 min, 90 min | Ex | 49 | 17 |
| Yousef et al. (1984) | 14 | 12 | 50-88 | — | 43 | 48 | 17-49 | — | 60 min | Ex | Desert | — |
| Miescher and Fortney (1989) | 7 | 0 | 61-67 | 64 | 6 | 0 | 21-29 | 26 | 240 min | Rest | 45 | 25 |
| Gonzalez et al. (1980) | 7 | a | 65-67 | — | 11 | 8 | 16-50 | — | 55 min | Rest | 50 | Dry |
| Schoenfeld et al. (1978) | 13 | 4 | 46-63 | — | 20 | 21 | 18-45 | — | 10 min | Rest | 80-90 | 3-4 |
| *Limb immersion* | | | | | | | | | | | | |
| Ohnishi et al. (1989) | 11 | 19 | 61-81 | — | 17 | 27 | 20-30 | — | 2 h | Leg | 42-43 | |
| Crowe and Moore (1974) | 9 | 0 | 70-82 | — | 4 | 0 | 16-20 | — | 1 h | Hand | 42.5 | |
| Fennell and Moore (1973) | 10 | 0 | 65-89 | — | 8 | 0 | 20-24 | — | 1 h | Hand | 42 | |
| Foster et al. (1976) | 28 | 18 | 70-94 | 79 (M)/85 (F) | 13 | 8 | 18-65 | 34 (M)/22 (F) | Variable | Feet, knees | 43.5 | |

aSex not stated, sample size given under M (males).

b"Desert" temperature and humidity not stated.

cAge distribution not stated.

dInfer same as Collins et al. (1977).

[ ] 2nd–3rd time sample listed in this table; Ex = exercise test; RH = relative humidity; F = females; min = minutes; h = hours.

Increased forearm blood flow measures vasodilation in response to heat stress. Vasomotor dysfunction is reported for older adults exposed to heat, consistent with the findings under cold exposure described above. A portion (7%) of a group with an average age of 74 years completely failed to vasodilate (Collins et al., 1977). Most studies report that older samples have lower forearm blood flow under thermoneutral conditions and during work and rest in heat and a smaller increase in forearm blood flow per degree change in body temperature (Collins et al., 1980; Shiraki et al., 1987; Tankersley et al., 1987; Kenney, 1988; Sagawa et al., 1988; Richardson, 1989). Hypertension and arteriosclerosis, prevalent at older ages, hamper vasodilation (Collins, 1987; Kenney and Hodgson, 1987). Lower blood flow transfers less heat from the deep body to the skin and could partly account for the higher deep body temperatures in older adults exposed to heat.

In contrast, several samples of older individuals actually have higher forearm blood flows during rest and heat exposure while reporting what seems inconsistently higher deep body temperatures (Hellon et al., 1956; Hellon and Lind, 1958; Wagner et al., 1972). One possible reason is a better "natural" state of acclimatization in the young sample: age differences in blood flow have been virtually eliminated after a period of acclimatization (Wagner et al., 1972). Another possible reason is the low average age (just 43 and 48 years) of the "older" samples.

Following a relatively poor vasomotor response, the older samples may take longer to initiate the sweating response, as much as 40% longer while resting in hot humid environments (Sagawa et al., 1988), 190% longer during exercise in a hot humid environment (Hellon and Lind, 1958), and during hand immersion in hot water (Crowe and Moore, 1974). Sweating thus begins at a significantly higher deep body temperature, i.e., further away from baseline values in older adults (Fennel and Moore, 1973; Crowe and Moore, 1974; Foster et al., 1976; Collins et al., 1977; Ohnishi et al., 1989).

The sweating response fails completely in a significant proportion of the elderly. One study found that only half the older sample sweat during a 46 minute heat exposure while all the young did so (Collins et al., 1977). Response to a chemical stimulus that elicits maximum sweating was absent in 14 of 19 people aged 70+ compared with just five of the 16 young controls of unspecified age (Ellis et al., 1976). Response was similarly absent in seven of 18 people aged 70+ compared with two of 14 young controls in another study (Foster et al., 1976). The latter study confirmed this response to artificial stimulus by reporting a significant portion of elderly, particularly women, failed to sweat during immersion of feet and legs in hot water.

A marked degeneration with age in the morphology and innervation of sweat glands of 80-year-olds (Abdel-Rahman et al., 1992) undoubtedly accounts partly for age differences in the sweating response. The sweating response may be analyzed on the basis of the rate, the volume, the time course of response, and the chemical composition of the sweat. Age differences in sweat rate appear to depend upon the heat stimulus. Figure 13-4 (from Kenney and Hodgson, 1987, 452) summarizes nine studies that reveal a pattern of substantially lower sweat rates in older samples measured under hot dry

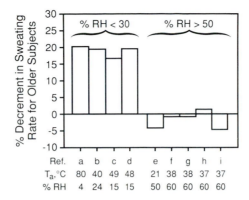

**Figure 13-4**  Percentage decrement in sweating response of older compared with younger individuals in hot humid and hot dry environments. From Kenney and Hodgson (1987: 452); reproduced with permission of AIDS Press.

conditions and little age difference in sweat rates under hot humid conditions. One study in humid heat subsequent to that review conforms to the pattern (Sagawa *et al.*, 1988), while one in dry heat reports no age deficit in sweat rate at rest and does not conform to the pattern (Miescher and Fortney, 1989).

The hypothesis that age differences in sweat rate depend upon the type of heat stress was tested comparing samples of women from 52 to 62 and 20 to 30 years old matched for body size, physical fitness, and heat acclimatization (Anderson and Kenney, 1987; Kenney and Hodgson, 1987; Kenney and Anderson, 1988). Older women had sweat rates similar to the young women in the hot humid environment but had lower sweat rates in the hot dry environment. This was because the older women had the same rates in the two environments whereas the young women attained higher rates in the hot dry than the hot humid environment. The older sample responded maximally relatively early during the heat exposure, while the younger sample responded incrementally throughout exercise in the hot dry environment and achieved a higher rate. Apparently the older sample did not have the reserve capacity to further increase sweating above the rate attained in the hot humid environment, or changes in the older skin may physically interfere with sweating (hydromeiosis) in the older sample (Collins, 1988b). While this offers an explanation for the lower sweat rate and the higher rise of deep body temperature among older adults in hot dry conditions, it does not explain the similarly higher body temperature rise in hot humid conditions.

Other evidence of disruption in the sweating response is the finding of a shorter duration of sweating and a smaller loss of sweat among older men in humid heat (Sagawa *et al.*, 1988). This suggests that future work investigating the response to heat stress should consider several parameters of sweating, such as the rate, duration, and total loss, and also examine the prevalence and the characteristics of non-responders. It appears that the sweating response is less efficient in older samples, although the particular aspects of sweating affected may differ depending upon the environmental conditions.

Despite the similar or smaller sweat rate, older individuals' plasma volumes tend to decrease more during heat exposure and return more slowly to baseline (Kenney and Anderson, 1988; Miescher and Fortney, 1989).

Similarly, salt loss in sweat is greater among older people and age differences may increase after acclimatization (Dill *et al.*, 1966a; Drinkwater *et al.*, 1982; Pandolf *et al.*, 1988; Ohnishi *et al.*, 1989) and thus there is a higher risk of the deleterious consequences of salt depletion.

Seasonal variation in sweat rate (Ohnishi *et al.*, 1989) and cardiovascular response to work (Henschel *et al.*, 1968) indicate that natural acclimatization through repeated exposure in everyday life occurs in older individuals. Several studies report the results of artificial acclimatization protocols involving repeated exposure to heat. A longitudinal study described above reported a very similar course of acclimatization changes during a week's exposure to work in the heat, although deep body temperature was slightly higher when the men were 44–60 than when they were 23–39 years old (Robinson *et al.*, 1965). Cross-sectional studies confirm that older men and women exhibit the same classic signs of acclimatization but there is slightly less improvement in homeostasis in the older groups. For example, there is less reduction in deep body temperature and less improvement in evaporation rate (Wagner *et al.*, 1974) and sweat gland output (Ohnishi *et al.*, 1989).

Hellon and Lind (1956) described the adaptive response of older adults to heat as "sluggish" relative to young adults. This seems apt in the light of subsequent findings of a more labile deep body temperature upon exposure to a hot environment, smaller vasodilation, and delayed and disordered sweating response. These age differences in biological adaptive responses in conjunction with the poorer thermal discrimination of older adults suggest that they may be more susceptible to hyperthermia, heatstroke, and other heat-associated disease.

Elderly mortality rates increase with increasing environmental temperatures above about 20°C. For example, Figure 13-3 demonstrates an upward inflection point in myocardial infarction mortality at about that temperature. Higher morbidity and mortality due to all causes is observed during heat waves (Bridger *et al.*, 1976; Jones *et al.*, 1982). The number of deaths during a New York City heat wave in 1948 was double the number observed during the same months in other years (Ellis, 1976). Vulnerable sub-populations experience an even larger increase. Mortality rates nearly quintupled in a California nursing home, among people over 65 years of age, during a 4-day heat wave with temperatures above 38°C (Ellis, 1976). Deaths due to heat-aggravated illnesses are more common than those due solely to heat illnesses themselves (Ellis, 1976). Causes of death during heat waves are mainly ischemic heart disease (Ellis *et al.*, 1975) and cerebrovascular accident (Schuman *et al.*, 1964).

Figure 13-5 (calculated from Bridger *et al.*, 1976, 40) presents a measure of "excess mortality" during the July 1966 heat wave in St Louis, Missouri, USA, when temperatures were consistently above 32°C and often above 38°C. "Excess mortality" is the death rate for that July less the annual average in the previous year. The inference is that these "excess deaths" are attributable to heat stress. The excess deaths in Figure 13-5 increase each decade, sharply so

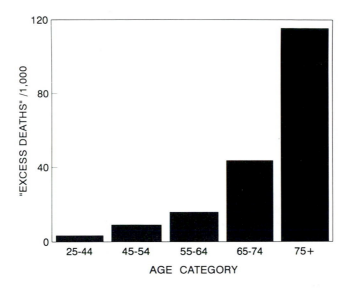

**Figure 13-5** "Excess mortality" rate/1,000 population during a St Louis heat wave, July 1966. Calculated from Bridger *et al.* (1976: 40).

after 64 years. The death rate at ages 65–74 is roughly triple that of ages 55–64 and the death rate at ages 75+ is roughly triple that of 65–74. This seems to indicate a steeper rise with age than the hypothermia death rates presented in Figure 13-2. A similar pattern of very sharp rise with age in deaths attributable to hyperthermia has been observed in several other states in the United States (Shattuck and Hilferty, 1932).

There is large intrapopulation variation in "excess death" rates. For example, among those 65–74 years old, "White" males and females have intermediate "excess death" rates while "other" males have the lowest excess mortality rate and "other" females the highest (four times higher).

Analysis of heatstroke morbidity during a more recent heat wave in St Louis and nearby Kansas City found that those over 65 years of age had 35–45-fold greater heatstroke prevalence (fatal and non-fatal) than those 19–44 years of age. It also found that the "other" population had a 3–7-fold higher heatstroke prevalence than the "White" and that the poorest district had 6–7-fold higher prevalence of heatstroke than the richest (Jones *et al.*, 1982). A case-control study of risk factors for heatstroke identified a number of factors associated with greater or lesser risk, and suggests several reasons why the older population is more vulnerable (Kilbourne *et al.*, 1982). For example, the use of alcohol and major tranquilizers was associated with greater risk while the ability to care for oneself, spend time in air-conditioned places, and drink extra fluids were all associated with lesser risk. These risk factors are all associated with poor health or lower socioeconomic status, both more prevalent at older ages. These findings emphasize that factors in addition to biological aging raise the heat-related mortality of older adults.

Several aspects of impaired biological thermoregulatory processes of older adults may be linked to morbidity and mortality associated with hyperthermia. Failure to sweat or sweating at a lower rate will permit deep-body temperature to rise to hyperthermic and possible lethal levels. Salt depletion and dehydration may increase the risk of morbidity. Loss of plasma volume can lead to increased blood viscosity and reduced blood flow and strain the cardiovascular system.

To conclude this discussion of age differences in adaptation to heat stress, elevated morbidity and mortality among older adults during heat waves is accounted for by a variety of factors. These include socioeconomic status and strain on the cardiovascular systems resulting from less effective thermoregulatory responses, as well as changes in the thermoregulatory process which permit body temperatures to rise further before initiating the less effective responses. It is important to obtain better information on thermoregulation above the age of 70 when mortality rates increase sharply. As was the case with cold adaptation, it is not clear to what extent chronological age, rather than health and socioeconomic status, accounts for the age differences in adaptation to heat. However, the evidence that sweating response becomes poorer with increasing age, even in healthy people, seems strong and this may indeed be a "true aging" phenomenon.

Further studies of populations with well-described chronic lifelong exposure will provide useful information on the universality of aging differences in response to heat stress. Similarly, studies of heat response in populations maintaining good cardiovascular health will be useful.

## HYPOXIC STRESS

Normal adaptive responses to hypoxia identified from studies of young adults, rely upon enhanced function of the respiratory and hematologic systems to extract and transport relatively more oxygen. Table 13-3 summarizes studies with information relevant to adult age differences in adaptation to hypoxia. While about 4,000 people are included in the table, the number is misleading because studies with some 3,000 men do not provide enough age information to determine how many "older" adults are in the sample. Likewise, two studies of "aging" include 4-year-old children and no one above the age of 46. About 700 people over 50 years of age appear to have been studied. Exposures range from clinical tests using acute transient hypoxic stress to lifelong chronic hypoxic stress due to residence at high altitudes.

A measure of adaptation to acutely experienced transient hypoxia is hypoxic ventilatory response. The brief (usually less than half hour) stress test consists of breathing gas mixtures with progressively less oxygen and the response is an increase in ventilation. Three studies report a smaller increase in ventilation in older adults who as a result had lower ventilation at any given level of hypoxemia and therefore would be expected to remain hypoxemic longer (Kronenberg and Drage, 1973; Peterson *et al.*, 1981; Tafil-Klawe *et al.*,

1989). For example, under baseline conditions ventilation of one sample of older men was 74% of the ventilation of young men, while under the most hypoxic conditions ventilation of the older men was just 25% that of the young men because the ventilation increase was much smaller in the older men (Kronenberg and Drage, 1973). However, two studies report the opposite, that older adults had roughly 50–75% greater hypoxic ventilatory response than the young controls (Chapman and Cherniack, 1987; Kawakami et al., 1981). The reason for this discrepancy is not known.

Evidence from another type of study suggests that older adults' adaptive response to acutely experienced transient hypoxia is less effective, consistent with the hypothesis of a decrease in hypoxic ventilatory response. Breathing a 10% oxygen–90% nitrogen mixture produced a greater drop in arterial oxygen saturation, i.e., a move further away from baseline, in a sample of men 52–66 years of age than in a control group 18–37 years of age (Simonson, 1962).

Acute short-term exposure of sea-level natives to high-altitude hypobaric hypoxia for periods of several days to several weeks illustrates that the respiratory and hematological changes of men 58–71 years old are in some senses the reverse of those of younger men and the same men measured 27 years earlier. Six male physiologists who had studied themselves at 3,600–5,300 metres altitude, restudied themselves 27 years later at the ages of 58–71 at 3,090–4,340 metres altitude. None had severe altitude sickness, although their subjective evaluation was that abatement of symptoms was slower during the later exposure (Dill, 1963; Dill et al., 1964). Vital capacity decreased by 20% or more in five of six older men during the first week at high altitudes yet it changed negligibly in young adult men (review in Dill et al., 1980). Similarly, hemoglobin concentration decreased in five of the six older physiologists and in all four men aged 46–77 in another study but increased in acutely exposed young men (Dill et al., 1969). Apparently this is due to an increase in plasma volume resulting in hemodilution in older individuals and a decrease in plasma volume resulting in hemoconcentration in the young individuals (Dill et al., 1966). Older adults respond qualitatively differently than young adults to acute short-term high-altitude hypoxia.

"Natural experiments" involving high-altitude populations who are chronically exposed to hypoxic stress provide a contrast to these short-term experiments. Research into adult age differences in adaptation to lifelong hypoxia has been stimulated by the hypothesis that chronic mountain sickness, a disease attributed to loss of altitude adaptation, is an inevitable concomitant of aging at high altitudes. Chronic mountain sickness is hypothesized to result from excess erythrocytosis secondary to aging processes in the respiratory system (Whittembury and Monge, 1972; Sime et al., 1975).

This hypothesis directs attention toward the respiratory and hematological systems. The effectiveness of the respiratory system at transferring oxygen to the blood has been measured as the percentage of arterial blood that is saturated with oxygen. Figure 13-6 contrasts the percentage arterial oxygen saturation in adults less than 50 years with that measured in older adults 50 and older in four high-altitude samples. Three of the four older samples have lower

**Table 13-3** Summary of participants and exposures used in studies with information relevant to adult age differences in adaptation to hypoxic stress.

| Source | Older | | | | Younger | | | | Exposure type | Response measure |
|---|---|---|---|---|---|---|---|---|---|---|
| | # M | # F | Mean age | Age range | # M | # F | Mean age | Age range | | |
| *Acute, transient* | | | | | | | | | | |
| Chapman and Cherniack (1987) | 5 | 5 | 69 | 64–76 | 6 | 4 | 22 | 18–31 | Progressive | HVR |
| Kronenberg and Drage (1973) | 8 | 0 | 70 | 64–73 | 8 | 0 | 26 | 22–30 | Progressive brief | HVR |
| Kawakami et al. (1981) | 10 | 0 | 71 | — | 15 | 0 | 30 | — | Progressive brief | HVR |
| Peterson et al. (1981) | 4 | 6 | 73 | 65–79 | 4 | 5 | 24 | 22–29 | Progressive brief | HVR |
| Tafil-Klawe et al. (1989) | | | | | | | | | | |
| Normal | 8 | [a] | 48 | 41–60 | 25 | [a] | — | 20–40 | Not stated | HVR |
| High BP | 8 | [b] | 49 | 41–60 | 18 | 8 | — | — | Not stated | HVR |
| Simonson (1962) | 68 | 0 | — | 52–66 | 59 | 0 | — | 18–37 | 10 min 10% $O_2$–90% $NO_2$ | Change in $O_2$ saturation |
| *Acute, short term* | | | | | | | | | | |
| Dill et al. (1963) | 6 | — | — | 58–71 | | | — | | 35 days, 3,090–4,343 m | Hemoglobin concentration |
| Dill et al. (1969) | 4 | 0 | 57 | 46–77 | 8 | 0 | 29 | 18–36 | 14–72 days, 3,800 m | Hemoglobin concentration |
| Dill et al. (1980) | 1[b] | 0 | — | 73 | 1 | 0 | — | 34 | 7 days, 3,800 m | Plasma volume |

*Chronic, long term*

| Study | M | F | | Age | M | F | | Age | Elevation / residence | Variable |
|---|---|---|---|---|---|---|---|---|---|---|
| Regensteiner and Moore (1985) | 195 | [a] | — | 60+ | 150 | [a] | — | 40–59 | Life, 2,456 m | Migration |
| Beall and Reichsman (1984) | 28 | 39 | — | 50–79 | 98 | 105 | — | 20–49 | Life, 3,250–3,450 m | Hemoglobin concentration |
| Guenard et al. (1984) | | | | | | | | <35 | Lifelong, 3,600–4,000 m | |
|   Sick | 22 | 1[c] | — | 35–70 | 22 | 1[c] | — | | | |
|   Sick | 4 | 1[c] | — | — | 40 | 1[c] | — | | | |
|   Control | 17 | 0 | — | 15–60 | | | — | | | |
| Beall et al. (1990) | 156 | 73 | — | 18–74 | 58 | 0 | — | 4–46 | Lifelong; 3,800 m | Hemoglobin concentration |
| Whittembury and Monge (1972) | 0 | 0 | — | — | | | — | — | Lifelong, 3,800–4,500 m | Hematocrit |
| Monge et al. (1990) | 2,892 | — | — | 20–69 | | | — | — | Not stated; 4,300 m | Hemoglobin concentration |
| Velarde et al. (1990) | [2,877] | — | — | 20–69 | | | — | — | Not stated; 4,300 m | Hemoglobin concentration |
| Sime et al. (1975) | 0 | 0 | — | — | 21 | [a] | — | 4–41 | Lifelong, 4,540 m | HVR, ventilation |
| Beall et al. (1992) | 16 | 0 | — | 47–68 | 17 | 0 | — | 22–35 | Lifelong, 3,500–4,100 m | Hemoglobin concentration, $O_2$ saturation |
| Chiodi (1978) | 8 | 0 | — | 45–57 | 34 | 0 | — | 22–44 | 1–22 years, 4,515 m | Hemoglobin concentration |
| Beall et al. (1987) | 47 | 56 | — | 16–82 | 79 | [d] | — | — | Lifelong, 4,850–5,450 m | Hemoglobin concentration |
| Beall and Goldstein (1990) | 24 | [d] | — | 50–79 | 63 | [d] | — | 20–49 | Lifelong, 4,850–5,450 m | $O_2$ saturation |
| | 25 | [d] | — | 50–79 | 56 | [d] | — | 20–49 | Lifelong; 4,545 m | $O_2$ saturation |
| | 19 | [d] | — | 50–79 | | | — | 20–49 | Lifelong; 3,939 m | $O_2$ saturation |
| Garruto (1976) | 38 | 0 | — | — | | | — | — | Lifelong, 4,000 m | Hemoglobin concentration |

[a] Sex not stated, sample size given under M (males).

[b] Individual listed elsewhere.

[c] Female of unknown age in sample.

[d] No sex difference.

F = female; HVR = hypoxic ventilatory response; [ ], inferred to be the same sample as listing just above.

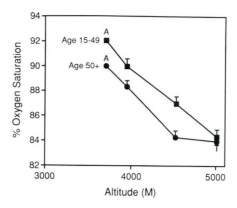

**Figure 13-6** Age differences in percentage oxygen saturation of native residents of three altitudes in Tibet (T) and one in the Andes (A). From Beall and Goldsten (1990: 64); reproduced with permission of B. C. Decker, Inc.

percentage oxygen saturations. For unknown reasons, the population under the greatest hypoxic stress is the one that does not exhibit age differences. A different measure of oxygenation is the alveolar partial pressure of oxygen, this did not vary between the ages of 15 and 60 in one study of healthy people, although it decreased with age in overweight people and those ill with chronic mountain sickness (Guenard *et al.*, 1984).

The ability of the blood to transport oxygen is often measured as the hemoglobin concentration, which is generally moderately increased at high altitude. Excessively high hemoglobin concentration is a symptom of chronic mountain sickness. However, the point at which this presumed adaptive response becomes a disease symptom is not clear. Most studies report no adult age differences in hemoglobin concentration at altitudes above 3,200-metres, indicating that these populations retain the ability to adapt hematologically by maintaining a hemoglobin concentration above that of sea level populations (Garruto, 1976; Chiodi, 1978; Beall and Reichsman, 1984; Tufts *et al.*, 1985; Beall and Goldstein, 1990; Beall *et al.*, 1990). Just one study reports a lower hemoglobin concentration in an older sample of healthy men at 3,600 metres (Beall *et al.*, 1992). This is analogous to the finding of lower hemoglobin concentration upon acute exposure of older men. However, the estimated arterial oxygen content of this older sample is within the normal sea-level range despite the lower hemoglobin concentration. It is not clear whether hemoglobin concentration, or estimated arterial oxygen content, or another parameter is the appropriate measure of adaptive responses.

In contrast are two earlier reports of a progressively greater and ultimately pathological hematological response to high altitude throughout adulthood (Whittembury and Monge, 1972; Sime *et al.*, 1975). These two studies extrapolated the childhood and adolescent increase in hemoglobin concentration (their sample ranged in age from 4 to just 46 years of age) into middle age and older adulthood and inferred that it would continue throughout adulthood, an inference that is probably unwarranted. Another report describes an age-related increase in hemoglobin concentration of unspecified amount among high-altitude miners 20–69 years of age (Monge *et al.*, 1990). This study cannot be adequately evaluated because the age distribution and actual values of hemoglobin concentration are not provided.

Overall, it appears that healthy male and female high-altitude natives may become less effective at oxygenating the blood with increasing age, while retaining equal ability to respond hematologically to the stress of high altitude, at least through the eighth decade of life.

Morbidity and mortality data could provide insight into age differences in adaptive responses to high-altitude hypoxia. Unfortunately there are no epidemiological studies of chronic mountain sickness. There is evidence that chronic mountain sickness is more prevalent among middle-aged than young adult men but no evidence is available that it is yet more prevalent among old men (Heath and Williams, 1989). One study statistically defines a condition of pathologically high hemoglobin concentration, "excess erythrocytosis" and reports that the prevalence in miners rises from 7% at age 20–29 to 33% at age 60–69 (Leon-Valarde *et al.*, 1990). Because no excess erythrocytosis was found in several hundred rural non-miners between 3,250 and 5,450 metres (Garruto, 1976; Beall and Reichsman, 1984; Beall *et al.*, 1987, 1990) and only a very low prevalence was found in nearly 600 urban non-miners (Tufts *et al.*, 1985), it seems that these findings indicate an interaction between age and some characteristic of miners. This could be a sub-clinical occupational condition that exacerbates high-altitude and age-related hypoxia and stimulates a pathological hematological response. Additional evidence that high-altitude residence exacerbates disease processes is provided by one study reporting that high-altitude residents of 60+ with heart or lung diseases are likely to move to lower altitudes and to experience an improvement in symptoms (Regensteiner and Moore, 1985).

Age differences in adaptation to hypoxia have not been as thoroughly studied as those of thermoregulation. To summarize this discussion of age differences in adaptation to hypoxia, the nature of age differences appears to depend greatly upon the type of exposure. The reversal of hematological response of older sea-level natives exposed to high altitude requires confirmation. The completely contradictory findings regarding age differences in hypoxic ventilatory response need to be reconciled. The role of age differences in hypoxic ventilatory response of high-altitude natives has not been investigated. This could explain the age differences in the percentage oxygen saturation of arterial blood in some groups. The epidemiology of chronic mountain sickness and its risk factors remain to be investigated. Hypoxic exacerbation of diseases whose prevalence increases with age also requires further study. Information relating poor hypoxic ventilatory response, or poor oxygen saturation, or unusually high or low hemoglobin concentration to morbidity and mortality would provide insight into the consequences of any age-related differences in adaptive response to hypoxia.

## THEORETICAL IMPLICATIONS AND FUTURE RESEARCH

The information reviewed above demonstrates adult age changes and age differences in biological adaptive responses to the stresses of cold, heat, and hypoxia. Adaptation to thermal stress in older persons remains qualitatively the same but is less efficient and the loss of efficiency may depend upon the type of heat stress. The prevalence of individuals with complete or near complete failure of one or more components of the thermoregulatory response increases with age yet some older individuals differ little from young adults. The larger range of variation in the direction of more individuals with poorer adaptive capacity and the increased prevalence of individuals with a failure of some component of the adaptive response suggest the hypothesis of relaxed natural selection at older ages. Research findings of age differences in adaptation to hypoxia are not consistent. However, the intriguing finding that adaptation to acute high-altitude stress may be qualitatively reversed in older adults while that to chronic lifetime high-altitude stress seems qualitatively unchanged offers tentative support for a hypothesis that natural selection may operate to maintain adaptive capacity in chronically exposed populations.

The greater heterogeneity of older samples could reflect genetic or environmental heterogeneity or disease; their relative contributions have not been studied. An informative step toward understanding this heterogeneity would be to ascertain whether those with failure of response, e.g., the non-constrictors, non-dilators, or non-sweaters, are distinct sub-populations or whether they represent one end of a distribution shifted in the direction of poor response. Another informative step would be to identify risk factors for these failures of responses.

Age differences in the human biology of adaptation to the environment seems to exemplify the theoretical model of a "failing but reinsured system of feedback" (Comfort, 1979, 257). According to the model, "the magnitude of the swings to be corrected by a given primary process may increase, the failure threshold of the primary process may decrease, or both" and the increased swing places more strain on the secondary processes (Comfort, 1979, 257). In the case of thermoregulation, the first (vasomotor) line of response seems prone to failure thus placing added emphasis on the second (metabolic and sweating) lines of response which also change with age and sometimes fail. These changes may reflect less effective integration of thermoregulation by the autonomic nervous system (Collins, 1983a). It is not known whether there is a similar increase in the prevalence of failure to adapt to hypoxic stress.

Identifying "true aging" processes, due to the passage of time rather than disease, requires improved understanding of the role of disease in adaptation. To some extent the increase in morbidity and mortality related to thermoregulation is influenced by the population's disease pattern. Diseases whose prevalence increases with age can influence the adaptive response in ways that predispose to failure. For example, hypertension reduces blood flow during heat exposure (Kenney and Hodgson, 1987) and drugs treating a variety of conditions interfere with thermoregulation (Collins, 1983a). Diseases whose prevalence increases with age can act to increase morbidity and mortality associated with adaptation to stress by altering the effect of the adaptive response on other organ systems. For example, the greater change in blood pressure or increased blood viscosity during cold exposure may strain weakened or diseased cardiovascular systems and contribute to higher mortality. Because the cardiovascular system and its diseases figure so prominently in these adaptive responses, future prospective studies of samples with and without cardiovascular disease or in populations with little cardiovascular disease will be useful for disentangling the independent effects of aging and disease on adaptive capacity.

More attention to the age range above 70 years when morbidity and mortality rates rise sharply is necessary. Few of the studies reviewed here sampled this rapidly increasing and apparently vulnerable age group.

Few studies, particularly few thermoregulatory studies, sampled outside modern industrial temperate latitude societies. Behavioral adaptations such as central heating and air-conditioning are important in reducing morbidity and mortality in these societies. It seems likely that older adults in traditional and developing societies with extreme environmental temperatures may have fewer options for behavioral adaptations because of lack of technology, knowledge, or income. If so, they rely more on biological than behavioral adaptive responses. Future studies of age differences in thermoregulation in these populations will provide information on aging changes in populations with lifelong exposures. A lower prevalence of the non-constricting response to cold or non-sweating response to heat my be hypothesized. Similarly, a low prevalence of poor hypoxic ventilatory response among high-altitude natives might be hypothesized.

It has not been possible in this review to answer the question of poorer rather than different adaptation to the environment at older ages. It has been possible to identify some of the issues that will have to be tackled in order to address this question. Broadly stated, these questions center on understanding the respective roles of social factors, disease, and dysfunctional biological aging changes in influencing the adaptation of older adults to the environment.

## REFERENCES

Abdel-Rahman, T. A., Collins, K. J., Cowen, T. and Rustin, M. (1992) Immunohistochemical, morphological and functional changes in the peripheral sudomotor neuro-effector system in elderly people. *Journal of the Autonomic Nervous System* **37**, 187–198.

Anderson, R. K. and Kenney, W. L. (1987) Effect of age on heat-activated sweat gland density and flow during exercise in dry heat. *Journal of Applied Physiology* **63**, 1089–1094.

Baker, P. T. and Weiner, J. S. (1966) *Human Adaptability*. Oxford: Clarendon Press.

Beall, C. M. and Goldstein, M. C. (1990) Hemoglobin concentration, percent oxygen saturation and arterial oxygen content of Tibetan nomads at 4,850–5,450 m. In: *Hypoxia. The Adaptations* (eds Sutton, J. R., Coates, G. and Remmers, J. E.). Toronto: B.C. Decker, pp. 59–65.

Beall, C. M. and Reichsman, A. R. (1984) Hemoglobin levels in a Himalayan high altitude population. *American Journal of Physical Anthropology* **63**, 301–306.

Beall, C. M., Goldstein, M. C. and the Tibetan Academy of Social Sciences (1987) Hemoglobin concentration of Tibetan nomads permanently resident at 4850–5450 m. *American Journal of Physical Anthropology* **73**, 433–438.

Beall, C. M., Brittenham, G. M., Macuaga, F. and Barragan, M. (1990) Variation in hemoglobin concentration among samples of high altitude natives in the Andes and the Himalayas. *American Journal of Human Biology* **2**, 639-651.

Beall, C. M., Strohl, K. P., Gothe, B., Brittenham, G. M., Barragan, M. and Vargas, E. (1992) Respiratory and hematological adaptations of young and older Aymara men native to 3600 m. *American Journal of Human Biology* **4**, 17–26.

Bernstein, L. M., Johnston, L. C., Ryan, R., Inouye, T., Hick, F. K. (1956) Body compositionn as related to heat regulation in women. *Journal of Applied Physiology* **9**, 241–256.

Brennan, P. J., Greenberg, G., Miall, W. E. and Thompson, S. G. (1982) Seasonal variation in arterial blood pressure. *British Medical Journal* **285**, 919–923.

Bridger, C. A., Ellis, F. P. and Taylor, H. L. (1976) Mortality in St. Louis, Missouri during heat waves in 1936, 1954, 1955 and 1966. *Environmental Research* **12**, 38–48.

Bull, G. M. and Morton, J. (1978). Environment, temperature and death rates. *Age and Ageing* **7**, 210–224.

Chapman, K. R. and Cherniack, N. S. (1987) Aging effects on the interaction of hypercapnia and hypoxia as ventilatory stimuli. *Journal of Gerontology* **42**, 203–209.

Chiodi, H. (1978) Aging and high-altitude polycythemia. *Journal of Applied Physiology* **45**, 1019–1020.

Collins, K. J. (1983a) Autonomic failure and the elderly. In: *Autonomic Failure* (ed. Bannister, R. G.). Oxford: Oxford University Press, pp. 489–507.

Collins, K. J. (1983b) *Hypothermia. The Facts.* Oxford: Oxford University Press.

Collins, K. J. (1987) Effects of cold on old people. *British Journal of Hospital Medicine* **38**, 506–514.

Collins, K. J. (1988a) Hypothermia in the Elderly. *Health Visitor* **61**, 50–51.

Collins, K. J. (1988b) Autonomic control of sweat glands and disorders of sweating. In: *Autonomic Failure* (ed. Bannister, R.). Oxford: Oxford University Press, pp. 748–765.

Collins, K. J. and Exton-Smith, A. N. (1981) Hypothermia: thermoregulation, thermal perception and thermal comfort in the elderly. In: *Hypothermia. Ashore and Afloat* (ed. Adam, J. M.). Aberdeen: Aberdeen University Press, pp. 158–176.

Collins, K. J. and Exton-Smith, A. N. (1986) Effects of Ageing on Human Homeostasis. In: *The Biology of Human Ageing* (ed. Bittles, A. H. and Collins, K. J.). Cambridge: Cambridge University Press, pp. 261–275.

Collins, K. J. and Hoinville, E. (1980) Temperature requirements in old age. *Building Services Engineering Research and Technology* **1**, 165–172.

Collins, K. J., Doré, C., Exton-Smith, A. N., Fox, R. H., Macdonald, I. C. and Woodward, P. M. (1977) Accidental hypothermia and impaired temperature homeostasis in the elderly. *British Medical Journal* **1**, 353–356.

Collins, K. J., Exton-Smith, A. N., James, M. H. and Oliver, D. J. (1980) Functional changes in autonomic nervous responses with ageing. *Age and Ageing* **9**, 17–24.

Collins, K. J., Exton-Smith, A. N. and Doré, C. (1981) Urban hypothermia: preferred temperature and thermal perception in old age. *British Medical Journal* **282**, 175–177.

Collins, K. J., Easton, J. C. and Exton-Smith, A. N. (1982) The ageing nervous system: impairment of thermoregulation. In: *Advanced Medicine* (ed. Sarner, M.). Bath: Pitman Medical, pp. 250–257.

Collins, K. J., Easton, J. C., Belfield-Smith, H., Exton-Smith, A. N. and Pluck, R. A. (1985) Effects of age on body temperature and blood pressure in cold environments. *Clinical Science* **69**, 465–470.

Collins, K. J., Durnin, C. J. A. and Pluck, R. A. (1986) Peripheral venous compliance and vasomotor responses to cooling and warming in young and elderly subjects. *Journal of Physiology* **382**, 27P.

Collins, K. J., Sacco, P., Easton, J. C., Abdel-Rahman, T. A. (1989) Cold Pressor and trigeminal cardiovascular reflexes in old age. In: *Thermal Physiology 1989* (ed. Mercer, J. B.). Amsterdam: Excerpta Medica, pp. 587–592.

Comfort, A. (1979) *Physiology, Homeostasis, and Ageing*, 3rd edn. Amsterdam: Elsevier.

Crowe, J. P. and Moore, R. E. (1974) Physiological and behavioural responses of aged men to passive heating. *Journal of Physiology* **231**, 43p–44p.

Damon, A. (1975) *Physiological Anthropology*. Oxford: Oxford University Press.

Davis, B. B. and Wood, W. G. (1985) Preface. In: *Homeostatic Function and Aging* (eds Davis, B. B. and Wood, W. G.). New York: Raven Press, pp. vii.

Dawson, J. A. (1987) A case-control study of accidental hypothermia in the elderly in relation to social support and social circumstances. *Community Medicine* **9**, 141–145.

Dill, D. B. (1963) Reunion at high altitude. *The Physiologist* **6**, 40–43.

Dill, D. B. (1964) *Handbook of Physiology,* Section 4: *Adaptation to the Environment.* Washington, DC: American Physiological Society.

Dill, D. B. and Consolazio, C. F. (1962) Responses to exercise as related to age and environmental temperature. *Journal of Applied Physiology* **17**, 645–648.

Dill, D. B., Terman, J. W. and Hall, F. G. (1963) Hemoglobin at high altitude as related to age. *Clinical Chemistry* **7**, 710–716.

Dill, D. B., Forbes, W. H., Newton, J. L. and Terman, J. W. (1964) Respiratory adaptations to high altitude as related to age. In: *Relations of Development and Aging* (ed. Birren, J. E.). Springfield, IL: Charles C. Thomas, pp. 62–73.

Dill, D. B., Hall, F. G. and Van Beaumont, W. (1966a) Sweat chloride concentration: sweat rate, metabolic rate, skin temperature, and age. *Journal of Applied Physiology* **21**, 99–106.

Dill, D. B., Hall, F. G., Hall, K. D., Dawson, C. and Newton, J. L., (1966b) Blood, plasma and red cell volumes, age, exercise and environment. *Journal of Applied Physiology* **21**, 597–602.

Dill, D. B., Horvath, S. M., Dahms, T. E., Parker, R. E. and Lunch, J. R. (1969) Hemoconcentration at altitude. *Journal of Applied Physiology* **27**, 514–518.

Dill, D. B., Hillyard, S. D. and Miller, J. (1980) Vital capacity, exercise performance, and blood gases at altitude as related to age. *Journal of Applied Physiology* **48**, 6–9.

Drinkwater, B. L. and Horvath, S. M. (1979) Heat tolerance and aging. *Medicine and Science in Sports* **11**, 49–55.

Drinkwater, B. L., Bedi, J. F., Loucks, A. B., Roche, S. and Horvath, S. M. (1982) Sweating sensitivity and capacity of women in relation to age. *Journal of Applied Physiology* **53**, 671–676.

Ellis, F. P. (1976) Heat illness I. Epidemiology. *Transactions of the Royal Society of Tropical Medicine and Hygiene* **70**, 402–411.

Ellis, F. P., Nelson, F. and Pincus, L. (1975) Mortality during heat waves in New York

City July, 1972 and August and September, 1973. *Environmental Research* **10**, 1–13.

Ellis, F. P., Exton-Smith, A. N., Foster, K. G. and Weiner, J. S. (1976) Eccrine sweating and mortality during heat waves in very young and very old persons. *Israel Journal of Medical Sciences* **12**, 815–817.

Fennell, W. H. and Moore, R. E. (1973) Responses of aged men to passive heating. *Journal of Physiology* **231**, 118P–119P.

Foster, K. G., Ellis, F. P., Dore, C., Exton-Smith, A. N. and Weiner, J. S. (1976) Sweat responses in the aged. *Age and Ageing* **5**, 91–101

Fox, R. J., Woodward, P. M., Exton-Smith, A. N., Green, M. F., Donnison, D. V. and Wicks, M. H. (1973) Body temperatures in the elderly: a national study of physiological, social and environmental conditions. *British Medical Journal* **1**, 200–206.

Frisancho, A. R. (1985) *Human Adaptation. A Functional Interpretation.* Ann Arbor, MI: University of Michigan Press.

Garruto, R. M. (1976) Hematology. In: *Man in the Andes* (eds Baker, P. T. and Little, M. A.). Stroudsburg: Dowden, Hutchinson and Ross, pp. 98–114.

Gonzalez, R. B., Berglund, L. G. and Stolwijk, S. (1980) Thermoregulation in humans of different ages during thermal transients. In: *Contributions to Thermal Physiology* (eds Szelenyi, Z. and Szekely, M.). New York: Pergamon, pp. 357–361.

Gonzalez, R. R. and Pandolf, K. B. (1989) Thermoregulatory competence during exercise transients in a group of heat-acclimated young and middle-aged men is influenced more distinctly by maximal aerobic power than age. In: *Thermal Physiology 1989* (ed. Mercer, J. B.). Amsterdam: Excerpta Medica, pp. 335–340.

Guenard, H., Vargas, E., Villena, M. and Carras, P. M. (1984) Hypoxemia et hematocrite dans la polyglobulie pathologique d'altitude. *Bulletin European Pathophysiologie Respiratoire* **20**, 319–324.

Heath, D. and Williams, D. R. (1989) *High-altitude Medicine and Pathology.* London: Butterworths.

Hellon, R. F. and Lind, A. R. (1956) Observations on the activity of sweat glands with special reference to the influence of aging. *Journal of Physiology* **133**, 132–144.

Hellon, R. F. and Lind, A. R. (1958) The influence of age on peripheral vasodilatation in a hot environment. *Journal of Physiology* **141**, 262–272.

Hellon, R. F., Lind, A. R. and Weinder, J. S. (1956) The physiological reactions of men of two age groups to a hot environment. *Journal of Physiology* **133**, 118–131.

Henschel, A. M., Cole, B. and Oyczkowskyj, O. (1968) Heat tolerance of elderly persons living in a subtropical climate. *Journal of Gerontology* **23**, 17–22.

Horvath, S. M., Radcliffe, C. E., Hutt, B. K. and Spurr, G. B. (1955) Metabolic responses of old people to a cold environment. *Journal of Applied Physiology* **8**, 145–148.

Jones, T. S., Liang, A. P., Kilbourne, E. M., Griffin, M. R., Patriarca, P. A., Wassilak, S. G. F., Mullan, R. J., Herrick, R. F., Donnel, H. D., Choi, K. and Thacker, S. B. (1982) Morbidity and mortality association with the July 1980 heat wave in St. Louis and Kansas City, Mo. *Journal of the American Medical Association* **247**, 3327–3331.

Kawakami, Y. T. Y., Shida, A., and Asanuma, Y. (1981) Relationships between hypoxia and hypercapnic ventilatory responses in man. *Japanese Journal of Physiology* **31**, 357–368.

Keating, W. R., Coleshaw, S. R. K., Cotter, F., Mattock, M., Murphy, M. and

Chelliah, R. (1984) Increases in platelet and red cell counts, blood viscosity, and arterial pressure during mild surface cooling: factors in mortality from coronary and cerebral thrombosis in winter. *British Medical Journal* **289**, 1405–1408.

Kenney, W. L. (1988) Control of heat-induced cutaneous vasodilatation in relation to age. *European Journal of Applied Physiology* **57**, 120–125.

Kenney, W. L. and Anderson, R. K. (1988) Responses of older and younger women to exercise in dry and humid heat without fluid replacement. *Medicine and Science in Sports and Exercise* **20**, 155–160.

Kenney, W. L. and Hodgson, J. L. (1987) Heat tolerance, thermoregulation and ageing. *Sports Medicine* **4**, 446–456.

Kilbourne, E. M., Choi, K., Jones, S., Thacker, S. B. and The Field Investigation Team (1982) Risk factors for heatstroke. A case-control study. *Journal of the American Medical Association* **247**, 3332–3336.

Krag, C. L. and Kountz, W. B. (1950) Stability of body function in the aged. I. Effect of exposure of the body to cold. *Journal of Gerontology* **5**, 227–235.

Kronenberg, R. S. and Drage, C. W. (1973) Attenuation of the ventilatory and heart rate responses to hypoxia and hypercapnia with aging in normal men. *Journal of Clinical Investigation* **52**, 1812–1819.

LeBlanc, J., Cote, J., Dulac, S. and Dulong-Turcot, F. (1978) Effects of age, sex, and physical fitness on responses to local cooling. *Journal of Applied Physiology* **44**, 813–817.

Leon-Velarde, F., Monge, C., Arregui, A. and Stanley, C. (1990) Increased prevalence of excessive erythrocytosis with aging in healthy high altitude miners. In: *Hypoxia. The Adaptations* (eds Sutton, J. R., Coates, G., Remmers, J. E.). Toronto: B.C. Decker, pp. 280.

Macmillan, A. L., Corbett, J. L., Johnson, R. H., Crampton Smith, A., Spalding, J. M. K. and Wollner, L. (1967) Temperature regulation in survivors of accidental hypothermia of the elderly. *Lancet* **2**, 165–169.

MacPherson, R. K., Ofner, F. and Welch, J. A. (1967) Effect of the prevailing air temperature on mortality. *British Journal of Preventive and Social Medicine* **21**, 17–21.

Mathew, L. Purkayastha, S. S., Singh, R. and Gupta, J. S. (1986) Influence of aging in the thermoregulatory efficiency of man. *International Journal of Biometeorology* **30**, 137–145.

Miescher, E. and Fortney, S. M. (1989) Responses to dehydration and rehydration during heat exposure in young and older men. *American Journal of Physiology* **257**, R1050–R1056.

Monge, C., Bonavia, D., Leon-Velarde, F. and Arregui, A. (1990) High altitude populations in Nepal and the Andes. In: *Hypoxia. The Adaptations* (eds Sutton, J. R., Coates, G. and Remmers, J. E.). Toronto: B.C. Decker, pp. 53–58.

Ohnishi, N., Ogawa, T., Sugenoya, J., Natsume, K., Yamashita, Y., Imamura, R. and Yousef, M. K. (1989) Effect of aging on adaptability of sweating capacity in association with heat acclimatization. In: *Thermal Physiology 1989* (ed. Mercer, J. B.). Amsterdam: Excerpta Medica, pp. 475–480.

Pandolf, K. B., Cadarette, B. S., Sawka, M. N., Young, A. J., Francesconi, R. P. and Gonzalez, R. R. (1988) Thermoregulatory responses of middle-aged and young men during dry-heat acclimation. *Journal of Applied Physiology* **65**, 65–71.

Peterson, D. D., Pack, A. I., Silage, D. A. and Fishman, A. P. (1981) Effects of aging on ventilatory and occlusion pressure responses to hypoxia and hypercapnia. *American Review of Respiratory Disease* **124**, 387–391.

Poehlman, E. T. and Horton, E. S. (1990) Regulation of energy expenditure in aging humans. *Annual Reviews of Nutrition* **10**, 255–275.

Rango, N. (1985) The social epidemiology of accidental hypothermia among the aged. *Gerontologist* **25**, 424–430.

Regensteiner, J. G. and Moore, L. G. (1985) Migration of the elderly from high altitudes in Colorado. *Journal of the American Medical Association* **253**, 3124–3128.

Richardson, D. (1989) Effects of age on cutaneous circulatory reponse to direct heat on the forearm. *Journal of Gerontology* **44**, M189–M194.

Robinson, S., Belding, H. S., Consolazio, F. C., Horvath, S. M. and Turrell, E. S. (1965) Acclimatization of older men to work in heat. *Journal of Applied Physiology* **20**, 583–586.

Sagawa, S., Shiraki, K., Yousef, K. M. and Miki, K. (1988) Sweating and cardiovascular responses of aged men to heat exposure. *Journal of Gerontology* **43**, M1–M8.

Schoenfeld, Y., Udassin, R., Shapiro, Y., Ohri, A. and Sohar, E. (1978) Age and sex difference in response to short exposure to extreme dry heat. *Journal of Applied Physiology* **44**, 1–4.

Schuman, S. H., Anderson, C. P. and Oliver, J. T. (1964) Epidemiology of successive heat waves in Michigan. *Journal of the American Medical Association* **189**, 733–735.

Shattuck, G. C. and Hilferty, M. M. (1932) Sunstroke and allied conditions in the United States. *American Journal of Tropical Medicine* **12**, 223–245.

Shiraki, K., Sagawa, S., Yousef, M. K., Konda, N. and Miki, K. (1987) Physiological responses of aged men to head-up tilt during heat exposure. *Journal of Applied Physiology* **63**, 576–581.

Sime, F., Monge, C. and Whittembury, J. (1975) Age as a cause of Chronic Mountain Sickness (Monge's Disease). *International Journal of Biometeorology* **19**, 93–98.

Simonson, E. (1962) Effect of age on hypoxia tolerance. In: *Aging Around the World (Vol. 4): Medical and Clinical Aspects of Aging* (ed. Blumenthal, J. T.). New York: Columbia University Press, pp. 40.

Tafil-Klawe, M., Raschke, F., Kublik, A., Stoohs, R. and von Wichert, P. (1989) Attenuation of augmented ventilatory response to hypoxia in essential hypertension in the course of aging. *Respiration* **56**, 154–160.

Tankersley, C., Smolander, J. and Fortney, S. (1987) Skin blood flow (SkBF) responses in Young (YM) and older men (OM) during exercise in the heat. *Federation Proceedings* **46**, 1440.

Thomas, R. B. (1975) The ecology of work. In: *Physiological Anthropology* (ed. Damon, A.). Oxford: Oxford University Press, pp. 59–79.

Tufts, D. A., Haas, J. D., Beard, J. L. and Spielvogel, H. (1985) Distribution of hemoglobin and functional consequences of anemia in adult males at high altitude. *American Journal of Clinical Nutrition* **42**, 1–11.

Wagner, J. A. and Horvath, S. M. (1985a) Influences of age and gender on human thermoregulatory responses to cold exposure. *Journal of Applied Physiology* **58**, 180–186.

Wagner, J. A. and Horvath, S. M. (1985b) Cardiovascular reactions to cold exposures differ with age and gender. *Journal of Applied Physiology* **58**, 187–192.

Wagner, J. A., Robinson, S., Tzankoff, S. P. and Marino, R. P. (1972) Heat tolerance and acclimatization to work in the heat in relation to age. *Journal of Applied Physiology* **33**, 616–622.

Wagner, J. A., Robinson, S. and Marino, R. P. (1974) Age and temperature regulation of humans in neutral and cold environments. *Journal of Applied Physiology* **37**, 562–565.

Weiner, J. S. and Edholm, O. G. (1981) Thermal physiology. In: *The Principles and Practice of Human Physiology* (eds Edholm, O. G. and Weiner, J. S.). London: Academic Press, pp. 111–190.

Whittembury, J. and Monge C. C. (1972). High altitude, haematocrit and age. *Nature* **238**, 273–274.

Yoshimura, H. and Iida, T. (1951–1952) Studies on the reactivity of skin vessels to extreme cold. Part II. Factors governing the individual difference of the reactivity, or the resistance against frost-bite. *Japanese Journal of Physiology* **2**, 177–185.

Yousef, M. K., Dill, D. B., Vitez, T. S., Hillyard, S. D. and Goldman, A. S. (1984) Thermoregulatory responses to desert heat: age, race and sex. *Journal of Gerontology* **39**, 406–414.

# IV
## METHODS FOR AGING RESEARCH AND ONGOING PROGRAMS

# 14

# Modeling the Variability in Longitudinal Patterns of Aging

## LARRY J. BRANT AND JAY D. PEARSON

There is no general pattern of aging that applies to all performances, all organ systems, or all individuals.
(Nathan Shock)

## INTRODUCTION

Human population biologists and biological anthropologists have often been concerned with establishing developmental norms, describing the range of normal and pathological variation from those norms, identifying the sources of the variability, and studying adaptive responses to change (Little and Haas, 1989). These are also topics of great interest to gerontologists because of the ongoing debate concerning "normal" aging versus disease (Rowe and Kahn, 1987; Fozard et al., 1990) and the desire for effective interventions to slow or arrest age-related disease processes. Human biologists' interests in variability and adaptation are also linked to gerontology by the observations that aging is characterized by increased phenotypic variability (Bourlière, 1970) and reduced adaptive capacity (Shock et al., 1984). In essence, all of these research questions hinge on the effective study of individual differences in patterns of change over time.

The validity of the concept of age norms depends both on the ability to identify average patterns of age-related change and on the relative amount of variation from those norms in the population. Ideally, an age norm should summarize the longitudinal pattern of change in the population and the rate of change and shape of the trend would be similar in most individuals (Figure 14-1A). In such a case, the interindividual differences in the elderly would be the result of individual differences in initial level of function, although most individuals would track on a similar course of aging. More commonly, the heterogeneity in the elderly is a result of both interindividual differences in initial level of function as well as in the patterns (i.e., rate and shape) of change (Figure 14-1B). It has almost become an axiom in gerontology that aging is a "highly individual phenomenon" (Shock et al., 1984:169). For many

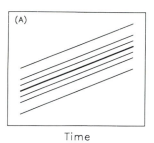
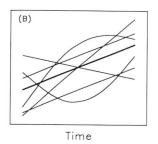
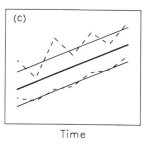

**Figure 14-1** Hypothetical examples of relationships between variability and patterns of aging (population average represented by heavy solid line). (A) The rate and shape of the patterns of aging may be similar in most individuals, differing only in initial level of function. (B) Individuals can differ in both rate and shape of pattern of aging. (C) Individuals vary in amount of fluctuation around their overall pattern of aging.

functions, some individuals maintain function quite well, others experience sharp declines, while function actually improves with age in a small percentage of individuals (Costa and Andres, 1986). In addition to interindividual differences in initial level and patterns of change, longitudinal fluctuations around an individual's overall trend also contribute to the heterogeneity in the population (Figure 14-1C). If these intraindividual fluctuations are large, they may obscure the general trend and reduce the usefulness of an age norm for individual-level counseling or research. Thus, examining the variability in longitudinal patterns of change helps guard against developing age norms that may describe such a small proportion of the population as to be misleading and contribute to inaccurate stereotypes.

In addition to their value at a descriptive level, individual differences in patterns of aging may also allow the identification of factors which affect various age-related phenomena and the ability to adapt to age-related changes. Anecdotal evidence indicates that there is a tremendous amount of variability in the natural history of aging. One of the challenges of gerontology is to identify the genetic, environmental, and life-style factors which allow some individuals to maintain, or even improve, function with increasing age. Studies of individual differences in patterns of aging may provide epidemiological evidence to help guide more detailed research at the molecular, cellular, systems, and societal levels.

In this chapter, we will introduce and discuss the use of individual differences in longitudinal patterns of aging as individual-level natural experiments. We also describe recent methodological advances which make studies of longitudinal patterns of change feasible as research strategies. Finally, we present examples drawn from a longitudinal study of changes in hearing thresholds in order to illustrate the methodological and substantive benefits of using studies of longitudinal variability in patterns of aging as a research tool in human biology, biological anthropology, and gerontology.

## NATURAL EXPERIMENTS AND LONGITUDINAL STUDIES

Human biologists and biological anthropologists have relied to a great extent on observational rather than experimental studies. Frequently, they have used natural experimental designs where the characteristics of naturally occurring groups are used to provide quasi-experimental control of genetic, environmental, and sociocultural factors (Baker, 1977). Natural experiments are generally conducted primarily at the population level where groups are chosen based on contrasts in their climate, physical environment, social class, sociocultural heritage, genetic background, or migrant status (Garruto *et al.*, 1989). However, natural experiments also occur at the individual level when over the course of a lifetime, individuals begin to differ in their histories of exposure to environmental agents, sociocultural phenomena, risk factors, and pathogens. Sometimes individuals also make conscious efforts to modify their behavior as they adapt to, or attempt to prevent, some event. Thus, each person's longitudinal pattern of aging can be viewed as an individual-level natural experiment where various exposures and interventions occur naturally over the course of a lifetime.

Since longitudinal studies are the only direct method of measuring change, they are the only method of studying longitudinal patterns of aging. Longitudinal studies are necessary to determine how many individuals within a population maintain stable functional abilities over time, how many improve, and how many decline. Longitudinal studies are also necessary to determine the degree of tracking or channeling of development and aging, and for measuring long-term flunctuations in function and risk-factor levels.

Despite the importance of longitudinal studies, there are certain limitations, such as selective attrition and volunteer bias which have been reviewed extensively (Botwinick, 1964; Shapiro *et al.*, 1969; Busse, 1970; Shock *et al.*, 1984). In this chapter, we will limit our discussion to problems of data analysis. Standard multi-variate procedures are usually not flexible enough to be applied to many longitudinal studies because they cannot accommodate unequally spaced points of observation, missing data, attrition, and time-dependent co-variates. These are all problems arising in the study of individuals over time. One strategy to avoid the limitations of standard multi-variate procedures might be naively to lump all the observations together and use standard regression techniques while ignoring the correlation between each individual's repeated measurements. However, this strategy is not advisable since it is likely to lead to biased estimates of the rates of change and their variability, and increases the chance of false inferences regarding statistical significance (Feldman, 1988). Since our primary interest is the study of change, a model which helps to account for the correlation among repeated measurements is of fundamental importance (Brant *et al.*, 1992b, 1993). Recent models for longitudinal data analysis have contributed greatly to the study of individual patterns of change by incorporating techniques to model the natural heterogeneity in the population while allowing unbalanced designs and missing data, and modeling the correlation between repeated observations for an individual.

Longitudinal studies of aging are characterized by repeated observations collected on a group of individuals over a period of years. Such data allow for comparisons in response between individuals of different ages (cross-sectional differences) and comparisons in response at different ages for a single individual (longitudinal differences). If we model the average responses as a function of age without distinguishing between the cross-sectional and longitudinal differences, then we effectively assume that the cross-sectional and longitudinal effects of aging are equal. However, these two effects need to be treated with separate parameters which measure the effects of age on the initial observation and on the changes in response over time. Otherwise, the estimates of the cross-sectional and longitudinal effects may be biased.

Several methods of data analysis have been proposed for the study of serial or repeated measurements. We briefly discuss three types of models—multi-variate, mixed-effects and autoregressive—that have been used to account for the co-variance structure in longitudinal investigations. When each individual in the study has been observed at the same time points, a multi-variate general linear model with a simple co-variance structure can be used (Johnson and Wichern, 1988). This method of analysis works well when there are few missing observations, if missing values can be replaced with estimated values or individuals with missing values can be removed from the analysis without affecting the results. However, when the data set is highly unbalanced (e.g., individuals observed at different times of observation, or incomplete with missing data) the resulting co-variance structure is more complicated and is handled more effectively by mixed-effects or autoregressive models.

Mixed-effects and related models with random effects for longitudinal data analysis have contributed greatly to the study of individual patterns of change (Rao, 1965; Harville, 1977; Laird and Ware, 1982; Strenio et al., 1983; Zeger and Liang, 1986; Lindstrom and Bates, 1988). The concept of a mixed-effects model with both fixed and random effects is not new. What is new is the use of random effects to estimate individual differences in patterns of change, and the recent availability of estimation procedures for data with unequal periods of observation between individuals, missing values, and so forth. These are all problems arising in the study of different individuals over time. Thus, it is currently possible to study situations where individuals have different patterns of change, and identify factors which may affect the pattern of change. The fixed effects in mixed-effects models represent the population averages for the intercept and slopes, while the random effects allow each individual to have an initial level or rate of change that is different from the average intercept or slope. In statistical terms, these random effects are terms for persons and interactions between persons and other variables in the model (Laird et al., 1987). The random effects are assumed to be independent of the statistical error term but the random effects are allowed to be correlated with one another.

The mixed-effects model assumes that the correlation among the repeated measurements of an individual is due to some latent characteristic of the individual that gives him or her a higher or lower than average intercept or slope. For example, it may be reasonable to assume that some individuals start

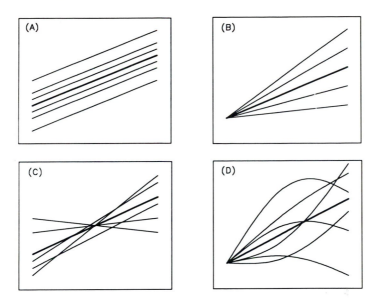

**Figure 14-2** Various mixed-effects models of the variability in patterns of aging. (A) Random intercept model: interindividual differences in initial level. (B) Random slope model: interindividual differences in rate of change. (C) Random intercept and slope model: interindividual differences in both initial level and rate of change. (D) Random non-linear term: interindividual differences in shape of pattern of change.

out with better hearing sensitivity than others or that hearing may change more rapidly in some individuals than in others. Thus, mixed-effects models are able to model a variety of sources of variability in the population. By placing random effects on the intercept, slope, and/or non-linear terms in the model, it is possible to model a wide variety of patterns of aging (Figure 14-2A–D). The random effects allow the observed variability in the sample to be partitioned between the usual unexplained or statistical error and the random effects which describe the natural heterogeneity in the population. Not only does this provide increased statistical power, but the random effects themselves may be of interest to human biologists, biological anthropologists, and gerontologists since they estimate the amount of variability in the population and summarize intraindividual patterns in a way that can be used for exploratory analyses.

Mixed-effects analyses can be conducted using either a two-stage approach (Feldman, 1988) or using unified estimation procedures (Laird and Ware, 1982; Lindstrom and Bates, 1988). Two-stage mixed-effects analyses consist of estimating regression parameters for each individual separately in the first stage and then analyzing between-individual variation in the second stage. The main advantages of the two-stage approach are that it is conceptually simple and that it can be performed using almost any statistical computing package. However, the two-stage approach may produce biased results since it does not take into account the co-variance structure of the random effects, such as the possibility that individuals with higher than average initial levels may also tend to have higher (or lower) rates of change. The two-stage approach also tends to produce slightly biased estimates of the variance components. The unified approaches to mixed-effects analysis take into account correlations among the random effects and provide less biased estimates of the variance components.

Autoregressive models have also been used to describe the co-variance structure in longitudinal data (Box and Jenkins, 1970; Anderson, 1971). These models were originally developed for a single long time series where successive measurements are correlated with each other. Asthma attacks are an example of an autoregressive phenomena since a recent asthma attack increases the probability of an asthma attack on several subsequent days (Hasselblad, 1978).

The proper choice of a model for the correlation between repeated measurements is usually based on *a priori* knowledge about the phenomenon or from an examination of autocorrelation functions. If one examines the degree of correlation between repeated measurements, an autoregressive correlation structure usually exhibits a decline in the correlation between repeated measurements as the time between measurements increases. In contrast, a mixed-effects correlation structure exhibits a constant correlation between repeated measurements regardless of time between measurements. While considerable progress has been made in the application of autoregressive (Kowalski and Guire, 1974; Rosner and Munoz, 1988), time-series (Reinsel *et al.*, 1981), transition (Korn and Whittemore, 1979), and discrete outcome models (Zeger *et al.*, 1988; Vonesh, 1990), we will limit our discussion to mixed-effects regression models because they are more directly relevant to our interests in studying patterns of change with age.

## HEARING LOSS AND AGING

In order to illustrate some of the concepts and methods discussed earlier, we examine the example of age-related changes in hearing thresholds. In industrialized societies, men and women suffer a progressive decline in hearing sensitivity as they age, particularly for high frequency sounds (Corso, 1963). Figure 14-3 presents average hearing sensitivities for 18–24-year-old and 59–65-year-old men showing the loss of hearing sensitivity in the high frequencies. As Figure 14-3 shows, data from an audiogram can be summarized efficiently by the function

$$y = S_0 + S_1 \ln x + S_2 \ln^2 x \qquad (14\text{-}1)$$

where $y$ represents the sound-pressure level in decibels (dB SPL) required to detect audio frequency $x$ (kHz) and ln is the natural logarithm (Brant and Fozard, 1990). This function will be referred to as the *frequency-intensity function* in the analyses described later.

The decline in hearing sensitivity with age has been termed *presbycusis (presbyacusia)* and has generally been described as a normal aging phenomenon. However, studies by Rosen and colleagues with the Mabaan tribe in the Sudan did not detect presbycusis in elderly individuals (Rosen *et al.*, 1962,

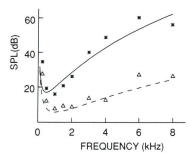

**Figure 14-3** Presbycusis is characterized by a loss of hearing sensitivity for high-frequency sounds. Thus, the average hearing thresholds (sound pressure level in dB) for 59–65-year-old (*) men are higher than for 18–24-year-old (△) men, especially at high audio frequencies (Corso, 1958). The lines indicate the frequency–intensity function for 18–24-year-old (dashed line) and 59–65-year-old (solid line) male BLSA participants (Brant and Fozard, 1990).

1964). Thus, Rosen's cross-cultural research demonstrated that presbycusis is not a universal aspect of normal aging. The greatly reduced amount of presbycusis in the Mabaan has been attributed to some combination of a noise-free environment, genetic factors, and the absence of arteriosclerosis, hypertension, and cardiovascular disease (Rosen et al., 1962, 1964, 1970; Rosen and Olin, 1965). As a result, the term *sociocusis* was coined to indicate the potential importance of general societal factors such as ambient noise levels, infection, ototoxic drug use, and trauma (Glorig and Nixon, 1962).

Current evidence suggests that the pattern of hearing decline observed with age may be the combined effect of normal aging and an accumulation of damage from a variety of extrinsic sources. Extrinsic factors which may produce variability in the timing and severity of an individual's hearing decline include noise exposure (Henderson et al., 1976), use of ototoxic drugs such as streptomycin, neomycin, and kanamycin (Bergstrom and Thompson, 1976), possibly arteriosclerosis or hypertension (Fabinyi, 1931; Bochenek and Jachowska, 1969; Rosen et al., 1970), and numerous diseases such as otitis media, measles, mumps, scarlet fever, otosclerosis, Meniere's disease, and stroke with aphasia.

## LONGITUDINAL PATTERNS OF HEARING LOSS

We now illustrate the use of the general multi-variate model and the mixed-effects model to examine the variability in hearing loss in men who participated in a longitudinal study of normal human aging. The longitudinal analyses described here draw from data collected during the Baltimore Longitudinal Study of Aging (BLSA), the primary study of human aging conducted by the intramural program of the National Institute on Aging. The BLSA is a multi-disciplinary study established in 1958 by Nathan Shock as an open panel of reasonably healthy, community-dwelling volunteers who would return for "thorough and repeated testing over a major portion, if not the remainder, of their lives" (Shock *et al.*, 1984:45). Participants return to the Gerontology Research Center at approximately two-year intervals for 2½ days of medical, physiological, psychological, and sociological testing. BLSA participants represent a select segment of the US population. They are predominantly White (95%), generally well educated (over 75% have a bachelor's degree), middle- and upper-class, and financially comfortable (82%). Over 1,400 men have participated in the study with an average of almost seven visits and 16 years of participation. Women were first recruited into the BLSA in 1978. Since that time, approximately 575 women have participated in the study with an average of over three visits and seven years of follow-up. Due to the shorter period of follow-up for women, longitudinal patterns of change in the hearing levels of women are not described here. Audiometric examinations have been conducted since 1968 in a soundproof chamber using a Bekesy audiometer with continuous pure tones as the stimulus.

## Longitudinal and Cross-sectional Change in Hearing Sensitivity

A recent BLSA study reported the largest and longest series of longitudinal measurements of hearing sensitivity published to date (Brant and Fozard, 1990). The study utilized a general multi-variate approach to longitudinal data analysis using the general linear model procedure of the Statistical Analysis System (SAS, 1985). The results of this analysis provide estimates of:

1. the average longitudinal pattern of change in hearing thresholds with increasing age;
2. the difference between longitudinal and cross-sectional estimates of change; and
3. the relative magnitude of various sources of variability in hearing thresholds.

The data consisted of repeated measurements of hearing thresholds obtained on 813 males ranging in age from 20 to 95 years. Information from medical histories and physical examinations were used to screen for individuals with possible otological disease as well as participants with subjective hearing complaints. The study participants were placed in one of seven age groups in which they had the majority of hearing tests performed during the study (20–35, 30–45, 40–55, 50–65, 60–75, 70–85, and 80–95 years of age). Each subject could have between two and six repeated measurements. Table 14-1 gives the number of subjects tested in each of the age groups along with the average number of repeated tests for each group.

An analysis of the longitudinal data for each of the seven age groups was carried out using a least squares regression approach which made use of a random-effects component to estimate the between-persons variance. Compared to methods which ignore the between-persons variance, this approach gives a more precise measure of the longitudinal change in hearing thresholds

**Table 14-1**   Sample sizes and number of repeated measurements for a longitudinal study of hearing loss in the BLSA men.

|  | Age group | | | | | | |
|---|---|---|---|---|---|---|---|
|  | 20 | 30 | 40 | 50 | 60 | 70 | 80 |
| Number of individuals tested | 72 | 136 | 155 | 173 | 127 | 118 | 32 |
| Average times tested | 3.5 | 3.8 | 4.1 | 4.3 | 3.8 | 3.4 | 2.8 |

and tests of the independent effects of age, frequency of pure tone and ear by effectively controlling for the large interindividual variance in hearing thresholds among persons of the same age. Also, cross-sectional differences in hearing thresholds were estimated by performing a regression analysis over all ages in the study. A small number of thresholds were missing at certain frequencies and were replaced with estimates of the missing values.

Figure 14-4 shows the modeled frequency-intensity functions, using the ln, $\ln^2$ equation described earlier, at 3-year intervals starting at the ages of 20, 40, 60 and 80 years. The four panels of Figure 14-4 show the extent of the longitudinal changes within each age group and the extent of the cross-sectional differences between the different age groups. As expected, hearing sensitivity declined faster at high frequencies than low frequencies among young and middle-aged men. However, after age 70, hearing sensitivity declined faster at lower frequencies than high frequencies. The faster hearing loss at the lower frequencies in the elderly is reflected in the disappearance of the "hook" at the left side of the hearing-intensity function curves for the 80s age group in Figure 14-4. This pattern of accelerated change in the low and speech frequencies in the elderly had not been noted previously in cross-sectional studies. The interpretation of this pattern is not yet clear. However, it is possible that the early and rapid rate of decline at high frequencies begins to approach a ceiling around age 70 while hearing sensitivity at low frequencies starts to decline more rapidly later in life.

The longitudinal analysis also suggests that the cross-sectional rates of change in hearing thresholds seriously underestimate the actual longitudinal rates of change (Figure 14-5). The estimates of the longitudinal rates are 0.91, 0.77, 0.73, 0.69, 0.74, 0.73, and 1.68 dB per year, respectively, for the 20–80-year-old groups, while the cross-sectional rate of change was only 0.59 dB per year. This illustrates how cross-sectional studies can provide biased estimates of change in aging studies.

Although Figure 14-5 effectively illustrates the average amount of change in hearing thresholds, it does not show the large amount of individual variability that exists between different individuals in the same age group. Examining the proportion of the total variance or effect size attributable to different variables entered in the model is one method of comparing the relative magnitude of various sources of variability (Camp and Maxwell, 1983). The proportion of the total variance attributable to age changes and between-subjects variability

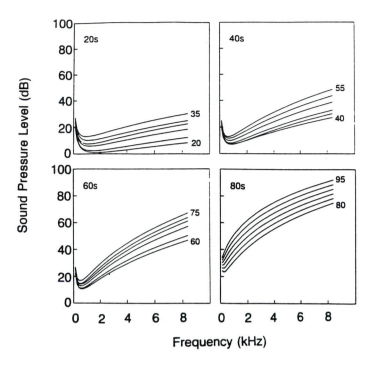

**Figure 14-4** Longitudinal changes in hearing thresholds in four cross-sectional age groups. The lines in each panel show the longitudinal change in the frequency-intensity function at 3-year intervals starting at the ages of 20, 40, 60, and 80 years. The lines are diverging in the panels for the 20-, 40-, and 60-year-olds, thus indicating that hearing sensitivity is declining faster at high frequencies than low frequencies. However, in the 80-year-olds, the hook in the frequency–intensity function at low frequencies disappears indicating that low frequencies start to decline faster than high frequencies among the elderly.

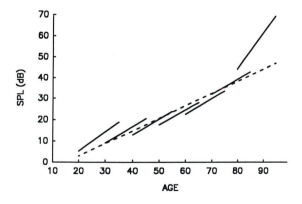

**Figure 14-5** Cross-sectional estimates of the rate of change in hearing sensitivity (dashed line) underestimate the longitudinal estimates of the rate of change in each age group (solid lines), especially in the oldest age group.

382

was 12.1% and 11.3% of the total variance whereas the unexplained within-subject variance was 15.0% on average. Thus, longitudinal change with age and interindividual differences in hearing level accounted for nearly equal amounts of the total variation in hearing sensitivity, while unexplained fluctuations around an individual's overall pattern represented approximately 15% of the total variability.

## Individual Variability in Hearing Loss Among the Elderly

Although the general multi-variate approach to longitudinal analysis described in the previous section was effective in describing average patterns of longitudinal change and in estimating the relative magnitude of various sources of variability, it was not very effective in revealing the variability in individual patterns of change in hearing sensitivity. Figure 14-6 illustrates the individual variability in hearing thresholds that exists in 70-year-old male BLSA participants. For pure tones greater than 1 kHz, there was as much as a 60 dB difference between individuals tested at a given frequency. The mixed-effects model is more effective in studying individual differences in patterns of change because it generates estimates of each individual's deviation from the population average.

Mixed-effects models are also more effective in handling missing data and unequal intervals between observations. Figure 14-6 shows that hearing threshold values may be missing at certain frequencies for some individuals. If there are substantial amounts of missing data, a least squares multi-variate model can perform poorly (Cook and Ware, 1983). Besides the problem of missing threshold values at certain frequencies, additional concerns arise because individuals may be observed at unequal intervals or have different numbers of repeated visits. However, the mixed-effects model, and the maximum likelihood procedures used for the model, effectively handle the

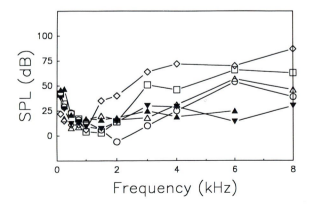

**Figure 14-6** Average trends often obscure the high degree of natural heterogeneity in the population. This figure shows the individual variability in hearing thresholds of six 70-year-old male BLSA participants.

correlation between repeated measurements and differing numbers of observations between individuals.

To illustrate the use of a mixed-effects model to study individual variability in patterns of aging, we consider 268 elderly male BLSA participants whose first audiograms were obtained at approximately age 70 (Morrell and Brant, 1991). This analysis demonstrates the use of mixed-effects models to:

1. investigate the effect of hearing impairment on rate of change in hearing sensitivity;
2. use the estimates of the random effects to examine individual outliers; and
3. generate individual-level estimates of longitudinal patterns of change.

If $y_{ij}$ represents the $j$th hearing threshold of participant $i$, the mixed-effects model for each observation can be written as

$$
\begin{aligned}
y_{ij} = {} & (\beta_0 + b_{i0}) + \beta_1 \, \text{Age1} + (\beta_2 + b_{i2}) \, \text{Time} + (\beta_3 + b_{i3}) \, \text{Time}^2 \\
& + (\beta_4 + b_{i4} + \beta_5 \, \text{Age}) \ln(\text{Freq.}) + (\beta_6 + b_{i6} + \beta_7 \, \text{Age} + \beta_8 \, \text{Impair}) \\
& \ln^2(\text{Freq.}) + \beta_9 \, \text{Impair} + e_{ij}.
\end{aligned}
\tag{14-2}
$$

Besides a fixed-effect term for the intercept or average hearing loss represented by $\beta_0$, the other fixed effects are age at first visit (Age1), linear and quadratic terms for length of time in the study (Time, Time$^2$), linear and quadratic terms for the natural logarithm of frequency (ln(Freq.), ln$^2$(Freq.)), presence of hearing impairment (Impair), and interaction terms for age at testing (Age) and ln(Freq.), Age and ln$^2$(Freq.), and Impair and ln$^2$(Freq.). The fixed-effects, covariance structure, and random effects for each individual are estimated using maximum likelihood and restricted maximum likelihood estimators. Details of the maximum likelihood and restricted maximum likelihood estimation procedures are given in Morrell and Brant (1991) and more generally in Lindstrom and Bates (1988).

The random terms in the model allow different estimates of the intercept and partial slopes for each person. The $\beta$ terms represent the "average" intercept and slopes, while the $b_i$ terms are the deviations from these averages for individual $i$. Thus, the model allows us to study individual differences more effectively by providing estimates of the intercept $(\beta_0 + b_{i0})$, growth curve or time components $(\beta_2 + b_{i2}, \beta_3 + b_{i3})$ and shape or frequency components $(\beta_4 + b_{i4}, \beta_6 + b_{i6})$ for each of the individuals in the study. The random effects account for natural heterogeneity in hearing in the population and are also useful in detecting "outlying" subjects.

Impaired individuals were found to have a hearing threshold of 15.6 dB greater than unimpaired individuals at 1 kHz (Table 14-2, Figure 14-7). As mentioned earlier, the use of a quadratic function in ln(Freq.) models the J-shaped or U-shaped relationship between frequency and threshold that audiograms typically follow. The Age $\times$ ln(Freq.) and Age $\times$ ln$^2$(Freq.) interaction terms were significant, thus indicating the frequency–intensity function had different shapes at different ages. The Impair $\times$ ln$^2$(Freq.) interaction term was also significant, indicating that the frequency–intensity

**Table 14-2** Fixed effects estimates from a multi-variate linear mixed-effects model analysis of hearing loss in the elderly.

| Effect | Estimate[a] | Standard error | Z-ratio |
|---|---|---|---|
| Constant or average ($\beta_0$) | −113.12 | 9.79 | −11.55 |
| Age 1 ($\beta_1$) | 1.81 | 0.13 | 13.92 |
| Time ($\beta_2$) | 1.05 | 0.21 | 5.00 |
| Time$^2$ ($\beta_3$) | 0.08 | 0.02 | 4.00 |
| ln (Freq.) ($\beta_4$) | −15.80 | 1.95 | −8.10 |
| Age × ln (Freq.) ($\beta_5$) | 0.35 | 0.02 | 17.50 |
| ln$^2$ (Freq.) ($\beta_6$) | 25.00 | 1.55 | 16.13 |
| Age × ln$^2$ (Freq.) ($\beta_7$) | −0.25 | 0.02 | −12.50 |
| Impair × ln$^2$ (Freq.) ($\beta_8$) | −1.97 | 0.86 | −2.29[b] |
| Impair ($\beta_9$) | 15.56 | 3.67 | 4.42 |

[a]Restricted maximum likelihood estimates of fixed-effects parameters.
[b]$P$ value is less than 0.05, all other Z-ratios have $P$ values less than 0.001.

function had a different shape in the impaired and non-impaired groups. This can be seen in Figure 14-7 where the frequency–intensity function is more bowed in the impaired subjects. Surprisingly, there was no evidence that individuals with hearing impairments lose their hearing at a different rate than individuals without an impairment since the interaction terms for Time × Impair and Time$^2$ × Impair were not statistically significant.

In addition, note that Age = Age1 + Time. Thus, the Age1 term (in years) models cross-sectional differences in hearing thresholds of subjects of different

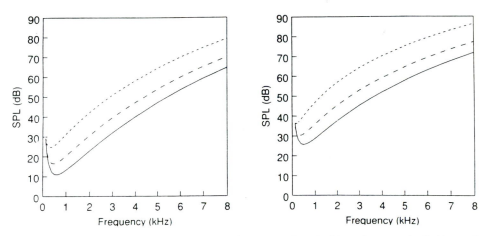

**Figure 14-7** Longitudinal change in hearing thresholds of normal (left) and impaired (right) 70-year-old BLSA participants as estimated by a mixed-effects regression analysis (Morrell and Brant, 1991). Impaired individuals do not lose hearing sensitivity faster than normal individuals, but the shape of the frequency–intensity curve is more bowed in impaired individuals. — = 70-year-old; -- = 5 years later; ---- = 10 years later.

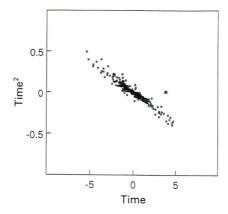

**Figure 14-8**　Bivariate plot of the random effects terms for time and time$^2$. One individual (*) falls outside the bivariate-normal elliptical region. Inspection of the data for this individual revealed an invalid hearing test for one of his repeated visits.

ages, while the Time and Time$^2$ terms (in years) model the longitudinal age changes in the thresholds for each individual.

Estimates of the random effects for each individual provided useful information in the study of the natural heterogeneity or individual variability. For example, a bivariate plot of the individual random effects terms for Time and Time$^2$ shows a high negative correlation ($-0.97$) between these two variables (Figure 14-8). This is not surprising as it indicates that the rate of change in hearing sensitivity tends to accelerate more slowly in those individuals whose hearing was changing fastest at the beginning of the study. Notably, one individual (denoted by an asterisk) had a Time and Time$^2$ random effect estimate outside the region containing the other estimates. Since the random effects are assumed to be normally distributed, the region containing the individual points on the graph should be circular or elliptical. Upon checking the data, the individual with the outlying random effects was found to have one invalid hearing test in five repeated visits. Although this outlier was an example of a technical problem, outliers are often a source of useful information. Additional investigation of outliers may reveal new information regarding disease states, environmental exposures, genetic predispositions, or other biological phenomena.

The estimated values for the fixed and random effects can also be substituted into the model to give the predicted hearing-intensity functions for each individual. Figure 14-9 shows fitted or predicted hearing thresholds for the six 70-year-old males given in Figure 14-6. These curves clearly show the between-individual variability in hearing thresholds, and as individualized predictions of hearing loss, they are potentially useful for individualized counseling.

Table 14-3 gives the restricted maximum likelihood estimate of the components of the variance–covariance matrix of the random effects and their correlations. The term in the table for between-persons variance ($\hat{\sigma}_p^2 = 212.16$)

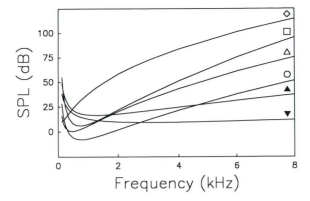

**Figure 14-9** Individualized estimates of hearing–frequency functions for the 70-year-old men shown in Figure 14.6. The ability of mixed-effects models to produce individualized estimates of patterns of change allows the description of the diversity of patterns of aging, and are useful for individualized counseling.

**Table 14-3** Restricted maximum likelihood estimates of the variances and co-variances of the random effects (upper triangular region) and the correlation between the random effects (lower triangular region).

| Random effect | Constant | Time | Time$^2$ | ln(Freq.) | ln$^2$(Freq.) |
|---|---|---|---|---|---|
| Constant | 212.16 | −4.09 | 0.28 | 18.01 | −32.49 |
| Time | −0.12 | 5.88 | −0.47 | −0.35 | −1.51 |
| Time$^2$ | 0.10 | −0.97 | 0.04 | 0.08 | 0.10 |
| ln(Freq.) | 0.27 | −0.03 | 0.09 | 20.90 | 1.50 |
| ln$^2$(Freq.) | −0.71 | −0.20 | 0.16 | 0.10 | 9.81 |

Estimate of error variance is $\hat{\sigma}_e^2 = 155.33$.

indicates a large difference between participants in hearing sensitivity. This estimate is somewhat larger than the estimate of the error variance $\hat{\sigma}_e^2 = 155.33$. Thus, the natural heterogeneity in hearing sensitivity in the population is greater than the statistical or measurement error in the model.

## OVERVIEW AND DISCUSSION

This chapter has focused primarily on issues related to variability in longitudinal patterns of aging and on recent methodological advances which make it easier to address these issues despite the complexities of longitudinal data sets.

The methodological advances are significant for several reasons. For the first time, they provide an integrated approach to estimating the average longitudinal patterns of aging in the population as well as variation from the average trends. This may encourage a more comprehensive description of the diversity in patterns of aging rather than an oversimplified view of "normal" aging. Since these methods directly model change, they also encourage a more dynamic approach to studying the process of aging. Furthermore, mixed-effects models provide methods of estimating cross-sectional and longitudinal effects in the same analysis. Finally, the ability of mixed-effects models to provide estimates of each individual's pattern of aging is an important step toward using an individual's pattern of aging as an individual-level natural experiment. Since these estimates are individualized, they are also useful for individual-level counseling.

These new methods of studying individual variability in longitudinal patterns of aging may be useful as descriptive tools, diagnostic tools, and epidemiologic tools. At the descriptive level, the ability to study individual patterns of aging will provide a better description of the aging process in all its diversity. A recent BLSA study used mixed-effects models to describe the natural history of normal and pathological growth of the prostate gland (Carter et al., 1992a; Pearson et al., 1994).

As a diagnostic tool, longitudinal patterns of change may provide clues as to current disease status and future outcomes. The BLSA prostate study also demonstrated that the longitudinal rate of change in prostate-specific antigen was significantly greater in individuals with prostate cancer than in individuals with benign prostatic hyperplasia or normal prostates, and that rates of change in prostate-specific antigen may be more useful as a screening tool than single prostate-specific antigen levels (Pearson et al., 1991b; Carter et al., 1992b).

As an epidemiologic tool, research focusing on the sources of individual differences in patterns of aging, and on the causes of sudden changes in an individual's pattern of aging, may allow investigators to tease apart the intrinsic and extrinsic factors which affect aging. In one recent study mixed-effects models were used to identify intrinsic and extrinsic factors which affect the longitudinal patterns of adaptation to nursing home living (Brant et al., 1992a). In another case, the results from a BLSA study suggest that sudden declines in pulmonary function may predict future cardiovascular events as strongly as the established cardiovascular risk factors (Rampal et al., 1989; Tockman et al., 1994). Evidence from the BLSA and other studies also suggests that long-term estimates of exposure to traditional cardiovascular risk factors may be better predictors of cardiovascular risk than baseline measurements (MacMahon et al., 1990; Pearson and Brant, 1990; Pearson et al., 1991a). One of the challenges facing the epidemiology of chronic diseases will be to adopt a life span perspective to study the role of the lifetime history of exposure to established risk factors and to determine if risk factors have different effects at different ages (Fozard et al., 1990; Brant et al., 1994).

One of the fundamental goals of gerontology is to describe the normal aspects of human aging and to distinguish them from the effects of disease.

Yet, it is difficult to define "normal" aging without a basic knowledge of the range and sources of variation in aging phenomena. Remarkably little is known about the variability in aging, either on a worldwide scale, within populations, or within individuals. However, the results of studies in non-Western populations have revealed counter-examples to some aging phenomena previously believed to be universal such as presbycusis (Rosen *et al.*, 1962) and increasing blood pressure with age (Huizinga, 1972; Page *et al.*, 1974; Friedlaender and Page, 1989). Biological anthropologists and human biologists have begun to use a combination of evolutionary, biosocial, and cross-cultural approaches to contribute to the understanding of variation in human aging (Beall, 1984; Beall and Weitz, 1989; Pearson and Crews, 1989; Crews, 1990). Historically some developmental psychologists (e.g., Baltes and Nesselroade, 1973; Buss, 1974) and biomedical scientists (e.g., Shock *et al.*, 1984; Costa and Andres, 1986) have also been interested in variability issues in Western populations. However, methodological advances now make it more feasible to study the variability in longitudinal patterns of aging. Viewed as a collection of individual-level natural experiments, these longitudinal patterns of aging may contribute to our understanding of the heterogeneous process of aging.

## REFERENCES

Anderson, T. W. (1971) *The Statistical Analysis of Time Series*. New York: John Wiley & Sons Inc.

Baker, P. T. (1977) Problems and strategies. In: *Human Population Problems in the Biosphere: Some Research Strategies and Designs* (ed. Baker, P. T.) Man and the Biosphere Technical Notes 3, Paris: UNESCO, pp. 11–32.

Baltes, P. B. and Nesselroade, J. R. (1973) The developmental analysis of individual differences on multiple measures. In: *Life-Span Developmental Psychology: Methodological Issues* (eds Nesselroade, J. R. and Reese, H. W.) New York: Academic Press, pp. 219–251.

Beall, C. M. (1984) Theoretical dimensions of a focus on age in physical anthropology. In: *Age and Anthropological Theory* (eds Kertzer, D. I. and Keith, J.) Ithaca: Cornell University Press, pp. 82–95.

Beall, C. M. and Weitz, C. A. (1989) The human population biology of aging. In: *Human Population Biology: A Transdisciplinary Science* (eds Little, M. A. and Haas, J. D.) New York: Oxford University Press, pp. 189–200.

Bergstrom, L. and Thompson, P. (1976) Ototoxicity. In: *Hearing Disorders* (ed. Northern, J. L.) Boston: Little, Brown and Company, p. 138.

Bochenek, Z. and Jachowska, A. (1969) Atherosclerosis, accelerated presbyacusis, and acoustic trauma. *International Audiology* **8**, 312–316.

Botwnick, J. (1964) Research problems and concepts in the study of aging. *The Gerontologist* **4**, 121–129.

Bourlière, F. (1970) *The Assessment of Biological Age in Man*. Public Health Papers No. 37. Geneva: World Health Organization.

Box, G. E. P. and Jenkins, G. M. (1970) *Time-Series Analysis: Forecasting and Control*. San Francisco: Holden-Day.

Brant, L. J. and Fozard, J. L. (1990) Age changes in pure-tone hearing thresholds in a longitudinal study of normal human aging. *Journal of the Acoustical Society of America* **88**, 813–820.

Brant, L. J., German, P. S., Rovner, B. W., Burton, L. C., Pearson, J. D. and Clark, R. D. (1992a) A longitudinal approach to modeling outcomes in a Nursing Home Study. *The Gerontologist* **32**, 159–163.

Brant, L. J., Pearson, J. D., Morrell, C. H. and Verbeke, G. N. M. (1992b) Statistical methods for studying individual change during aging. *Collegium Antropologicum* **16**, 359–369.

Brant, L. J., Pearson, J. D., Morrell, C. H., Metter, E. J., Fozard, J. L. and Fleg, J. L. (1993) Longitudinal methods for assessing vulnerability. In: *Autonomy and Well-Being in the Aging Population: Concepts and Design of the Longitudinal Study of Amsterdam* (eds Deeg, D. J. H., Knipscheer, C. P. M. and van Tilburg, W.). Bunnik, The Netherlands: Netherlands Institute of Gerontology, pp. 185–197.

Brant, L. J., Fozard, J. L. and Metter, E. J. (1994) Age differences in biological markers of mortality. In: *Practical Handbook of Human Biologic Age Determination* (ed. Balin, A.) Cleveland: CRC Press, Inc. (in press).

Buss, A. R. (1974) A general developmental model for interindividual differences, intraindividual differences, and intraindividual changes. *Developmental Psychology* **10**, 70–78.

Busse, E. W. (1970) Administration of the interdisciplinary research team. In: *Normal Aging* (ed. Palmore, E.). Durham, North Carolina: Duke University Press, pp. 7–17.

Camp, C. J. and Maxwell, S. E. (1983) A comparison of various strength of association measures commonly used in gerontological research. *Journal of Gerontology* **38**, 3–7.

Carter, H. B., Morrell, C. H. Pearson, J. D., Plato, C. C., Metter, E. J., Chan, D. W., Fozard, J. L. and Walsh, P. C. (1992a) Estimation of prostatic growth using serial prostate specific antigen measurements in men with and without prostate disease. *Cancer Research* **52**, 3323–3328.

Carter, H. B., Pearson, J. D., Metter, E. J., Brant, L. J., Chan, D. W., Andres, R., Fozard, J. L. and Walsh, P. C. (1992b) Longitudinal evaluation of prostate specific antigen levels in men with and without prostate disease. *Journal of the American Medical Association* **267**, 2215–2220.

Cooke, N. R. and Ware, J. H. (1983) Design and analysis methods for longitudinal research. *Annual Reviews of Public Health* **4**, 1–23.

Corso, J. F. (1958) Proposed laboratory standard of normal hearing. *Journal of the Acoustical Society of America* **30**, 14–23.

Corso, J. F. (1963) Age and sex differences in pure-tone thresholds. *Archives of Otolaryngology* **77**, 385–405.

Costa, P. T., Jr and Andres, R. (1986) Patterns of age changes. In: *Clinical Geriatrics*, 3rd edn (ed. Rossman, E.) New York: J. P. Lippincott Co., pp. 23–30.

Crews, D. E. (1990) Anthropological issues in biological gerontology. In: *Anthropology and Aging: Comprehensive Reviews* (ed. Rubenstein, R.). Dordrecht: D. Reidel, pp. 11–38.

Fabinyi, G. (1931) Regarding morphological and functional changes in the internal ear arteriosclerosis. *Laryngoscope* **4**, 663–670.

Feldman, H. A. (1988) Families of lines: random effects in linear regression analysis. *Journal of Applied Physiology* **64**, 1721–1732.

Fozard, J. L., Metter, J. L. and Brant, L. J. (1990) Next steps in describing aging and disease in longitudinal studies. *Journal of Gerontology* **45**, P116–127.

Friedlaender, J. S. and Page, L. B. (1989) Population biology and aging: the example of blood pressure. *American Journal of Human Biology* **1**, 355–365.

Garruto, R.M., Way, A. B., Zansky, S. and Hoff, C. (1989) Natural experimental models in human biology, epidemiology, and clinical medicine. In: *Human Population Biology: A Transdisciplinary Science* (eds Little, M. A. and Haas, J. D.). New York: Oxford University Press, pp. 82–109.

Glorig, A. and Nixon, H. L. (1962) Hearing loss as a function of age. *Laryngoscope* **27**, 1596–1610.

Harville, D. A. (1977) Maximum likelihood approaches to variance component estimation and to related problems. *Journal of the American Statistical Association* **72**, 320–338.

Hasselblad, V. (1978) *Comparison of Methods for the Analysis of Panel Studies*. Report of the United States Environmental Protection Agency, EPA-600/1-78-043, Research Triangle Park, North Carolina.

Henderson, D., Hammernik, A., Dosanjh, D. and Mills, J. (eds) (1976) *Effects of Noise on Hearing*. New York: Raven Press.

Huizinga, J. (1972) Casual blood pressure in populations. In: *Human Biology of Environmental Change* (ed. Vorester, D. J. M.) London: International Biological Programme, pp. 164–169.

Johnson, R. A. and Wichern, D. W. (1988) *Applied Multivariate Statistical Analysis*. Englewood Cliffs, NJ: Prentice Hall.

Korn, E. L. and Whittemore, A. S. (1979) Methods for analyzing panel studies of acute health effects of air pollution. *Biometrics* **35**, 795–802.

Kowalski, C. J. and Guire, K. E. (1974) Longitudinal data analysis. *Growth* **38**, 131–169.

Laird, N. M., Lang, N. and Stram, D. (1987) Maximum likelihood computations with repeated measures: application of the EM algorithm. *Journal of the American Statistical Association* **82**, 97–105.

Laird, N. M. and Ware, J. H. (1982 Random-effects models for longitudinal data. *Biometrics* **38**, 963–974.

Lindstrom, M. J. and Bates, D. M. (1988) Newton-Raphson and EM algorithms for linear mixed-effects models for repeated-measures data. *Journal of the American Statistical Association* **83**, 1014–1022.

Little, M. A. and Haas, J. D. (eds) (1989) *Human Population Biology: A Transdisciplinary Science*. New York: Oxford University Press.

MacMahon, S., Peto, R., Cutler, J., Collins, R., Sorlie, P., Neaton, J., Abbott, R., Godwin, J., Dyer, A. and Stamler, J. (1990) Blood pressure, stroke, and coronary heart disease: Part 1, prolonged differences in blood pressure: prospective observational studies corrected for the regression dilution bias. *The Lancet* **335**, 765–774.

Morrell, C. H. and Brant, L. J. (1991) Modelling hearing thresholds in the elderly. *Statistics in Medicine* **10**, 1–12.

Page, L. B., Damon, A. and Mooellering, R. C., Jr (1974) Antecedents of cardiovascular disease in six Solomon islands societies. *Circulation* **49**, 1132–1146.

Pearson, J. D. and Brant, L. J. (1990) Baseline measurements are not reliable estimates of chronic levels of risk factors. *The Gerontologist* **30** (Special Issue), 3A (abstract).

Pearson, J. D. and Crews, D. E. (1989) Evolutionary, biosocial, and cross-cultural perspectives on the variability in human biological aging. *American Journal of Human Biology* **1**, 303–306.

Pearson, J. D., Brant, L. J., Fleg, I. L. and Morrell, C. H. (1991a) Longitudinal variability causes baseline measurements to underestimate risk from chronic exposure to risk factors. *American Journal of Human Biology* **3**, 66–67 (abstract).

Pearson, J. D., Kaminski, P., Morrell, C. H., Carter, H. B., Metter, E. J., Fozard, J. L. and Brant, L. J. (1991b) Modeling longitudinal rates of change in prostate specific antigen during aging. *Proceedings of the Social Statistics Section of the American Statistical Association*, Washington, DC, pp. 580–585.

Pearson, J. D., Morrell, C. H., Landis, P. K., Carter, H. B. and Brant, L. J. (1994) Mixed-effects regression models for studying the natural history of prostate disease. *Statistics in Medicine* (in press).

Rampal, K., Tockman, M., Fleg, J. and Fozard, J. (1989) Pulmonary function as a predictor of myocardial perfusion defects on exercise thallium 201 myocardial perfusion scintography in the Baltimore Longitudinal Study of Aging. *The Gerontologist* **29** (Special Issue), 39A (abstract).

Rao, C. R. (1965) The theory of least squares when the parameters are stochastic and its application to the analysis of growth curves. *Biometrika* **52**, 447–458.

Reinsel, G., Tiao, G. C., Wang, M. N., Lewis, R. and Nychka, D. (1981) Statistical analysis of stratospheric ozone data for the detection of trends. *Atmospheric Environment* **15**, 1569–1577.

Rosen, S. and Olin, P. (1965) Hearing loss and coronary heart disease. *Archives of Otolaryngology* **82**, 236–243.

Rosen, S., Bergman, M., Plester, D., El-Mofty, A. and Satti, M. H. (1962) Presbycusis study of a relatively noise-free population in the Sudan. *Annals of Otology* **71**, 727–743.

Rosen, S., Plester, D., El-Mofty, A. and Rosen, H. V. (1964) High frequency audiometry in presbycusis: a comparative study of the Mabaan tribe in the Sudan with urban populations. *Archives of Otolaryngology* **79**, 34–48.

Rosen, S., Olin, P. and Rosen, H. V. (1970) Dietary prevention of hearing loss. *Acta Otolaryngology* **70**, 242–247.

Rosner, B. and Munoz, A. (1988) Autoregressive modelling for the analysis of longitudinal data with unequally spaced examinations. *Statistics in Medicine* **7**, 59–71.

Rowe, J. W. and Kahn, R. L. (1987) Human aging: usual and successful. *Science* **237**, 143–149.

Shapiro, S., Weinblatt, E. and Densen, P. (1969) Longitudinal vs. crosssectional approaches in studying prognostic factors in coronary heart disease. *Journal of Chronic Disease* **19**, 935–945.

Shock, N. W., Greulich, R. C., Andres, R., Arenberg, D., Costa, P. T., Lakatta, E. G. and Tobin, J. D. (1984) *Normal Human Aging: The Baltimore Longitudinal Study of Aging*. Washington, DC: US Government Printing Office, Publication 84-2450.

Statistical Analysis System (1985) *SAS Users Guide: Statistics, Version 5 Edition*. Cary, NC: Statistical Analysis System Institute Inc.

Strenio, J. F., Weisberg, H. I. and Byrk, A. S. (1983) Empirical Bayes estimation of individual growth-curve parameters and their relationship to covariates. *Biometrics* **39**, 71–86.

Tockman, M., Pearson, J., Fleg, J., Metter, E., Cruise, L., Rampal, K. and Fozard, J. (1994) Accelerated longitudinal decline in pulmonary function: A new risk factor for mortality due to coronary heart disease. *American Review of Respiratory Disease* (in press).

Vonesh, E. F. (1990) Modelling peritonitis rates and associated risk factors for individuals on continuous ambulatory peritoneal dialysis. *Statistics in Medicine* **9**, 263–271.

Zeger, S. L. and Liang, K. (1986) Longitudinal data analysis for discrete and continuous outcomes. *Biometrics* **42**, 121–130.

Zeger, S. L., Liang, K. Y. and Albert, P. S. (1988) Models for longitudinal data: a generalized estimating equation approach. *Biometrics* **44**, 1049–1060.

# 15

# Morphological Indicators of Skeletal Aging: Implications for Paleodemography and Paleogerontology

## SUSAN R. LOTH AND MEHMET YAŞAR İŞCAN

## INTRODUCTION

Paleogerontology, simply stated, is the scientific study of aging ancients. One of the most pressing of many questions paleogerontologists face is determining if, indeed, there is anything to study at the senescent phase of the life span. Moreover, if only a few extinct forms did reach extreme old age, will any be found? If no fetal or infant skeletons were ever recovered, we can still safely assume that this stage of life existed in all hominids, but we cannot make the same assumption at the other end of the life cycle, let alone precisely delineate its absolute maximum for pre-modern humans. Finally, assuming elderly specimens are excavated, will scientists be able to recognize and interpret senescence in the remains? That is where skeletal biologists must provide paleodemographers with the knowledge they need.

The signs of post-maturity aging are clear in the living or newly deceased. In bones, however, the manifestations of age are subtle, irregular, variable characteristics that are often confusing, sometimes contradictory, and always a challenge to interpret accurately. Therefore, this chapter will focus on the recognition and interpretation of the manifestations of age in the adult skeleton by critically analyzing, and discussing the most current morphological methods. This information is vital to human biologists and researchers on aging because skeletal remains provide our only direct look at an organism from the past. Comparing the appearance of archaeological material with that of known individuals is the primary mode of elucidating the effects of the aging process.

It is no secret that paleodemographers face great difficulties attempting to reconstruct extinct or extant populations on the basis of skeletal evidence, especially when dealing with fragmentary groupings of prehistoric individuals. In the first place, one can rarely be certain if the bones in question are truly representative of the populace as a whole or if they derive from "specialized" burial areas. At times the ratio of males and females is impossibly skewed.

Often, "populations" are found that appear to lack, for example, infants, children, or anyone over age 30. Decades of heated debate and great frustration led Bocquet-Appel and Masset (1982) to bid "farewell to paleodemography." However, as they also indicated, valuable information can be gleaned from estimating the age of the individuals who comprise the archaeological and fossil records of humankind.

Understanding the aging process in an evolutionary context may lead to the reconstruction of the life history of human ancestors—an issue of utmost importance to biological anthropologists and human population biologists. As Smith (1991:157) states "human evolution is an important test case for . . . theories of growth and aging". Angel (1969) deemed adult longevity to be the best single indicator of general health in earlier populations.

Estimating age at death from the adult skeleton is one of the most important and at the same time most difficult evaluations that must be undertaken. The basic overall form and proportion of the modern human skeleton can be traced to *Homo erectus* (Poirier, 1990). However, there continue to be changes such as increasing secular trends in height (e.g., Tanner, 1962) accompanied by a "general trend towards gracilization of the skeleton [including the masticatory apparatus], a structural reduction of size and robusticity . . . since the Upper Paleolithic" (Henneberg, 1988:402). Furthermore, such factors as maturation rate, disease, diet, culture, the environment, inter- and intra-populational admixture and variation, and levels of physical activity have changed considerably. All of these can leave their imprint on the rate of developmental and remodeling processes going on within the bones, and it is upon these processes that the estimation of age at death is based. The inevitable changes that have occurred in many, if not all, of these variables can affect the accuracy of techniques used to establish demographic profiles.

One of many elements that make adult age assessment particularly difficult is the great variation that exists in the aging process itself as well as in how it is reflected in the human body. This is the controversy over chronological versus biological or physiological age (Angel *et al.*, 1986; Borkan, 1986). There are always individuals who appear considerably older or younger than one would expect at a given age. Physiologically, a 50-year-old man might be judged to have the heart of a 25-year-old. The same situation exists in the skeleton. It is not uncommon to find bones that just do not show the morphological features usually found in a given age range. Some of these differences have been linked to conditions as disparate as education levels, marital status, general health, and heredity (Angel, 1984; Borkan, 1986).

There is also the question of changes in both the age of onset of the post-maturity aging process and its manifestations in temporally diverse populations. Schranz (1959:227) questioned the use of current standards on ancient humans, and declared that "differences may increase as we go back in time, just as today [variation exists] among peoples living under different circumstances." Differences have been uncovered between people of today and those as recently as the turn of the century. Variation in rates of maturation can be problematic because the formations noted are based on time elapsed since the cessation of growth at that site. Tanner (1962:143) stated that "During the last 100 years there has been a very striking tendency for the time of adolescence . . . to become earlier" especially after 1930. It is now two years earlier than at the turn of the century (Bogin, 1988). Since adult aging techniques are based on post-maturity metamorphoses, this may result in underaging—especially if the trend began early in hominid evolution.

## EVOLUTION OF THE HOMINID LIFE SPAN

Researchers have now traced hominid origins back over 3 million years to the genus *Australopithecus*, and a myriad of theories and phylogenetic pathways of evolutionary progress have been published and compiled (e.g., Smith and Spencer, 1984; Poirier, 1990; Brace, 1991). Chronologically, the primitive Australopithecines gave way to the first members of the genus *Homo* (*H. habilis*) roughly 2 million years ago. Early *H. erectus* followed about 1.8 m.y.a. in Africa with later forms persisting until approximately 300,000 years ago in Europe and Asia. At this point in time, both dating and taxonomic assignment become more difficult and controversial, but the first Archaic *Homo sapiens* is thought to have appeared some 200,000–300,000 years ago. If one "averages" the varied array of dates for the appearance and disappearance *H. sapiens neanderthalensis*, an acceptable range might be from about 100,000–35,000 years ago. Most experts do agree that the only hominid in existence for the past 30,000–35,000 years is anatomically modern *H. sapiens sapiens*.

Determining the life span of fossil man has been of major importance to human population biologists and biological anthropologists since the first pre-modern hominids were unearthed (Crews, 1990). This is reflected in Weidenreich's (1939) study of *H. erectus* in China. He pronounced three individuals to be 40–50 years old and found "small fragments" of a female skull he deemed to be "really old . . . over 50 . . . or even 60 years of age" (Weidenreich, 1939:35), and concluded that there is "evidence of *H. erectus* reaching the stage of senescence—real or relative when compared with that of modern man. . . [and] the attainment of an advanced age cannot be merely the effect of an artificially cultivated and undisturbed life under modern conditions" (Weidenreich, 1939:38). Although he based his findings on only one, notoriously unreliable age estimation method, cranial suture closure, his conclusion about longevity—at least in late *H. erectus*—is proving to be sound.

The most recent research in this area has taken a different direction. Rather than relying solely on determining the age at death of the relatively few specimens recovered, efforts focused on extrapolating maximum life span from such factors as rates of dental development and brain to body ratio (Smith, 1991). Extensive research of her own and careful consideration of others has led Smith (1991:171) to conclude that

> [T]he unique rate and pattern of human development are not of ancient origin . . . evidence suggests that small-brained, small-bodied *Australopithecus* possessed a life history similar to that of the great apes and that the life history of

early *Homo* [*habilis* and early *erectus*] matched no living primate species. Far from the idea that evolution of growth and aging ended in Pliocene *Australopithecus*, I suggest that a synergism of evolving life history and increasing complexity of behavior continued to operate throughout the evolution of the genus *Homo*.

Few would disagree that the increase in size (and complexity) of the brain is the single most important anatomical change underlying both human biological and behavioral evolution. Considering the evidence presented by Smith (1991) it would not be unreasonable to conclude that this is also the most significant factor leading to the increase observed in the human life span. Figure 15-1

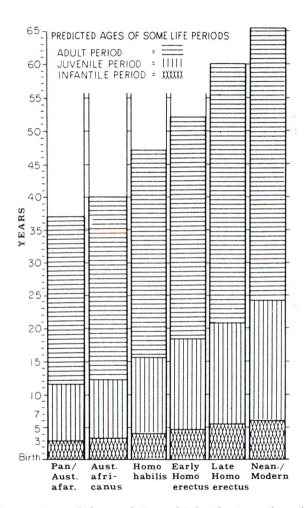

**Figure 15-1** Comparison of the evolution of infantile, juvenile, adult stages, and longevity of hominids as predicted from dental development and brain and body weight estimates for fossil species (including *Pan* "to suggest equivalency with *A. afarensis*"). The past 3+ million years of evolution have seen an increase of 3 years in infancy, an added 10 years to the juvenile period, and a jump of 30 years in the life span. Modified from Smith (1991: 170), Figure 6.

succinctly illustrates the evolution of the hominid life span, including estimations for the relative timing of infancy, adolescence, adulthood, and longevity.
The past 3+ million years of evolution have seen an increase of three years in
the duration of infancy, an added ten years to the juvenile period, and a jump
of 30 years in the life span. Of particular interest is the placement of
Neandertals in the same longevity range (65+ years) as modern humans. This
should help put to rest earlier suggestions that "significant postreproductive
survival was rare among Neandertals" (Trinkaus and Thompson, 1987:123)—it
is much more likely that this form did, indeed, survive beyond the age of 40.

An excellent, in-depth source of the latest research and thinking in this
avenue of inquiry is the special issue of the *American Journal of Physical
Anthropology* (1991, Vol. 86) devoted to the Dental Anthropology Associa-
tion-sponsored Primate Tooth Formation Symposium.


## HISTORICAL PERSPECTIVE

The switch from historical demography to paleodemographic assessment based
on the analysis of skeletal remains was ushered in by Todd's development and
publication of the first systematic, data-based aging techniques in the 1920s
(Acsádi and Nemeskéri, 1970). Nearly 40 years later, Vallois (1960) stated that
the two "processes" that can be used for individuals past the age of 20 years,
dental wear and cranial suture closure, are much more irregular than the signs
of age in sub-adults. He further noted that "modifications of certain parts of
the bones may be added, but these . . . are still badly understood and
insufficiently systematized" (Vallois, 1960:187). Howells' discussion of Vallois'
presentation provides an assessment of the state of the art of age determination
at that time—5 July 1959 (Howells, 1960:205–208):

> Dr Vallois' paper deals with the very important matter of age determination
> based upon skeletal material . . . [he] correctly points out that [tooth wear] is
> quite variable and therefore relatively unreliable, particularly for early man like
> the Neandertalers . . . [In my own experience] the use of the teeth for aging can
> be treacherous in the modern population as well . . . It seems to me that the teeth
> can be used [only] as a way of avoiding gross error . . . [when] the rest of the
> skeleton [of an older individual] doesn't show marked signs of aging.
>
> [As for cranial sutures] Cobb . . . found these very unsatisfactory . . . [and]
> Stewart . . . concluded that [suture closure] is quite irregular and a poor guide to
> conditions of adult life.

Howells (1960:207) went on to note that it is often difficult to use Todd's
(1920) pubic symphyseal types and, although McKern and Stewart's (1957)
component system may have better addressed variability, "the variation is very
great, and any correlation with age is, at best, only an approximation."

Age estimation accuracy has been improved by the addition of innovative
techniques from new skeletal sites, revisions of existing ones, and a better
understanding of both internal and external factors that can affect the
manifestations of age. However, many of the same problems noted by Howells
over 30 years ago have yet to be resolved. Therefore, the present paper

elaborates how skeletal biologists discern the aging process in the skeleton, and discusses and evaluates the latest methodological advances from anatomical sites in the pelvis, cranium, dentition, and ribs. This chapter also includes the first report of preliminary results of tests of the rib phase technique on the archaeological Spitalfields cemetery population, and the first publication of this method's efficacy on Neandertals. The upper limits of current technology are highlighted because of their importance for estimating longevity and life expectancy during earlier phases of human evolution. The chapter concludes with an overview and future research perspectives in biological anthropology and human population biology.

## ELABORATION OF THE AGING PROCESS IN THE SKELETON

Unlike the well-defined, regular series of events (culminating in an easily recognizable terminal morphology) that characterize the growth and development periods, post-maturity aging is irregular, and highly variable, both on the individual and group levels. Skeletal biologists must look at the interaction of a number of diverse processes—normal remodeling, bony build-up through periosteal deposition or arthritic thickening or osteophytosis, thinning via endosteal resorption or osteoporotic deterioration. To make matters worse, all of these conditions are affected by numerous physiological and environmental factors as noted previously. Furthermore, each part of the skeleton may show the effects of age at different rates within the same person (Loth and İşcan, 1989).

By conducting systematic research on numerous specimens, we can see certain general formations and patterns emerging. Separated into "components," or grouped into "stages" or "phases" of progression and statistically associated with age, these become the standards for age assessment.

For the better part of this century, skeletal biologists have been working on the formidable task of recognizing age-related changes in adult bones, correlating them with actual chronological age and then developing reliable, widely applicable methods for estimating age at death (see İşcan, 1989). Yet, despite the years devoted to research in this area since the 1920s, experts today still have no foolproof way of making this determination with pinpoint accuracy in every case. Human variation is inherent and inescapable, so that even under the best of conditions, i.e., a complete, undamaged skeleton, one must rely on standards that reflect the more typical manifestations of the aging process in a given population at a particular point in time. Experience is extremely helpful (Angel, 1984)—it gives a better "feel" for the material—but does not eliminate all the other sources of error.

Another problem is the fact that the accuracy of age assessment decreases as age increases. Angel (1984:165) noted that the precision of age estimation decreases "slowly but logarithmically from adolescence to old age." He conducted a study using his own considerable skills to monitor this decline in a sample of complete cases whose ages at death were known. From ages 20–29 years, he averaged a deviation of only 1.7 years and increased by a few years per decade reaching a maximum of 10.4 in the 70 and over range. He concluded that deviations can be traced to each "individual's personal physiological resistance at the various joints and surfaces . . . we use in aging and . . . [one's] retardation or acceleration with respect to calendar age"—and these may reach 10–20 years in the elderly (Angel, 1984:165). This problem can be frustrating to human population biologists studying aging who are concerned with determining the upper limits of the life span.

As in all scientific sub-disciplines, this field has evolved its own specialized terminology, resources, and shorthand. For example, in the phrase "aging a skeleton," aging is short for "estimating age at death." If an estimate is older than actual age, it is referred to as "overaging" and the opposite situation is labeled "underaging." Since age assessment is dependent on other factors such as sex, the term "sexing" is used because it takes up much less room than repeating "determining the sex of" a skeleton. Although skeletons are sometimes "mis-sexed," they are never "oversexed" or "undersexed" . . .

In order to develop standards for determining demographic characteristics from the skeleton, researchers must rely primarily on the study of known individuals. In the United States, there are two major skeletal collections: the Terry Collection (TC) at the Smithsonian Institution, and the Hamann–Todd Collection (HTC) at the Cleveland Museum of Natural History. Both contain thousands of complete skeletons from known subjects, most of whom were born before the turn of the century (İşcan, 1990). Unfortunately, legal constraints have limited collections to a few sections of different bones from individuals autopsied at medical examiner's offices. Although the documentation on recent forensic cases is often superior to that accompanying the TC and HTC, piecemeal assemblages make it difficult to get the entire picture of skeletal aging.

## CURRENT AGE ASSESSMENT TECHNIQUES

After many years of relative inactivity, the 1980s saw a resurgence of research and publications in the area of age determination. Many of these efforts were aimed at "retooling" and testing standards from the pubic symphysis, cranial sutures, and dentition (İşcan and Loth, 1989). More significant was the introduction of methods from two new sites, the sternal extremity of the rib, by the authors in 1984 (İşcan et al., 1984a, 1984b), and the auricular surface of the ilium, by Lovejoy and co-workers (1985a). A number of books dealing with the skeleton as a whole such as Krogman and İşcan (1986) and Ubelaker (1989) contain chapters that present most available methods for sub-adults and adults along with recommendations about their use.

A comprehensive description and critical evaluation of adult age estimation studies and techniques from the end of the last century through the 1980s can be found in İşcan and Loth (1989). A recent book, *Age Markers in the Human Skeleton*, edited by İşcan (1989), concentrates on the interpretation of skeletal evidence of aging from the fetus throughout the entire life span. It contains chapters written by experts who discuss all available methods including morphological and invasive skeletal and dental analyses, radiography, and histomorphometry (not covered in the present paper).

Besides improving overall accuracy, the research of the 1980s has resulted in techniques that have expanded the range of efficacy of age assessment to include the most long-lived members of human populations. Significantly, the upper end range for some new systems has increased from the fifth decade to past the seventh. The following section touches upon older methods still in use and focuses on newer ones introduced in the last decade.

## Pelvis

### Pubic Symphysis

Using the pubic symphysis, Todd (1920) introduced the first systematic data-based technique for age estimation. He discovered that age-related events at the symphysis could be grouped into ten phases of progression beginning by age 20 and ending by age 50. This part of the skeleton is still an important locus in archaeological populations because it often survives fairly well and is more reliable than cranial sutures. Although Todd's White male derived "all purpose" age phases have been criticized for years, his basic scheme of age-related changes is still being used, either in its original form or in one of its "reincarnations" (Brooks, 1955; Nemeskéri et al., 1960; Angel, 1980; Meindl et al., 1985; Katz and Suchey, 1986). The component systems for males (McKern and Stewart, 1957) and females (Gilbert and McKern, 1973) developed to counteract the so-called static nature of the typological phases are, on the other hand, no longer considered viable (Lovejoy et al., 1985b; Meindl et al., 1985; Pfeiffer, 1985; Katz and Suchey, 1986; Masset, 1989). Part of the problem for paleodemographic study can be traced to the attenuated age range of the Korean War dead sample (Masset, 1989) that yields survivorship curves in which it appears that no one lived to the ripe old age of 50 years (e.g., Pfeiffer, 1985).

The most recent modifications of Todd's phases have been offered within the last decade. In 1985, Meindl et al. condensed the original ten phases into five that they thought would better account for variation. Their reference sample was drawn from the HTC. One problem that they determined could not be corrected for in their standards was biological variability at the symphysis. Size was also found to be a factor in the rate of aging—larger bones show less change, and thus will be underaged. Conversely, in females, small ones were often overaged as opposed to larger ones that followed the male pattern more closely.

Like the other recent techniques this group published, it is difficult to apply—even by seasoned experts. Statements such as "the above description should not be applied in too strict a fashion . . . judgment should be made on the overall maturity of the [symphyseal] face, not on the singular presence or absence of defined criteria" (Meindl et al., 1985:38) may reflect the true situation one faces in age assessment; however, too many exceptions can only lead to confusion and a rather subjective analysis.

Since many of the exceptions and deviations were related (by Meindl et al.,

1985) to "being female," it seems apparent that accuracy could be improved with sex-specific standards. Along with others, such as Gilbert and McKern (1973) who uncovered gender-based variation in morphology and maturation rates, Brooks and Suchey (1990) have found definite differences between the sexes. Dorsal lipping, for example, is not directly age-related in females, but is more likely to arise from pregnancy or other factors. On the other hand, age-related changes are seen in the ventral aspects of females, but not in males. Although tests by Meindl and associates do not show significant differences between sexes or races, the matter of sex or race variation should be examined before, not after, standards are produced. Testing after the fact is not truly valid because enough characteristics from each group will be included so that most differences will not register as significant. In our experience, generalized standards cannot account for proven differences (between sexes and races) in the age of onset, and rates of skeletal and physiological maturation. Furthermore, mixing the differences from all groups can only increase the range of variation that must be accounted for in each phase. This often results in unwieldy or meaninglessly large age ranges (e.g., Katz and Suchey, 1989).

In 1986, Katz and Suchey offered yet another modification of Todd. The six, sex-specific Suchey–Brooks phases were developed from a very large, carefully documented, recent forensic sample that was not separated by race. It is fairly easy to match most bones with the symphyseal casts. The major drawback is that variability at the symphysis results in extremely large 95% confidence ranges for most of the phases. Table 15-1 illustrates this problem in contrast to the narrower ranges for the rib phases. Some of the variation was traced to their use of mixed-race standards, because a subsequent re-evaluation of their sample revealed significant differences in rates of aging across racial groups (Katz and Suchey, 1989). Independent testers of these casts along with those of McKern and Stewart (1957) and Gilbert and McKern (1973) concluded that all of these techniques "proved disappointing in . . . both accuracy and precision . . . and in no cases did the proportion of cases falling within a designated interval . . . even closely approach the proportion expected from the original database samples (Klepinger et al., 1992:767).

A comparison by Meindl et al. (1990) shows clearly that these two sets of standards simply represent different groupings of Todd's original phases. Obvious distinctions lie in such areas as temporally diverse base samples and sample selection procedures, separation by sex (or lack of it), number of phases, and age assignments. In response to criticism of their use of the Hamann–Todd Collection because of known problems in documentation of age (by Katz and Suchey, 1989), Meindl's group tested the Suchey–Brooks phases on a "restructured" sample drawn from that collection. Using a series of "powerful" statistical procedures, they concluded that the criticism that their original sample selection resulted in reduced age variances was unfounded. They characterize the Suchey–Brooks phases as a "purely mechanical . . . 'handbook' styled approach for simple forensic application by inexperienced investigators" (Meindl et al., 1990:352,356). Meindl et al. (1990:356) stated that interobserver error was not their primary concern and, although their standards are more difficult to apply, they represent a "biological assessment

**Table 15-1** A comparison of mean ages and 95% intervals of the rib phases and Suchey–Brooks public symphyseal phases.

| | Rib[a] | | Public symphysis[b] | |
|---|---|---|---|---|
| | 95% | | 95% | |
| Phase | Mean | Range | Mean | Range |
| *Males* | | | | |
| 1 | 17.3 | 16.5–18.0 | 18.5 | 15–23 |
| 2 | 21.9 | 20.8–23.1 | 23.4 | 19–34 |
| 3 | 25.9 | 24.1–27.7 | 28.7 | 21–46 |
| 4 | 28.2 | 25.7–30.6 | 35.2 | 23–57 |
| 5 | 38.8 | 34.4–42.3 | 45.6 | 27–66 |
| 6 | 50.0 | 44.3–55.7 | 61.2 | 34–86[c] |
| 7 | 59.2 | 54.3–64.1 | | |
| 8 | 71.5 | 65.0–78.0[c] | | |
| *Females* | | | | |
| 1 | 14.0 | | 19.4 | 15–24 |
| 2 | 17.4 | 15.5–19.3 | | 19–40 |
| 3 | 22.6 | 20.5–24.7 | 30.7 | 21–53 |
| 4 | 27.7 | 24.4–31.0 | 38.2 | 26–70 |
| 5 | 40.0 | 33.7–46.3 | 48.1 | 25–83 |
| 6 | 50.7 | 43.3–58.1 | 60.0 | 42–87[c] |
| 7 | 65.2 | 59.2–71.2 | | |
| 8 | 76.4 | 70.4–82.3[c] | | |

[a]Modified from İşcan *et al.* (1984a, 1985).
[b]Modified from Brooks and Suchey (1990).
[c]Terminal phase age ranges are open ended.

. . . [that] provides more information [for] the estimation of chronological age . . . than comparison matching a specimen to a series of discrete archetypes." At present, it appears that both techniques could use some "fine tuning."

For years, many Europeans have relied on the five-stage symphyseal standards of Nemeskéri and associates (1960) as part of their complex method. Although these standards have never found favor in the US, they were recommended by the Workshop of European Anthropologists (1980) as recently as 1980. However, a comparison of these stages (as they appear in Acsádi and Nemeskéri, 1970) with the Suchey–Brooks phases raised a number of questions about their potential for accuracy (Brooks and Suchey, 1990). These ranged from the uneven distribution of the base sample (it contained very few young individuals) and ignoring certain morphological changes, to a lack of correspondence with modern age ranges for symphyseal formations. They found no support for the use of the Nemeskéri *et al.* (1960) standards. Although a number of valid points were made, it is difficult to agree with their specious conclusion that "methods that do not apply to modern human remains cannot be expected to be useful for age determination on past skeletal material" (Brooks and Suchey, 1990). This flies in the face of evidence that modern populations show more variation than the normally homogeneous archaeological ones (Howells, 1960; Lovejoy *et al.*, 1985b).

Of evolutionary interest is "Lucy"—an unusually complete *Australopithecus afarensis* (the earliest, most primitive hominid) dating from more than 3 million years ago. Meindl *et al.* (1985) observed that her well-preserved symphyseal face exhibited the morphological development of a 40-year-old even though the rest of the skeleton points to an age much closer to 20 years. The pelvis was the focus of many forces during evolution—adjustments to bipedalism, and enlargement of the birth canal to accommodate brain expansion. Therefore, it is not unexpected that there have been "considerable physiological maturational changes" in the pubic symphysis over the last 2 million years of evolution (Meindl *et al.*, 1985).

## Auricular Surface of the Ilium

The 1980s also saw the introduction of the auricular surface of the ilium as a new site for age estimation by Lovejoy and co-workers (1985a). Changes at this site were found to have a good correlation with age and the structure itself had the advantage of being well preserved in archaeological cases. Moreover, these authors claim that detectable changes at this site continue well beyond the age of 50 (unlike the pubic symphysis). Another built-in advantage of this technique for paleodemographic study might be the fact that specimens from the prehistoric Libben site were included in the standards rather than only Hamann–Todd individuals.

One of the developers of this method used it (as part of a summary age analysis) to assess the paleodemography of the Late Archaic (3,000–4,500 years BP) Carlston Annis site in Kentucky (Mensforth, 1990). Through principal component analysis, it was determined that, of the indicators used (auricular surface, pubic symphysis, proximal femur, clavicle, and dental wear), the auricular surface had the highest correlation with age.

On the other hand, many colleagues have found these highly complex series of changes difficult to work with. It is often impossible, for example, to distinguish the appearance of "build-up" from "break-down." In response to this criticism, the authors produced a set of slides (presented by Bedford *et al.*, 1989) containing examples of auricular surfaces with descriptions to help clarify some of the pertinent features set forth by Lovejoy *et al.* (1985a) in the original article. A recent test indicated that, although its mixed sex standards were not a significant problem, the auricular surface was not suitable for modern forensic application (Murray and Murray, 1991).

## Cranial Sutures

The first systematic technique for age estimation from cranial suture closure was published by Todd and Lyon (1924, 1925). Using specimens from the HTC, they based their stages of progression on Broca's scheme. However, years of frustration with their inaccuracy led to a great deal of criticism (e.g., Singer, 1953; McKern and Stewart, 1957). Singer (1953) found fault with Todd and Lyon's research design and interpretation of their material. The extreme variability encountered within the range of normalcy led him to state unequivocally that age determination from the cranial sutures is "hazardous and unreliable" (Singer, 1953). McKern and Stewart (1957) warned that sutural closure is so erratic that almost any pattern can be found at any age.

Despite the many obvious problems, researchers were not ready to abandon cranial sutures. Nemeskéri and associates (1960) published a five-phase system for evaluating closure in the vault. However, this was not meant to stand alone—but rather to be used (along with the pubic symphysis and proximal epiphyses of the humerus and femur) as part of their complex method, which represented the first set of standards for multiregional skeletal age assessment.

In 1985, Meindl and Lovejoy returned to the HTC to re-evaluate suture closure. They reasoned that many of the problems with age estimation at this site could be traced to the methodological misjudgments of Todd and Lyon (1924, 1925) who "culled" their sample to eliminate "anomalous" specimens. To remedy this situation, all observed variations were included in the four stages (0–3) used to judge closure at specific 1 cm sites on all ectocranial sutures (Meindl and Lovejoy, 1985). The scores from each segment in a specified groups of sutures were added, and age ranges were calculated for all possible total scores. As in their other techniques, tests of these mixed sex/race standards did not reveal significant errors based on these factors. Despite their findings that correlation with age was inferior to most other methods, these authors indicated that suture closure can be of value if used along with other skeletal age indicators (Meindl and Lovejoy, 1985).

The most recent effort by Masset (1989) is particularly relevant because it was expressly designed for the purpose of increasing the accuracy of paleo-demographic assessment of archaeological populations. Using a mathematical approach, Masset traced systematic statistical errors to a number of causes, such as sex differences not accounted for in existing methods. An even more serious problem arose from discrepancies between the age structure of the reference population (from which age standards were derived) and the sample to be analyzed. Error from this source was magnified by the inherent variability of suture closure. This was borne out by tests conducted on a large sample of early 20th century individuals from Lisbon and Coimbra (Masset, 1989).

Finally, Masset observed a phenomenon he called "attraction of the middle." This "attraction" results when individual estimates are built into an age structure for a given population, in which case they tend to accumulate in the middle age range. While agreeing that the cranial sutures cannot be used for precise individual age estimation, he advocates their usefulness in revealing major demographic shifts over time in a particular cemetery. Masset (1989) suggests that statistical manipulations such as the probability vector method can eliminate may systematic errors (e.g., sampling error), but cautions that the age distribution cannot essentially deviate from that of the reference population from which the age estimation standards were derived. One cannot assume that population distribution remained static over time. This may be an important issue for studies on the evolution of aging and changing life parameters.

Masset (1989, 1990) makes it clear that even if a cemetery population may exhibit the same morphological features as the aging system used to analyze it, that does not mean that they are indicative of the same age because the means and ranges of the standards reflect the distribution of the reference population, not the archaeological assemblage. There may be considerable differences, especially in suture closure. Masset used the example of how results will differ if standards developed from different known collections are used. The use of standards from the Korean War dead sample used by McKern and Stewart (1957) with a mean age of 23.5 years and Nemeskéri's hospital sample with a mean age of 57.5 may produce very dissimilar probability profiles for the same cemetery population.

Due to the survivability of the skull, colleagues relentlessly re-examine cranial suture closure hoping that "perfect" methodology will somehow overcome the intrinsic irregularity of this process. Although such efforts are admirable and refinements have been offered, it is unlikely that suture closure can ever be used as more than a technique of last resort. Problems extend beyond the extreme, inherent variability that characterizes the process itself to environmental conditions such as acidic soil. Singer (1960) noted that the "variability of suture closure is so tremendous that . . . you couldn't be quite certain [if] the individual was 25 or 45." He further pointed out that "acid soils, which will allow fossilization . . . will also open up sutures," and this may be the reason that so many fossil skulls appear to be those of "fairly young men" (Singer, 1960).

## Dentition

Broca was the first to capitalize on the association between tooth wear and age by introducing a five-stage rating scale nearly 100 years ago (Lovejoy, 1985). Essentially, the studies that followed were modifications of his system. At present, it is likely that the most frequently applied adult standards were charted by Brothwell (1981).

After 1972, research in this area consisted primarily of tests of factors affecting dental attrition (Brothwell, 1989). Sex differences ranged from nonexistent to slight (but not statistically significant) (Lovejoy, 1985). Researchers have found that tooth-wear rates and patterns show considerable inter-population variation and can be affected by diet, jaw size, and chewing stresses (Miles, 1962; Molnar, 1971; Brothwell, 1981). Although significant correlations were made with other age indicators (Nowell, 1978; Lovejoy et al., 1985b), this method is not considered effective beyond age 50 (Brothwell, 1989).

The latest standards were published by Lovejoy in 1985. Derived from the archaeological Libben population, they were found to be very highly correlated with age. The observed patterns were quite similar to those Murphy (1959) obtained from Australian aborigines. Brothwell (1989) cautioned that standards specific to various populations must be based on the wear rates for a sub-adult sample within each racial, ethnic, or temporally diverse group. Lovejoy was aware of this problem and realized the significance of his findings that the Libben standards were effective despite the geographic diversity of the HTC collection and the fact that he had to base wear rates on adult seriation (because there were not enough sub-adults from which to create population specific standards). This unexpected success led him to predict even better results from homogeneous archaeological populations.

The reputation of this age indicator has not been much better than that of cranial suture closure, but as with the latter, dentition is one of the sites most likely to withstand the ravages of time. Therefore, it would be of great value if, as Lovejoy and associates (1985b:12) assert, of the sites they tested, dental wear is the "best single indicator of age at death in skeletal populations . . . [it] is consistently without bias and probably presents the highest accuracy." This is a good example of what can arise from Howells' (1960) suggestion to use complete archaeological collections to study earlier morphological patterns.

## Rib

The sternal extremity of the rib is one of the most recent additions as a site for age determination. It is the first new osteological site from which a reliable system with manageable age ranges was developed since the 1920s. The male rib phase technique was introduced by the authors in 1984 and the female phases were published the following year (İşcan et al., 1984a, 1985).

Advancing age in the rib is marked by two processes—periosteal deposition as well as deterioration (Epker et al., 1965). One of the advantages of the costochondral junction of the rib is that these processes continue to create detectable changes (divided into Phases 0 through 8) that can be followed throughout life (İşcan et al., 1984a, b). Therefore, the rib phase method is one of the few that can effectively reach beyond the 50s. The oldest phase (8) separates individuals over 65–70 years and is one of the most accurate for contemporary White males and females (Loth et al., 1990). The rib also displays a number of age markers that are well confined to specific age ranges. In males, for example, a well-developed scalloping pattern on the margin is most frequently found in the early 20s and has not been noted in individuals over 30. The same goes for the "V-shaped" pit where the rib articulates with the cartilage. In both sexes, a fragile paper-thin bone is always classified as a Phase 8, no matter what its morphology.

Significant differences were found not only between the sexes, but also between American Whites and Blacks (İşcan et al., 1987). Blacks displayed the effects of periosteal ossification much earlier than Whites. This made them appear older than their White counterparts by the 30s. Osteometric analysis supports the contention that adult periosteal deposition occurs much more rapidly in Blacks (Loth and İşcan, 1991). This may also partially explain the observation that ribs of Blacks remained more firm and solid throughout life, rarely showing the extreme thinning and deterioration found in Whites— especially females. Although there were many Blacks in the Terry Collection in their 70s, 80s, and 90s, few even approached the appearance of a White Phase 8 (Loth, 1990a).

Intercostal variation is a concern because the phase method standards were derived from the fourth rib, and it is not always possible to be certain of rib position—especially in archaeological cases. Therefore, systematic studies were conducted to quantify differences between ribs 3, 4, and 5 (Loth, 1990b; Loth et al., 1994). Nearly 90% of ribs 3 and 5 from contemporary Whites and TC Blacks were in the same phase, and the rest did not deviate more than 1 phase of the fourth rib. A chi-square test of association applied in a test of ribs 2–9 from both cadaveral and archaeological remains revealed no significant differences (Dudar, 1990).

Tests using blind study protocols have supported the rib phase method's accuracy, ease of application, and negligible interobserver error based on experience (İşcan and Loth, 1986a, 1986b; Loth et al., 1990). The authors also conducted tests comparing age estimates from the rib with those from the pubic symphysis of the same individuals (Loth et al., 1990; İşcan et al., 1992). These tests, conducted on a large sample of modern forensic cases not in the reference population, revealed that the ribs were correctly judged twice as often as the pubis. Overall, for both sexes, the rib was within one phase in nearly 94% of cases with no bias, while the pubis averaged only 57% with a much greater degree of deviation and a pronounced tendency to underage.

## EFFICACY OF THE RIB PHASES ON ARCHAEOLOGICAL REMAINS

Although the rib phases have been successful in modern individuals, there were concerns about applicability to temporally diverse populations. Of the methods discussed here, only the rib phases have not been widely tested on archaeological populations. Therefore, the ribs of the Spitalfields cemetery population and the Tabun 1 and Kebara 2 Neandertals were assessed using the phase method. The following sections present preliminary results of these analyses. The Spitalfields profiles appear for the first time in this chapter; the Neandertal analysis was first reported at the 1992 meeting of the American Association of Physical Anthropologists (Loth, 1992).

### Spitalfields

One of the primary problems in paleodemographic age assessment is uncertainty about the applicability of techniques whose standards are based on people who died as recently as the 1980s. Although there is no sure way of documenting the ages of prehistoric remains or those from societies without writing, we are occasionally afforded the opportunity to go back hundreds of years through the excavation of cemeteries that have good church records. The Spitalfields sample is an excellent example of this. According to Theya Molleson, curator of these remains (personal communication), Spitalfields is a London cemetery population (of French Huguenots) dating from the 16th to 18th centuries with church documentation of dates of birth and death, and is currently housed at the Museum of Natural History, London.

The analysis was carried out (by S. R. Loth) using only the ribs or rib fragments without access to the rest of the skeleton or knowledge of their gender or actual age. The ribs had been painstakingly separated from the rest of the bones and placed in plastic bags (identified only with case numbers) by the museum staff. Because the rib phases are sex specific, the investigator attempted to ascertain sex morphologically from the ribs. She was found to have achieved 85% accuracy with no bias when the records were compared by Molleson.

This preliminary report presents a simple comparison and explanation of male and female demographic profiles constructed using the best age estimates from the rib and the actual profile based on church records. A more detailed breakdown and analysis of the results is underway.

A total of 111 cases were deemed adequately intact for this analysis, even if rib position could not be determined exactly in some cases. Individuals below the age of 20 ($N$=15) were all classified as such, and of these, all who had not reached skeletal maturity at this site were correctly identified. The remaining adults (aged 20 years and older) were included in the histograms in Figures 15-2 and 15-3. Males ($N$=46) and females ($N$=49) were analyzed separately using the appropriate sex-specific standards.

Males were slightly, but consistently, underaged—the added individuals in the first two age intervals in Figure 15-2 were actually older males that conformed with standards for younger ones. Overaging was relatively infrequent and equaled, but never surpassed, underaging in the third and fourth intervals. Interestingly, the phenomenon was limited to only those intervals covering the 43–64-year age range. The age intervals used in the histograms were slightly expanded from the 95% confidence intervals of the original rib standards to cover the small gaps where they were not continuous (see Loth and İşcan, 1989). As Figure 15-2 indicates, the discrepancy between the actual

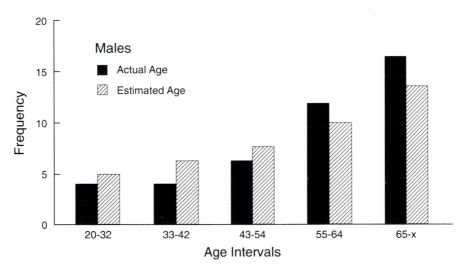

**Figure 15-2** Actual age distribution of the Spitalfields males compared with profile estimated from the rib.

age distribution of the males and that obtained from the rib phases averaged about two individuals per interval. Overall, the rib estimates yielded a fairly good approximation of the range and distribution of the Spitalfields sample.

The consistent underaging may reflect temporal or populational differences in the rate of the aging process at this site, because as noted earlier, tests using modern specimens have revealed no bias in either direction and the best results were obtained in the oldest and youngest phases (Loth *et al.*, 1990). One source of known error in the present sample was the effects of disease, however this contributed to overaging. Where overaging did occur, a number of these specimens were later noted to be suffering from what Molleson diagnosed as diffuse idiopathic skeletal hypertosis (commonly known as DISH disease). This gives the ribs the appearance of extreme old age because it produces extensive ossification of the costochondral junction and costal cartilage. Time constraints limited Loth to re-examining only a few of the aberrant specimens, but while those were eliminated from this analysis, the remainder contributed to the results presented.

Females showed much more variability than males. Many failed to show the degree of morphological progression expected at a given age. Interestingly, as Figure 15-3 clearly illustrates, the most problematic ages (33–58) are those covered by Phases 5 and 6. These phases also exhibited the most variation in the modern reference and test samples.

Another source of error was mis-sexing. Of the six females classified as males, half were incorrectly aged by more than one phase. The remaining three were correctly assigned. The effect was hardly noticeable in males—five out of seven males assessed as females were aged exactly, and the remaining two were within one phase. Males fared considerably better overall including the fact that only one male was underaged into the under 20 group while this was the case for four females.

As mentioned earlier, underaging may be traced in part to the fact that maturity was reached at later ages several hundred years in the past. One must also consider that in Britain the average age of menarche is, even today, slightly older than in the United States (Tanner, 1962). Lovejoy *et al.* (1985b) suggested that error tends to be in the direction of underaging, because the pace of skeletal change is more likely to be slower than the rate of chronological aging. In this particular case, another consideration is the investigator's observation that although there was obvious thinning, the bones of many older individuals "felt" more firm and solid than similarly aged contemporary Whites. This becomes a factor because the criterion of bone quality is an important and sensitive age marker in modern Whites. For numerous specimens, notations such as "rib looks Phase 8, but feels younger" were made during age estimation indicating that the texture and density of the bone make it feel younger than it looks. When such conflicting observations occur with modern ribs, the authors' experience has shown that the firmness of the bone is significant and justifies assigning a younger phase despite older morphology. However, the results of this analysis indicate that this strategy should not be used on archaeological specimens. On the other hand, there are many cases when a "young looking" rib is very thin and frail. These are

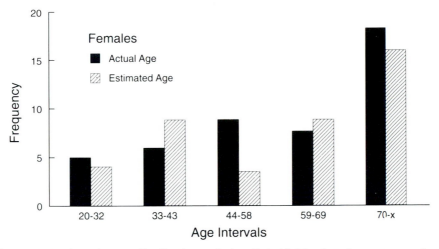

**Figure 15-3**  Actual age distribution of the Spitalfields females compared with profile estimated from the rib.

routinely and almost always correctly assessed as Phase 8 (65–70 and over), in both recent forensic cases and the Spitalfields skeletons. Finally, it must be kept in mind that many of the individuals with "paper-thin" ribs (especially characteristic of modern White females) were among those eliminated from this analysis because of their extremely fragmented condition (they looked like bags of "rib chips") and destruction of the costochondral junction.

There was evidence of intercostal variation. However, it was usually limited to ±1 phase. In this population, the best estimates (used for this preliminary analysis) were obtained primarily from the fourth and fifth ribs (and occasionally the third) — in a number of cases the fifth was best because it often looked older than the fourth. Rib 2 was consistently young, but was included when the other ribs could not be used. Individuals who were judged from an unidentified rib (where the bones were fragmented, but many rib ends were intact) were included only when all available rib ends were clearly in the same phase.

Overall, the results of this first archaeological test of the rib phase method indicate that it can yield accurate age estimates and a good approximation of the demographic profiles of earlier "White" populations. No doubt further testing on other samples will lead to adjustments of the technique if consistent trends are detected. The rib seems to have the rather unique advantage of being most effective in the oldest and youngest adult categories [no problem here with what Masset (1989) refers to as "attraction of the middle"]. The mid-age range was where the rib was least effective here, and in contemporary samples (Loth *et al.*, 1990).

No doubt the results would likely have been influenced by the appearance of other bones (had they been available) and some errors probably would have been avoided in equivocal cases that had a mix of older and younger features. Therefore, as with all skeletal assessments—the authors recommend a careful examination and consideration of the entire skeleton—not just bags of ribs.

## Neandertals and Mousterian Hominids

*Homo sapiens neanderthalensis*—the Neandertal—who lived from about 100,000–35,000 years ago, was the immediate chronological predecessor of modern humans. They were more robust than moderns, but post-cranially were very similar. The most obvious differences were in the long and low skull with heavy brow ridges, very large noses, pronounced alveolar prognathism, lack of menton (in most specimens), and the largest anterior teeth of any hominid. The Neandertal brain was as large if not larger than that of modern man, but was proportioned somewhat differently. Although we know a great deal about these pre-modern humans, leading authorities disagree on the nature of their relationship to *H. sapiens sapiens*. The more popular interpretation of the data is that Neandertals were our direct ancestors or a race of modern humans, while some paleontologists think that Neandertals were not in our phylogenetic line and simply became extinct (see Poirier, 1990).

The Tabun 1 Neandertal is a particularly robust female specimen dating from *ca.* 50,000 years ago (Wolpoff, 1980). Examination (by S. R. Loth) of what Arthur Keith determined to be the fourth rib at the Natural History Museum, London, revealed a striking similarity to the authors' 22-year-old White female Phase 3 prototype specimen shown in Figure 15-4. Assuming a comparable age of maturation, the age of this individual would be about 21–25 years. This is compatible with recent estimates based on dental wear by Wolpoff (personal communication). The superior–inferior dimension of the costochondral junction was close to the mean for modern White females, however, the anterior–posterior dimension was much wider (Trinkaus, 1984; İşcan, 1985).

The Kebara 2 skeleton dates from about 60,000 years ago and was originally designated as a Neandertal (Arensburg *et al.*, 1985; Rak and Arensburg, 1987; Valladas *et al.*, 1987). Some researchers such as Bar-Yosef (1989) and Shea (1990) still classify the Kebara find as Neandertal, but Arensburg (1989:170) now prefers the term "Mousterian hominid" because this extremely robust specimen contains a "mosaic of characteristics . . . found in modern populations [and] also to some extent in Middle Paleolithic or even earlier groups." Casts of the sternal ends of several ribs were comparable to modern males in their late 20s. Figure 15-5 shows the fourth rib cast of Kebara 2 along with the sternal ends of the ribs of two White male forensic cases in the authors' collection chosen for their similarity to the casts — one was 28 years old, the other, 29. This estimate falls into the 25–35-year age range arrived at by Arensburg (personal communication) after studying all the bones recovered. Again, it must be kept in mind that the interpretation of the age-related features is based on years since the cessation of growth at a particular site.

It was interesting to note that although Kebara 2 is described as "so robust that the robust skeletons . . . from Shanidar seem almost gracile by comparison" (Arensburg, 1989:170), this was not reflected in the costochondral dimensions. This may lend some support to Arensburg's opinion that Kebara 2 shows a mix of features and may not be a "true" Neandertal. Unlike Tabun 1,

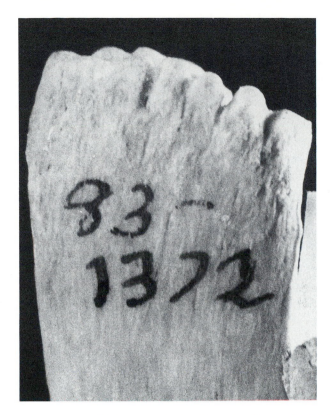

**Figure 15-4**   Recent 22-year-old White female rib end with a striking resemblance to the rib of the Tabun 1 Neandertal.

the fourth rib of Kebara 2 fits comfortably into the range obtained for both dimensions of modern White males. Blacks, on the other hand, have significantly smaller rib dimensions (Loth, 1990a, 1990b).

With all the variation observed between modern populations, it was enlightening to note that these two fossils—Tabun 1 and Kebara 2—exhibit aging patterns identical to modern Whites. It was also somewhat unexpected to find that there was apparently less difference between modern Whites and the few Neandertal ribs examined than between contemporary Whites and Blacks! Obviously, this finding in itself does not settle the question of the phylogenetic status of Neandertals, but it does add to the growing body of the evidence that supports a close relationship to present day humans.

## OTHER CLUES TO AGE

Other parts of the skeleton have been investigated to determine their value as age indicators. Further details on these less commonly used sites can be found in the sources listed earlier in this chapter. Stewart has probably been one of

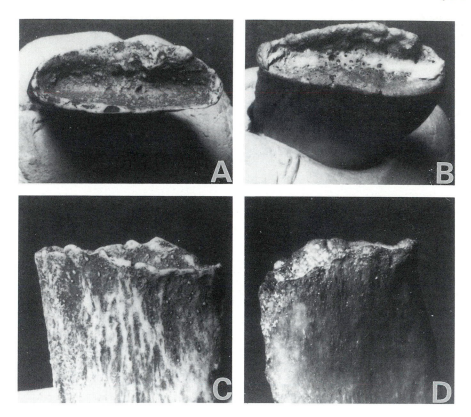

**Figure 15-5**   Comparison of the Kebara 2 specimen (A and C) with recent White males, 29 (B) and 28 (D) years old, respectively.

the most active in combing the skeleton from vertebral osteophytosis to sternal fusion for this purpose (Stewart, 1954, 1958, 1976; McKern and Stewart, 1957). Although no reliable systems based on direct morphological analysis have as yet arisen from skeletal sites other than those already discussed, they can be helpful in assessing the overall aging process and giving a sense of, for example, if an individual is over or under the age of 40, and offering a general indication of wear and tear. Lovejoy *et al.* (1985b) make use of several such of these features in what they term "clinical age"—statistically weighting modifications based on "minor" criteria such as degenerative joint disease and osteophytosis.

## THE UPPER AGE LIMITS OF CURRENT TECHNOLOGY: A SUMMARY

An important concern of researchers in human population biology and aging is longevity. However, attempts to determine the life span of extinct populations are limited to the maximum reaches of age estimation methodology. Prior to the 1980s the "ceiling" for state of the art reliability was the 50s. As can be seen in the synopsis below, we have extended our reach 20 years with revisions of old techniques and the addition of new ones.

## Pubic Symphysis

Terminal phases for the pubic symphysis have been increased from Todd's (1920) "50 and over" years to 60+ for Suchey–Brooks phases. Only Angel (1980) attempted to separate individuals 65 years and older by adding an extra phase (characterized by extreme deterioration) to Todd's system. However, in a recent study we found that only one of nine males and two of four females over age 65 were correctly assigned to the terminal phase (Loth *et al.*, 1990). The gains in range are offset by considerable variability that increases noticeably with age. For example, Suchey–Brooks end-phase morphology is about as likely to be found in a 40-year-old as an 80-year-old. Meindl and associates (1985) calculated an approximate 16-year inaccuracy and bias in the direction of underaging for Todd's phases and reduced that figure to about ten years with their modifications. However, they do not include a "modal age" range for their terminal stage, but indicate that it begins at 40 years, with differentiations that extend it to age 55+.

## Auricular Surface of the Ilium

The terminal modal age for this site is "60+" with an inaccuracy of 7.2 years and a bias (underaging) of about 6 years.

## Cranial Sutures

Even with the improvements offered by Meindl and Lovejoy (1985), similar patterns of suture closure can be found in individuals from 33 to 76 years. They also found completely open sutures persisting to age 50. Their oldest grouping of composite scores (11–14) had a mean age of 56.2 years, and they reported inaccuracy and bias (underaging) of nearly 17 years.

## Dental Wear

Lovejoy's (1985) terminal phase for functional attrition covers 40–50 years for the maxilla and 45–55 years for the mandible. Reported inaccuracy approached 11 years, but bias was very low — only +2 years in the 50–59 range, but climbed to –8.2 for individuals over 60.

## Rib

The rib-phase technique can consistently and accurately separate individuals over 70 years of age. Differences in the early end of the terminal ranges for males (65 years) and females (70 years) result from the differences in the age ranges of the respective samples. The mean ages for Phase 8 (the terminal phase) are 71.5 years for males and 76.2 for females. In the original research,

82% of males and 73% of females classified as Phase 8 (the terminal phase) were over 70. In tests on a new sample, 11 of the 12 specimens over 70 years of age were correctly assigned to Phase 8 (the other rib was underaged by just one phase) (Loth et al., 1990). (In contrast, the same study revealed that only three of 12 pubic symphyses of the same individuals yielded correct assessments— and most were underaged by several phases.) Loth (1993) calculated inaccuracy of six years and bias (underaging) of about five years in the Spitalfields sample.

## OVERVIEW AND FUTURE RESEARCH PERSPECTIVES

It should be kept in mind that age estimation is only one facet of paleodemography. The scope of this discipline encompasses many other characteristics of earlier populations including those of interest to human population biologists, such as fertility, mortality, and longevity. Practitioners, for example, gather data from whatever remains can be found and extrapolate population profiles in an attempt to reconstruct longevity during previous phases of hominid evolution. However, three major factors: the fragmentary nature of the data, in terms of both quantity and quality; the methodological limitations of skeletal biology and stochastic analysis; and as Weiss (1976:371) suggests, the lack of "sound biodemographic theory" have resulted in a "tide of untrammeled speculation."

"Refinements in methods" for aging skeletal materials is one of the ten categories Weiss (1976) contends are necessary to improve paleodemographic evaluation. In that regard, this chapter focusses on the interpretation of age indicators in the actual skeletal remains themselves rather than the speculation about characteristics of the skeletons that are not unearthed. The evaluation and interpretation of age indicators is one matter—implications drawn from them are another. Even Masset (1990) sees improvements in age assessment techniques (introduced since his "Farewell. . .") as *motifs d'espérer*—signs of hope for paleodemographic research, but reiterates his warning that one must acknowledge deficiencies in the available data.

When, for example, no elderly individuals are found, several factors must be considered, since it is widely accepted that the maximum *potential* life span was not shorter in early humans than it is today (Molleson, 1986)—or at least beginning with the *H. erectus* stage (Smith, 1991). It is probably true that few individuals lived to age 70 and beyond. Furthermore, the bones of those who did survive to such extreme ages would be in a relatively weakened condition and thus less likely than those of individuals under 50 to survive the rigors of being subjected to millennia of taphonomic forces. This can also explain, in part, the inability to find the remains of delicate fetal or infant skeletons. This was irrefutably demonstrated by Walker and associates (1988) in a comparison of skeletal remains with cemetery records. Therefore, one can neither assume that extreme old age was never attained nor fault all methodologies for skeletal age assessment.

Since age estimation is more difficult when one is dealing with fossil remains, we must be prepared to glean as much information as possible from every bone because the discovery of complete undamaged skeletons is the exception rather than the rule. For the most part one must deal with fragmentary remains and commingled ossuary sites. In those cases where multi-regional "summary" methods (e.g., Lovejoy *et al.*, 1985b) can not be used, it is necessary to rely on single bone estimates (Ubelaker, 1974). Thus, knowing which site is most reliable becomes paramount.

The ravages of time also take their toll on accuracy. Poor preservation can sometimes mimic the signs of deterioration noted at advanced ages. Osteologists are also hampered by the differential preservation of skeletal remains and may not always have the most definitive or reliable sites for age estimation. Despite the fact that cranial sutures are notoriously unreliable, in many cases this site becomes the primary source for age assessment simply because of the hardiness of the cranium. The reverse is true for the rib. Masset (1990) states that the sternal end of the rib is one of the best indicators of age, but expresses concern that the fragility of this structure may limit its value for paleodemography. On the other hand, extinct hominid forms had more robust skeletons than modern humans, and this might confer better resistance to damage. Even upon attainment of *H. sapiens sapiens* status, the trend of a decline in robusticity appears to have continued gradually over time (Henneberg, 1988). This may be one reason why recently developed aging techniques have a tendency to underage the oldest specimens from even historic archaeological sites. The unexpected firmness of many of the ribs in the Spitalfields sample dating from 200–400 years ago caused a number of individuals to be judged younger than their years. Other evidence, such as a noticeable decrease in sternal rib end dimensions between turn of the (20th) century Terry Collection Blacks and recent forensic cases (despite a secular trend of increasing height) provides ongoing support for Henneberg's (1988) gracilization theory (Loth, 1990a, 1990b).

Another phenomenon that should be addressed is intraskeletal variation among different bones. There are many possible explanations, such as relative functional stress and differential use. There is considerable evidence of bone's sensitivity to mechanical forces (e.g., Murray, 1936; Semine and Damon, 1975; Ortner and Putschar, 1981) that can ultimately affect the registration of age changes (Klepinger *et al.*, 1992). With the possible exception of the first rib, true ribs, for example, are exposed to much less direct stress with less individual variance than the pelvis.

It has been suggested that archaeological populations were more homogeneous than those of today (Howells, 1960; Lovejoy, 1985), yet a range of variation between populations has always existed. This variation has been documented by human population biologists and biological anthropologists studying the aging process in diverse groups (e.g., Beall and Weitz, 1989; Crews, 1990). To further complicate matters, this variation shifts over time and continues to be a problematic source of inaccuracy. Masset (1989) uncovered significant variation in cranial suture closure patterns from one cemetery population to another. We have demonstrated significant variation in the manifestations of the aging process in the sternal end of the rib between the sexes and races.

Brooks and Suchey's (1990:237) contention that because their technique is based on a "large multi-racial sample . . . [with] diverse socioeconomic backgrounds . . . it should be appropriate . . . [for] prehistoric studies," is not sound. In paleodemography, the question of temporal variation is paramount and cannot be simply answered in terms of modern population diversity—one is a horizontal consideration, the other vertical. Similarities in the progression of the morphological manifestations of the aging process are what determines the suitability of a technique for cross-temporal usage—even if the exact rate of these transformations may not be assessable. This is one reason Meindl and Lovejoy (1989) stressed the value of seriating a skeletal assemblage before attaching ages. Masset (1990) finds merit in the work of Lovejoy and associates (especially on the auricular surface), but thinks that they did not go far enough—they merely "recalibrated" methods without really trying to understand the cause of deviations.

The new methodological advances of the 1980s should be seized upon and tested at every opportunity on both new and existing skeletal assemblages and fossil remains. The rib phases are proving to be applicable for modern forensic, historic, and prehistoric remains. They are also effective where accuracy in the assessment of a single individual is needed (such as in fossil man). Furthermore, the technique is easy to apply and boasts little interobserver error. The auricular surface (along with modifications of other "summary age" sites presented by Lovejoy and his teams as noted above) was designed specifically to improve paleodemographic census results at least in part through the practice of seriation. Concerns that mitigate against their use in modern, case by case forensic application (e.g., İşcan and Loth, 1989; Katz and Suchey, 1989; Murray and Murray, 1991) may be balanced by their potential for producing improved mortality profiles for skeletal populations (Lovejoy et al., 1985b). Even our objections to mixed sex/race standards must be tempered by the realization that more generalized prototypes may be advantageous in the many archaeological specimens where even sex cannot be determined with certainty (Weiss, 1972; Krogman and İşcan, 1986).

Although the auricular surface has the advantage of longevity by virtue of its protected position if found in situ, the difficulty of using standards from that site (as well as, for example, from their pubic symphyseal phases) and complexity of the summary method as a whole cannot be ignored. In discussing their pubic symphyseal standards, Meindl and associates (1990) clearly state that easy application and low interobserver error are not among their priorities. However, in our opinion, ease of application and manageable interobserver error are important for two reasons: high interobserver error limits comparability of results, and no matter how "biologically accurate" a method is, its value becomes questionable if few experts besides its developers can use it. There must be balance.

At present, the fossil record can only be interpreted in terms of contemporary documented populations. The question of the accuracy of these standards for past populations still remains and "particular care must be taken before we draw conclusions as to age or rate of maturation in earlier peoples" (Molleson, 1986:96). This does not mean we should ignore the temporal differences that undoubtedly exist, but can not be precisely quantified. It does mean that it can be of value to be able to say that Neandertals (or early "moderns"), for example, follow a similar pattern of aging to that seen today, even if it might not have occurred at the exact same mean age. However, there is no reason to believe that a particular stage of age-related progression does not lie within a similar range. The morphological similarities in themselves may even be phylogenetically significant.

Finally, even though great strides have been made in age-estimation methodology, this does not completely solve the problems of this aspect of demographic assessment. Researchers are still faced with not being able to find the great majority of individuals who resided in a given locale, or knowing if the remains that are found are representative. It is most frustrating to recognize that in many cases we will never be able to document our findings or look up the answers, or even precisely quantify and predict the patterns of temporal, racial, and geographic variation. The words of Acsádi and Nemes-kéri (1970:57) still ring true today: "successful paleodemographic research is subject to methodological conditions seldom met in the past and may not be invariably fulfilled in the future." For now, paleodemography continues to be an exercise in statistical manipulation and stochastic analysis, improved, of course, by each additional find and every new technique for the estimation of age at death from the skeleton. This means that until (and if) remains of the oldest individuals are found, age profiles of ancestral hominid populations must be reconstructed by combining data skeletal biologists have gathered from the fossil record with extrapolations of life span calculated from a growing body of knowledge of the evolutionary relationship between dental development, somatic growth, and the primate life cycle.

In the future, research may be much more fruitful if the paradigm is shifted from symptomology to causality. Beyond quantifying the increase in life span, we must investigate the adaptive and evolutionary significance of protracted postreproductive survival. In developing age-assessment methodology, attention has been focused on the commonalties, yet more answers may be found by concentrating on the differences. Undoubtedly, one of the keys to interpreting the aging process lies in understanding variation and its myriad causes. If the point on the continuum where normal variation ends and true age-related change begins can be discovered, we may, indeed, be able to pinpoint age at death from the skeleton. This knowledge will also go a long way toward elaborating the cause and effect of aging.

## ACKNOWLEDGMENTS

We are very grateful to Theya Molleson of the Museum of Natural History, London, for giving SRL access to the Spitalfields ribs. Robert Kruszynski's assistance in preparation for (with help from L. Scheuer) and during her visit to the museum was very much appreciated. The Spitalfields excavation was made possible through funding from the English Heritage and Nuffield Foundations. We thank also Chris Stringer for the opportunity to examine Tabun 1 at the Museum of Natural History, London, and Baruch Arensburg for preparing and sending casts of the Kebara 2 ribs.

We also appreciate the efforts of Douglas Crews and Ralph Garruto for giving us the opportunity to contribute to this volume. The original rib studies were supported by FAU Sponsored Research grants to MYI and a Smithsonian Institution grant to SRL. SRL appreciates the generosity of Thelma L. Wexler for a grant to cover travel expenses to London, and the hospitality of D. P. Loth and T. Plotz while there.

# REFERENCES

Acsádi, G. and Nemeskéri, J. (1970) *History of Human Life Span and Mortality*. Budapest: Akadémiai Kiadó.

Angel, J. L. (1969) The bases of paleodemography. *American Journal of Physical Anthropology* **30**, 427–437.

Angel, J. L. (1980) Physical anthropology: determining sex, age, and individual features. In: *Mummies, Disease, and Ancient Cultures* (eds Cockburn, A. and Cockburn, E.). Cambridge: Cambridge University Press, pp. 241–257.

Angel, J. L. (1984) Variation in estimating age at death of skeletons. *Collegium Antropologicum* **2**, 163–168.

Angel, J. L., Suchey, J. M., İşcan, M. Y. and Zimmerman, M. R. (1986) Age at death from the skeleton and viscera. In: *Dating and Age Determination in Biological Materials* (eds Zimmerman, M. R. and Angel, J. L.). London: Croom Helm, pp. 179–220.

Arensburg, B. (1989) New skeletal evidence concerning the anatomy of Middle Palaeolithic populations in the Middle East: the Kebara skeleton. In: *The Human Revolution: Behavioural and Biological Perspectives on the Origins of Modern Humans* (eds Mellars, P. and Stringer, C.). Edinburgh: University Press, pp. 165–171.

Arensburg, B., Bar-Yosef, O., Chech, M., Goldberg, P., Laville, H., Meignen, L., Rak, Y., Tchernov, E., Tillier, A. M. and Vandermeersch, B. (1985) Une sépultre neandertalienne dan la grotte de Kébara (Israël). *Compte-Rendus de l'Academie des Sciences, Paris* **300**, 227–230.

Bar-Yosef, O. (1989) Geochronology of the Levantine Middle Paleolithic. In: *The Human Revolution: Behavioural and Biological Perspectives on the Origins of Modern Humans* (eds Mellars, P. and Stringer, C.). Edinburgh: University Press, pp. 589–610.

Beall, C. M. and Weitz, C. A. (1989) The human population of aging. In: *Human Population Biology: A Transdisciplinary Science* (eds Little, M. A. and Haas, J. D.). New York: Oxford University Press, pp. 189–200.

Bedford, M. E., Russell, K. F. and Lovejoy, C. O. (1989) The utility of the auricular surface aging technique. *American Journal of Physical Anthropology* **78**, 190–191 (abstract).

Bocquet-Appel, J. P. and Masset, C. (1982) Farewell to paleodemography. *Journal of Human Evolution* **11**, 321–333.

Bogin, B. (1988) *Patterns of Human Growth*. Cambridge: Cambridge University Press.

Borkan, G. A. (1986) Biological age assessment in adulthood. In: *The Biology of Human Ageing* (eds Bittles, A. H. and Collins, K. J.). Cambridge: Cambridge University Press, pp. 81–94.

Brace, C. L. (1991) *The Stages of Human Evolution*. Englewood Cliffs, NJ: Prentice-Hall.

Brooks, S. T. (1955) Skeletal age at death: reliability of cranial and pubic age indicators. *American Journal of Physical Anthropology* **13**, 567–597.

Brooks, S. T. and Suchey, J. M. (1990) Skeletal age determination based on the os pubis: a comparison of the Acsádi–Nemeskéri and Suchey–Brooks methods. *Human Evolution* **5**, 227–238.

Brothwell, D. R. (1981) *Digging Up Bones*. Ithaca: Cornell University Press.

Brothwell, D. R. (1989) The relationship of tooth wear to aging. In: *Age Markers in the Human Skeleton* (ed. İşcan, M. Y.). Springfield, IL.: Charles C. Thomas, pp. 303–316.

Crews, D. E. (1990) Anthropological issues in biological gerontology. In: *Anthropology and Aging: Comprehensive Reviews* (eds Rubinstein, R. L. with Keith, J., Shenk, D. and Wieland, D.). Dordrecht: Kluwer, pp. 11–38.

Dudar, J. C. (1990) An investigation of intercostal variation in adult sternal rib ends. *Canadian Society of Forensic Science Journal* **23**, 139 (abstract).

Dudar, J. C. (1992) An evaluation of the sternal rib end age at death estimation technique. *American Academy of Forensic Sciences Program*, 162 (abstract).

Epker, B. N., Kelin, M. and Frost, H. M. (1965) Magnitude and location of cortical bone loss in human rib with aging. *Clinical Orthopedics* **41**, 198–203.

Gilbert, B. M. and McKern, T. W. (1973) A method for aging the female os pubis. *American Journal of Physical Anthropology* **38**, 31–38.

Henneberg, M. (1988) Decrease in human skull size in the Holocene. *Human Biology* **60**, 395–405.

Howells, W. W. (1960) Discussion of "Vital statistics in prehistoric population as determined from archaeological data" by H. Vallois. In: *The Application of Quantitative Methods in Archaeology* (eds Heizer, R. F. and Cook, S. F.). Chicago: Viking Fund Publications 28, Quadrangle Books, pp. 186–222.

İşcan, M. Y. (1985) Osteometric analysis of sexual dimorphism in the sternal end of the rib. *Journal of Forensic Sciences* **30**, 1090–1099.

İşcan, M. Y. (ed.) (1989) *Age Markers in the Human Skeleton*. Springfield, IL: Charles C. Thomas.

İşcan, M. Y. (1990) A comparison of techniques on the determination of race, sex and stature from the Terry and Hamann–Todd Collections. In: *Skeletal Attribution of Race: Methods for Forensic Anthropology* (eds Gill, G. W. and Rhine, J. S.). Albuquerque: University of New Mexico, Maxwell Museum of Anthropology Papers No. 4. pp. 73–81.

İşcan, M. Y. and Loth, S. R. (1986a) Determination of age from the sternal rib in white males: a test of the phase method. *Journal of Forensic Sciences* **31**, 122–132.

İşcan, M. Y. and Loth, S. R. (1986b) Determination of age from the sternal rib in white females: a test of the phase method. *Journal of Forensic Sciences* **31**, 990–999.

İşcan, M. Y. and Loth, S. R. (1989) Osteological manifestations of age in adults. In: *Reconstruction of Life from the Skeleton* (eds İşcan, M. Y. and Kennedy, K. A. R.). New York: A. R. Liss, pp. 23–40.

İşcan, M. Y., Loth, S. R. and Wright, R. K. (1984a) Age estimation from the rib by phase analysis: white males. *Journal of Forensic Sciences* **29**, 1094–1104.

İşcan, M. Y., Loth, S. R. and Wright, R. K. (1984b) Metamorphosis at the sternal rib end: a new method to estimate age at death in white males. *American Journal of Physical Anthropology* **65**, 147–156.

İşcan, M. Y., Loth, S. R. and Wright, R. K. (1985) Age estimation from the rib by phase analysis: white females. *Journal of Forensic Sciences* **30**, 853–863.

İşcan, M. Y., Loth, S. R. and Wright, R. K. (1987) Racial variation in the sternal extremity of the rib and its effect on age determination. *Journal of Forensic Sciences* **32**, 452–466.

İşcan, M. Y., Loth, S. R. and Scheuerman, H. S. (1992) Age assessment from the sternal end of the rib and pubic symphysis. *Anthropologie* **30**, 41–44.

Katz, D. and Suchey, J. M. (1986) Age determination of the male os pubis. *American Journal of Physical Anthropology* **69**, 427–435.

Katz, D. and Suchey, J. M. (1989) Race differences in pubic symphyseal aging patterns in the male. *American Journal of Physical Anthropology* **80**, 167–172.

Klepinger, L. L., Katz, D., Micozzi, M. S. and Carroll, L. (1992) Evaluation of cast methods for estimating age from the os pubis. *Journal of Forensic Sciences* **37**, 763–770.

Krogman, W. M. and İşcan, M. Y. (1986) *The Human Skeleton in Forensic Medicine.* Springfield, IL: Charles C. Thomas.

Loth, S. R. (1990a) *A comparative analysis of the manifestations of age, sex and race in the sternal extremity of the rib: a consideration of human skeletal variation.* M.A. thesis, Florida Atlantic University, Boca Raton.

Loth, S. R. (1990b) A comparative analysis of the ribs of Terry Collection blacks. *Adli Tip Dergisi [Journal of Forensic Medicine],* Istanbul **6**, 119–127.

Loth, S. R. (1992) Age assessment from the sternal end of the rib in the Tabun I and Kebara 2 Neandertals. *American Journal of Physical Anthropology* **14** (Suppl.), 113 (abstract).

Loth, S. R. (1993) Age assessment of the Spitalfields cemetery population based on rib phase analysis. *American Journal of Physical Anthropology* **16** (Suppl.), 135 (abstract).

Loth, S. R. and İşcan, M. Y. (1989) Morphological assessment of age in the adult: the thoracic region. In: *Age Markers in the Human Skeleton* (ed. İşcan, M. Y.). Springfield, IL: Charles C. Thomas, pp. 105–136.

Loth, S. R. and İşcan, M. Y. (1991) Discriminant function assessment of race from the sternal end of the rib. *American Journal of Physical Anthropology* **12** (Suppl.), 119 (abstract).

Loth, S. R., İşcan, M. Y. and Scheuerman, E. H. (1990) A systematic comparison of the accuracy of age estimation from the rib and pubis. *American Journal of Physical Anthropology* **81**, 260 (abstract).

Loth, S. R., İşcan, M. Y. and Scheuerman, E. H. (1994) Intercoastal variation at the sternal end of the rib. *Forensic Science International* **64** (in press).

Lovejoy, C. O. (1985) Dental wear in the Libben population: its functional pattern and role in the determination of adult skeletal age at death. *American Journal of Physical Anthropology* **68**, 47–56.

Lovejoy, C. O., Meindl, R. S, Pryzbeck, T. R. and Mensforth, R. P. (1985a) Chronological metamorphosis of the auricular surface of the ilium: a new method for the determination of age at death. *American Journal of Physical Anthropology* **68**, 15–28.

Lovejoy, C. O., Meindl, R. S., Mensforth, R. P. and Barton, T. J. (1985b) Multifactorial determination of skeletal age at death: a new method with blind tests of its accuracy. *American Journal of Physical Anthropology* **68**, 1–14.

Masset, C. (1989) Age estimation on the basis of cranial sutures. In: *Age Markers in the Human Skeleton* (ed. İşcan, M. Y.) Springfield, IL: Charles C. Thomas, pp. 71–103.

Masset, C. (1990) Ou en est la paléodémographie? *Bulletin et Mémoires de la Société d'Anthropologie de Paris* **2**, 109–122.

McKern, T. W. and Stewart, T. D. (1957) *Skeletal Age Changes in Young American Males. Analysed from the Standpoint of Age Identification*. Environmental Protection Research Division (Quartermaster Research and Development Center, US Army, Natick, MA), Technical Report No. EP-45.

Meindl, R. S. and Lovejoy, C. O. (1985) Ectocranial suture closure: a revised method for the determination of skeletal age at death and blind tests of its accuracy. *American Journal of Physical Anthropology* **68**, 57–66.

Meindl, R. S. and Lovejoy, C. O. (1989) Age changes in the pelvis: implications for paleodemography. In: *Age Markers in the Human Skeleton* (ed. İşcan, M. Y.) Springfield: Charles C. Thomas, pp. 137–168.

Meindl, R. S., Lovejoy, C. O., Mensforth, R. P. and Walker, R. A. (1985) A revised method of age determination using the os pubis, with a review and tests of accuracy of other current methods of pubis symphyseal ageing. *American Journal of Physical Anthropology* **68**, 29–45.

Meindl, R. S., Russell, K. F. and Lovejoy, C. O. (1990) Reliability of age at death in the Hamann–Todd Collection: validity of subselection procedures used in blind tests of the summary age technique. *American Journal of Physical Anthropology* **83**, 349–357.

Mensforth, R. P. (1990) Paleodemography of Carlston Annis (Bt-5) Late Archaic skeletal population. *American Journal of Physical Anthropology* **82**, 81–99.

Miles, A. E. W. (1962) Assessment of the ages of a population of Anglo-Saxons from their dentitions. *Proceedings of the Royal Society of Medicine* **55**, 881–886.

Molleson, T. (1986) Skeletal age and paleodemography. In: *The Biology of Human Ageing* (eds Bittles, A. H. and Collins, K. J.) Cambridge: Cambridge University Press, pp. 95–118.

Molnar, S. (1971) Human tooth wear, tooth function and cultural variability. *American Journal of Physical Anthropology* **34**, 175–190.

Murphy, T. (1959) The changing pattern of dentine exposure in human tooth attrition. *American Journal of Physical Anthropology* **17**, 167–178.

Murray, K. A. and Murray, T. (1991) A test of the auricular surface aging technique. *Journal of Forensic Sciences* **36**, 1162–1169.

Murray, P. D. F. (1936) *Bones*. Cambridge: Cambridge University Press.

Nemeskéri, J., Harsányi, L. and Acsádi, G. (1960) Methoden zur diagnose des lebensalters von skelettfunden. *Anthropologischer Anzeiger* **24**, 70–95.

Nowell, G. W. (1978) An evaluation of the Miles method of ageing using the Tepe Hissar dental sample. *American Journal of Physical Anthropology* **49**, 261–276.

Ortner, D. J. and Putschar, W. G. J. (1981) *Identification of Pathological Conditions in Human Skeletal Remains*. Washington, DC: Smithsonian Institution Press.

Pfeiffer, S. (1985) Comparison of adult age estimation techniques, using an ossuary sample. *Canadian Review of Physical Anthropology* **4**, 13–17.

Poirier, F. E. (1990) *Understanding Human Evolution*. Englewood Cliffs, NJ: Prentice Hall.

Rak, Y. and Aresberg, B. (1987) Kebara 2 Neandertal pelvis: first look at a complete inlet. *American Journal of Physical Anthropology* **73**, 227–231.

Schranz, D. (1959) Age determination from the internal structure of the humerus. *American Journal of Physical Anthropology* **17**, 273–278.

Semine, A. A. and Damon, A. (1975) Costochondral ossification and aging in five populations. *Human Biology* **47**, 101–116.

Shea, J. J. (1990) A new perspective on Neandertals from the Levantine Mousterian. *AnthroQuest* (L. S. B. Leakey Foundation) pp. 14–18.

Singer, R. (1953) Estimation of age from cranial suture closure: a report on its unreliability. *Journal of Forensic Medicine* **1**, 52–59.

Singer, R. (1960) Discussion of "Vital statistics in prehistoric population as determined from archaeological data" by H. Vallois. In: *The Application of Quantitative Methods in Archaeology* (eds Heizer, R. F. and Cook, S. F.). Chicago: Viking Fund Publications 28, Quadrangle Books, pp. 186–222.

Smith, B. H. (1991) Dental development and the evolution of life history in Hominidae. *American Journal of Physical Anthropology* **86**, 157–174.

Smith, F. H. and Spencer, F. (eds) (1984) *The Origins of Modern Humans*. New York: Alan R. Liss.

Stewart, T. D. (1954) Metamorphosis of the joints of the sternum in relation to age changes in other bones. *American Journal of Physical Anthropology* **12**, 519–536.

Stewart, T. D. (1958) The rate of development of vertebral osteoarthritis in American whites and its significance in skeletal age identification. *Leech* **28**, 114–151.

Stewart, T. D. (1976) Sacro-iliac osteophytosis. *American Journal of Physical Anthropology* **44**, 210 (abstract).

Tanner, J. M. (1962) *Growth at Adolescence*. Oxford: Blackwell Scientific Publications.

Todd, T. W. (1920) Age changes in the pubic bone: I. The male white pubis. *American Journal of Physical Anthropology* **3**, 285–334.

Todd, T. W. and Lyon, D. W., Jr (1924) Endocranial suture closure, its progress and age relationship: Part I. Adult males of white stock. *American Journal of Physical Anthropology* **7**, 325–384.

Todd, T. W. and Lyon, D. W., Jr (1925) Cranial suture closure, its progress and age relationship: Part II. Ectocranial closure in adult males of white stock. *American Journal of Physical Anthropology* **8**, 23–45.

Trinkaus, E. (1984) Western Asia. In: *The Origins of Modern Humans* (eds Smith, F. H. and Spencer, F.). New York: Alan R. Liss, pp. 251–294.

Trinkaus, E. and Thompson, D. D. (1987) Femoral diaphyseal histomorphometric age determinations for the Shanidar 3, 4, 5, and 6 Neandertals and Neandertal longevity. *American Journal of Physical Anthropology* **72**, 123–129.

Ubelaker, D. H. (1989) *Human Skeletal Remains*. Washington, DC: Taraxacum.

Ubelaker, D. H. (1974) *Reconstruction of Demographic Profiles from Ossuary Skeletal Samples*. Washington, DC: Smithsonian Institution Press.

Valladas, H., Joron, J. L., Valladas, B., Arensburg, B., Bar-Yosef, O., Belfer-Cohen, A., Goldberg, P., Laville, H., Meignen, L., Rak, Y., Tchernov, E., Tillier, A. M. and Vandermeersch, B. (1987) Thermoluminescence dates for the Neanderthal burial site at Kebara in Israel. *Nature* **330**, 159–160.

Vallois, H. V. (1960) Vital statistics in prehistoric population as determined from archaeological data. In: *The Application of Quantitative Methods in Archaeology* (eds Heizer, R. F. and Cook, S. F.). Chicago: Viking Fund Publications 28, Quadrangle Books, pp. 186–204.

Walker, P. L., Johnson, J. R. and Lambert, P. M. (1988) Age and sex biases in the preservation of human skeletal remains. *American Journal of Physical Anthropology* **76**, 183–188.

Weidenreich, F. (1939) The duration of life of fossil man in China and the pathological lesions found in his skeleton. *Chinese Medical Journal* **55**, 34–44.

Weiss, K. M. (1972) On the systematic bias in skeletal sexing. *American Journal of Physical Anthropology* **37**, 239–250.

Weiss, K. M. (1976) Demographic theory and anthropological inference. *Annual Reviews of Anthropology* **5**, 351–381.

Wolpoff, M. (1980) *Paleoanthropology*. New York: Alfred A. Knopf.

Workshop of European Anthropologists (1980) Recommendations for age and sex diagnosis of skeletons. *Journal of Human Evolution* **9**, 517–549.

# 16

# Role of the National Institute on Aging

PHYLLIS B. EVELETH

## INTRODUCTION

The National Institute on Aging (NIA) of the National Institutes of Health (NIH) conducts and supports biomedical and behavioral research and research training related to the aging process, and to diseases and other special problems and needs of older people. This is done through various funding mechanisms (research project grants, career development awards and contracts) to universities and other research institutions, as well as in NIA laboratories and clinics in Bethesda and Baltimore, Maryland. NIA's programs are dedicated to a broad range of aging research encompassing basic, clinical, behavioral, social, epidemiological, and demographic studies. There is also some applied research on interventions in common problems, such as urinary incontinence, falls, and osteoporosis, and problems of older drivers. Integrative and cross-disciplinary approaches to health problems are encouraged. Of equal importance is the role the NIA plays in the support of training and career development of research gerontologists and geriatricians. Details of all programs of the NIA are given in *NIH Extramural Programs: Funding for Research and Research Training* (NIH, 1992). This chapter contains information only in those areas that are of potential interest for anthropologists.

The worldwide increase in the proportion of the population in the upper age groups is the success story of the 20th century. The projections for the 21st century make it imperative to expand research in aging in order to meet the health demands of the unprecedented increase in the older population. It follows that dissemination and application of research results to meet health and societal requirements is also needed. Moreover, the increase in numbers of older people is not limited to the industrialized nations. It is believed that the population growth rate for persons 55 years and over is three times as high in developing as in developed countries (Kinsella, 1988; Kinsella and Taeuber, 1992). However, because of the burden of numerous other health issues in developing countries, the problems of an aging population have not yet received much attention.

It is important to examine hereditary and environmental risk factors that may be managed to reduce the risk of degenerative conditions and to optimize the potential for retaining functional ability at older ages. This requires a developmental approach to gene–environmental interactions across the life span, and encompasses behavioral and social factors that are important to well-being.

## INTERNATIONAL ACTIVITIES

The NIA supports and participates in a wide range of international activities (NIH, 1990). Among these are cross-national studies to identify risk factors for various diseases and their interactions. It is recognized that differences among populations and groups in disease prevalence might be partially explained, at least, by cultural, environmental, or genetic differences.

### WHO Special Program for Research on Aging

The NIA and World Health Organization (WHO) are collaborating in four priority scientific areas: age-associated dementias, osteoporosis, determinants of healthy aging, and immune function. A cross-national study is planned to ascertain the incidence of hip fractures in participating countries, to identify risk factors for hip fractures and for the decrease of bone mass, and to determine the distribution of bone density in different populations by race, age, and sex.

### Honolulu Heart Study Extension

NIA has established an Asia-Pacific Office of the Epidemiology, Demography, and Biometry Program to conduct research on dementia and aging among the participants in the long-running Honolulu Heart Study that has been sponsored by the National Heart, Lung and Blood Institute. The sample consists of approximately 6,000 Japanese–American men, aged 70–90 years, living in Hawaii. Japanese researchers are planning to conduct parallel studies in Japan.

### International Data Base on Aging

This data base, which is available to researchers studying aging, includes extensive tables of demographic and sociological information on aging popula-tions in 42 countries. The Center for International Research of the US Bureau of Census, working with the NIA, has compiled and will distribute the data upon request. The data also are available from the University of Michigan's National Archive for Computerized Data on Aging.

## BIOLOGY OF AGING

This is one of four programs within the NIA and includes areas ranging from molecular biology to immunology to nutrition and metabolism. The overall objectives of the program are related to understanding normal functions and alterations in them that can be induced by interaction with the environment and disease processes as aging proceeds. Both normal and abnormal changes in age-related disease states are included.

## Genetics

Specific areas of interest are in isolating and identifying the molecular basis for age-related changes and for onset of age-related diseases. Research in classical and evolutionary genetics of aging and senescence includes identification of longevity assurance genes and cellular senescence genes.

## Immunology

The program supports research on the decline of the immune potential with age, as manifested by decreases in antibody formation, cell-mediated immunity and immune surveillance against tumors. There is interest in the immune response to infectious agents, vaccines, tumors, and also studies of autoimmunity and immunopathology in senescence.

## Endocrinology

The aging female and male reproductive systems are areas in need of research. The processes leading to menopause are important, including the effects of estrogen loss on osteoporosis, cardiovascular disease and dementia and the long-term effects of estrogen replacement in women and growth hormone in men and women.

## Nutrition

In the area of nutrition there is interest in nutrient requirements in old age and the relationships that may exist between dietary components and chronic diseases of old age. Current dietary recommendations are based upon research on younger people and may not necessarily apply to individuals over 65 years. Aging changes in energy metabolism related to thermogenesis, glycolysis, and body composition is another area of importance. The interaction of ethnic group, gender, and age presents additional opportunities for study in the relationship of body composition, obesity, and chronic diseases. There is controversy over whether the positive association of obesity with mortality or morbidity declines after 50 years of age. Another controversial area is whether low body weight in old age is a risk factor for mortality. Studies are needed on adult-onset diabetes and risk factors, such as fat distribution in different ethnic groups, and causes of these differences in the development and extent of complications.

## Caloric Restriction

It has been known for years that caloric restriction without malnutrition extends life and slows the rate of aging in laboratory animals. It is not known whether aging processes are delayed in primates on low-calorie diets, although NIA is currently carrying out such a study on rhesus and squirrel monkeys. There is interest in supporting more research from institutions outside NIH in this area.

## Gender Differences

Gender differences in longevity, disease patterns, and functioning of older men and women continue to be emphasized by both this program and the Behavioral and Social Research Program. It is not clear that specific risk factors have the same importance for older women as for older men or whether there are different risk factors involved. In addition, studies are sought about biological and psychological consequences of menopause and the effects of menopause on risk factors.

## Animal Models

In addition, the Biology of Aging Program provides aging animals to investigators at a reasonable cost and explores the development of new animal models. Currently, NIA supports rat, mouse and non-human primate colonies, including a rodent colony that is calorically restricted. A biomarkers of aging initiative has been underway to develop and test biomarkers that can be used in assessing future interventions in the aging process.

## GERIATRICS

This program supports research on clinical problems that occur predominantly among older persons or that are associated with increased morbidity and mortality in older people. Areas of interest include cardiovascular–pulmonary diseases, infectious diseases, osteoporosis, digestive diseases, and physical function and performance. Age-related cardiovascular changes and changes in risk factors with age, especially in different ethnic groups, are areas of interest.

## Physical Performance

Questions about how aging affects human adaptability and responses to both acute and long-term physical activity need to be answered. There is some preliminary evidence that long-term training in older individuals is successful in promoting health, reducing bone loss, and improving strength and balance. An NIA program studying various interventions to improve functional capacity in old and frail persons is collecting information at several sites across the country. NIA objectives are not only to increase length of life, but also quality of life throughout the entire life span.

## Osteoporosis

Due to its public health importance in old age, osteoporosis and associated fractures are areas of major emphasis. Interest is in all aspects: bone loss, falls, prevention, and interventions. Research is encouraged in both Type I and Type II osteoporosis—whether they have different etiological mechanisms and risk factors, since prevalence differs by gender and age. There are few longitudinal studies of male osteoporosis and little is known about differences and similarities between the genders. Some recognized racial differences may be explored to suggest mechanistic explanations of Type II osteoporosis. There also is interest in the severity and progression of chronic degenerative conditions, such as diabetes and osteoporosis in different minority populations.

## BEHAVIORAL AND SOCIAL RESEARCH

This program focuses on understanding how psychological and social aging interact with biomedical aging processes, how older people relate to social institutions, such as the family and health care systems, and the antecedents and consequences of demographic changes in the population. It encourages comparisons among persons of different racial, cultural, and socioeconomic backgrounds, and among countries that vary in life style and standard of living. Areas of special interest for anthropologists are how health behaviors and life styles lead to particular health outcomes, on dynamic inter-relationships between health behaviors and aging, and on psychosocial and physiological aspects of aging among women, including studies on menopause and cross-cultural perspectives of menopause.

## Demography

Demographic research is encouraged on the changing structure of societies, on international comparisons, world patterns of migration, and urban–rural population differences. A major focus is the study of the effects of population aging in both industrialized and developing countries. The impact of population aging on the infrastructure and economy of third world countries needs to be examined, as well as determinants of labor force participation among older workers employed in physical labor and the financing of health care systems. The International Database on Aging provides an important framework for comparative studies (see p. 427).

NIA supports some major data resources, such as the National Long-Term Care Survey, the National Nursing Home Followup Survey, the Baltimore Longitudinal Study of Aging, the Health and Retirement Survey, and part of the Panel Study of Income Dynamics. These longitudinal surveys provide data for national forecasting of the nature, levels, and changes over time of the health and care needs of older persons.

## Human Factors

Interest in human factors research on older people relates design of environments (residences and devices) to the skills, activities, and functioning of older people. The objective of this area is to generate a knowledge base in human engineering that permits improving environments, tasks, and equipment in order to increase independence in older people. One special area of interest deals with older drivers.

# NEUROSCIENCE AND NEUROPSYCHOLOGY OF AGING

## Dementias

Alzheimer's disease and other dementias of aging continue to be the centerpiece of this program. The dementias of later life are the most common cause of cognitive disorder and are projected to become increasingly important as the number of older people in the population grows. There is a need for cross-national and cross-cultural studies on the incidence and prevalence of age-related dementias to examine differences with geographic, genetic, ethnic, and socioeconomic characteristics. There is interest in whether incidence and prevalence rates vary with gender, education, dietary habits, and trauma. Familial–genetic aspects of Alzheimer's disease should be investigated through common environment and pedigree studies with establishment of family registries. Isolated communities which have a high degree of consanguinity may be useful in studies of familial Alzheimer's disease. In addition to heredity, external factors, such as toxins or infections, may play a role. A major aim is to develop tests of cognitive function that are unbiased by culture, education, or native language.

## Sleep Disorders

Sleep disturbances affect a large number of older people. It is not known whether these disorders reflect underlying pathologies or normal maturation of the aging nervous system, nor whether psychosocial and environmental conditions contribute to these changes.

In sum, the research at the NIA is targeted toward improving and maintaining the health of older people. Knowledge about the basic nature of aging processes is intended to improve individual lives and society generally. Unprecedented demographic shifts in the population will have a major impact on society in the 21st century when an even greater increase in population aging will occur. Individual life expectancy may continue to increase and, thanks to modern science, prevalence of some diseases will change. Moreover, the way in which an individual lives, his or her culture and habits, may assume an even greater role in health in the future than it does now.


## GRANT APPLICATION PROCESS

There are many mechanisms at the NIH to support research and research training, the most common being the research project grant (R01). Other common mechanisms are program project and center grants, conference grants, institutional training grants, postdoctoral fellowships, and various career development awards. A detailed application must be submitted which is then referred to an initial review group (study section) for technical and scientific review and to an institute, division, or center for possible funding. A second review by the council or advisory board of the institute occurs to consider the appropriateness of the scientific review and the relevancy of the proposed research to the goals of the institute. Advance planning is needed since the entire process from receipt of application to award takes approximately ten months (fellowships, six months). There are specific deadlines three times during the year.

There are several articles by NIH staff that give helpful advice on preparation of grant applications (Eaves, 1984; Novello, 1985; Murphy and Dean, 1986) and inform the community about the peer review process (Henley, 1977; Eaves, 1982). Reprints of these papers are available from the Office of Grants Inquiries, NIH, Westwood Building, Room 449, Bethesda, Maryland, 20892. Institute staff can also be consulted about grant mechanisms, program interests, budgets, and preparing the application itself.

Scientific areas of special interest to the NIA change as the science changes. These are made known through program announcements and requests for applications published in the *NIH Guide to Grants and Contracts*. A compilation of these announcements is available from the Office of Extramural Affairs, NIA, Gateway Building, Suite 2C218, Bethesda, Maryland 20892.

In the past, anthropologists have been successful applicants at the NIA and NIH. Although no current data are available, in 1978 NIH awarded 37 grants to principal investigators who were biological anthropologists (Eveleth, 1980). This represented almost 6% of the membership of the American Association of Physical Anthropologists. It can be assumed that many more were supported as co-investigators on research projects, a category that NIH does not track. At that time the NIA had no grants to anthropologists. However, last year there were 10–12. This is a reflection of the significant growth of the Institute and wider program interests.


## REFERENCES

Eaves, G. N. (1982) Review of research grant applications at the National Institute of Health. Proceedings from *Workshop on Thinking and Writing Clearly*, pp. 3–11.

Eaves, G. N. (1984) Preparation of the research-grant application: Opportunities and pitfalls. *Grants Magazine* **7**, 151–157.

Eveleth, P. B. (1980) Physical anthropology and research programs at the National Institutes of Health. *American Journal of Physical Anthropology* **54**, 573–577.

Henley, C. (1977) Peer review of research grant applications at the National Institute of Health. *Federation Proceedings* **36**, 2066–2068, 2186–2190, 2335–2338.

Kinsella, K. (1988) *Aging in the Third World.* Washington, DC: US Department of Commerce, Bureau of the Census.

Kinsella, K. and Taeuber, C. M. (1992) *An Aging World II.* Washington, DC: US Department of Commerce, Bureau of the Census.

Murphy, D. G. and Dean, D. J. (1986) Biomedical research and research training support by the National Institutes of Health. *Nutrition International* **2**, 38–44.

NIH (1990) *Annual Report of International Activities, Fiscal Year 1989.* NIH publication no. 90–62.

NIH (1992) *NIH/ADAMHA Extramural Programs: Funding for Research and Research Training.* US Department of Health and Human Services, NIH publication no. 91–33.

Novello, A. C. (1985) The peer review process: how to prepare research grant applications to the NIH. *Mineral Electrolyte Metabolism* **11**, 281–286.

# Epilogue: Human Aging—The Scientific Relevance of Transdisciplinary Approaches

## RALPH M. GARRUTO AND DOUGLAS E. CREWS

The chapters in this volume clearly illustrate that biological anthropologists and human population biologists have the potential to build on their already substantial contributions to the field of aging research and to make greater (even landmark) contributions to the field in years to come. The common challenge facing biological anthropologists and gerontologists is to bridge the gap between reductionist biological and medical models, and broader-scale ecological, evolutionary, and sociocultural research designs, which dramatically influence both the progression and spread of disease and the aging process *per se*. However, if this potential is to materialize, it is imperative that biological anthropologists seek to understand not only population biology, but also basic functional processes at the cellular and molecular level. By combining basic biology with epidemiological, evolutionary and sociocultural perspectives, in both field and laboratory settings, a synthesis between biological anthropology and gerontology will truly occur. Biological anthropologists and human population biologists can no longer assume an isolated scientific role in unravelling the mysteries of aging. Instead, they must utilize their expertise and multi-disciplinary knowledge in conjunction with biomedical scientists from other disciplines.

It is, therefore, not surprising that two of the proposed scientific initiatives in the National Institutes of Health Strategic Plan, a vision designed to catapult health research into the 21st century, include population based studies (Fogle, 1992). The first scientific initative is designed to "explore normal variations in biological, behavioral and social factors within and between racial and ethnic, gender and age groups". . . and to evaluate specific chronic disease conditions. This initiative represents the central focus of the transdisciplinary endeavors of biological anthropology and human population biology. The second initiative is to "study environmental effects on genes and gene products and on integrated biological systems and study individual susceptibility to environmentally caused diseases and dysfunctions." Examining such gene–environment interactions has long been a fundamental cornerstone of biological anthropology and human population biology in the quest to understand the interactive mechanisms by which variation occurs in the human phenotype.

The application of these initiatives to a further understanding of human biological variation across the life span is obvious. The incredible ability of our species to adapt to diverse physical and cultural environments demonstrates our great plasticity and ability to change. Human aging is also a transitional process. Although essentially a temporal one—a transition from young to old—what we term human aging is part of the health transition (Ruzicka and Kane, 1990), where the majority of human populations worldwide are changing from semi-isolated traditional life styles to modern ones that include new biological consequences and rising life expectancies (Baker and Garruto, 1992). Our current and future research strategies will, by necessity, address how specific gene–environment interactions in conjunction with cultural–behavioral factors, operate to produce intra- and inter-population variability in the aging human phenotype.

The contributors to this volume articulate but a few of the new directions age-related research may take, using research strategies designed around traditional bioanthropological methods such as comparative, cross-cultural, longitudinal, and holistic approaches. These approaches provide a more informed and realistic measure of "normative" variation (biodiversity) in human aging and of the polar extremes of this continuum, "delayed and pathological" aging. Indeed, the importance of some of these concepts and the promise they hold for understanding the biology and evolution of human aging have been recently recognized by the gerontological community (e.g., cross-cultural aging including non-Western populations, see Eveleth, this volume). While both natural and experimental models of non-primate aging are enormously important to our overall understanding of the aging process, there can no longer be substitutes or excuses for not using the thousands of linguistically, culturally, and biologically diverse human populations world-wide, in an attempt to understand the aging process in our own species.

Even before this volume was conceived we were certainly aware of the kinds of contributions biological anthropologists and human population biologists were making and could make to the study of "normative" aging. However, we were somewhat surprised by the numerous serious and often innovative attempts such individuals were making to solve the mysteries of "pathologic" aging and toward an understanding of age-related disorders. While this latter component is not a traditional area for our discipline, it represents yet another new perspective on human biological variation and aging.

Finally, whether an anthropological perspective will continue to enrich this new emphasis on human variation in biological gerontology is to a very great extent in the hands of the traditional gerontological community and their willingness to allow "outsiders" to penetrate their ranks and contribute toward policy issues, program development, and training and to share the shrinking number of biomedical dollars available for research. We believe the outlook is quite hopeful, because of the multi-disciplinary history of gerontology. But it is up to biological anthropologists to demonstrate the relevance of their concepts and methods, indeed their discipline, to the gerontological community. It has not gone unnoticed that social and cultural anthropologists a number of years ago seized the opportunity to help develop the field of social gerontology. It remains unknown, however, whether the ever-growing contingent of biological anthropologists will seize presently existing and future opportunities to contribute in a major way to the development of a synthesis between disciplines. As we enter the 21st century we can only imagine what a world of predominantly aged individuals would be like without major breakthroughs in resolving the enormous social, economic, biomedical, and quality of life issues that this segment of society faces.

## REFERENCES

Fogle, S. (1992) NIH strategic plan pitches "War on Illness". *Journal of NIH Research* **4**, 24–25.

Baker, P. T. and Garruto, R. M. (1992) Health transition: examples from the western Pacific. *Human Biology* **64**, 785–789.

Ruzicka, L. and Kane, P. (1990) Health Transition: the course of morbidity and mortality. In: *What We Know About Health Transition: The Cultural, Social and Behavioral Determinants of Health* (eds Caldwell, J., Findley, S., Caldwell, P., Santow, G., Cosford, W., Braid, J. and Broers-Freeman, D.). Canberra: Australian University Press.

# Index